DM Entrance Examination
CARDIOLOGY

Dr. Jamal Yusuf

Dr. Mohit D Gupta

Dr. Saibal Mukhopadhyay

Department of Cardiology

G.B. Pant Hospital

New Delhi

PEEPEE

PUBLISHERS and DISTRIBUTORS (P) LTD.

DM Entrance Examination Cardiology

Published by
Pawaninder P. Vij

Peepee Publishers and Distributors (P) Ltd.
Head Office: 160, Shakti Vihar, Pitam Pura, Delhi 110 034 (India)

7/31, Ansari Road, Daryaganj, Post Box-7243
New Delhi 110002 (India)
Ph: 55195868, 9811156083
e-mail: peepee160@yahoo.co.in
e-mail: peepee160@rediffmail.com

First Edition: **2005**

ISBN: 81-88867-35-7

Creatives by: Monica Gupta and Nitin Yadav

Printed at
Lordson, C-5/19, Rana Pratap Bagh, Delhi-110 007

Dedicated
to
Almighty

Preface

In this era of super-specialization, almost every post-graduate student harbors a desire of acquiring training in a specialized way. One of the most fascinating branches to students of medicine is cardiology. Though there are many books of multiple choice questions for postgraduate entrance compiling questions of various institutes, there is no such book for DM entrance. Further the pattern of questions for *DM Entrance Examination in Cardiology* varies in different institutes. So we took up this task of providing post graduate students aspiring for super-specialization in cardiology to have an idea of the pattern of questions asked in different prestigious institutes like GB Pant, AIIMS, PGI Chandigarh, SGPGI Lucknow, Srichitra-to name a few. Apart from compiling questions of various examinations, we have also included a miscellaneous section trying to cover areas not well represented in the papers or on recent topics from which questions are likely to be asked.

The questions are authentic and the answer of each and every question has been checked from various standard textbooks. We have not mentioned the references to avoid complexity.

Every effort has been made to minimize grammatical errors and spelling mistakes. We hope that you would pardon us for any inadvertent error.

Finally we would like to know your opinion about the book and are looking forward to your suggestions to make it more useful.

Wishing you all the best!!!

Dr. Jamal Yusuf

Dr. Mohit D Gupta

Dr. Saibal Mukhopadhyay

Please email to us at: Dr.mohitgupta@yahoo.com

Acknowledgements

We sincerely acknowledge unconditional support from *Dr. Ajay Raj, Dr. P Nanda Kishore, Dr. Praloy Chakraborty, Dr. Sunandan Sikdar, Dr. Naveen Bhamri, Dr. Sanjeev Kathuria, Dr. Manish Sharma, Dr. Ashutosh Sahu, Dr. B S Vivek, Dr. Asit Khanna, Dr. Dinesh Raj, Dr. Praveen Singh, Dr. Himanshu Dabral, Dr. Srinivasan N, Dr. Milind Shrivastav, Dr. Sanjeev Kumar* for their help during preparation of this book.

Contents

Section I
1. GB Pant 2004 .... *1*
2. GB Pant 2003 .... *8*
3. GB Pant 2002 .... *15*
4. GB Pant 2001 .... *22*
5. GB Pant 2000 .... *27*
6. GB Pant 1999 .... *32*
7. GB Pant 1998 .... *38*
8. GB Pant 1997 .... *44*
9. GB Pant 1996 .... *49*
10. GB Pant 1995 .... *54*

Section II
11. AIIMS June 2004 .... *58*
12. AIIMS December 2003 .... *65*
13. AIIMS June 2003 .... *71*
14. AIIMS December 2002 .... *77*
15. AIIMS June 2002 .... *85*
16. AIIMS December 2001 .... *91*
17. AIIMS June 2001 .... *98*
18. AIIMS December 2000 .... *104*
19. AIIMS June 2000 .... *111*
20. AIIMS December 1999 .... *118*
21. AIIMS June 1999 .... *124*
22. AIIMS 1998 .... *131*
23. AIIMS December 1997 .... *137*
24. AIIMS June 1997 .... *143*
25. AIIMS 1996 .... *149*
26. AIIMS 1995 .... *155*
27. AIIMS 1994 .... *161*
28. AIIMS 1993 .... *168*

Section III
29. SGPGI December 2003 .... *174*
30. SGPGI June 2003 .... *181*
31. SGPGI December 2002 .... *188*
32. SGPGI June 2002 .... *195*
33. SGPGI 2001 .... *202*
34. SGPGI December 2000 .... *209*
35. SGPGI June 2000 .... *216*
36. SGPGI 1999 .... *223*
37. SGPGI 1998 .... *229*

Section IV
38. Srichitra 2004 .... *237*
39. Srichitra 2003 .... *245*
40. Srichitra 2002 .... *253*
41. Srichitra 2001 .... *261*

Section V
42. BHU 2004 .... *269*
43. BHU 2003 .... *277*
44. BHU 2002 .... *285*
45. BHU 2001 .... *293*
46. BHU 2000 .... *301*

Section VI
47. PGI 2004 .... *309*
48. PGI December 2003 .... *316*
49. PGI June 2003 .... *323*
50. PGI December 2002 .... *330*
51. PGI June 2002 .... *335*
52. PGI 2001 .... *343*
53. PGI December 2000 .... *350*
54. PGI June 2000 .... *354*
55. PGI 1999 .... *361*
56. PGI 1998 .... *365*

Section VII
57. Jaipur 2004 .... *371*
58. Jaipur 2003 .... *378*
59. Jaipur 2002 .... *385*
60. Jaipur 2001 .... *392*
61. Jaipur 2000 .... *398*
62. Jaipur 1999 .... *405*

Section VIII
63. UPDM 2003 .... *410*
64. UPDM 2001 .... *418*
65. UPDM 2000 .... *422*

Section IX
66. CMC Vellore 2004 427
67. CMC Vellore 2002 436
68. CMC Vellore 2001 443
69. CMC Vellore 2000 450

Section X
70. Jayadeva 2002 458

Section XI
71. Miscellaneous 465

GB Pant 2004

1. **Feature of typical angina:**
   - A. Relieved by antacids
   - B. Left precordial pain
   - C. Caused by emotional exertion
   - D. Prolonged, repeated

2. **In NYHA classification following is not a symptom:**
   - A. Angina
   - B. Cyanosis
   - C. Dyspnea
   - D. Palpitation

3. **Phasic ejection click of aortic valve is seen in:**
   - A. PS
   - B. TOF
   - C. Systemic hypertension
   - D. AS

4. **Wide split second heart sound is seen in:**
   - A. LV pacing
   - B. PDA
   - C. LVOT obstruction (severe)
   - D. LSVC to LA with intact septum

5. **Wide pulse pressure is seen in:**
   - A. PDA with PR
   - B. Severe hypertensive TR
   - C. Adult TOF
   - D. AS with MR

6. **Early systolic murmur is seen in all *except:***
   - A. MVP with MR
   - B. Small VSD
   - C. Acute severe MR
   - D. Normotensive TR

7. **Normotensive TR is seen in all *except:***
   - A. Carcinoid
   - B. MS with functional TR
   - C. IE
   - D. Tricuspid valve prolapse

8. **BP in lower limbs is significantly more than in upper limb:**
   - A. Takayasu arteritis
   - B. Coarctation of aorta with AR
   - C. Femoral AV fistula
   - D. Bilateral RAS

9. **Cannon "a" wave is seen in:**
   - A. VVI
   - B. DDD
   - C. Severe TS
   - D. PSVT

10. **Effort syncope is seen in:**
    - A. Severe LMCA stenosis
    - B. Straight back syndrome
    - C. Pulmonary AV fistula
    - D. Persistent LSVC to LA

11. **Syncope is not a characteristic manifestation of:**
    - A. HOCM
    - B. Severe PS
    - C. CoA
    - D. MS

12. **Nocturia is seen in all *except:***
    - A. Diabetes Mellitus
    - B. CHF
    - C. Hypertension
    - D. VSD

1 C 2 B 3 B 4 A 5 A 6 A 7 B 8 A 9 A 10 A 11 C 12 D

13. R in V1 is seen in all *except:*
A. VSD
B. Duchenne's muscular dystrophy
C. Posterior wall MI
D. Situs inversus with dextrocardia

14. ACE-inhibitors cause abrupt increase in Serum Creatinine in:
A. Hypotension B. CHF
C. B/L RAS D. All of the above

15. True about ACE-Inhibitors is all *except:*
A. Increase renin
B. Increase angiotensin-1
C. Decrease renal blood flow
D. Increase bradykinin

16. Digoxin toxicity is seen in all *except:*
A. Hypokalemia
B. Acidosis
C. Hypomagnesemia
D. Decrease intravascular volume

17. Digoxin level is increased in all *except:*
A. Phenytoin B. Amiodarone
C. Erythromycin D. Verapamil

18. Cardioselective beta blocker is:
A. Sotalol B. Bisoprolol
C. Nadolol D. Pindolol

19. RV impulse is prominent in:
A. MS with severe PAH
B. Ebstein's anomaly
C. Tricuspid atresia
D. TOF with pulmonary atresia

20. K^+ channel activator is:
A. Adenosine B. Amiodarone
C. Labetalol D. Sotalol

21. Drug to be given in first 24 hours of MI:
A. ACE-inhibitor B. CCB
C. Statin D. Digoxin

22. Drug beneficial in mortality in CHF:
A. Digoxin
B. Spironolactone
C. Oral anticoagulants
D. All of the above

23. Antioxidant effect is seen with all *except:*
A. Carvedilol B. Vitamin D
C. Allopurinol D. Probucol

24. Statin may cause all *except:*
A. Decreased stent thrombosis
B. Stablizes plaque
C. Decrease senile osteoporoisis
D. Improves endothelial function

25. Smoking causes atherogenesis by all *except:*
A. Antioxidant effect
B. Decreased HDL
C. Increased platelet aggregation
D. Endothelial dysfunction

26. Anterolateral papillary muscle is supplied by
A. LAD and LCx B. LAD
C. LCx D. RCA

27. Not a branch of RCA:
A. OM B. Acute marginal
C. Conus D. PDA

28. Vein draining into RA through coronary sinus are all *except:*
A. Thebesian vein
B. Small cardiac vein
C. Anterior cardiac vein
D. Vein of Marshall

29. Vein used for LV pacing:
A. Posterolateral vein
B. Anterior cardiac vein
C. Small cardiac vein
D. Thebesian vein

13 A 14 D 15 C 16 D 17 A 18 B 19 A 20 A 21 A 22 B 23 B 24 A 25 A
26 A 27 A 28 A 29 A

30. Most common stenotic valve (Aortic) at birth is:
A. Unicuspid B. Bicuspid
C. Tricuspid D. Quadricuspid

31. Spontaneous contrast in LA is seen in:
A. RCMP B. Acute MI
C. Severe TS D. RA myxoma

32. Superior axis deviation is seen in all *except:*
A. RSOV to RV
B. TOF with large inlet VSD
C. ECD
D. Tricuspid atresia

33. Coronary AV fistula most commonly drain in:
A. RV B. RA
C. LV D. Pulmonary artery

34. Penetrating injury most commonly affects:
A. RV B. LV
C. RA D. IVS

35. Bisferins pulse best felt in:
A. Carotid
B. Brachial
C. Abdominal aorta
D. Radial

36. Cyanosis with decreased blood flow is seen in:
A. Ebsteins anomaly
B. Tricuspid atresia with nonrestrictive VSD without PS
C. Taussig Bing anomaly
D. TGA

37. Pulsus paradoxus is seen in:
A. COPD
B. HOCM
C. Cardiac tamponade with AR
D. Severe TR

38. Enlarged LA is seen in:
A. Lutembacher's syndrome
B. ASD-OS
C. Corpulmonale
D. Ebstein's anomaly

39. Oxygen step up in RV is seen in:
A. PDA with PR
B. RSOV into LA
C. Sinus venosus ASD
D. Cortriatriatum

40. Adult survival is expected in:
A. PS
B. TGA
C. Ostium primum ASD
D. TOF with pulmonary atresia

41. Down's syndrome: most commonly associated with:
A. ECD
B. TOF
C. PS
D. Pulmonary artery stenosis

42. Which of the following is an incorrect match:
A. AS-Ross
B. TGA-Banding PA
C. TOF-BT
D. Pulmonary atresia-Unifocalisation

43. CHF in first week of life is seen in all *except:*
A. Severe MR
B. Coarctation of aorta
C. VSD
D. Congenital MS

44. WPW in congenital heart disease is associated with:
A. RSOV B. TGA
C. Ebstein's D. Uhl's anomaly

45. Markers of myocardial infarction are all *except:*
A. Troponin C B. Myosin light chain
C. LDH D. CK-MB

30 A 31 A 32 A 33 A 34 A 35 A 36 A 37 A 38 A 39 A 40 A 41 A 42 B
43 C 44 C 45 A

46. RVMI: true is all *except:*
A. Increased RA pressure
B. Normal PA pressure
C. Increased PCWP
D. Increased RV diastolic pressure

47. CHF: true is all *except:*
A. Reduced norepinephrine
B. Reduced Co P
C. Increased arteriovenous difference (oxygen)
D. Increased filling pressure

48. Pericarditis is seen with:
A. Methysergide
B. Lithium
C. Protamine
D. Indomethacin

49. In diabetes mellitus: Goal of Anti-lipid therapy is (without CAD):
A. LDL <100 and TG <150 mg%
B. LDL <100 and TG <200 mg%
C. LDL <130 and TG <200 mg%
D. LDL <160 and TG <150 mg%

50. MVA in echo is assessed by all *except:*
A. Gorlin's formula B. PISA
C. Planimetry D. PHT

51. True in echo for aortic valve disease:
A. Velocity of 2.5 m/s s/o mild AS
B. Peak instantaneous pressure in echo has good correlation with peak to peak pressure in cath
C. Mean aortic pressure in echo is invariably lower than that in cath
D. Gradual deceleration in gradient indicates severe AR

52. True in echo is all *except:*
A. Fractional shortening is 50-60%
B. PLAX for coronary artery
C. RV systolic function assessed by tricuspid annular velocity
D. LA contrast in mitral stenosis

53. Acute severe AR: true are all *except:*
A. Absent S4
B. Austin flint murmur
C. Absent peripheral signs
D. Soft S1

54. Which of the following is true:
A. Diastolic murmur graded from 1 to 6
B. Gallavardin phenomenon is seen in noncalcific AS
C. Carvallo's sign in TR with RVF
D. Austin flint murmur is absent in mild AR

55. Pregnancy: following are suggestive of heart disease:
A. Diastolic murmur at apex
B. LVS3
C. Systolic murmur-grade2/6 in pulmonary area
D. Edema

56. Poor prognosis in pregnancy is seen in:
A. PPH B. CoA
C. OS-ASD D. MR

57. Most dangerous coronary anomaly:
A. ALCAPA
B. Left coronary from right aortic sinus with interarterial course
C. LAD from right aortic sinus with retroaortic route
D. RCA from Lt aortic sinus

58. Amyl nitrate inhalation increases murmur of:
A. HOCM B. TOF
C. PDA D. MR

59. Cyanotic spell is maximum in TOF:
A. Less than 2 month B. 2-6 months
C. > 6 months D. 1-2 years

46 C 47 A 48 A 49 A 50 A 51 A 52 B 53 A 54 D 55 A 56 A 57 B 58 A 59 B

60. Treatment of cyanotic spell is all *except:*
- A. Morphine
- B. Esmolol
- C. Phenylephrine
- D. Frusemide

61. SCD in athlete: most common cause is:
- A. HOCM
- B. CAD
- C. Coronary abnormality
- D. Idiopathic ventricular tachycardia

62. Pacing: true is:
- A. Pacemaker mediated tachycardia is seen in VVI pacing
- B. DDD pacing causes less of atrial arrhythmia than VVI
- C. Biventricular pacing in HOCM is beneficial
- D. VVI is useful in CHF

63. Atrial fibrillation: true is:
- A. Risk of thromboembolism is more in non-valvular than valvular
- B. Biatrial pacing is useful in prevention of intermittent AF
- C. Rhythm control is definitely better than rate control
- D. Aspirin and warfarin are equally efficacious in preventing stroke

64. Infective endocarditis: Highest risk is associated with:
- A. Bicuspid aortic valve
- B. Ebstein's anomaly
- C. PPH
- D. OS-ASD

65. IE: indication for surgery are all *except:*
- A. Unstable prosthesis
- B. Intractable CHF
- C. NVE relapse after optimal antimicrobial treatment
- D. Vegetation > 10 mm with embolic phenomenon

66. Myocardial viability is assessed with all *except:*
- A. SAECG
- B. PET
- C. Dobutamine stress
- D. Stress Thallium

67. Findings in stress thallium s/o multivessel CAD are all *except:*
- A. Transient LV dilatation
- B. Increase RV uptake
- C. Uptake lung/heart <0.45
- D. Defect in more than 2 coronary artery territory

68. Which of the following findings are suggestive of strongly positive TMT:
- A. Exercise duration less than 8 min
- B. Exercise induced LBBB
- C. Recurrent sustained symptomatic VT
- D. Peak exercise BP more than 180 mm Hg

69. Not an indication of TMT:
- A. Advanced CHB
- B. Congenital asymptomatic CHB
- C. To diagnose IHD in chest pain patient
- D. Final assessment in valvular heart disease

70. BMV balloon size:
- A. Height of person in cm/10 + 10 mm
- B. Height of person in cm/10 + 5 mm
- C. Height of person in mts + 10 mm
- D. Height of person in cm/8 + 10 mm

71. IABP: Absolute contraindication:
- A. Severe AR
- B. Cardiogenic shock with aortic aneurysm
- C. Acute MI with VSD
- D. Severe MR

72. Characteristic pathology in Marfan's in aorta:
- A. Cystic medial necrosis
- B. Annuloaortic ectasia
- C. Fibrinoid degenration
- D. Plexiform arteriopathy

73. Primary hyperaldosteronism: true are all *except:*
- A. Urine K < 30 meq
- B. Hypertension
- C. Hypokalemia
- D. Decreased renin

60 D 61 A 62 B 63 B 64 A 65 C 66 A 67 C 68 C 69 A 70 A 71 A 72 A 73 A

74. Primary prevention trial is:
A. AFCAPS
B. 4S
C. CARE
D. LIPID

75. Indication of thrombolysis in pulmonary embolism:
A. Paradoxical emboli
B. LV dysfunction
C. RV dysfunction/hypokinesia/hypotension
D. All of the above

76. Familial myxoma: true are all *except:*
A. Endocrine disorder
B. Present in elderly
C. Multiple
D. Biatrial

77. Mechanism of hemoptysis in MS are all *except:*
A. Acute pulmonary edema
B. Chest infection
C. Recurrent laryngeal nerve paralysis
D. Pulmonary thromboembolism

78. Most common complication of catheterization:
A. Local vascular complications
B. Azotemia
C. Ventricular tachycardia
D. Acute MI

79. Cyanosis is seen in:
A. Common atrium
B. RSOV to RV
C. VSD with AR
D. Coronary AV fistula

80. Lp(a): true are all *except:*
A. Important risk factor in Asian Indians
B. Inhibit endogenous fibrinolysis
C. Homologous to fibrinogen
D. Decreased by niacin

81. All are true about ARVD *except:*
A. Familial incidence
B. LV almost always spared
C. RFA often unsuccessful
D. Male predominance

82. Eplerenone is:
A. Aldosterone antagonist
B. Endothelin antagonist
C. Cholesterol absorption inhibitor
D. Phosphodiesterase 3 inhibitor

83. Laser is used in:
A. Instent restenosis
B. Calcified lesions
C. Thrombus
D. Bifurcation lesion

84. All are true about type B lesions *except:*
A. 15 mm
B. Ostial
C. Thrombus containing
D. Concentric

85. Pulmonary artery develops from which arch:
A. Arch 3
B. Arch 4
C. Arch 5
D. Arch 6

86. Eruptive xanthomas are seen in:
A. Type 1 hyperlipidemia
B. Type 2 hyperlipidemia
C. Type 3 hyperlipidemia
D. Type 4 hyperlipidemia

87. CPK MB is present in all *except:*
A. Pancreas
B. Liver
C. Tongue
D. Prostate

88. All are cardioselective beta blocker *except:*
A. Bucindolol
B. Acebutalol
C. Bisoprolol
D. Butoxalol

89. All are trials related to carvedilol *except:*
A. MOCHA
B. COMET
C. CIBIS-1
D. COPERNICUS

90. All are true about adenosine *except:*
A. Can revert VT
B. Post ablation success checking
C. Terminate atrial flutter
D. I/v bolus 3 mg

74 A 75 C 76 B 77 C 78 A 79 A 80 C 81 B 82 A 83 A 84 D 85 D 86 A
87 B 88 D 89 C 90 C

91. LV aneurysm: most common symptom is:
A. Arrhythmia
B. Angina
C. Dyspnea
D. Thromboembolism

92. ST elevation is seen in all *except:*
A. Hypothermia
B. Hyperkalemia
C. Hypocalcemia
D. Early repolarisation

93. All are true about TMT *except:*
A. Smoking reduces exercise tolerance
B. Heparin decreases exercise tolerance
C. Hyperkalemia-gives false positive
D. Negative TMT in a patient on digoxin is a valid response

94. Counterclockwise QRS is seen in all *except:*
A. DORV
B. Tricuspid atresia
C. Pulmonary atresia
D. ECD

95. Intravascular ultrasound used in all *except:*
A. Instent restenosis
B. Thrombus
C. Myocardial viabililty
D. Aortic dissection

96. Advanced case of CCP has all *except:*
A. Kussumal's sign
B. S3 gallop
C. Diffuse inspiratory rales
D. Ascites

97. True about amyloidosis on echo are all *except:*
A. Increase LA size
B. Increase LV thickness
C. Increase LV volume
D. Pericardial effusion

98. Coronary artery on echo is seen in which view:
A. PLAX
B. Short Axis view
C. Apical 4 chamber view
D. Subcostal view

99. All are Framingham major criteria *except:*
A. CVP of 14 cm of water
B. Circulation time of 30 msec
C. Cardiomegaly
D. Hepatojugular reflux

100. Continuous murmur is seen in all *except:*
A. Truncus arteriosus
B. Lutembacher syndrome
C. Severe RVOT obstruction
D. Arteriovenous fistula

91 C 92 C 93 B 94 C 95 C 96 C 97 C 98 B 99 A 100 A

GB Pant 2003

1. **Bifid T waves can be seen in all *except:***
   A. Congenital heart disease
   B. Cerebrovascular accident
   C. Long QT syndrome
   D. Hypertension

2. **In Mason-Likar modification, all are true *except:***
   A. Q waves appears in aVL
   B. Voltage increases in inferior leads
   C. Absent q waves in inferior leads
   D. There is left axis deviation

3. **Most reliable marker of ischemia is seen in which lead:**
   A. II, V5 **B.** I, V5
   C. II, V4 **D.** II, V3

4. **In TMT, all are poor prognostic *except:***
   A. Ventricular tachycardia
   B. Early ST depression
   C. Severe hypertension
   D. Multiple lead involvement

5. **Following reliably differentiate SVT from VT *except:***
   A. Capture beat
   B. Fusion beat
   C. VA association
   D. Carotid sinus massage

6. **QT prolongation is seen with:**
   A. Hypercalcemia
   B. Hypomagnesemia
   C. Hyperkalemia
   D. Digitalis

7. **In three lead system, best to see ischemia is:**
   A. MCL1 **B.** CM5
   C. CB5 **D.** CC5

8. **Reverse redistribution is seen with:**
   A. Thallium
   B. Tc-tetrafosmin
   C. Indium^{111} labelled antimyosin antibodies
   D. Tc-sestamibi

9. **Which is used within 48 hours of myocardial injury:**
   A. Indium-111 labelled antimyosin Ab
   B. Thallium 201
   C. Tc-tetrafosmin
   D. Tc-sestamibi

10. **For perfusion imaging with PET, all of the following compounds are used *except:***
    A. Rb^{82}
    B. H_2O^{15}
    C. N^{13} ammonia
    D. FDG

1 D 2 D 3 A 4 C 5 C 6 B 7 A 8 A 9 A 10 D

11. Microvascular integrity is best seen with:
A. TEE
B. PET
C. Myocardial contrast echocardiography
D. Scintigraphy

12. RF ablation is indicated in all *except:*
A. Brugada syndrome
B. Verapamil responsive VT
C. AVNRT
D. WPW syndrome

13. Pacemaker mediated tachycardia is seen in all *except:*
A. AAIR **B.** VDD
C. DDD **D.** VVR

14. Gated blood gas pool imaging is useful in all *except:*
A. LVEF
B. RVEF
C. Cardiotoxicity especially drug induced
D. Myocardial reserve in CAD

15. Worst prognosis arrhythmia that may be due to acquired/congenital LQTS:
A. Torsades de pointes
B. Ventricular tachycardia
C. Ventricular fibrillation
D. Monomorphic ventricular tachycardia

16. Poor prognosis in exercise imaging are indicated by all *except:*
A. Reduced lung uptake
B. Large defect
C. LV dilatation
D. None of the above

17. Poor prognosis in exercise imaging are indicated by all *except:*
A. Reduced gall bladder uptake
B. Large defect
C. LV dilatation
D. Increased lung uptake

18. Valve area is calculated by all *except:*
A. Gorlin's formula
B. Simpson's formula
C. Continuity equation
D. 2-D echo

19. Calcium in coronary artery is best seen by:
A. Cine CT **B.** Fluoroscopy
C. MRI **D.** 2D echo

20. LV diastolic dysfunction is seen with:
A. E > A **B.** A >E
C. A absent **D.** E absent

21. MS in M-mode is seen by:
A. Decreased EF slope
B. Posterior movement of PML
C. Paradoxical septal movement
D. SAM

22. EPSS is consistently increased in:
A. DCMP
B. RCMP
C. CCP
D. Tamponade

23. Spontaneous contrast echo is seen in all *except:*
A. HOCM **B.** RCMP
C. MS **D.** LA myxoma

24. Findings of HOCM are all *except:*
A. SAM
B. ASH
C. Mid systolic closure of aortic valve
D. E > A

25. ASH is not seen with:
A. RVH **B.** AS
C. PWMI **D.** LVH

11 C 12 A 13 A 14 D 15 C 16 A 17 A 18 B 19 A 20 B 21 A 22 A 23 A
24 D 25 C

26. Best zone for PA catheter is:
A. West lung zone 1
B. West lung zone 2
C. West lung zone 3
D. West lung zone 4

27. PA catheter on AP chest X ray; correct position is within 2 cm of:
A. Cardiac silhouette
B. LPA
C. RPA
D. Pulmonary conus

28. Thermodilution method used for determining cardiac output is:
A. Stewart Hamilton equation
B. Fick's principle
C. Mc Donald's formula
D. None of the above

29. Reading from intrathoracic intravenous catheter are best recorded in:
A. End expiration B. End inspiration
C. Mid inspiration D. Mid expiration

30. 7-3 formula is for:
A. RAP B. PAP
C. CVP D. None of the above

31. Decrease amplitude in fast flushing method for measurement of invasive intraarterial pressure indicates:
A. High damping coefficient with low systolic BP
B. High damping coefficient with high systolic BP
C. Low damping coefficient with low systolic BP
D. Low damping coefficient with high systolic BP + Diastolic BP

32. All catheters have end holes *except:*
A. Pigtail B. NIH
C. Cournard D. GL catheter

33. False is:
A. JL-4 is designed for left coronary angiogram
B. Amplatz can be substituted for Judkins catheter
C. CAG should be done before left ventriculography
D. Sones is designed for transbrachial approach

34. RCA is viewed in all *except:*
A. RAO 30° B. LAO 60°
C. Right lateral D. Left lateral

35. Pulmonary catheter in Lung zone 2—seen is:
A. a and v waves are not seen
B. Accurately measures LA pressures
C. Inspiratory and expiratory changes will be marked
D. Damping

36. Hamilton Stewart equation is used for calculation of:
A. Cardiac output B. Blood volume
C. Chamber pressure D. Valve area

37. Stroke volume is:
A. 50-90 ml B. 20-50 ml
C. 90-120 ml D. 100 ml

38. Balloon in PA catheter is filled with:
A. 1 cc air B. 1 cc water
C. 5 cc air D. 5 cc saline

39. Which of the following is not seen in atrium:
A. Eustachian valve
B. Thebasian valve
C. Pectinate muscle
D. Ligament of Marshall

40. In RV, all are true *except:*
A. Pulmonic valve is below aortic valve
B. Anterior cusp of tricuspid valve is smallest
C. Trabeculae carnae are seen
D. Conical inbfundibulum leads to PA

26 C 27 A 28 A 29 A 30 C 31 A 32 B 33 C 34 C 35 C 36 A 37 A 38 A 39 D 40 A

41. Conotruncal anomalies are seen in all *except:*
A. DORV
B. TOF
C. D-TGA
D. Inlet VSD

42. In Ebstein's anomaly, true about septal leaflet displacement is:
A. 8 mm/m^2
B. 5 mm/m^2
C. 2 mm/m^2
D. 5 mm/cm^2

43. Heart failure in 1st week of life may be seen in all *except:*
A. Mitral atresia
B. Hypoplastic left heart syndrome
C. D-TGA
D. Large VSD

44. LAD in VSD is seen in:
A. Multiple VSD
B. Pulmonary HTN
C. LV to RA shunt
D. Muscular VSD

45. Indications of pacing in CHB are all *except:*
A. Day time heart rate < 70/min
B. LA enlargement
C. Cardiomegaly
D. LV dysfunction on Echo

46. Pulsus alterans is seen in all *except:*
A. AS
B. RCMP
C. DCMP
D. Ischemia

47. Pulsus bisferians is best felt in:
A. Brachial
B. Femoral
C. Radial
D. Carotid

48. Square wave response in valsalva is seen in all *except:*
A. MS
B. ASD
C. AR
D. Heart Failure

49. All are seen in cardiac tamponade *except:*
A. Pericardial rub
B. Prominent y descent
C. Pulsus paradoxus
D. Electrical alternans

50. Cardiac tamponade: JVP findings is:
A. Prominent x descent
B. Prominent y descent
C. V-y collapse
D. a = v

51. Paradoxical split in S2 is seen in:
A. WPW Type B
B. VSD
C. Pulmonary embolism
D. ASD

52. Paradoxical split S2 is seen in all *except:*
A. LV dysfunction
B. AS
C. MR
D. Pulmonary embolism

53. Hepatojugular reflux is seen in all *except:*
A. LVF
B. RV failure
C. TS
D. Raised PCWP

54. Intermittent canon a wave is seen in all *except:*
A. AF
B. CHB
C. AIVR
D. VT

55. H wave in JVP correlates with:
A. Isovolumic relaxation
B. Diastasis
C. Isovolumic contraction
D. Plateau phase

56. Phasic ejection click is heard in all *except:*
A. TOF
B. AS
C. PS
D. Truncus arteriosus

57. Amyl nitrate inhalation decreases all murmurs *except:*
A. MR
B. AR
C. MS
D. VSD

41 D 42 A 43 D 44 A 45 A 46 B 47 D 48 C 49 B 50 A 51 A 52 C 53 C
54 A 55 B 56 B 57 C

58. Post PVC murmur increases in all *except:*
A. HOCM B. AS
C. MR D. PS

59. Super statin is:
A. Atorvastatin B. Rosuvastatin
C. Simvastatin D. Lovastatin

60. Role of beta blocker in CHF is all *except:*
A. Down regulation of beta receptors
B. Decrease catecholamine toxicity
C. Anti-apoptotic effect
D. Electrolyte imbalance correction

61. Beta blocker with vasodilation are all *except:*
A. Labetelol B. Nebivolol
C. Carvedilol D. Bisoprolol

62. Heparin in dilution for ABG use causes proportional decrease in:
A. pH B. pCO_2
C. pO_2 D. SaO_2

63. Platelet count decreased by which of the following drug:
A. Ticlopidine B. Eptifibatide
C. Lovastatin D. Ezitimibe

64. Digoxin does not cause:
A. Second degree AV block
B. Mobitz Type 2 block
C. Sinus arrest
D. CHB

65. Canadian Cardiovascular society scale includes:
A. Angina B. Palpitation
C. Dyspnea D. All of the above

66. A 45 year old male presenting with acute ASMI. Treatment of choice would be:
A. Aspirin + Reopro + PTCA/stent
B. Aspirin + Reopro + LMWH
C. Aspirin + Reopro + tenecteplase
D. Aspirin + PTCA/stent + Clopidogrel

67. Angiogenesis is not done by:
A. Gamma interferon
B. TNF-α
C. TGF-β
D. VEGF

68. Thrombolysis is absolutely contraindicated in all *except:*
A. Day 1 of menses
B. Hemorrhagic stroke/ICH
C. Intracranial neoplasm
D. Aortic dissection

69. In RVMI, not found is:
A. TR
B. ↑RV systolic pressure and ↑PA pressure
C. ↑RAP
D. ↑Cardiac enzymes

70. Major criteria for CHF are all *except:*
A. Nocturnal cough
B. Increased JVP/CVP
C. ↑Abdominojugular reflux
D. Cardiomegaly

71. Jones criteria: true is all *except:*
A. Used for chronic RHD
B. Nodules associated with carditis
C. Erythema marginatum is rare
D. Arthritis is most common

72. Prosthetic valve: All are true *except:*
A. Some stenosis is common/acceptable
B. Early endocarditis is treated by surgery
C. Mild regurgitation is common
D. Bioprosthetic valve is preferred if pregnancy is contemplated

73. BAV is not indicated in which of the following:
A. Elective AVR in patients with critical AS
B. Severe calcific AS as a bridge over
C. In pregnancy
D. Cardiogenic shock in AS

58 C 59 B 60 A 61 D 62 A 63 A 64 B 65 A 66 D 67 A 68 A 69 B 70 A
71 A 72 B 73 A

74. PCWP and LVEDP in AR is:
A. PCWP > LVEDP
B. PCWP < LVEDP
C. PCWP = LVEDP
D. No correlation

75. BPV; true are all *except:*
A. Has replaced surgery
B. Immediate secondary subpulmonic PS regresses spontaneously
C. Mild PR common
D. Outcome is not related to duration and severity

76. Acute AR; all are true *except:*
A. S4 is consistently present
B. Absent peripheral signs
C. Presystolic accentuation is present
D. LV dilatation is absent

77. Which of the following is not seen in pregnancy:
A. Mild axis deviation
B. Sinus bradycardia
C. Occasional VPC's
D. ST depression mimicking ischemia

78. In females, which is not true:
A. MI is less common
B. Increase repolarization abnormalities
C. Increase vasospastic angina
D. SPECT has more specificity

79. Takayasu arteritis; True is:
A. Subclavian artery is not involved
B. AR is never present
C. DCM is never seen
D. Coronary ostium may be involved

80. All are poor prognostic factors in HOCM *except:*
A. Apical HOCM
B. Severe LVH
C. Recurrent syncope in young
D. Malignant family history

81. True about HOCM is:
A. Digoxin increases the gradient and murmur
B. Valsalva decreases the murmur
C. Isoproterenol + squatting increases the murmur
D. Amylnitrate decreases the murmur

82. Radiation causes all *except:*
A. LV aneurysm
B. Acute pericarditis
C. Chronic constrictive pericarditis
D. Occlusive CAD

83. All are true about PPH treatment *except:*
A. Ventricular assist device
B. Vasodilators
C. Prostaglandins
D. Biatrial septostomy

84. Features of pulmonary embolism are all *except:*
A. Pneumothorax
B. Paradoxical embolism
C. Syncope
D. Pulmonary infarct

85. Surgery in aortic dissection is indicated in all *except:*
A. Proximal aortic dissection
B. Isolated arch dissection
C. AR
D. Marfans syndrome

86. End tidal pCO_2 < arterial pCO_2 indicates:
A. Pulmonary shunt
B. Increase dead space
C. Ventilation insufficiency
D. Pneumothorax

87. Lowering of freezing point principle is used in calculating:
A. Osmolality
B. Oxygen saturation
C. Urine creatinine
D. Serum sodium

74 B 75 B 76 C 77 B 78 D 79 D 80 A 81 A 82 A 83 A 84 A 85 B 86 B 87 A

88. Oxygen index used in ECMO therapy is calculated by:
A. FiO_2 × mean pressure/PaO_2
B. FiO_2 × peak pressure/PaO_2
C. FiO_2 × peak pressure/$PaCO_2$
D. FiO_2 5 mean pressure/$PaCO_2$

89. Oxygen flux is best measured by:
A. Pulse oximetry
B. Cardiac output
C. Mixed venous oxygen saturation
D. Pulmonary venous oxygen saturation

90. Inhalation of 100% oxygen in normal person causes:
A. Proportional increase in SaO_2 + PaO_2 + Venous oxygen saturation
B. Proportional increase in SaO_2 + PaO_2 but not Venous oxygen saturation
C. Proportional increase in SaO_2 + but not paO_2 and Venous oxygen saturation
D. Proportional increase in paO_2 but not SaO_2

91. Special pre-operative cardiac evaluation is required in:
A. Known CAD with unknown functional status
B. Stable class II angina
C. Poor functional status with no risk factor for CAD
D. Patient with family history of CAD

92. Best guide for coagulation monitoring during surgery is:
A. Complete coagulogram
B. Thromboelastogram
C. Fluoroscene labeled flow cytometry
D. Turbidometric assay

93. In life support to increase aortic pressure and cerebral blood flow:
A. Interposed abdominal compression
B. Counter abdominal compression
C. Phasic abdominal compression
D. Active compression and decompression

94. Ability to detect true negativity is:
A. Sensitivity
B. Specificity
C. Predictive value
D. Accurate assay

95. IVC filter is not indicated in:
A. Cancer chemotherapy
B. Bleeding diathesis
C. Hemorrahagic stroke
D. Recurrent emboli in patient on antiplatelet

96. Urgent surgery in infective endocarditis is indicated in all *except:*
A. Fungal endocarditis
B. Refractory CHF
C. Prosthetic valve malfunction
D. Intravenous drug abusers

97. Wide pulse pressure is seen in:
A. PDA with PR
B. Severe hypertensive TR
C. Adult TOF
D. AS with MR

98. Pulmonary capillary pressure configuration in myocardial ischemia; critical change will be:
A. Prominent a and v waves
B. Disappearance of a waves
C. Disappearance of v waves
D. None of the above

99. Characteristic feature of ECG in c TGA is:
A. Absent q in I, aVL, V5 and V6
B. Varying degree blocks
C. Tall R in V1
D. Increase P wave amplitude

100. End systolic pressure volume relationship signifies:
A. LV compliance
B. LV afterload
C. LV contractility
D. None of the above

88 A 89 C 90 D 91 A 92 B 93 A 94 B 95 D 96 D 97 A 98 A 99 A 100 C

GB Pant 2002

1. Most common side effect of bretylium:
A. Postural hypotension
B. Parotid pain
C. Pancreatitis
D. Hypertension

2. Commonest side effect of enalapril:
A. Cough
B. Hypotension
C. Rash
D. Alteration of taste

3. Acute MI: which of the following drug is not beneficial in reducing mortality:
A. I/v metoprolol
B. Oral atenolol
C. I/v enalapril
D. Oral ramipril

4. MVP with thickened and redundant valve with mild MR on echo. IE prophylaxis for dental extraction is:
A. Oral amoxicillin
B. I/v Ampi + Genta
C. Vancomycin
D. None of the above

5. Abciximab is:
A. Monoclonal antibody
B. Polypeptide
C. Non-peptide
D. Hexameric molecule

6. Coarctation of aorta in infancy: most common ECG presentation is:
A. RVH
B. LVH
C. LAE
D. LAHB

7. Ideal time for operation in CoA is:
A. 0-3 years
B. 3-5 years
C. 5-8 years
D. 10-12 years

8. Arterial switch operation is carried out in:
A. TGA
B. Single ventricle
C. DORV
D. Ebstein's anomaly

9. Five year old female came with dyspnea, severe cyanosis, clubbing. On physical examination: normal S1, single S2, seesaw murmur at base. Which of the following is the correct diagnosis:
A. TOF with absent pulmonary valve
B. TOF with PDA
C. PS with PR
D. PDA with eisenmenger

10. Kussumal's sign is seen in:
A. Tamponade
B. CCP
C. Pneumothorax
D. Asthma

11. Abdominojugular reflux: true is:
A. Sustained rise of 5 cm is normal
B. Pressure for 30 sec in right lumbar region
C. Can be seen in RVF and LVF
D. Examination during deep inspiration

1 A 2 A 3 C 4 A 5 A 6 A 7 B 8 A 9 A 10 B 11 C

12. Thrity-three year old male presenting with retrosternal chest pain, sweating, orthopnea, hepatomegaly, raised JVP: most likely diagnosis is:

A. Acute MI
B. RSOV
C. Aortic dissection
D. Oesophageal rupture

13. RSOV is most commonly associated with:

A. Bicuspid aortic valve
B. PDA
C. CoA
D. VSD

14. TOF is least likely associated with:

A. Right aortic arch
B. CoA
C. ASD
D. Absent pulmonary valve

15. Least likely in Ebstein's anomaly:

A. Split S1 B. Split S2
C. S3 D. S4

16. Triple ripple at apex is seen in:

A. RCM B. HOCM
C. DCM D. AS with AR

17. Mechanical valve prosthesis is associated with all *except:*

A. Hemolytic anemia
B. Intracranial hemorrhage
C. Berry aneurysm
D. IE

18. Young male presenting with sudden onset of palpitations. On examination, respiratory rate is 18/mt, BP is 120/80 mm Hg, ECG shows wide QRS, no p waves, varying R-R interval. Drug of choice is:

A. Adenosine B. Procainamide
C. Lidocaine D. Digoxin

19. Osborn waves is seen in:

A. Hypercalcemia B. Alkalosis
C. Hyperthyroidism D. Hypothermia

20. Negative U waves are seen in all *except:*

A. Hypokalemia
B. CAD
C. Hypertension
D. Intracranial hemorrhage

21. All are seen in hyperkalemia *except:*

A. Absent p wave B. Broad QRS
C. ST depression D. Sine wave pattern

22. Digoxin toxicity is precipitated by all *except:*

A. Hypothyroidism
B. Hypercalcemia
C. Hypoxia
D. Hyperparathyroidism

23. Acute MI: indication of i/v amiodarone is:

A. Atrial infarction with persistent AF
B. VPC's more than 10/hour
C. NSVT
D. VF after one hour of thrombolysis

24. Coronary artery aneurysm is not seen in:

A. Fibromuscular dysplasia
B. Syphilis
C. Atherosclerosis
D. Lupus

25. Syphilis: which of the following is not found:

A. Saccular aneurysm of ascending aorta
B. Dissection of descending aorta
C. Coronary ostial narrowing
D. Perivascular inflammation

26. Rotational atherectomy is not done in which of the following:

A. Thrombosed graft
B. Calcified lesions
C. Ostial lesions
D. Instent restenosis

12 B 13 D 14 B 15 D 16 B 17 C 18 B 19 D 20 A 21 C 22 C 23 A 24 A 25 B 26 A

27. Type A lesion: which of the following is not a feature:
A. Size less than 10 mm
B. Ostial lesions
C. Angulation less than 45
D. Concentric lesions

28. Atherosclerotic renal artery stenosis: most common site is:
A. Segmental B. Lobar
C. Ostial D. Midsegment

29. CABG showed consistently improved result over PTCA in:
A. Diabetics B. Age > 65
C. Smoker D. Males

30. PTCA is preferred over thrombolysis in:
A. Cardiogenic shock
B. Diabetes
C. Elderly
D. Women

31. Features of Tangier's disease are all *except:*
A. Autosomal recessive
B. Decreased HDL
C. Cholesterol deposition in peripheral tissues
D. Xanthomas

32. Lipoprotein 'a' reducing drugs are all *except:*
A. Estrogens B. Atorvastatin
C. Nicotinic acid D. Bezafibrate

33. HOCM inheritance is:
A. AD B. AR
C. X linked-dominant D. X linked recessive

34. Syncopal attack in 65 year old male lying on a couch is due to:
A. Sclerodegenrative CHB
B. Neurocardiogenic syncope
C. Carotid sinus hypersensitivity
D. HOCM

35. Indication of surgery in HOCM when basal LV gradient is:
A. 10 mm Hg
B. 20 mm Hg
C. 30 mm Hg
D. 50 mm Hg

36. Transient occlusion of both carotid artery leads to:
A. Vasodilation
B. Hypertension
C. Increased stimulus from carotid sinus
D. Reduced venous return

37. Temporal areteritis: not true is:
A. Intracranial artery involvement
B. Steroids for treatment
C. Greater in males
D. Granulomatous lesions

38. Takayasu's arteritis: not involved is:
A. Aorta
B. Carotid
C. Subclavian
D. Inferior mesenteric artery and left external iliac

39. IMA is a branch of:
A. Descending thoracic aorta
B. Common carotid artery
C. Subclavian
D. Thyrocervical trunk

40. Cardiogenic shock: percentage of myocardium involved is:
A. 15% B. 25%
C. 40% D. 75%

41. Anatomically right combination:
A. LAD-OM
B. LAD-sinus nodal artery
C. LCx-Diagonal
D. RCA-acute marginal

---

27 B 28 C 29 A 30 A 31 A 32 B 33 A 34 A 35 D 36 B 37 C 38 D 39 C
40 C 41 D

42. Ischemia is seen most commonly in:
A. Single coronary artery
B. LCx from right sinus of valsalva
C. Coronary artery fistula
D. LAD and LCx from other sinuses

43. Truncus arteriosus: most common murmur heard is:
A. Pansystolic murmur
B. Diastolic murmur
C. Midsystolic murmur
D. Wide split S2

44. Uncommon feature of subvalvular AS is:
A. Diastolic murmur
B. Long systolic murmur
C. Increased velocity across the valve
D. Non ejection click

45. HOCM: which of the following echo findings is not present:
A. Aortic valve doming
B. SAM
C. Notch on aortic valve on M mode
D. Increased echoes on basal septum

46. Normal blood flow is seen in:
A. Stunned myocardium
B. Hibernating myocardium
C. Myocardial bridges
D. Infarcted myocardium

47. Myocardial bridges is most common in:
A. RCA B. OM
C. LAD D. PDA

48. Which of the following is a phosphodiesterase inhibitor?
A. Digoxin
B. Milrinone
C. Dobutamine
D. Dopamine

49. Mortality is not reduced after MI:
A. Monotrate
B. Aspirin
C. Betablockers
D. Enalapril

50. Syncope in MS is not due to:
A. AF with fast ventricular rate
B. AF with slow ventricular rate
C. Peripheral pulmonary embolism
D. PAH

51. Verapamil is not given in:
A. AVNRT
B. Antidromic conduction
C. Orthodromic conduction
D. AF with WPW

52. AV node not involved in reentry in:
A. AVRT
B. AVNRT
C. Atrial flutter
D. Junctional reciprocating tachycardia

53. Temporary pacing in MI is not indicated in:
A. CHB
B. Bifascicular block
C. LPHB
D. Type II second degree block

54. IABP: absolute contraindication is:
A. Severe AS
B. Severe AR
C. Carotid artery stenosis
D. Severe MR

55. Propranalol decreases the ischemia in acute MI by:
A. Decrease oxygen requirement
B. Decreased contractility
C. Decrease BP
D. Coronary dilatation

42 C 43 A 44 D 45 A 46 A 47 C 48 B 49 A 50 C 51 D 52 C 53 C 54 B
55 A

56. Not an alpha blocker is:
- **A.** Carvedilol
- **B.** Terazosin
- **C.** Labetolol
- **D.** Bisoprolol

57. Dual chamber pacing is not beneficial in:
- **A.** CHB
- **B.** Sick sinus syndrome
- **C.** HOCM
- **D.** DCM

58. ICD is most beneficial in which of the following groups in DCM:
- **A.** EF 40-50%
- **B.** EF > 50 %
- **C.** EF 25-40%
- **D.** EF < 25%

59. Bicuspid aortic valve with severe AS with AF and worsening NYHA Class and gradient of 140 mm Hg; which of the following will not be seen:
- **A.** Increased apico-carotid delay
- **B.** Sustained apical impulse
- **C.** Presystolic impulse
- **D.** Syncope

60. Which is true:
- **A.** Percussion wave usually not palpated
- **B.** Tidal wave usually palpated
- **C.** Bifid pulse seen in dynamic LVOT obstruction
- **D.** Bisferians pulse seen in static LVOT

61. Pregnancy: abnormal finding:
- **A.** Pedal edema
- **B.** S3
- **C.** MDM at apex
- **D.** Distended neck veins

62. Lunula and nodule are seen in:
- **A.** AV valve
- **B.** Semilunar valve
- **C.** RA
- **D.** LA

63. Not a part of RV:
- **A.** Crista terminalis
- **B.** Moderator band
- **C.** Trabeculae carnii
- **D.** Papillary muscle

64. Gerbode defect is defect in:
- **A.** AV septum
- **B.** Septum primum
- **C.** Septum pellucidum
- **D.** Septum trabeculam

65. Five year old child with recurrent respiratory tract infection on examination, pansystolic murmur at lower left sternal border, MDM at apex, with normal S1, S2 and S3 present, LVH present. Diagnosis is:
- **A.** Supracristal VSD
- **B.** Inlet VSD
- **C.** RHD with MS and MR
- **D.** MVP with MR

66. Young male with abdominal pain, pedal edema, prominent x and absent y. Next line of management is:
- **A.** Pericardiocentesis
- **B.** I/v fluids
- **C.** I/v NTG
- **D.** I/v lasix

67. ASH is not seen in:
- **A.** HOCM
- **B.** AS
- **C.** PWMI
- **D.** TGA

68. Patient with heart rate of 140/mt, normal BP, chest clear, wide QRS tachycardia. Lidocaine is given in dose of:
- **A.** 60 mg over 3 minutes
- **B.** 60 mg bolus
- **C.** 60 mg in 100 ml Normal saline @ 2 ml/mt
- **D.** 10 mg

69. Young male with breathlessness, RA pressure 6 mm Hg, RV-45/9, PA –50/12, PCWP-20 mmHg, LV 112/8, aorta 120/85. Differential diagnosis is all *except:*
- **A.** DCMP
- **B.** Pulmonary veno-occlusive disease
- **C.** MS
- **D.** Cortriatriatum

56 D 57 D 58 C 59 C 60 C 61 C 62 B 63 A 64 A 65 B 66 A 67 C 68 B 69 A

70. Viability of myocardium: most sensitive is:
A. PET B. Stress Echo
C. Thallium D. MRI

71. Increased lung uptake in stress thallium indicates:
A. LV dysfunction
B. MR
C. Pulmonary embolism
D. COPD

72. Raised PA pressure is seen in all *except:*
A. Pneumonia with COPD
B. High altitude
C. Post single lung pneumectomy
D. Moderate CHF

73. Non Q MI: not beneficial:
A. Tirofiban B. Reteplase
C. Beta blocker D. Clopidogrel

74. TAPVC; true is all *except:*
A. Oxygen saturation is equal in all 4 chambers
B. Snowman's heart
C. Operation best at the age of 10-12 years
D. Pulmonary venous obstruction most common with infradiaphragmatic variety

75. Wide split S2 is heard with all *except:*
A. Severe MR
B. Severe AS
C. RV Dysfunction
D. Pulmonary hypertension

76. Rheumatic TS is associated with all *except:*
A. MS
B. TR
C. Pulmonary hypertension
D. AF

77. Balloon valvotomy gives most beneficial long term results for which of the following condition:
A. MS B. TS
C. PS D. AS

78. Forty-five year old male with MVP and MR, EF 50%, grade III systolic murmur; Best long term results are seen with:
A. MV repair B. Homograft
C. Tilting disc D. Ball valve

79. Prosthetic valve endocarditis: which of the following drug is not useful:
A. CP B. Vancomycin
C. Gentamicin D. Rifampicin

80. Which arrhythmia is least common in chronic constrictive pericarditis:
A. AF B. APC
C. VT D. Sinus tachycardia

81. Commonest cause of CCP in India:
A. Secondaries B. Uremia
C. Tuberculosis D. Idiopathic

82. Most common malignancy of heart is:
A. Rhabdomyosarcoma
B. Mesothelioma
C. Secondaries
D. Angiosarcoma

83. One day neonate with R-R interval of 1000 msec P-P interval of 400 msec, narrow QRS complexes. Investigation of choice is:
A. Anti-Ro-SSA
B. Anti-Ro-SSB
C. Anti-rubella
D. Howell Jolley bodies

84. Echocardiography in acute myocarditis. All are true *except:*
A. Thickening of LV
B. Thinning of LV
C. Dilated chambers
D. LV dysfunction

70 A 71 A 72 C 73 B 74 C 75 B 76 C 77 C 78 A 79 A 80 C 81 C 82 C
83 A 84 B

85. Best predictor of mortality in MI is:
A. Ejection fraction
B. Anatomy of coronary artery by angiography
C. Left ventricular end diastolic dimension
D. Left ventricular end systolic volume

86. Predictor of restenosis are all *except:*
A. Ostial lesions
B. LCx
C. Chronic total occlusion
D. Calcification

87. PA saturation more than aorta is seen in:
A. TOF
B. Taussig Bing anomaly
C. VSD
D. Pulmonary atresia

88. Atrial flutter with 2:1 block with heart rate 180/min, atrial rate 360/min. Normal BP. Treatment of choice is:
A. I/v procainamide
B. I/v lidocaine
C. DC shock (synchronized)
D. I/v digoxin

89. Warfarin effect is decreased by:
A. OC pills
B. Rifampicin
C. Aspirin
D. Phenylbutazine

90. Torsades de pointes is not caused by:
A. Ranitidine
B. Haloperidol
C. Terfanedine
D. Erythromicin

91. Plateau phase of action potential corresponds with which segment of ECG?
A. ST
B. QRS
C. T
D. QT

92. High output state is not seen with:
A. Thiamine deficiency
B. Hypothermia
C. Hyperparathyroidism
D. None of the above

93. Difference between SVT with aberrancy and VT is all *except:*
A. A-V association
B. Left axis deviation
C. QRS > 0.16 ms
D. Monomorphic QRS in chest leads

94. Stroke volume in a normal adult is:
A. 50-74 ml
B. 75-90 ml
C. 91-104 ml
D. 105-120 ml

95. Defect is Marfan's syndrome is due to:
A. Elastin
B. Collagen
C. Fibrillin
D. Myotroponin

96. MVP with sudden death is most common in:
A. Familial form
B. Severe MR
C. Accessory pathway
D. Acquired MVP

97. All of the following are useful in decreasing the rate of reinfarction *except:*
A. ACE-I
B. Aspirin
C. Beta blocker
D. Isosorbide

98. Window period for thrombolysis in pulmonary embolism is:
A. 6 hours
B. 12 hours
C. 7 days
D. 14 days

99. Earliest sign of pulmonary venous hypertension is:
A. Perihilar cuffing
B. Cephalization of pulmonary vessels
C. Kerley B lines
D. Kerley A lines

100. Most common drug causing cardiomyopathy is:
A. Doxorubicin
B. Cyclophsphamide
C. Cisplatin
D. Vincristine

85 A 86 B 87 B 88 C 89 B 90 A 91 A 92 B 93 A 94 B 95 C 96 A 97 D
98 D 99 B 100 A

GB Pant 2001

1. The most anterior valve of the human heart is:
A. Mitral
B. Tricuspid
C. Aortic
D. Pulmonary

2. The crux of the heart is located on which surface?
A. Apical
B. Anterobasal
C. Posterbasal
D. Lateral

3. A wide split second heart sound is found in all *except:*
A. Massive pulmonary embolism
B. Operated ASD
C. LBBB
D. Left ventricular paced beat

4. Stroke volume in a normal adult is:
A. 50-74 ml
B. 75-90 ml
C. 91-104 ml
D. 105-120 ml

5. Elecrocardiographic manifestations of hypermagnesaemia includes:
A. Increased PR and QRS,SA and AV block
B. Increased PR and narrow QRS
C. Short PR and broad QRS
D. Short PR and narrow QRS

6. Syncope is least common in:
A. Mitral stenosis (MS)
B. Mitral regurgitation (MR)
C. Aortic stenosis (AS)
D. Aortic regurgitation (AR)

7. Patients with chronic heart failure have:
A. Oliguria
B. Polyuria
C. Oliguria during day and Polyuria during night
D. Anuria

8. Third heart sound is not heard in:
A. Chronic constrictive pericarditis
B. Ventricular aneurysm
C. malignant hypertension
D. Critical AS

9. Pulsus bisferians is not found in:
A. Fever
B. Hypertrophic cardiomyopathy
C. Non obstructive cardiomyopathy with amylnitrite inhalation
D. Aortic regurgitation with heart failure

10. Branham's sign is:
A. Bradycardia due to carotid sinus massage
B. Bradycardia due to compression of feeder artery in AV fistula
C. Tachycardia due to decreased preload
D. Tachycardia due to decreased blood pressure

11. Acrocyanosis refers to:
A. Cyanosis due to methaemoglobinaemia
B. Transient cyanosis in ASD
C. Persistent cyanosis of periphery due to cold intolerance
D. Cyanosis due to carbon monoxide

1 D 2 C 3 C 4 B 5 A 6 B 7 C 8 D 9 D 10 B 11 C

12. **S4 is usually present in:**
A. Mitral stenosis
B. Chronic mitral regurgitation
C. Left ventricular aneurysm
D. Amyloid heart disease

13. **Wide splitting of Ist heart sound (S1)is found in:**
A. Severe calcific mitral stenosis
B. Left bundle branch block
C. Left atrial myxoma
D. Ebstein's anomaly

14. **A2-OS interval in a patient of mitral stenosis may vary from:**
A. 60-120 msec B. 120-240 msec
C. 200-320 msec D. 300-400 msec

15. **The timing of S3 in a normal person lies within which interval after S1?**
A. 60-120 msec B. 120-240 msec
C. 200-320 msec D. 300-400 msec

16. **Congential heart diseases associated with more than 5 mm Hg pressure difference between the two arms:**
A. Tetralogy of Fallot
B. Supravalvular aortic stenosis
C. D-Transposition of great arteries
D. Hypertrophic obstructive cardiomyopathy

17. **All of the following diseases may be associated with pulsus paradoxus *except:***
A. Pericardial effusion
B. Chronic obstructive lung disease
C. Chronic constrictive pericarditis
D. Cardiac tamponade

18. **Which of the following produce wide splitting of second heart sound?**
A. Left bundle branch block
B. Moderate mitral regurgitation
C. Severe aortic stenosis
D. Left ventricular dysfunction

19. **Which of the following is not usually associated with digitalis administration?**
A. Bluish vision B. Yellow vision
C. Gynecomastia D. Scotomas

20. **Which of the following is not seen in patient with severe pulmonary stenosis with congestive heart failure?**
A. Loud pulmonary closure sound
B. Delayed pulmonary closure sound
C. Large a wave in JVP
D. RVS3

21. **Warfarin limits the carboxylation of all the following proteins *except:***
A. Protein C B. Protein S
C. Factor II D. Factor VIII

22. **Polyarteritis nodosa may be associated with any of the following *except:***
A. Acute myocardial infarction
B. Congestive cardiac failure
C. Mononeuritis multiplex
D. Aortic root dilatation

23. **Mitral stenosis patients will have loud first heart sound if there is:**
A. Prolonged flow through mitral valve
B. Ist degree heart block
C. heavy calcification
D. Immobility of the valve

24. **Which of the following does not occur in primary pulmonary hypertension?**
A. Anginal chest pain
B. Tricuspid regurgitation
C. Raised LV end diastolic pressure
D. Right atrial hypertrophy

25. **Following streptococcal infection which of the following suggest rheumatic fever?**
A. Erythema nodosum
B. Erythema multiforme
C. Erythema marginatum
D. Short PR interval on electrocardiogram

---

12 C 13 D 14 A 15 D 16 B 17 A 18 B 19 A 20 A 21 D 22 D 23 A 24 C
25 C

26. Coronary artery disease is associated with all the following diseases *except:*
A. Amyloidosis
B. Rheumatoid arthritis
C. Hurlers syndrome
D. Homocysteinuria

27. The correct way to demonstrate outflow gradient in case of hypertrophic obstructive cardiomyopathy is:
A. Two catheters in LV through RA→LA → LV and second from Ao → LV
B. Two catheters, one in LV and another in LVOT
C. Pullback from LV to AO with pigtail catheter
D. Pullback from LV to AO with Cournand catheter.

28. Myocardial sarcoidosis may present with any of the following *except:*
A. Pericardial effusion
B. Heart block
C. Ventricular aneurysms
D. G6-PD deficiency

29. LEOPARD syndrome is associated with:
A. Pulmonary stenosis
B. Aortic stenosis
C. Mitral regurgitation
D. Pericardial constriction

30. One of the following is most common in patients having Tricuspid atresia with VSD and pulmonary stenosis:
A. RVS3
B. Cyanotic spells
C. Loud pulmonic component of second heart sound
D. LVS4

31. In patient of critical aortic stenosis, the three symptoms given below can be arranged in order of worsening prognosis as:
A. Failure > Angina > Syncope
B. Syncope > Failure > Angina
C. Angina < Syncope < Failure
D. Angina < Failure < Syncope

32. Conditions predisposing to cerebrovascular accidents (Strokes) in patients with congential heart disease include all of the following *except:*
A. Age < 4 years B. Age > 7 years
C. Iron deficiency D. Dehydration

33. A patient is admitted to the emergency with recurrent ventricular tachycardia, normal LV size and contractility. His holter shows pause dependent mechanism for his ventricular tachycardia. His QT is prolonged. The treatment of choice for his patient would be:
A. Magnesium B. Cardiac pacing
C. Xylocaine D. Amiodarone

34. Causes of step up of oxygen at the RA level includes:
A. Aortopulmonary window
B. VSD with tricuspid regurgitation
C. Patent ductus arteriosus
D. Eisenmenger syndrome

35. The survival of a population in years is given below. What is the median survival of this population. (2, 3, 3, 4, 4, 4, 4, 5, 5, 6, 6, 7, 8, 8, 9)
A. 4 years B. 4.7 years
C. 5 years D. 5.2 years

36. Electrocardiogram of a patient with athletic heart syndrome may show:
A. Increased QRS amplitude
B. prominent u wave
C. Shortened QT interval
D. Sinus bradycardia

37. Plain X-ray chest in a 2 years old child with coarctation of aorta not in CHF, which of the following radiological signs would be seen?
A. Rib notching B. Cardiomegaly
C. E sign D. Normal heart size

26 A 27 B 28 D 29 A 30 B 31 C 32 B 33 B 34 B 35 C 36 D 37 D

38. **Which of the following changes is not observed in patient with hypothermia?**
A. Osborne waves
B. J point elevation
C. Sinus bradycardia
D. Ventricular tachycardia

39. **A 25 year old young lady is admitted to the emergency with tight mitral stenosis, 24 wks pregnancy and atrial fibrillation which started two hours back. Which of the following best modality of treatment in the patient?**
A. Electrical cardioversion
B. Quinidine IV
C. Therapeutic abortion
D. Verapamil IV

40. **Which of the following is an abnormal finding in pregnancy?**
A. Wide splitting of first heart sound
B. Third heart sound
C. Fourth heart sound
D. Extra cardiac murmur

41. **Which of the following help in differentiating mitral insufficiency from tricuspid insufficiency?**
A. Increase in inspiration
B. Associated mitral stenosis
C. Radiation to base of the heart
D. Opening snap

42. **A 27 year old lady with the following hemodynamic data will have a differential diagnosis of all the following *except:***

AO 110/90 (96 mean)	**PA 40/23 (30 mean)**
PAW a27 v28 (26 mean)	**RA a25 V v26 (22 mean)**
LV 110/25ed	**RV 40/24 ed**

Cardiac Index = 2.1 Lit/min/m2

A. Tight mitral stenosis
B. Pulmonary embolism
C. Endomyocardial fibrosis
D. Chronic constrictive pericarditis

43. **Ebstein's anomaly is characterized by downward deviation of septal leaflet by more than:**
A. 6 mm/m2 BSA
B. 8 mm/m2 BSA
C. 10 mm/m2 BSA
D. 11 mm/m2 BSA

44. **In a patient known to have secundum ASD, atrial septal aneurysms are characterized by:**
A. Disappearance with age
B. Right ventricular inflow obstruction
C. Left ventricular inflow obstruction
D. Pulmonary arterial hypertension

45. **Arterial switch procedure in d-TGA is done within:**
A. 2 weeks of life
B. 4 weeks of life
C. 6 weeks of life
D. 8 weeks life

46. **Most common aortic arch anomaly in Taussig-Bing anomaly is:**
A. Interrupted Aortic arch type A
B. Interrupted Aortic arch type B
C. Co-arctation of aorta
D. Double aortic arch

47. **Procedure which has replaced surgery in congenital heart disease:**
A. Balloon pulmonary valvoplasty
B. Balloon angioplasty of RVOT in TOF
C. Balloon angioplasty of co-arctation of aorta in neonates
D. VSD closure by devices

48. **Newer risk factors for CAD includes all of the following *except:***
A. Fibrinogen
B. Homocysteinemia
C. Lipoprotein(a)
D. Calcium

49. **STEP II AHA diet lowers serum cholesterol by:**
A. 5%-10%
B. 10%-20%
C. 20%-30%
D. 40%

38 D 39 A 40 C 41 C 42 A 43 B 44 A 45 A 46 C 47 D 48 D 49 B

50. Drugs shown to reverse endothelial dysfunction are all *except:*
A. Estrogen
B. Progesterone
C. ACE inhibitors
D. Lovastatin

51. As compared to mortality of 75% with conservative management, mortality associated with primary PTCA in cardiogenic shock is:
A. 10%
B. 20%
C. 30-40%
D. 60%

52. 52 year old male diabetic, hypertensive suffered Ac. Inferior wall MI complicated by 2:1 AV block on day 2. Recovery was uneventful. Best modality for risk stratification would be:
A. Pre-discharge TMT
B. TMT at 6 weeks
C. Coronary angiogram before discharge
D. Coronary angiography

53. Risk of CAD in woman equals that of man by:
A. 55 years
B. 65 years
C. 75 years
D. 85 years

54. Murmurs heard posteriorly–include all *except:*
A. Pulmonary A-V fistula
B. Bronchial collateral vessels
C. Systemic collateral murmurs
D. PDA

55. Which is not an example of continuous murmur?
A. RSOV
B. Coronary A-V fistula
C. VSD-AR
D. PDA

56. Restenosis rate in Aortic stenosis after valvuloplasty in adults is:
A. 75% at 6 months
B. 100% at 6 months
C. 25% at 6 months
D. 50% at 6 months

57. Best management of Atrial Flutter in a patient with 32 week pregnancy is:
A. Digoxin
B. Verapriamil
C. DC shock
D. Beta blockers

58. Spontaneous dissection of the following artery is typically described in pregnancy:
A. Aorta
B. Coronary
C. Carotid
D. Pulmonary

59. Inferior vena cava filters are indicted in a case with pulmonary thromboembolism when:
A. Calf vein thrombus is present
B. Repeated PTE occurs despite anticoagulation
C. Large areas of V/Q mismatch demonstrated
D. Large thrombus is present in pulmonary Artery

60. 4 year male child with recurrent VT-most likely diagnosis:
A. Cardiac fibromyxoma
B. Rhabdomyosarcoma
C. Arrythmogenic dysplasia of right ventricle
D. Uhl's anomaly

50 B 51 C 52 A 53 B 54 D 55 C 56 D 57 C 58 B 59 B 60 B

GB Pant 2000

1. Right isomerism is characterized by all *except:*
- **A.** Bilateral morphologic Right Bronchi
- **B.** wandering spleen
- **C.** Howel jolly bodies
- **D.** Asplenia

2. Most important EKG feature of c-TGA is:
- **A.** q-wave absent in I, avL, v5, v6
- **B.** q-wave absent in II, III, avF
- **C.** Equiphasic complexes in midprecordial leads
- **D.** 2:1 heart block

3. Most accepted indication of balloon angioplasty in coarctation of aorta is:
- **A.** Restenosis after surgical repair
- **B.** Restenosis after angioplasty
- **C.** Co-arctation in infants
- **D.** Co-arctation

4. Brugada's syndrome is characterized by:
- **A.** ST elevation in V1 with rsR pattern
- **B.** ST elevation in V1 with qR pattern
- **C.** ST depression on V1 with rsR pattern
- **D.** ST elevation in V2 with rsR pattern

5. Indication of AICD implantation:
- **A.** Atrial fibrillation with fast ventricular rate
- **B.** Ventricular tachycardia with hemodynamic compromise
- **C.** Incessant ventricular tachycardia
- **D.** Primary ventricular tachycardia

6. Drugs shown to reverse endothelial dysfunction are all *except:*
- **A.** Estrogen
- **B.** Progestrone
- **C.** ACE-inhibitors
- **D.** Lovastatin

7. Which infection has not been related to atherosclerosis?
- **A.** CMV
- **B.** Herpes
- **C.** H Pylori
- **D.** Chlamydia

8. ACEI should be started after Ac MI after:
- **A.** as soon as patient stabilizes
- **B.** 10 hrs
- **C.** 24 hrs
- **D.** 48 hrs or more

9. Right atrial enlargement with LAD in a cyanotic heart disease is characterized by:
- **A.** Ebstein anomally
- **B.** Pulmonic stenosis with R-L shunt
- **C.** Pulmonary atresia with VSD
- **D.** Tricuspid atresia

10. Probable cure for Eisenmenger syndrome is:
- **A.** Heart lung transplant
- **B.** Cardiac transplantation
- **C.** Lung transplantation
- **D.** Not possible

1 B 2 A 3 A 4 A 5 B 6 B 7 B 8 A 9 D 10 A

11. Newer risk factors for CAD include all of the following *except:*
A. Fibrinogen
B. Homocysteinemia
C. Lipoprotein (a)
D. Calcium

12. Use of Simvastatin in 4S study increased HDL levels by:
A. 2% B. 20%
C. 8% D. 30%

13. Best echo view for pulmonary valve is:
A. PLAX B. Apical 4-C
C. PSAX D. Suprasternal

14. Differential diagnosis of linear echo in LA includes all *except:*
A. Dilated Coronary sinus
B. TAPVC
C. Cortriatriatum
D. Left pulmonary artery

15. ELITE trial compared ..... in CCF patients:
A. Losartan with Felodipin
B. Enalapril with Quinapril
C. Losartan with captopril
D. Digoxin with Diuretics

16. VAQWISH Trial concluded that in patients with Non Q-MI:
A. Angioplasty is superior to medical therapy
B. Medical (conservative) treatment is better than radical
C. CABG is superior to angioplasty
D. Stress thallium is must before coronary angiography

17. Features in M-mode indicating raised LVEDP include all *except:*
A. B-bump
B. Premature closure of MV
C. Early appearance of A-point
D. Increased EPSS

18. Which feature is most important in distinguishing CCP from RCM:
A. Atrial Fibrillation
B. Respiratory variation in mitral inflow velocity
C. LV dysfunction
D. Mitral/tricuspid regurgitation

19. I year survival in patient with cardiac transplant:
A. > 85% B. > 70%
C. > 50% D. > 40%

20. ATLAS trail concluded:
A. Low dose lisinopril is more effective than high dose in reducing mortality in patients with CCF
B. High does lisinopril is more effective than low dose in reducing mortality in patients with CCF
C. No difference in mortality rates with use of different doses of lisinopril in patients with CCF.
D. High dose lisinopril is effective in reducing mortality in elderly with CCF but not in the young

21. Spontaneous dissection of the following artery is typically described in pregnancy:
A. Aorta B. Coronary
C. Carotid D. Pulmonary

22. Inferior vena cava filters are indicated in a case with pulmonary thromboembolism when:
A. Calf vein thrombus is present
B. Repeated PTE occurs despite anticoagulants
C. Large areas of V/Q mismatch demonstrated
D. Large thrombus is present in Pulmonary Artery

23. 4 year male child with recurrent VT-most likely diagnosis:
A. Cardiac fibromyxoma
B. Rhabdomyosarcoma
C. Arrythmogenic dysplasia of roght ventricle
D. Uhl's anomaly

11 D 12 C 13 C 14 D 15 C 16 B 17 C 18 B 19 A 20 B 21 B 22 B 23 B

24. Ebstein's anomaly is characterized by downward deviation of septal leaflet by more than:
A. 6 mm/m^2 BSA
B. 8 mm/m^2 BSA
C. 10 mm/m^2 BSA
D. 11 mm/m^2 BSA

25. Small Aorta with small PA is a cardiological feature of:
A. Criss Cross heart B. Home's heart
C. Ebstein's heart D. Cretinism

26. Arterial switch procedure in d-TGA is done within:
A. 2 wks of life B. 4 wks of life
C. 6 wks of life D. 8 wks of life

27. Gerbode's defect refers to:
A. Coronary sinus ASD
B. LV-RA communication
C. Partial absence of pericardium
D. Perforation of mitral valve

28. Drug contra indicated in pregnancy–3rd trimester:
A. ACE I B. Lignocaine
C. Phenytoin D. Warfarin

29. Indicators of surgery in a patient with aortic regurgitation with no symptoms:
A. NYHA II B. LVESD > 45 mm
C. LVEF < 70% D. LVEDD > 52 mm

30. Restenosis rate in aortic stenosis valvupalsty in adults:
A. 75 % at 6 months B. 100 % at 6 months
C. 25 % at 6 months D. 50 % at 6 months

31. Drug which has been shown to retard progression of aortic regurgitation conclusively is:
A. Digoxin B. Enalapril
C. Nifedipine D. Prazosin

32. Procedure of choice of mitral valvuloplasty in pregnancy is:
A. CMV B. OMV
C. BMV D. MVR

33. Absolute contra-indication to pregnancy:
A. Severe AS in NYHA I
B. Severe AR
C. Eisenmenger's syndrome
D. Severe MR

34. Best management of atrial flutter in a patient with 32 wks pregnancy:
A. Digoxin B. Verapamil
C. DC shock D. β blockers

35. Cause of paradoxical splitting of S2:
A. LV dysfunction
B. Severe MR
C. Large VSD
D. Severe TR

36. Sqaure wave response with valsalva maneuver seen in:
A. ASD
B. HCM
C. MR-MVP
D. Pericardial effusion

37. Incidence of involvement of plumonary Valve in RHD is less than …….in autopsy series:
A. 1% B. 2%
C. 3% D. 7%

38. 52 years old male diabetic, hypertensive, suffered Ac, inferior wall MI complicated by 2: 1 AV block on day 2, recovery was uneventful. Best modality for risk stratification would be:
A. Pre discharge TMT
B. TMT at 6 weeks
C. Coronary angiogram before discharge
D. Coronary angiography and EPS before discharge

24 B 25 C 26 A 27 B 28 D 29 B 30 D 31 C 32 C 33 C 34 C 35 A 36 A
37 C 38 A

39. 45 years old male diabetic, hypertensive for 10 years, developed severe acute retrosternal chest pain with EKG showing ST depression from VI-V4; Best management is:
A. Coronary angiography and angioplasty
B. Medical management only
C. Medical management followed by revascularization if symptoms not controlled
D. Immediate thrombolysis

40. Drug shown to provide mortality benefits in chronic stable angina does not include:
A. B blockers
B. Ca channel blockers
C. Lipid lowering agents
D. Dispirin

41. BARI trial showed that CABG is superior to PTCA in:
A. All patients
B. Diabetics
C. Patients with two vessel disease and LV dysfunction
D. Patient with high lipids

42. In coarctation of aorta, cause of death includes all *except:*
A. Rupture of aorta
B. Infective endocarditis
C. Cerebral hemorrhage
D. Myocardial infraction

43. Incidence of toxemia in patients with Coarctation of aorta (as comapared to general population):
A. Highest B. Same
C. Lower D. Invariably present

44. In a patient known to have Secundum ASD, atrial septal aneurysms are characterized by:
A. Disappearance with age
B. Right ventricular inflow obstruction
C. Left ventricular inflow obstruction
D. Pulmonary arterial hypertension

45. Left axis deviation in a case of VSD is seen in:
A. Multiple VSD's
B. VSD with AR
C. VSD with Plumonary hypertension
D. VSD with MR

46. Absolute indication of closure of VSD is:
A. Large VSD in neonate
B. Moderate sized VSD in 6 months old child
C. VSD with AR
D. VSD with mild PS

47. Which statement is false regarding VSD with acquired PS?
A. Occurs in 7-15% cases of VSD
B. Was first described by Gasul
C. Usually due to infundibular hypertrophy
D. PS is valvular in location

48. BT shunt is indicated as an emergency procedure in:
A. TOF with hypoplastic pulmonary arteries
B. TOF with recurrent spells
C. TOF with pulm atresia
D. TOF with endocardial cushion defect

49. Eisenmenger syndrome occurs in late adulthood in:
A. VSD
B. PDA
C. ASD
D. Endocardial cushion defect

50. Which is an oral GpIIb/IIIa inhibitor?
A. Lamifiban B. Xemilofiban
C. Tirofiban D. Eptifibatide

51. Restrictive physiology is defined by all of the following *except:*
A. LVEF 45% or more
B. Dip and plateau pattern on cardiac cath
C. Prominent x and y descent in JVP
D. Prominent "a" wave in mitral valve Doppler study

39 A 40 B 41 B 42 D 43 B 44 A 45 A 46 C 47 D 48 B 49 C 50 B 51 A

52. Interpret the following oxymetry data:

IVC = 55%	**RA = 82%**
SVC = 80%	**RV = 84%**
PA = 85%	**AO = 82%**

Diagnosis:

A. TAPVC
B. Sinus venosus ASD
C. Double outlet right ventricle
D. LV–RA shunt

53. SO_2 more in PA than in aorta is seen in all *except:*

A. d-TGA
B. Taussing Bing anomaly
C. Ebstein's anomaly
D. TAPVC with streaming

54. Sinoatrial node most commonly is supplied by branch of:

A. Right coronary artery
B. Left anterior descending artery
C. Left circumflex artery
D. Direct branch from left main artery

55. EPSS is markedly increased in:

A. HCM
B. Cardiac tamponade
C. DCM
D. c-TGA

56. Left axis deviation in pulmonary artery stenosis occurs in:

A. PS with rubella syndrome
B. PS with dysplastic valve
C. PS with Noonan's syndrome
D. PS with R-L shunt

57. STEP II AHA diet lowers serum cholesterol by:

A. 5%-10% B. 10%-20%
C. 20%-30% D. 40%

58. S-lip (a) levels can be decreased using:

A. ACE-I
B. Simvastatin
C. Niacin
D. Gemfibrozil

59. Most common aortic arch anomaly in Taussing-Bing anomaly is:

A. Interrupted aortic arch type A
B. Interrupted Aortic arch type B
C. Co-arctation of aorta
D. Double aortic arch

60. Gerbode's defect refers to:

A. Coronary sinus ASD
B. LV-RA communication
C. Partial absence of pericardium
D. Perforation of mitral valve

52 A 53 C 54 A 55 C 56 A 57 B 58 C 59 C 60 B

GB Pant 1999

1. **A2-OS interval in a patient of mitral stenosis may vary from:**
   A. 60-120 msec B. 120-240 msec
   C. 200-320 msec D. 300-400 msec

2. **The timing of S3 in a normal person lies within which interval after S1?**
   A. 60-120 msec
   B. 120-240 msec
   C. 200-320 msec
   D. 300-400 msec

3. **Which of the following coagulation factors is not Vitamin K dependent?**
   A. II B. VII
   C. IX D. XI

4. **Congenital heart diseases associated with more than 5 mm Hg pressure difference between the two arms is:**
   A. Tetralogy of Fallot
   B. Supravalvular aortic stenosis
   C. d-Transposition of great arteries
   D. Hypertrophic obstructive cardiomyopathy

5. **All of the following diseases may be associated with pulsus paradoxus *except:***
   A. Pericardial effusion
   B. Chronic obstructive lung disease
   C. Chronic constructive Pericarditis
   D. Cardiac tamponade

6. **All of the following may be associated with falsely lower systolic blood pressure measurement *except:***
   A. Rapid deflation of cuff
   B. Slow deflation cuff
   C. Venous congestion
   D. Use of a narrow cuff

7. **Which of the following would you use in phase IV of Korotkoff's sound as an index of diastolic blood pressure:**
   A. Aortic stenosis
   B. Riley-Day syndrome
   C. severe aortic regurgitation
   D. Mitral stenosis

8. **All of the following can result in an increase of pulse pressure *except:***
   A. Capillary vasodilatation
   B. Cardiac tamponade
   C. Paget's disease
   D. Decreased compliance of the arteries

9. **Beat to beat variation in blood pressure can be seen in all *except:***
   A. Polymorphic ventricular tachycardia
   B. Complete hear block
   C. Idio-ventricular rhythm
   D. Atrial fibrillation

1 A 2 D 3 D 4 B 5 A 6 D 7 C 8 B 9 C

10. Which of the following produce wide splitting of second heart sound ?
A. Left bundle branch block
B. Moderate mitral regurgitation
C. Severe aortic stenosis
D. Left ventricular dysfunction

11. Which of the following clinical signs would suggest that the patient is unsuitable for balloon mitral valvotomy?
A. Loud opening snap
B. LVS3
C. Wide A2-OS interval
D. Loud first heart sound

12. Which of the following is not usually associated with digitalis administration?
A. Bluish vision
B. Yellow vision
C. Gynecomastia
D. Scotomas

13. P2 component of second heart sound in tetralogy of Fallot may be audible with all of the following *except:*
A. Pink Fallot
B. Excessive bronco-pulmonary collaterals
C. Bilateral Pulmonary artery branch stenosis
D. Malposition of great arteries

14. Which of the following is not seen in a patient of severe pulmonary stenosis with congestive heart failure?
A. Loud pulmonary closure sound
B. Delayed pulmonary closure sound
C. Large a wave in JVP
D. RVS3

15. Which of the findings given below are abnormal in a 45 year old man ?
A. Grade I/III left parasternal heave
B. LVS3
C. A2 louder than P2
D. Absent pulmonary sound in mitral area

16. Warfarin limits the carboxylation of all the following proteins *except:*
A. Protein C
B. Protein S
C. Factor II
D. Factor VIII

17. A patient is admitted to the emergency with digitalis toxicity showing trifascicular block with a heart rate of 45/min. His serum potassium is 3.5 mEq/Liter and blood pressure is 90/60. His ejection fraction is 22%. His treatment measures should include all of the following *except:*
A. Potassium correction i/v
B. Inj Xylocaine i/v
C. Temporary cardiac Pacemaker
D. Stop digoxin

18. Polyarteritis nodosa may be associated with any of the following *except:*
A. Acute myocardial infarction
B. Congestive cardiac failure
C. Mononeuritis multiplex
D. aortic root dilatation

19. High altitude pulmonary edema is associated with:
A. Decreased pulmonary capillary permeability
B. Increased pulmonary artery wedge pressure
C. Normal LA pressure
D. Raised LV end diastolic pressure

20. Mitral stenosis patient will have loud first heart sound if there is:
A. Pronged flow through mitral valve
B. Ist degree heart block
C. Heavy calcification
D. Immobility of the valve

21. Primary pulmonary hypertension is not associated with:
A. Raised arterial CO_2 tension
B. Hoarseness of voice
C. Prominent a waves in the jugular venous pulse
D. Constant ejection click

10 B 11 B 12 A 13 B 14 A 15 B 16 D 17 A 18 D 19 C 20 A 21 A

22. Which of the following does not occur in primary pulmonary hypertension?
A. Anginal chest pain
B. Tricuspid regurgitation
C. Raised LV end diastolic pressure
D. Right atrial hypertrophy

23. During cardiac catheterization of a 3 year old child with VSD the following data are obtained:

Saturations PA 88%, AO 91%, RA60 %, pulmonary vein 90%, His arterial blood gases show PaO_2 = 67 $PaCO_2$ = 56 pH = 7.31.

Most likely cause of low aortic saturation is:
A. Right to left shunt at atrial level
B. Eisenmenger syndrome
C. Presence of chest infection
D. Sedative overdose

24. Following streptococcal infection which of the following suggests rheumatic fever ?
A. Erythema nodosum
B. Erythema multiform
C. Erythema marginatum
D. Short PR interval on electrocardiogram

25. Cardiac cath data of a 3 year old child with patent ductus arteriosus shows:

QP/QS ratio = 1.5; Aorttic pressure 115/60; PA pressure 35/15.

This patient should be operated to prevent:
A. Infective endocarditis
B. Congestive heart failure
C. Eisenmenger syndrome
D. Systemic embolism

26. Coronary artery disease is associated with all the following diseases *except:*
A. Amyloidosis
B. Rheumatoid arthritis
C. Hurlers syndrome
D. Homocysteinuria.

27. Which of the following is useful in the treatment of uncomplicated hypertrophic obstructive cardiomyopathy ?
A. Dual chamber pacing-Epicardial leads over LA and LV
B. Nitroglycerine
C. Digoxin
D. Dual chamber pacing-Endocardial Leads in RA and RV

28. The correct way to demonstrate outflow gradient in case of hypertrophic obstructive cardiomyopathy is:
A. Two catheters in LV through RA → LA → LV and second from Ao → LV
B. Two catheters, one in LV and another in LVOT
C. Pullback from LV to AO with pigtail catheter
D. Pullback from LV to AO with Cournand catheter

29. All the following may occur after digoxin over dosage *except:*
A. Wenckebach block
B. Complete heart block
C. 1st degree heart block
D. Ventricular tachycardia

30. Myocardial sarcoidosis may present with any of the following *except:*
A. Pericardial effusion
B. Heart block
C. Ventricular aneurysms
D. G-6PD deficiency

31. Cigarette smoking is not associated with:
A. Shift of oxygen dissociation curve to right
B. Mobilization of catecholamine
C. Increased risk of angina
D. Mobilization of free fatty acids

32. LEOPARD syndrome is associated with:
A. Pulmonary stenosis
B. Aortic stenosis
C. Mitral regurgitation
D. Pericardial constriction

22 C 23 D 24 C 25 A 26 A 27 D 28 B 29 C 30 D 31 A 32 A

33. Transoesophageal echocardiography is superior to Transthoracic echocardiography in assessment of all the following *except:*
A. Detection of LA appendage thrombi
B. Assessment of severity of Mitral stenosis
C. Emphysematous patient
D. Patients with poor ECHO window

34. Of the following, which is most common in patient having Tricuspid atresia with VSD and pulmonary stenosis?
A. RVS3
B. Cyanotic spells
C. Loud pulmonic component of second heart sound
D. LVS4

35. Class lll antirrhythmics according to Vaughen classification are:
A. Xylocaine B. Mexiletine
C. Amiodarone D. Bretylium

36. In patient of critical stenosis the three symptoms given below can be arranged in order of worsening prognosis as:
A. Failure > Angina > Syncope
B. Syncope < Failure < Angina
C. Angina < Syncope < Failure
D. Angina < Syncope > Failure

37. Components of situs solitus include all the following *except:*
A. Right atrium on right and left atrium on left side
B. Trilobed right lung with hyparterial bronchus
C. Right Sided vena cava
D. Bilobed left lung with hyparterial bronchus

38. Conditions predisposing to cerebrovascular accident (Stroke) in patient with congenital heart disease includes all of the following *except:*
A. Age < 4 years B. Age > 7 years
C. Iron deficiency D. Dehydration

39. All of the following cyanotic congenital heart disease are associated with increased pulmonary blood flow *except:*
A. d-Transposition of great arteries with intact ventricular septum
B. Tricuspid atresia Type IC
C. Truncus arteriosus
D. Patent ductus arteriosus

40. A patient is admitted to the emergency with recurrent ventricular tachycardia, normal LV size and contractility. His Holter shows pause dependent mechanism for his ventricular tachycardia. His QT is prolonged. The treatment of choice for this patient would be:
A. Magnesium
B. Cardiac Pacing
C. Xylocaine
D. Amiodarone

41. Heparin administration may be associated with all of the following *except:*
A. Osteoporosis
B. Thrombocytopenia
C. Increased level of factor V
D. Prolonged activated clotting time

42. Causes of stepup of oxygen at the RA level include:
A. Aortopulmonary window
B. VSD with Tricuspid regurgitation
C. Patent ductus arteriosus
D. Eisenmenger syndrome

43. 32 year old young man is admitted with intermitted sever sinus bradycardia and heart rate of 25/min. His TMT shows that he achieved 97% of his target heart rate with no ST-T changes. Electrophysiology showed HV=40 mscc at an atrial pacing of 150/min. The pacing modality of choice for this patient would be:
A. VVI B. VVIR
C. DDD D. AAI

33 B 34 B 35 D 36 C 37 D 38 B 39 D 40 B 41 C 42 B 43 D

44. The survival of a population in years is given below. What is the median survival of this population? (2, 3, 3, 4, 4, 4, 5, 5, 6, 6, 7, 8, 8, 9):
A. 4 years B. 4.7 years
C. 5 years D. 5.2 years

45. Drugs producing inhibition of clearance of S isomer of warfarin include all of the following *except:*
A. Phenylbutazone
B. Cotrimoxazole
C. Metronidazole
D. Omeprazole

46. Electrocardiogram of a patient with athletic heart syndrome may show:
A. Increased QRS amplitude
B. Prominent U wave
C. Shortened QT interval
D. Sinus bradycardia

47. Which of the following are true with respect to right aortic arch?
A. Associated congenital cardiac malformations in 95% cases
B. Occurs in 25% cases of Tricuspid atresia
C. Occurs in 5% cases of Tetralogy of Fallot
D. Occurs in 5% cases of Truncus arteriosus

48. Plain X-ray chest in a 2 year old child with coarctation of aorta not in CHF which of the following radiological signs would be seen?
A. Rib notching
B. Cardiomegaly
C. E sign
D. Normal heart size

49. Which of the following is not usually seen in patient with Eisenmenger syndrome?
A. Peripheral pruning of blood vessel on a chest X-ray
B. Syncope
C. Hemoptysis
D. Squatting

50. Which of the following changes is not observed in a patient with hypothermia ?
A. Osborne waves
B. J point elevation
C. Sinus bradycardia
D. Ventricular tachycardia

51. P_{50} of the oxygen dissociation curve is shifted to the left by:
A. Acidosis
B. Increase in pH
C. Increase in temperature
D. Increase in PCO_2

52. A 25 year old young lady is admitted to the emergency with tight mitral stenosis, 24 weeks pregnancy and atrial fibrillation which started two hours back. Which of the following is the best modality of treatment in this patient?
A. Electrial cardio version
B. Quinidine IV
C. Therapeutic abortion
D. Verapamil IV

53. Which of the following is not associated with increased incidence of fetal mortality?
A. Cardiopulmonary bypass
B. Oral coumarin
C. ACE inhibitors
D. Heparin anticoagulation

54. Which of the following is an abnormal finding in pregnancy?
A. Wide splitting of first heart sound
B. Third heart sound
C. Fourth heart sound
D. Extra cardiac murmur

55. All the following have pure R wave in electrocardiogram *except:*
A. Duchenne“s muscular dystrophy
B. True posterior wall infarction
C. Cor pulmonale
D. Ebsteins anomaly

44 C 45 D 46 D 47 A 48 D 49 D 50 D 51 B 52 A 53 D 54 C 55 D

56. Which of the following help in differentiating mitral insufficiency from tricuspid insufficiency:

A. Increase in inspiration
B. Associated mitral stenosis
C. Radiation to base of the heart
D. Opening snap

57. Rupture of chordae tendineae is seen in all the following *except:*

A. Aortic insufficiency
B. Rheumatic heart disease
C. Atrial septal defect
D. Idiopathic hypertrophic subaortic stenosis

58. Opening snap is not seen in which of the following ?

A. Primary pulmonary arterial hypertension
B. Atrial septal defect
C. Ebsteins anomaly
D. Pure mitral regurgitation

59. A 27 year old lady with the following hemodynamic data will have a differential diagnosis of all the following *except:*

AO 110/90 (96 mean) PA 40/23 (30 mean)
PAW a27 v28 (26 mean) RA a25 v26 (22mean)
LV 110/25 ed RV 40/24 ed
Cardiac Index =2.1 Lit/min/m2

A. Tight mitral stenosis
B. Pulmonary embolism
C. Endomycardial fibrosis
D. Chronic constructive pericarditis

60. A patient is admitted with the following hemodynamics:

Cardiac output 6.7 Lit/min/m2;
LVED 22 mm Hg PA wedge 23 mm
AO = 90/30 PA = 35/25
RA mean 14

Which of the following may lead to this state?

A. Mitral stenosis (Severe)
B. Aortic stenosis (Severe)
C. Paget's disease
D. Constrictive pericarditis

56 C 57 A 58 A 59 A 60 C

GB Pant 1998

1. **High altitude pulmonary edema is associated with:**
   A. Decreased pulmonary capillary permeability
   B. Increased pulmonary artery wedge pressure
   C. Normal LA pressure
   D. Raised LV end diastolic pressure

2. **All of the following may be associated with falsely lower systolic blood pressure measurement *except:***
   A. Rapid deflation of cuff
   B. Slow deflation cuff
   C. Venous congestion
   D. Use of a narrow cuff

3. **Which of the following clinical signs would suggest that the patient is unsuitable for balloon mitral valvotomy?**
   A. Loud opening snap
   B. LVS3
   C. Wide A2-OS interval
   D. Loud first heart sound

4. **The timing of S3 in a normal person lies within which interval after S1?**
   A. 60-120 msec B. 120-240 msec
   C. 200-320 msec D. 300-400 msec

5. **Which of the following is not usually associated with digitalis administration?**
   A. Bluish vision B. Yellow vision
   C. Gynecomastia D. Scotomas

6. **RV systolic pressure is greater than LV systolic pressure in:**
   A. PS with intact septum
   B. PDA-Eisenmenger's syndrome
   C. Subaortic VSD
   D. TOF with pulmonary atresia

7. **Warfarin limits the carboxylation of all the following proteins *except:***
   A. Protein C B. Protein S
   C. Factor II D. Factor VIII

8. **Which of the following would you use in phase IV of Korotkoff's sound as an index of diastolic blood pressure:**
   A. Aortic stenosis
   B. Riley-Day syndrome
   C. Severe aortic regurgitation
   D. Mitral stenosis

9. **A patient is admitted to the emergency with digitalis toxicity showing trifascicular block with a heart rate of 45/min. His serum potassium is 3.5 mEq/Liter and blood pressure is 90/60. His ejection fraction is 22%. His treatment measures should include all of the following *except:***
   A. Potassium correction i/v
   B. Inj Xylocaine i/v
   C. Temporary cardiac Pacemaker
   D. Stop digoxin

1 C 2 D 3 B 4 D 5 A 6 A 7 D 8 C 9 A

10. A2-OS interval in a patient of mitral stenosis may vary from:
A. 60-120 msec
B. 120-240 msec
C. 200-320 msec
D. 300-400 msec

11. Primary pulmonary hypertension is not associated with:
A. Raised arterial CO_2 tension
B. Hoarseness of voice
C. Prominent a waves in the jugular venous pulse
D. Constant ejection click

12. Which of the following coagulation factors is not Vitamin K dependent?
A. II B. VII
C. IX D. XI

13. During cardiac catheterization of a 3 year old child with VSD the following data are obtained:

Saturations PA 88%, AO 91%, RA60 %, pulmonary vein 90%, His arterial blood gases show $PaO_2 = 67$ $PaCO_2 = 56$ pH = 7.31.

Most likely cause of low aortic saturation is:
A. Right to left shunt at atrial level
B. Eisenmenger syndrome
C. Presence of chest infection
D. Sedative overdose

14. Mitral stenosis patient will have loud first heart sound if there is:
A. Pronged flow through mitral valve
B. Ist degree heart block
C. Heavy calcification
D. Immobility of the valve

15. Following streptococcal infection which of the following suggests rheumatic fever ?
A. Erythema nodosum
B. Erythema multiform
C. Erythema marginatum
D. Short PR interval on electrocardiogram

16. Polyarteritis nodosa may be associated with any of the following *except:*
A. Acute myocardial infarction
B. Congestive cardiac failure
C. Mononeuritis multiplex
D. Aortic root dilatation

17. Cardiac cath data of a 3 year old child with patent ductus arteriosus shows:

QP/QS ratio = 1.5; Aorttic pressure 115/60; PA pressure 35/15.

This patient should be operated to prevent:
A. Infective endocarditis
B. Congestive heart failure
C. Eisenmenger syndrome
D. Systemic embolism

18. Which of the following does not occur in primary pulmonary hypertension?
A. Anginal chest pain
B. Tricuspid regurgitation
C. Raised LV end diastolic pressure
D. Right atrial hypertrophy

19. Coronary artery disease is associated with all the following diseases *except:*
A. Amyloidosis
B. Rheumatoid arthritis
C. Hurlers syndrome
D. Homocysteinuria.

20. All of the following can result in an increase of pulse pressure *except:*
A. Capillary vasodilatation
B. Cardiac tamponade
C. Paget's disease
D. Decreased compliance of the arteries

10 A 11 A 12 D 13 D 14 A 15 C 16 D 17 A 18 C 19 A 20 B

21. The correct way to demonstrate outflow gradient in case of hypertrophic obstructive cardiomyopathy is:

A. Two catheters in LV through RA → LA → LV and second from Ao → LV
B. Two catheters, one in LV and another in LVOT
C. Pullback from LV to AO with pigtail catheter
D. Pullback from LV to AO with Cournand catheter

22. LEOPARD syndrome is associated with:

A. Pulmonary stenosis
B. Aortic stenosis
C. Mitral regurgitation
D. Pericardial constriction

23. All the following may occur after digoxin over dosage *except:*

A. Wenckebach Block
B. Complete heart block
C. 1st degree heart block
D. Ventricular tachycardia

24. Which of the following is useful in the treatment of uncomplicated hypertrophic obstructive cardiomyopathy ?

A. Dual chamber pacing-Epicardial leads over LA and LV
B. Nitroglycerine
C. Digoxin
D. Dual chamber pacing-Endocardial Leads in RA and RV

25. Myocardial sarcoidosis may present with any of the following *except:*

A. Pericardial effusion
B. Heart block
C. Ventricular aneurysms
D. G-6PD deficiency

26. Cigarette smoking is not associated with:

A. Shift of oxygen dissociation curve to left
B. Shift of oxygen dissociation curve to right
C. Decrease mobilization of free fatty acids
D. Reduce risk of angina

27. Transoesophageal echocardiography is superior to Transthoracic echocardiography in assessment of all the following *except:*

A. Detection of LA appendage thrombi
B. Assessment of severity of Mitral stenosis
C. Emphysematous patient
D. Patients with poor ECHO window

28. Congenital heart diseases associated with more than 5 mm Hg pressure difference between the two arms is:

A. Tetralogy of Fallot
B. Supravalvular aortic stenosis
C. d-Transposition of great arteries
D. Hypertrophic obstructive cardiomyopathy

29. Of the following, which is most common in patient having Tricuspid atresia with VSD and pulmonary stenosis?

A. RVS3
B. Cyanotic spells
C. Loud pulmonic component of second heart sound
D. LVS4

30. In patient of critical stenosis the three symptoms given below can be arranged in order of worsening prognosis as:

A. Failure > Angina > Syncope
B. Syncope < Failure < Angina
C. Angina < Syncope < Failure
D. Angina < Syncope > Failure

31. Causes of stepup of oxygen at the RA level include:

A. Aortopulmonary window
B. VSD with Tricuspid regurgitation
C. Patent ductus arteriosus
D. Eisenmenger syndrome

21 B 22 A 23 C 24 D 25 D 26 A 27 B 28 B 29 B 30 C 31 B

32. **Components of situs solitus include all the following *except:***
A. Right atrium on right and left atrium on left side
B. Trilobed right lung with hyparterial bronchus
C. Right Sided vena cava
D. Bilobed left lung with hyparterial bronchus

33. **Conditions predisposing to cerebrovascular accident (Stroke) in patient with congenital heart disease includes all of the following *except:***
A. Age < 4 years
B. Age > 7 years
C. Iron deficiency
D. Dehydration

34. **Beat to beat variation in blood pressure can be seen in all *except:***
A. Polymorphic ventricular tachycardia
B. Complete hear block
C. Idio-ventricular rhythm
D. Atrial fibrillation

35. **All of the following cyanotic congenital heart disease are associated with increased pulmonary blood flow *except:***
A. d-Transposition of great arteries with intact ventricular septum
B. Tricuspid atresia Type IC
C. Truncus arteriosus
D. Patent ductus arteriosus

36. **Class III antirrhythmics according to Vaughen classification are:**
A. Xylocaine B. Mexiletine
C. Amiodarone D. Bretylium

37. **Heparin administration may be associated with all of the following *except:***
A. Osteoporosis
B. Thrombocytopenia
C. Increased level of factor V
D. Prolonged activated clotting time

38. **A patient is admitted to the emergency with recurrent ventricular tachycardia, normal LV size and contractility. His Holter shows pause dependent mechanism for his ventricular tachycardia. His QT is prolonged. The treatment of choice for this patient would be:**
A. Magnesium B. Cardiac Pacing
C. Xylocaine D. Amiodarone

39. **The survival of a population in years is given below. What is the median survival of this population? (2, 3, 3, 4, 4, 4, 5, 5, 6, 6, 7, 8, 8, 9):**
A. 4 years B. 4.7 years
C. 5 years D. 5.2 years

40. **Drugs producing inhibition of clearance of S isomer of warfarin include all of the following *except:***
A. Phenylbutazone B. Cotrimoxazole
C. Metronidazole D. Omeprazole

41. **Which of the following are true with respect to right aortic arch?**
A. Associated congenital cardiac malformations in 95% cases
B. Occurs in 25% cases of Tricuspid atresia
C. Occurs in 5% cases of Tetralogy of Fallot
D. Occurs in 5% cases of Truncus arteriosus

42. **Which of the following is not associated with increased incidence of fetal mortality?**
A. Cardiopulmonary bypass
B. Oral coumarin
C. ACE inhibitors
D. Heparin anticoagulation

43. **Plain X-ray chest in a 2 year old child with coarctation of aorta not in CHF which of the following radiological signs would be seen?**
A. Rib notching
B. Cardiomegaly
C. E sign
D. Normal heart size

32 D 33 B 34 C 35 D 36 D 37 C 38 B 39 C 40 D 41 A 42 D 43 D

44. Most common complication following BMV is:
A. MR
B. Acute pulmonary oedema
C. Acute cardiac tamponade
D. Systemic embolization

45. Which of the following produce reverse splitting of second heart sound ?
A. Left bundle branch block
B. Moderate mitral regurgitation
C. MVP
D. Mitral stenosis

46. Which of the following changes is not observed in a patient with hypothermia ?
A. Osborne waves
B. J point elevation
C. Sinus bradycardia
D. Ventricular tachycardia

47. 32 year old young man is admitted with intermitted sever sinus bradycardia and heart rate of 25/min. His TMT shows that he achieved 97% of his target heart rate rate with no ST-T changes. Electrophysiology showed HV=40 mscc at an atrial pacing of 150/min. The pacing modality of choice for this patient would be:
A. VVI B. VVIR
C. DDD D. AAI

48. P_{50} of the oxygen dissociation curve is shifted to the left by:
A. Acidosis
B. Increase in pH
C. Increase in temperature
D. Increase in PCO_2

49. Electrocardiogram of a patient with athletic heart syndrome may show:
A. Increased QRS amplitude
B. Prominent U wave
C. Shortened QT interval
D. Sinus bradycardia

50. A 25 year old young lady is admitted to the emergency with tight mitral stenosis, 24 weeks pregnancy and atrial fibrillation which started two hours back. Which of the following is the best modality of treatment in this patient?
A. Electrial cardio version
B. Quinidine IV
C. Therapeutic abortion
D. Verapamil IV

51. P2 component of second heart sound in tetralogy of Fallot may be audible with all of the following *except:*
A. Pink Fallot
B. Excessive bronco-pulmonary collaterals
C. Bilateral Pulmonary artery branch stenosis
D. Malposition of great arteries

52. Which of the following is an abnormal finding in pregnancy?
A. Wide splitting of first heart sound
B. Third heart sound
C. Fourth heart sound
D. Extra cardiac murmur

53. Pulsus paradoxus is seen in:
A. Pericardial effusion
B. Chronic obstructive lung disease
C. Pulmonary stenosis
D. Tricuspid regurgitation

54. All the following have pure R wave in electrocardiogram *except:*
A. Duchenne's muscular dystrophy
B. True posterior wall infarction
C. Cor pulmonale
D. Ebsteins anomaly

55. Rupture of chordae tendineae is seen in all the following *except:*
A. Aortic insufficiency
B. Rheumatic heart disease
C. Atrial septal defect
D. Idiopathic hypertrophic subaortic stenosis

44 A 45 B 46 D 47 D 48 B 49 D 50 A 51 B 52 C 53 B 54 D 55 A

56. A patient is admitted with the following hemodynamics:

Cardiac output 6.7 Lit/min/m2;
LVED 22 mm Hg PA wedge 23 mm
AO = 90/30 PA = 35/25
RA mean 14

Which of the following may lead to this state?

A. Mitral stenosis (Severe)
B. Aortic stenosis (Severe)
C. Paget's disease
D. Constrictive pericarditis

57. Opening snap is not seen in which of the following ?

A. Primary pulmonary arterial hypertension
B. Atrial septal defect
C. Ebsteins anomaly
D. Pure mitral regurgitation

58. Which of the findings given below are abnormal in a 45 year old man?

A. Grade I/III left parasternal heave
B. LVS3
C. A2 louder than P2
D. Absent pulmonary sound in mitral area

59. Which of the following help in differentiating mitral insufficiency from tricuspid insufficiency:

A. Increase in inspiration
B. Associated mitral stenosis
C. Radiation to base of the heart
D. Opening snap

60. A 27 year old lady with the following hemodynamic data will have a differential diagnosis of all the following *except:*

AO 110/90 (96 mean) PA 40/23 (30 mean)
PAW a27 v28 (26 mean) RA a25 v26 (22mean)
LV 110/25 ed RV 40/24 ed
Cardiac Index =2.1 Lit/min/m2

A. Tight mitral stenosis
B. Pulmonary embolism
C. Endomycardial fibrosis
D. Chronic constructive pericarditis

56 C 57 A 58 B 59 C 60 A

GB Pant 1997

1. In a patient with right aortic arch and PDA, the PDA is found on:
A. Right side
B. Left side
C. Both side
D. Opposite innominate artery

2. Transoesophageal echocardiography is more useful than TTE in diagnosing all *except:*
A. Pulmonary venous embolism
B. LA appendage clot
C. Dissection of descending thoracic aorta
D. Pulmonary artery confluence

3. Color Doppler echo is most useful in diagnosis of:
A. Large ASD B. Large VSD
C. TAPVC D. LV to RA shunt

4. Cyanotic spell is precipitated by all *except:*
A. Fever
B. Polycythemia
C. Digoxin
D. Acidosis

5. In Acute rheumatic fever, the earliest murmur heard is that of:
A. MS B. MR
C. AR D. TR

6. MR in endocardial cushion defect is due to:
A. Cleft mitral leaflet
B. MVP
C. SAM
D. Non coaptation of mitral leaflet

7. Dressler's syndrome is treated with:
A. NSAID B. Aspirin
C. Corticosteroids D. Paracetamol

8. Carcinoid syndrome is characterised by all *except:*
A. Flushes B. Hypertension
C. Bronchitis D. Hypermotility

9. XY collapse is seen in:
A. CCP
B. Cardiac tamponade
C. TB
D. RV failure

10. Characteristic histopathological changes are seen in all *except:*
A. Doxorubicin toxicity
B. Myocarditis
C. DCMP
D. Amyloidosis

11. Balloon atrial septostomy is indicated in all *except:*
A. TGA
B. TOF
C. Complex cyanotic congenital heart disease
D. Pulmonary atresia

1 B 2 D 3 D 4 B 5 B 6 A 7 B 8 C 9 A 10 C 11 B

12. **Eisenmenger syndrome occurs earliest in:**
A. ASD B. VSD
C. PDA D. AP window

13. **Phasic ejection click occurs in:**
A. AS B. CoA
C. PS D. PAH

14. **Continous murmur is heard in all *except:***
A. RSOV
B. Pulmonary atresia
C. TAPVC (Supracardiac)
D. Fetal circulation

15. **Bounding femoral pulse in 1 day old baby is seen in:**
A. PDA
B. Hypoxia
C. Systemic A-V fistula
D. CoA

16. **Congestive heart failure in fetus occurs in:**
A. PDA B. Ebstein's anomaly
C. CoA D. ALCAPA

17. **Hypercholesterolemia occurs in all *except:***
A. Biliary obstruction
B. CRF
C. Pregnancy
D. Ulcerative colitis

18. **Gestational hypertesion: all of the following antihypertensives can be used *except:***
A. Methyldopa
B. Hydralazine
C. Betablockers
D. Diuretics

19. **All of the following are pulmonary vasodilators *except:***
A. Oxygen B. Nitrous oxide
C. PGE1 D. Acidosis

20. **Which complication is not seen in modified BT shunt:**
A. Infective endocarditis
B. Shortening of the arm
C. CHF
D. Obstruction of the shunt

21. **Continuous murmur is heard in all *except:***
A. TAPVC
B. BT Shunt
C. PDA with equalization of systemic and pulmonary pressure
D. Fetal circulation

22. **From the cardiac catheterization data of the child, RA O_2 sat: 67%, PA-71%, LA-69%, Aorta-70%; Probable diagnosis is:**
A. Tricuspid atresia
B. TAPVC
C. ASD
D. PAPVC

23. **Paradoxical movement of IVS is seen in all *except:***
A. PAH
B. Pulmonary embolism
C. Cardiac tamponade
D. RV MI

24. **Adverse effect of using bicarbonate in CPR is:**
A. Respiratory alkalosis
B. Hyperkalemia
C. Hypercalcemia
D. Respiratory acidosis

25. **Best way of diagnosing CAD in a patient with LBBB:**
A. TMT
B. Nuclear imaging
C. Dobutamine echo
D. Contrast echo

12 D 13 C 14 D 15 C 16 B 17 C 18 D 19 D 20 B 21 C 22 A 23 C 24 D
25 B

26. Congenital heart disease which presents with cyanosis at birth:

A. D-TGA
B. l-TGA
C. CoA
D. TOF with pulmonary atresia

27. Type of HDL which has antiatherosclerotic property is:

A. HDL-1 B. HDL-2
C. HDL-3 D. HDL-4

28. Dissection of aorta is associated with:

A. Marfan's syndrome B. Takayasu's disease
C. CoA D. Chest Trauma

29. Clinical features of CHF are all *except:*

A. ↑ A-V oxygen difference
B. Cyanosis
C. ↑ Filling pressures
D. Oliguria

30. Cardiac manifestation in HIV include:

A. Pericarditis B. Myocarditis
C. Malignancy D. All of the above

31. Child born with CHF: Probable diagnosis is:

A. TGA
B. Hypoplastic LV syndrome
C. CoA
D. Critical AS

32. Calcium is not used routinely in CPR because of:

A. Intracellular accumulation causing uncoupling of oxidative phosphorylation
B. Promotion of hypokalemia
C. Promotion of acidosis
D. Promotion of alkalosis

33. Following condition increases sensitivity to digoxin *except:*

A. Cor pulmonale B. Hypothyroidism
C. Hypothermia D. Hyperthermia

34. Beta blockers without ISA activity and membrane stabilizing action is:

A. Carvedilol B. Bucindolol
C. Acebutolol D. Pindolol

35. A-V dissociation in SVT rules out:

A. Intra-atrial reentry
B. SA nodal reentry
C. AV nodal reentry
D. AV nodal reentry through bypass tracts

36. Salient features regarding lipoprotein 'a' are:

A. Analogue of plasminogen
B. Responsible for increase incidence of CAD in Indians
C. Decrease by Niacin, Oestrogen, bezafibrate and stanozol
D. All of the above

37. Oxygen saturation in PA will be greater than aorta in:

A. d-TGA
B. DORV with subpulmonic VSD
C. DORV with subaortic VSD
D. Pulmonary atresia with VSD

38. Valsalva maneuver causes:

A. Widening of A2-OS gap
B. Narrowing of A2-OS gap
C. No effect on A2-OS gap
D. Paradoxical occurrence of A2-OS gap

39. Factors responsible for increased mortality in obesity:

A. Hyperinsulinemia
B. Hypertension
C. Hypertriglyceridemia
D. Hypercholesterolemia

40. Factor which does not reverse with weight reduction in obese subjects is:

A. PAH
B. Increased blood volume
C. Increased Cardiac output
D. LVH

26 A 27 B 28 A 29 B 30 D 31 B 32 A 33 D 34 A 35 D 36 D 37 A 38 B
39 A 40 A

41. Compensatory mechanism in shock are all *except:*
A. Increased ADH
B. Increased sympathetic flow
C. Increased renin
D. Increased ANP

42. The diagnosis of malignant pheochromocytoma is made by:
A. Abdominal CT Scan
B. ID 123 MIBG
C. Meta
D. Rapid

43. The commonest reperfusion arrhythmia in acute inferior wall MI is:
A. Sinus bradycardia B. CHB
C. PJRT D. AIVR

44. Which of the following contribute to changes in the contour of the arterial pulse, pressure wave as it is transmitted peripherally?
A. Difference in elastic behaviour and caliber of the arteries
B. Conversion of kinetic energy into potential or hydrostatic energy
C. Distortion and damping of components of the pulse wave
D. Amplification of reflected resonance or standard waves

45. Which is incorrect regarding rupture of IV septum following acute myocardial infarction:
A. Occurs most commonly 3-5 days after MI
B. Occurs more commonly at the apex in AWMI
C. Basal septum rupture is more common in IWMI
D. Apical rupture of the IVS is more fatal

46. Which is not true about electrolytes and urinary finding in primary hyperaldosteronism:
A. Hypokalemia
B. Alkalosis
C. Decreased specific gravity of urine
D. Hyponatremia

47. Drug not metabolized in liver is:
A. Amiodarone B. Diltiazem
C. Propranolol D. Adenosine

48. Pott's shunt is:
A. Ascending aorta with RPA
B. Descending aorta with LPA
C. Descending aorta with left subclavian
D. Descending aorta with MPA

49. Amyl-nitrite inhalation causes all *except:*
A. Decreased AR murmur
B. Decreased MR murmur
C. Decreased MS murmur
D. Increased MS murmur

50. Which of the statement about cardiac tamponade is not true?
A. Systemic venous pressure is elevated
B. Pulmonary venous pressure is elevated
C. Venous return to the right side falls during inspiration
D. Heart rate is increased

51. In a patient with acute arthritis, rheumatic fever is probable cause in all *except:*
A. ESR is raised
B. Erythema marginatum is present
C. Pericardial rub is present
D. Opening snap of mitral valve is present

52. All of the following are true with regard to pulse wave being transmitted to periphery *except:*
A. Initial stroke becomes steeper
B. Anacrotic shoulder increases
C. Systolic summit increases
D. Incisura is replaced by dicrotic notch

53. Which of the following is not a major factor in the determination of myocardial oxygen consumption:
A. Intramyocardial tension
B. Heart rate
C. Cardiac output
D. Contractile state of the heart

41 D 42 B 43 A 44 D 45 D 46 D 47 D 48 B 49 C 50 C 51 D 52 B 53 C

54. When an infarct occurs in a normal heart, how much myocardium must be lost before ventricular failure occurs:

A. 10% B. 15%
C. 25% D. 40%

55. Which is a true statement:

A. Asplenia usually has severe pulmonary stenosis or atresia and a high association with hepatic segment of IVC
B. Asplenia usually presents in older children and commonly has a right aortic arch
C. Polysplenia usually occurs in older children and frequently associated with absent hepatic segment of IVC
D. None of the above

56. ST elevation is seen in all *except:*

A. Acute MI
B. Normal Variation
C. Pericarditis
D. Spontaneous pneumothorax

57. When RV apex is paced, the Frontal plane axis is:

A. – 60°, RBBB B. + 60°, LBBB
C. – 60°, LBBB D. – 120°, LBBB

58. Digoxin absorption is affected by all *except:*

A. Amiodarone B. Cholestyramine
C. Antacids D. Neomycin

59. Which of the following drugs have been found to reduce mortality in post MI patients with LV dysfunction:

A. Amiodarone
B. Beta Blocker
C. Calcium channel blocker
D. Nitrates

60. Which of the following is not usually associated with digitalis administration?

A. Bluish vision B. Yellow vision
C. Gynaecomastia D. Scotomas

54 C 55 C 56 D 57 D 58 A 59 B 60 A

GB Pant 1996

1. ACE inhibitors in acute MI should be started:
A. As soon as patient stabilizes
B. Within 234 hours
C. Within 48 hours
D. Within 72 hours

2. Most sensitive indicator of myocardial ischemia is:
A. ST elevation B. ST depression
C. Chest pain D. Inverted u wave

3. Congenital CHB is seen with:
A. C-TGA B. D-TGA
C. Tricuspid atresia D. TOF

4. A beta blocker without ISA and membrane stabilizing action is:
A. Carvedilol B. Bucindilol
C. Acebutolol D. Pindolol

5. Following conditions increase sensitivity to digoxin *except:*
A. Cor pulmonale B. Hypothyroidism
C. Hyperthermia D. Hypothermia

6. AV dissociation in SVT rules out:
A. Intraatrial reentry
B. SA node reentry
C. AV node reentry
D. AV node reentry through a bypass tract

7. Commonest site of IVS rupture in AMI is:
A. Distal IVS B. Proximal IVS
C. Mid IVS D. None of the above

8. Freidwald's formula is:
A. LDL-C = T. cholesterol – HDL-C – Tg/5
B. LDL-C = T. cholesterol + HDL-C – Tg/5
C. LDL-C = T. cholesterol – HDL-C + Tg/5
D. None of the above

9. Salient features regarding lipoprotein "a" are:
A. More atherogenic than LDL-C
B. Responsible for increase in incidence of CAD in indians
C. Niacin can be used for treatment
D. All of the above

10. Following can be given in unstable angina *except:*
A. Thrombolysis B. Beta blockers
C. Aspirin D. Statins

11. Pott's shunt is:
A. Descending aorta to pulmonary artery
B. Ascending aorta to pulmonary artery
C. Subclavian artery to pulmonary artery
D. None of the above

12. A child born to a mother with SLE is most likely to have the following cardiac abnormality:
A. CHB B. IE
C. MR D. TOF

1 A 2 B 3 A 4 A 5 C 6 D 7 A 8 A 9 D 10 A 11 A 12 A

13. Oxygen saturation more in pulmonary artery than aorta will be found in:
A. d-TGA
B. Tausig Bing anomaly
C. DORV with subaortic VSD
D. TOF with pulmonary atresia

14. Reverse splitting of S2 is heard in all *except:*
A. LBBB B. MVP
C. AS D. HOCM

15. The normal A2-pericardial knock interval is:
A. 90-120 msec B. 120-150 msec
C. 70-90 msec D. 50-70 msec

16. Valsalva maneuver causes:
A. ↓A2-P2 interval, ↓coronary blood flow
B. ↑A2-P2 interval, ↑coronary blood flow
C. ↓A2-P2 interval, ↑coronary blood flow
D. ↑A2-P2 interval, ↓coronary blood flow

17. Amylnitrate inhalation has what effect on murmur of MS:
A. Increases B. Decreases
C. No effect D. None of the above

18. An agent which interferes with the scar formation in AMI is:
A. Corticosteroids B. Beta blockers
C. Interleukins D. NSAIDS

19. A pacing wire which is wrongly introduced into the CS and then into the great cardiac vein closely mimics being at the RV apex. The frontal plane QRS axis in this case is:
A. Superior, LBBB
B. Inferior, LBBB
C. Superior, RBBB
D. Inferior, RBBB

20. Pulsus alternans is characteristically seen in:
A. DCMP B. HOCM
C. CCP D. RCMP

21. Earliest elevation of which of the following will be seen in AMI:
A. CPK-MB B. CPK-MM
C. Troponin D. Myoglobin

22. Pulmonary oedema with normal PCWP is seen in:
A. HAPE B. MS
C. AS D. Cortriatriatum

23. Sudden death with exercise is seen with:
A. Origin of left coronary artery from right cusp with passage between aorta and pulmonary artery
B. Anomalous origin of LCx from RCA
C. Anomalous origin of coronary artery from pulmonary artery
D. None of the above

24. Treatment of choice for severe primary pulmonary hypertension is:
A. Heart lung transplantation
B. Heart transplantation
C. Bilateral lung transplantation
D. Single lung transplantation

25. The commonest reperfusion arrhythmia in acute IWMI is:
A. Sinus bradycardia B. CHB
C. Sustained VT D. PSVT

26. Reverse Splitting of S1 is heard in:
A. MS B. TS
C. TR D. PS

27. Normal AH and HV interval is:
A. 55-130 msec, 35-55 msec
B. 10-55 msec, 55-130 msec
C. 35-55 msec, 55-130 msec
D. 10-45 msec, 55-75 msec

28. Drug interfering with digoxin absorption is:
A. Beta blocker B. ACE inhibitor
C. Cholestyramine D. Lidocaine

13 A 14 B 15 A 16 A 17 A 18 A 19 C 20 A 21 D 22 A 23 A 24 C 25 A
26 A 27 A 28 C

29. Most common cause of MI in infant at 8 wks is:
A. ALCAPA
B. ARCAPA
C. Anomalous origin of LCx from RCA
D. TGA

30. A patient of MI presents on 7th day and cath findings are elevated RVEDP, elevated PA pressure and step up of oxygen upto 15% at RV level. The treatment of choice in this condition will be:
A. Immediate surgery
B. Routine management of MI
C. ACE inhibitor
D. None of the above

31. Maximum oxygen consumption is equal to:
A. HR × BP
B. SV × HR
C. Coronary blood flow × Coronary sinus oxygen content
D. CO × A-V oxygen difference

32. Cause of left AV valve regurgitation in c-TGA is:
A. Displacement of AV valve below annulus
B. A cleft in the septal leaflet
C. Dilatation of valve annulus
D. Intrinsic deformity of valve such as thickening of leaflet

33. Pacemaker sounds:
A. Are generated only when cardiac perforation by the pacing electrode occurs
B. Always indicate the need for electrode repositioning
C. Are generated by the left hemi diaphragm or intercostal muscle adjacent to the electrode tip
D. Are usually associated with failure of cardiac sensing and pacing

34. Laboratory findings in primary aldosteronism will show:
A. ↓Sodium, ↓potassium, ↓CO_2, ↑urine pH
B. ↑Sodium, ↓potassium, ↑CO_2, ↑urine pH, ↑PRA
C. Normal Sodium, ↓potassium, CO_2, ↑urine pH, ↑PRA
D. Normal Sodium, ↓potassium, ↑CO_2, ↑urine pH, ↓PRA

35. Which of the following contributed to changes in the contour of the arterial pulse pressure wave as it is transmitted peripherally:
A. Difference in elastic behaviour and calibre of the arteries
B. Conversion of kinetic energy into potential or hydrostatic energy
C. Distortion and clamping of components of the pulse wave
D. Amplification by reflected resonance or standard waves

36. Which of the following hemodynamic situation results in a decrease in the mean arterial blood pressure:
A. Elevated cardiac output with increase viscosity of blood
B. Increase blood viscosity with decrease net length of blood vessels
C. Peripheral vasoconstriction combined with decrease venous return
D. Diminish net vascular tone together with hemodilution

37. All of the following are true with regard to the pulse wave being transmitted to the periphery *except:*
A. The initial upstroke becomes steeper
B. The anacrotic shoulder increases
C. Systolic summit becomes increased
D. Incisura is replaced by a dicrotic notch

38. Which of the following is not a major factor in determination of myocardial oxygen consumption?
A. Intramyocardial tension
B. Heart rate
C. Contractile state of heart
D. Cardiac output

29 A 30 A 31 D 32 A 33 C 34 D 35 D 36 D 37 B 38 D

39. True statement regarding electrical defibrillation are:
A. Delivered energy is less than energy stored in the capacitor
B. Delivered output of commercially available defibrillators has increased over the past 5 years
C. Delivered waveform is altered by varying the impedance into which the defibrillator is discharged
D. All of the above

40. How much myocardium is lost before ventricular failure occurs in MI?
A. 10% B. 25%
C. 40% D. 50%

41. Application of magnet over a permanent pacemaker results is:
A. Total pacemaker inhibition so that underlying cardiac conduction may be evaluated
B. Reversion to the fixed rate mode
C. Ventricular fibrillation in normal patients
D. Loss of cardiac capture

42. The diagnosis of malignant pheochromocytoma is best by:
A. Presence of metastasis
B. Histologic criteria
C. Response to drug therapy
D. Rapid progression of the disease

43. Which of the following drug has prominent arteriolar dilating effect:
A. Hydralazine B. NTG
C. Prazosin D. Frusemide

44. Which of the following arterial pulses normally peaks nearly simultaneously when palpated simultaneously?
A. Carotid and brachial
B. Radial and femoral
C. Carotid and femoral
D. Brachial and femoral

45. Which of the following circulatory parameters does not appear to be reversible with weight reduction in obese subjects:
A. LVH
B. HTN
C. High cardiac output
D. Pulmonary hypertension

46. What 2 variables must be determined when blood velocity is calculated from doppler echocardiographic data ?
A. Cross sectional area and doppler frequency shift
B. Doppler frequency shift and doppler angle
C. Doppler frequency shift and cosine of Doppler angle
D. Doppler angle and crossectional area

47. The most important factor which determines the clinical manifestation of a penetrating cardiac wound is:
A. Type of weapon used for injusry: bullet or knife
B. Site of cardiac wound: atrial or ventricular
C. Size of wound: large or small
D. The state of pericardial wound: sealed or open

48. Following a transient ischemic stroke, the likelihood of ischemic stroke within 2 years is about:
A. 5% B. 20%
C. 40% D. 60%

49. Which of the following statements is false regarding M1 and T1 component of first heart sound:
A. Both occur 20-40 msec after pressure cross over of the respective ventricles and atria
B. In the normal subject M1 precedes T1 and is usually the dominant sound heard
C. M1 and T1 are coincident with the final closure point (C) of mitral and tricuspid valves on echocardiogram
D. There is always a direct correlation between the intensity of M1 and T1 and the peak Dp/Dt of the right and left ventricle respectively

39 D 40 B 41 B 42 A 43 A 44 B 45 D 46 C 47 D 48 B 49 D

50. **The most frequent complication of popliteal artery aneurysm is:**
A. Thromboembolism
B. Rupture
C. Pressure on surrounding structures
D. Infection

51. **Paradoxical interventricular septal motion is not seen in:**
A. CCP
B. Aortic stenosis
C. ASD
D. After MVR

52. **Which of the following is least sensitive in the diagnosis of right ventricular infarction?**
A. Radionuclide angiography
B. Hemodynamic monitoring
C. Tc^{99} pyrophosphate myocardial scintigraphy
D. Two dimensional echocardiography

53. **Which of the following is not an ECG manifestation of an athletes heart?**
A. RBBB
B. qS in V1-V3
C. Inverted T in V4-V6
D. Persistent juvenile T wave pattern

54. **A disease process producing pure AR which involves both aorta and valve is:**
A. Syphilis
B. Marfans syndrpme
C. Ankylosing spondylosis
D. Infective endocarditis

55. **Which of the following is not associated with a lower procedural success rate:**
A. Eccentric lesions
B. Calcified lesions
C. Concentric lesions
D. Long lesions

56. **Which is not a physical examination finding in trained athletes:**
A. Third heart sound
B. Fourth heart sound
C. Aortic ejection sound
D. Right ventricular hypertrophy

57. **What is the time interval between the onset of myocardial ischemia and initiation of glycolytic metabolism ?**
A. < 60 sec
B. 1-5 min
C. 5-10 min
D. > 10 min

58. **Indications for permanent pacing in chronic bundle branch block include:**
A. RBBB
B. LBBB
C. RBBB an LAHB
D. Bifascicular block with symptomatic second degree AV block

59. **Which of the following statement is correct:**
A. Higher frequency are more easily palpable than lower frequency
B. Lower frequencies are more easily audible than higher frequency
C. Phonocardiograms are obtained by attenuation of rapid changes of the primary displacement or pressure signal
D. Phonocardiograms are usually obtained by attenuation of lower frequencies of the primary displacement or pressure signal

60. **Which of the following is not an important feedback mechanism in shock:**
A. Increased activity of the sympathetic nervous system
B. Increased adrenal medullary synthesis of catecholamine
C. Decrease in oxygen utilization by vital organs
D. ADH release from the posterior pituitary

50 A 51 B 52 A 53 A 54 C 55 C 56 C 57 A 58 D 59 D 60 C

GB Pant 1995

1. Parameter used to assess the severity of AR in a case with AR plus MR is:
A. Situation of LV apex
B. S3
C. MDM
D. Type of split of S2

2. Myxedema is associated with all *except:*
A. Decrease heart rate
B. Low QRS
C. Type III hyperlipidemia
D. Preexcitation

3. Which is true statement about NTG?
A. May cause chest pain in HOCM
B. Primary mechanism by increase vasodilation
C. Commonly causes methemoglobinemia
D. Prolonged increase in receptors with continuous use

4. Aortic root angio leading to opacities in pulmonary artery is least likely in:
A. RSOV to RV
B. RSOV to LV
C. RSOV to RA
D. RSOV to PA

5. Commonest cause of IE in India is:
A. Sterptococcus viridians
B. Staphylococcus aureus
C. Staphylococcus albus
D. Chlamydia pneumonia

6. BP difference greater than 5 mm Hg in upper limbs is seen in all *except:*
A. PDA
B. Subvalvular AS
C. Origin of SCA from descending thoracic aorta
D. Coarctation of Aorta

7. Interstitial nephritis is associated with all *except:*
A. Hyperkalemia, hypercloremic acidosis
B. Increase anmmonia production and excretion
C. Fanconi's syndrome
D. None of the above

8. Increase chance of aortic dissection is seen in all *except:*
A. ASD B. CoA
C. PDA D. Congenital AS

9. Barter's syndrome; all are seen *except:*
A. Hypertension
B. Metabolic alkalosis
C. Oliguria
D. None of the above

10. Drug contraindicated in pregnancy is:
A. Enalapril B. Digoxin
C. Propanalol D. Heparin

11. Large tongue is seen in all *except:*
A. Hyperthyroidism B. Amyloidosis
C. Down's syndrome D. Hurler's syndrome

1 C 2 D 3 A 4 B 5 A 6 B 7 B 8 A 9 A 10 A 11 A

12. **Pompe's disease: all are seen *except:***
    A. Type II glycogen storage disease
    B. HCMP
    C. Phytanic acid storage
    D. Acid mutase deficiency

13. **Suprasystemic RV pressure is seen in:**
    A. PS with intact IVS
    B. Eisenmenger's syndrome
    C. TOF
    D. Pulmonary atresia

14. **Aortic oxygen 98% and PA oxygen saturation 58% is suggestive of:**
    A. Low cardiac output state
    B. High output state
    C. Right to left shunt
    D. Left to right shunt

15. **PA saturation greater the aortic saturation is seen in all *except:***
    A. Taussig Bing Anomaly
    B. DORV with doubly committed VSD
    C. TGA
    D. Pulmonary atresia

16. **Lipoprotein 'a'; all are true *except:***
    A. Bell shaped distribution in population
    B. Independent risk factor in population
    C. Niacin can be used for treatment
    D. Easily standardized assays

17. **Which of thew following are associated with increased effective PBF:**
    A. ALCAPA B. TGA
    C. TOF D. None of the above

18. **Following are the complications of a very small VSD *except:***
    A. IE
    B. Recurrent embolism from ventricular septal aneurysms
    C. Prolapse of aortic valve in outlet VSD
    D. Eisenmenger's syndrome

19. **Square root pattern of valsalva is seen with all *except:***
    A. ASD B. VSD
    C. CCF D. MS

20. **Features suggestive of impaired LV function in TMT is:**
    A. Failure of BP to rise
    B. ST depression
    C. Inadequate heart rate rise
    D. VPC's

21. **Wide split S2 is seen in all *except:***
    A. LBBB B. VSD
    C. ASD D. MR

22. **Absolute indication for stopping exercise testing is:**
    A. Giddiness
    B. ST depression in V1-V3
    C. Q in II, III, aVF
    D. Inverted U waves in V1-V6

23. **Half life of digoxin is:**
    A. 12 hours B. 24 hours
    C. 36 hours D. 48 hours

24. **Normal PCWP is upto:**
    A. 2 mm Hg B. 4 mm Hg
    C. 6 mm Hg D. 8 mm Hg

25. **Glenn's shunt is:**
    A. SVC to RPA B. IVC to RPA
    C. IVC to MPA D. SVC to LPA

26. **If velocity across aortic valve is 5 m/sec, then the gradient is:**
    A. 50 mm Hg B. 75 mm Hg
    C. 100 mm Hg D. 125 mm Hg

27. **Single second sound is heard in:**
    A. Eisenmenger complex
    B. Eisenmenger PDA
    C. TOF
    D. VSD

12 C 13 A 14 A 15 D 16 D 17 B 18 D 19 B 20 A 21 A 22 A 23 C 24 D
25 A 26 C 27 A

28. Which of the following is not seen in obesity:
A. Decreased oxygen consumption
B. Increased EDV
C. LVH
D. Increased QT

29. Which of the following is not seen in pregnancy:
A. S3
B. Increased PVR
C. Decreased PVR
D. Hyperkinetic circulation

30. Which of the following is not a CAD risk factor:
A. Decrease HDL
B. Diabetes mellitus
C. Smoking
D. Se Calcium levels

31. Renovascular hypertension is associated with all of the following findings in IVP *except:*
A. Early opacification
B. Delayed opacification
C. Early filling of kidney without renal artery stenosis
D. None of the above

32. Which of the following statement is true about TS:
A. End diastolic pressure of RV is normal
B. End diastolic pressure of RV decreases during expiration
C. End diastolic volume increases on expiration
D. None of the above

33. EPSS on echo is increased in:
A. DCMP B. HOCM
C. AS D. PS

34. Syndrome X is associated with all *except:*
A. Normal coronaries
B. Normal coronary reserve
C. Angina
D. More in women

35. Common virus causing myocarditis is:
A. Coxsackie B
B. Coxsackie A
C. HIV
D. Echo virus

36. Endocardial cushion defects include all *except:*
A. Ostium secundum ASD
B. Ostium Primum ASD
C. VSD
D. MR

37. H wave is seen in all *except:*
A. Restrictive CMP
B. CCP
C. Right ventricular infarction
D. Pulmonary embolism

38. Penetrating chest injury most commonly involves:
A. RV B. RA
C. LA D. LV

39. Cath data:

PCWP = LAP = RVEDP = PADP,
PA = RV 60/40 mm Hg,

is suggestive of:
A. MS B. PS
C. TR D. PR

40. Pulsus Parvus et tardus is seen in:
A. AS B. AR
C. MS D. MR

41. Apo B100 is associated with:
A. HDI B. LDL
C. Triglyceride D. None of the above

42. Kussumaul's sign is seen with all *except:*
A. CCP
B. RV failure
C. PS
D. Cardiac tamponade

28 A 29 B 30 D 31 A 32 A 33 A 34 B 35 A 36 A 37 D 38 A 39 A 40 A
41 B 42 D

43. Ten year old male with cyanosis and clubbing and normal ECG and normal Cardiovascular examination; diagnosis is:
A. Pulmonary AV fistula
B. TOF
C. cTGA VSD PS
D. Ebsteins anomaly

44. Right heart border is formed by all *except:*
A. SVC B. RA
C. IVC D. RV

45. Cobalt cardiomyopathy is:
A. DCMP B. RCMP
C. HCMP D. None of the above

46. Rarest type of RSOV is:
A. Into RA B. Into LV
C. Into RV D. Into PA

47. Intravenous propanalol produces:
A. Increase heart rate
B. Increase EDV
C. Increase oxygen consumption
D. Decrease oxygen consumption

48. Left dominant circulation is called when:
A. PDA arises from LCx
B. PDA arises from RCA
C. RV branch is very small
D. None of the above

49. Which is the shortest acting beta blocker:
A. Esmolol B. Propranolol
C. Bucindilol D. Timolol

50. In normotensive TR, pulmonary artery pressure is:
A. > 40 mm Hg B. 40-60 mm Hg
C. < 40 mm Hg D. More than 80 mm Hg

51. Paradoxical split of S2 is heard in all *except:*
A. LBBB B. AS
C. HOCM D. MVP

52. Most common cardiological presentation of PAN is:
A. CHF B. MI
C. IE D. RCMP

53. Obtuse marginal is a branch of:
A. LCx B. RCA
C. LAD D. Pulmonary artery

54. QT prolongation is seen with all *except:*
A. Amiodarone B. Quinidine
C. Lidocaine D. Flecainide

55. Earliest sign of hyperkalemia is:
A. Tall tented T waves
B. Widened QRS
C. Decrease P wave amplitude
D. None of the above

56. In Barlow's syndrome, the drug to be avoided is:
A. Nitrates B. Beta blockers
C. Aspirin D. Phenytoin

57. Urgent BT shunt is used for:
A. Hypoplastic pulmonary arteries
B. Child with recurrent cyanotic spells
C. Pink TOF
D. TOF with pulmonary atresia

58. Coronary vasodilator is:
A. Adenosine B. Nitrates
C. Acetycholine D. All of the above

59. Plexogenic changes are seen in all *except:*
A. PPH
B. Pulmonary embolism
C. Eisenmenger's syndrome
D. Left to right shunts

60. Cholesterol crystals in pericardial fluid are seen in:
A. Tubercular B. Ischemic
C. Traumatic D. Hypothyroidism

43 A 44 D 45 A 46 B 47 D 48 A 49 A 50 C 51 D 52 A 53 A 54 C 55 A
56 A 57 B 58 D 59 B 60 D

AIIMS 2004 (June)

1. **Hypertension is seen with all *except:***
   A. Low level of lead exposure
   B. Acute intermittent porphyria
   C. Reninoma
   D. Barter's syndrome

2. **Stroke with BP 170/100 mm Hg is mostly due to:**
   A. Preeclampsia
   B. CRF
   C. Coarctation
   D. Essential hypertension

3. **Young 30 year male present with worst ever headache with absent femoral and BP 170/100 most probable diagnosis is:**
   A. SAH
   B. Hypertensive encephalopathy
   C. Aortic dissection
   D. Temporal arteritis

4. **All of the following are common in women *except:***
   A. Hypertension
   B. Low HDL
   C. Diabetes
   D. Obesity

5. **Women compared to man have all *except:***
   A. More false positive stress test
   B. More mortality after MI
   C. More bleeding with thrombolytic
   D. Present more commonly as MI

6. **All are true about early systolic murmur *except:***
   A. VSD with severe PAH
   B. Small VSD
   C. TR due to MS
   D. Chordae rupture

7. **All are true about continuous murmur *except:***
   A. Cerebral AVM
   B. Peripheral pulmonary artery stenosis
   C. Small VSD with MS
   D. ALCAPA

8. **Graham Steel murmur all true *except:***
   A. TOF with absent pulmonary valve
   B. MS
   C. PDA
   D. Pulmonary embolism

9. **All are true about dicrotic pulse *except:***
   A. Sepsis
   B. Elderly hypertensive
   C. Hypovolemia
   D. CHF

10. **All are true about syncope *except:***
   A. Pulmonary embolism
   B. Cardiac tamponade
   C. Internal hemorrhage
   D. Carotid artery stenosis

1 D 2 C 3 A 4 B 5 D 6 C 7 C 8 A 9 B 10 D

11. All are true about hypersensitive carotid sinus syndrome all true *except:*
A. More in elderly
B. >3 sec pause
C. Precipitated by neck movements
D. Cure mostly by ventricular pacing

12. Incidence of VF is more in all *except:*
A. Malignant hyperthermia
B. WPW
C. Malignant neurocardiogenic syncope
D. Acute inferior MI

13. Dose of aspirin for prevention of vascular atherosclerosis:
A. 75-375 mg B. 50-150 mg
C. 150-1500 mg D. 10 mg/kg

14. Total pulmonary vascular resistance is:
A. 700-1600 B. 20-130
C. 10-300 D. 400-600

15. Increase arteriovenous oxygen difference with decreased mixed venous oxygen difference is seen in all *except:*
A. Strenuous exercise
B. Anaemia
C. Low cardiac output
D. Cyanide poisoning

16. 70 year old male with severe AS with chronic AF: all are true *except:*
A. Mechanical valve
B. Ross procedure
C. Tissue valve
D. Aortic valve repair

17. Asymptomatic adult patient with AR and LVEDD 55mm management is:
A. Aortic valve repair
B. Ross procedure
C. Nifedipine
D. Homograft

18. 10 year old boy comes with acute rheumatic fever; echo findings are all *except:*
A. MS B. MVP
C. AS D. TR

19. Acute IE is caused by all *except:*
A. β hemolytic streptococci
B. Pneumococci
C. Staph aureus
D. HACEK

20. All is true about serology of culture negative endocarditis *except:*
A. Bartonella B. Brucella
C. Coxiella D. Tuberculosis

21. 10 year old girl with total cholesterol 600 mg%, triglycerides 120 mg% diagnosis is:
A. Erruptive xanthoma
B. Bilateral xanthelesma
C. Tendon xanthoma
D. Tuberous xanthoma

22. All are true for Framingham major criteria for CHF *except:*
A. PND
B. S_3
C. Circulation time >25 sec
D. Bilteral ankle edema

23. In aldosteronism absence of edema explained by:
A. Decreased renin
B. Suppressed angiotension II receptors
C. Pressure natriuresis
D. Hypokalemia

24. All are true about A1 receptor of adenosine *except:*
A. SA node depression
B. AV node depression
C. Coronary vasodilation
D. Ischemic preconditioning

11 D 12 C 13 A 14 C 15 D 16 C 17 C 18 C 19 D 20 D 21 C 22 D 23 C
24 C

25. All are true about LVH on ECG *except:*
A. Less sensitive and more specific
B. Indicator of increased morbidity and mortality
C. Suggestive of myocardial mass 90 gm/m^2
D. False positive in children

26. All are true about critical limb ischemia *except:*
A. Absence of pulse with exercise
B. Rubor
C. Dependent edema
D. Rest pain

27. All are true about pseudoinfarction pattern *except:*
A. Emphysema
B. Myocardial sarcoid
C. HOCM
D. Post cardiopulmonary bypass

28. All are true about low voltage ECG all true *except:*
A. WPW
B. Normal variant
C. Extensive MI
D. Addison's disease

29. In CHF commonly seen electrolyte abnormality are all *except:*
A. Hypophosphotemia
B. Dilutional Hyponatremia
C. Hypouricemia
D. Hypomagnesemia

30. All are true about severity of AS *except:*
A. Cardiomegaly
B. Gradient velocity @ 4 m/sec
C. Valve calcification
D. LVH with strain

31. Severe AR on echo true is:
A. PHT <200 msec
B. AML fluttering
C. Aortic annulus >50 mm
D. LVEDD >55 mm

32. All are true about poor prognostic marker on TMT *except:*
A. Not increasing SBP to >120 mmHg
B. Angina at low work threshold
C. ST elevation
D. Rate pressure product >25,000

33. Relative indication for termination of TMT are all *except:*
A. Hypertensive response
B. SVT
C. Patient's desire to stop
D. Fatigue

34. All are features of Marfan syndrome *except:*
A. Aortic root dilatation
B. MVP/AR
C. Bicuspid aortic valve
D. Aortic dissection

35. All of the following have shown to decrease the symptoms/mortality in CHF *except:*
A. Digoxin
B. ACE inhibitors
C. β blockers
D. Dual chamber pacing

36. All are true about RVMI with CHB *except:*
A. IV fluids
B. AV sequential pacing
C. IABP
D. IV NTG

37. Which of the following catheter is not used for CAG:
A. Judkins
B. Sones
C. Amplatz
D. Cournard

38. Indication of surgery for treatment of true aneurysm are all *except:*
A. Tachyarrhythmia
B. Refractory angina
C. Rupture
D. Emboli

25 C 26 A 27 D 28 A 29 C 30 C 31 A 32 D 33 C 34 C 35 D 36 D 37 D 38 C

39. JNC 7 grade 1 hypertension treatment modalities include all *except:*
A. Lifestyle modification
B. Moderation of alcohol
C. Thiazide diuretics
D. K^+ sparing diuretics

40. LV wall stress measurement require all *except:*
A. Ventricular radius
B. Ventricular pressure
C. LV stress constant
D. Wall thickness

41. Diastolic function on echo are assessed by all *except:*
A. –ve dp/dt
B. Aortic closure to MV opening time (IVRT)
C. Tau index
D. Peak rate of LV wall thinning

42. Least half life is of:
A. Tenecteplase (TNK)
B. Reteplase
C. Alteplase
D. STK

43. Incidence of CHB in RFA is least in:
A. AVNRT
B. Atrial flutter
C. Posteroseptal/anteroseptal pathway
D. Left free wall pathway

44. Total electrical alternans is seen in:
A. Long QT syndrome
B. AVRT
C. Myocardial ischemia
D. Cardiac tamponade

45. Termination of atrial fibrillation; drug of choice for oral administration is:
A. Flecainide B. Digoxin
C. Dilzem D. Amiodarone

46. Drugs causing Torsade de pointes are all *except:*
A. Procainamide B. Sotalol
C. Mexiletine D. Amiodarone

47. Least common presentation of SLE is:
A. Pericarditis
B. PHT
C. Cardiac tamponade
D. MI

48. PGE_1 infusion is used to keep PDA patent in all *except:*
A. Pulmonary atresia with intact septum
B. Severe CoA
C. Corrected TGA
D. Hypertrophic pyloric stenosis

49. All true about brain abscess in congenital cyanotic heart disease *except:*
A. Low grade fever in 80%
B. Anticonvulsant to be given in all patient for 6 months
C. MRI for early diagnosis of cerebritis
D. Endocarditis not usually seen with brain abscess

50. Contrast nephropathy; all used for treatment/ prevention *except:*
A. Iso osmolar agent B. N acetyl/cysteine
C. IV frusemide D. Hemofiltration

51. Cyanotic spells in TOF is precipitated by all *except:*
A. Anemia
B. Winter
C. Ephedrine like substance
D. SVT

52. All true about reentrant tachycardia *except:*
A. Monomorphic VT in old MI
B. Atrial flutter
C. WPW with AVRT
D. PAT with block (digoxin induced)

39 D 40 C 41 D 42 C 43 D 44 D 45 A 46 C 47 C 48 C 49 A 50 C 51 C
52 D

53. QT dispersion is related to:
A. Bazetts formula
B. Risk of ventricular arrhythmia
C. Hypocalcemia
D. Filtered QRS duration

54. Fontan in a patient of PS is done in all *except:*
A. Tricuspid atresia
B. DORV with mitral atresia
C. TOF
D. Univentricular heart

55. Vmax least in phase 0 in:
A. Purkinje fibres
B. SA node
C. Papillary muscle
D. Ventricles

56. Restenosis with drug eluting stent:
A. 0-2% B. 4-8%
C. 10% D. 12%

57. True about mortality in MI are all *except:*
A. 30% mortality overall
B. 25% of MI die before reaching hospital
C. In MI survivor at 1 year mortality of 4%
D. 30% mortality in elderly at 1 year

58. True regarding thrombolysis are all *except:*
A. 7% bleeding in 70 year old male
B. tPA better TIMI3 flow than STK
C. Hemorrhagic stroke before 5 years absolute CI
D. 4-10% hypotension with STK

59. Following patient requires TPI during non cardiac surgery:
A. RBBB
B. CHB: 1 yr back IW MI
C. Old MI with RBBB
D. Alternate BBB

60. Myocardial bridges is most common in:
A. LAD B. LC_x
C. RCA D. PDA

61. Digital gangrene with preserved pulses is seen in:
A. DM
B. Leriche's syndrome
C. Burger's disease
D. Aortic aneurysm

62. All are true about β blocker with vasodilatation *except:*
A. Carvidilol B. Bisoprolol
C. Bucindolol D. Labetalol

63. In HIV least common cardiac presentation is:
A. Premature CAD
B. Primary Kaposi sarcoma
C. Asymptomatic pericardial effusion
D. DCMP

64. All are true about heparin induced thrombocytopenia *except:*
A. Type I is most common
B. Type II maximum at 4 days to 2 weeks
C. LMWH less incidence
D. Heparin to be omitted in all

65. Acute MI imaging:
A. Technitium 99 pyrophosphate scan
B. Indium scan
C. Rest thallium
D. MUGA

66. Tuberculosis with hemoptysis: approach should be:
A. Bronchial artery embolization
B. Pulmonary artery cauterization
C. Nd YAG laser
D. Thrombin

67. Reinfarction > 8 days of index event is diagnosed by:
A. Troponin B. CK-MB
C. Thallium D. Echo

53 B 54 C 55 B 56 B 57 B 58 A 59 D 60 A 61 D 62 B 63 B 64 D 65 B
66 A 67 B

68. Fetal echo can diagnose all *except:*
A. AV canal defects **B.** CHB
C. Ebstein's anomaly **D.** PDA

69. ABIOCOR is:
A. Total artificial heart
B. VAD
C. Anti apoptotic drug
D. VSD device

70. Which of the following drug is withdrawn from market?
A. Cerivastatin **B.** Lovastatin
C. Fluvastatin **D.** Gemfibrozil

71. Acute AR with IE is improved by all *except:*
A. Nitroprusside
B. NTG
C. IV Labetolol
D. Urgent Aortic valve replacement

72. All are true about chromosome 22 deletion all true *except:*
A. Truncus/thymic hypoplasia
B. Hypocalcemia
C. Ebstein's anomaly
D. Mild mental retardation

73. Erythropoietin level is increased in all *except:*
A. Lieomyoma
B. TOF
C. Polycythemia vera
D. Cerebellar hemangioma

74. Eosinophilia is caused by all *except:*
A. IL-2
B. Hydroxyurea
C. L-tryptophan ingestion
D. Loefflar's endocarditis

75. All are true about neurofibroma *except:*
A. Arises from Schwan cells
B. Ras oncogene over expression
C. In NF pheochromocytoma is most common cause of hypertension
D. Interferon treatment may regress NF in long term

76. In physiological changes of aging all are decrease *except:*
A. Renin **B.** Total body water
C. Haemoglobin **D.** GFR

77. IV bicarbonate treatment: true is all *except:*
A. Given if pH is < 7.1
B. Goal to reach pH of 7.4 in 30-40 minutes
C. Causes Hypokalemia
D. May precipitate acidosis

78. In respiratory alkalosis all are true *except:*
A. Hypokalemia
B. Bohr shifted to left
C. Cerebral vasodilatation
D. Hypocalcemia

79. All are true about asplenic patient *except:*
A. H. Influenzae **B.** Pneumococcal
C. N. Meningitis **D.** Candida

80. pH 7.4, PO_2 92, PCO_2 40, HCO_3 26, chloride 80 meq/L, K^+ 3.8 meq/L, Na^+ 135 meq/L interpretation is
A. Normal ABG
B. Mixed acid base imbalance
C. Compensated respiratory acidosis
D. Diuretic treatment

81. In early course of disease increased LVEDP is seen in all *except:*
A. Ischemia **B.** RCMP
C. HCMP **D.** Chronic MR

82. Metabolic syndrome X include all *except:*
A. Decreased HDL
B. Normal epicardial coronaries
C. Increased triglycerides
D. Insulin resistance

68 D 69 A 70 A 71 C 72 C 73 C 74 B 75 D 76 C 77 B 78 C 79 D 80 B
81 D 82 B

83. In classical DM lipid abnormalities are all *except:*

A. Decreased HDL
B. Increased triglycerides
C. Increased total cholesterol
D. Increased LDL

84. In atherosclerosis least commonly involved is:

A. Proximal LAD
B. Proximal renal artery
C. Middle cerebral artery
D. Carotid bifurcation

85. True in PPH are all *except:*

A. Nitric oxide
B. Endothelin
C. cAMP
D. Prostacyclin

86. Chorea is caused by all *except:*

A. Pregnancy
B. Hypoxic insult
C. Throtoxicosis
D. APLAS

87. All are true about prinzmetal angina *except:*

A. Smokers
B. Pain during Sleep
C. Precipitated by ergonovine
D. Poor prognosis

88. Large anterior wall MI with apical thrombus; drug to be given life long are all *except:*

A. Aspirin
B. β blockers
C. ACE inhibitors
D. Warfarin

89. Boundaries of Koch's triangle include all *except:*

A. Tendon of Todaro
B. Septal leaflet of tricuspid valve
C. Coronary sinus ostium
D. Limbus of Fossa ovalis

90. IABP is inflated by:

A. Air
B. Oxygen
C. Helium
D. Fluorine

83 D 84 C 85 B 86 B 87 D 88 D 89 D 90 C

AIIMS 2003 (December)

1. **Normal ECG on presentation in acute myocardial infarction is seen in:**
   A. 5% B. 10%
   C. 15% D. 20%

2. **Loss of Q waves 6-12 months post MI:**
   A. 5% B. 10%
   C. 20% D. 30%

3. **RCA dominance is seen in:**
   A. 50% B. 65%
   C. 85% D. 75%

4. **In LAD proximal stenosis all are seen *except:***
   A. Deep T inversion V_1 to V_4
   B. Pseudonormalization of T wave
   C. Ventricular bigeminy
   D. Inverted U waves on exercise

5. **TMT is not advisable in all *except:***
   A. Early post MI (14 days)
   B. Evaluation of CAD in valvular heart disease
   C. Routine screening of asymptomatic patient
   D. Routine follow up of PTCA

6. **RV identified on echo by all *except:***
   A. More apical tricuspid valve
   B. Moderator band
   C. Course septal trabeculation
   D. Origin of pulmonary trunk

7. **Most anteriorly placed valve is:**
   A. Tricuspid B. Aortic
   C. PV D. MV

8. **Hypoxia, normal $PaCO_2$, normal alveolar arterial gradient is suggestive of:**
   A. Decreased FiO_2
   B. Hypoventilation
   C. Shunt lesion
   D. V/Q mismatch

9. **DLCO is decreased in all *except:***
   A. PPH B. VSD
   C. Emphysema D. ILD

10. **Reynold number decreases with:**
    A. Radius of vessel
    B. Velocity of flow
    C. Viscosity of flow
    D. Length of vessel

11. **True about COPD are all *except:***
    A. Inhaled long acting β blockers better than short acting anticholinergic
    B. Glucocorticoids decrease recurrence
    C. Home oxygen treatment PaO_2 <60 mmHg reduces mortality
    D. Lung reduction surgery in non apical emphysema with relatively preserved exercise capacity

1 B 2 D 3 C 4 C 5 A 6 D 7 C 8 A 9 B 10 D 11 B

12. Ventilator associated pneumonia is reduced by all *except:*
A. Gastrointestinal decontamination
B. Frequent hand washing by ICU personnel
C. Frequent tube change
D. Nursing in semi recumbent position

13. True about diaphragmatic palsy are all *except:*
A. Hypoxemia in REM sleep
B. High cervical cord lesion–pacing effective (diaphragmatic)
C. Cause is usually not obvious
D. Can be seen after cardiac surgery

14. Early ischemic stroke is benefited with all *except:*
A. Admission to stroke unit
B. Aspirin
C. LMWH
D. Thrombolysis with rtPA

15. All causes chylous ascites *except:*
A. Filariasis B. Nephrotic syndrome
C. Cirrhosis D. Tuberculosis

16. PGE infusion causes all *except:*
A. Hypertrophic pyloric stenosis
B. Apnoea
C. Fever
D. Ductal aneurysm

17. Dengue haemorrhagic fever: all true *except:*
A. Case fatality rate in untreated person 10%
B. Type 2 is most dangerous
C. Immunological mechanism is responsible for pathogenesis
D. In Dengue shock syndrome myocardial depression occurs

18. Carnitine level may be decreased in all *except:*
A. Chronic renal failure (Fanconi syndrome)
B. Fatty acyl co enzyme A deficiency
C. Total parenteral nutrition
D. Vegetarian diet

19. Stem cell culture does not give rise to:
A. Pancreas B. Myocardium
C. Placenta D. Astrocytes

20. LV S3 likely to indicate LV dysfunction in:
A. VSD B. Anemia
C. CCP D. AR

21. Non infarction septal Q wave in V_5V_6 is seen in all *except:*
A. LBBB B. WPW
C. HOCM D. Hyperkalemia

22. Low voltage ECG is seen in all *except:*
A. Extensive MI
B. Addison's disease
C. Normal variant
D. Glycogen storage disease

23. Linked angina: all true *except:*
A. Caused by true myocardial ischemia
B. Precipitated by Gastrointestinal reflux
C. Seen after cardiac transplant
D. Found in normal coronaries

24. β-blocker-no mortality benefit in CHF:
A. Metoprolol B. Carvidelol
C. Bisoprolol D. Atenolol

25. In MI mortality benefit seen by all *except:*
A. Nitrate B. Aspirin
C. β-blocker D. ACE inhibitor

26. All of the following prolong survival in CHF *except:*
A. Thiazide B. Valsartan
C. Lisinopril D. Carvedilol

27. Increased arterio-venous oxygen difference seen in all *except:*
A. Septic shock
B. Carbon monoxide poisoning
C. Cyanide poisoning
D. Excessive exercise

12 C 13 B 14 C 15 C 16 A 17 A 18 D 19 D 20 D 21 A 22 D 23 C 24 D
25 A 26 A 27 C

28. According to JNC 7 1st drug of choice for hypertension:
A. Diuretics B. CCB's
C. β-blockers D. ACE inhibitors

29. Which of the following acts by prolonging phase 2 of action potential:
A. Digoxin B. Hypocalcemia
C. Quinidine D. Propranalol

30. Relative contra indication to cardiac transplant are all *except:*
A. DM
B. Age > 50 yrs
C. Recent pulmonary infarction
D. Increased PVR

31. All true about rheumatic chorea *except:*
A. 50% of the rheumatic chorea patient may develop MS
B. Secondary prophylaxis in isolated rheumatic chorea
C. Hemichorea
D. Pregnancy may precipitate chorea

32. Amyl nitrate increase intensity of murmur of all *except:*
A. TOF B. AS
C. TR D. HOCM

33. True about acute severe MR is all *except:*
A. Normal LA size B. Absent murmur
C. P2 may be normal D. CHF

34. All are true about MI free wall rupture *except:*
A. Elderly female B. HT
C. LV > RV D. Repeated infarction

35. Second left intercostal space with loud systolic murmur is heard in:
A. ASD with severe MS
B. ASD with PAH
C. RSOV to LV
D. Pulmonary AV fistula

36. All may occur in cirrhosis *except:*
A. PPH
B. Hypoxia
C. Pulmonary AV fistula
D. Hemoptysis

37. All are true about Pulmonary vasoconstriction *except:*
A. Hypoxia
B. Hypercarbia
C. Alkalosis
D. Endothelin involved

38. EDRF derived from:
A. L arginine B. Citruline
C. Tryptophan D. Melanin

39. Dicrotic pulse all true *except:*
A. Fever B. Cardiac tamponade
C. Hypertension D. Shock

40. All are poor prognostic markers of HOCM *except:*
A. Malignant genotype
B. Friedrich's ataxia
C. LVH >40 mm
D. Exercise induced hypotension

41. Cyanotic congenital heart disease all true *except:*
A. Hemostatic disturbances
B. Thrombotic stroke
C. High risk pregnancy (mother)
D. Thrombocytosis

42. Fetal death is seen in all *except:*
A. Ebstein B. d-TGA
C. PSVT D. CHB

43. Oxygenation is improved by all *except:*
A. CNS depression
B. Persistent fetal circulation
C. Pulmonary edema
D. Choanal atresia

28 A 29 B 30 B 31 A 32 A 33 C 34 D 35 A 36 D 37 C 38 A 39 C 40 B
41 D 42 B 43 B

44. Fetal circulation established by:
A. 23-28 days B. 40-42 days
C. 55-60 days D. 90 days

45. Hypotension is caused by all *except:*
A. IL-2
B. L dopa
C. Chlorpromazine
D. OCP's

46. Hypertension is caused by all *except:*
A. Brain tumors
B. Sleep apnea
C. Acute porphyria
D. Parkinsons disease

47. All are true about Atheroembolism *except:*
A. Arch thrombus does not embolise
B. Livedo reticularis
C. Renal failure especially after cath
D. Toe gangrene with preserved pulses

48. Right aortic arch is least common in:
A. Truncus arteriosus
B. TOF
C. Ebstein's anomaly
D. VSD with pulmonary atresia

49. Paradoxical septal motion is seen with all *except:*
A. ASD
B. CCP
C. Post cardiac surgery
D. RCM

50. Most sensitive for cardiac tamponade:
A. RA collapse
B. RV collapse
C. Pulmonary vein flow reversal
D. IVC collapse < 50%

51. Least common symptom of pheochromocytoma is:
A. Diaphoresis B. Headache
C. Dizziness D. Palpitation

52. All true about syncope *except:*
A. β-blocker may decrease vasovagal syncope
B. Repeated episodes of unconsciousness in a day is a sign of syncope but not seizures.
C. Basilar artery migraine may cause it
D. Cardiac tamponade may cause syncope

53. All are Cardiac growth promoters *except:*
A. Thyroxine B. TGF-β
C. Myo-D D. Growth hormone

54. Most common material used to make stent in PCI is:
A. Nitinol
B. Biodegradable plastic
C. Non degradable plastic
D. Stainless steel

55. Hyperhomocysteinemia seen in all *except:*
A. CRF
B. HRT
C. Cholesterol lowering drugs
D. Hypothyroidism

56. Insulin resistant syndrome is characterized by all *except:*
A. Increased Lp(a)
B. Increased VLDL
C. Decreased HDL
D. Post prandial lipaemia

57. All are true about β blocker *except:*
A. Bronchospasm B. Impotence
C. Increased TGS D. Hypokalemia

58. All are true *except:*
A. Warfarin increases both PT and aPTT
B. Addition of plasma in a patient of increased PT & aPTT which does not normalize is a sign of afibrinogenaemia.
C. PT determines extrinsic pathway
D. alpha-2 antiplasmin assays assess fibrinolytic system

44 A 45 D 46 D 47 A 48 C 49 D 50 A 51 C 52 B 53 C 54 D 55 B 56 A
57 D 58 B

59. Which of the following is not determined by PT and aPTT?
A. Prekallikrein B. HMW kininogen
C. Factor 13 D. Cascade factor 10

60. Least dependent on load is:
A. Circumferential fibre shortening
B. Ejection fraction
C. Dp/dt
D. End systolic pressure volume relationship

61. Janeway lesion is most commonly caused by:
A. S. viridans B. S. aureus
C. Fungus D. Pseudomonas

62. All are true about eclampsia *except:*
A. Methyldopa is a drug of choice
B. Fluid restriction may prevent eclampsia
C. ACE inhibitors are contraindicated
D. Sodium restriction is advised

63. Two day old infant with heart rate 230/min:
A. Sepsis B. AVNRT
C. AVRT D. VT

64. VSD in infant least likely:
A. Growth failure B. Increased PAH
C. RSV infection D. AR

65. Hypomagnesaemia all true *except:*
A. Increased PR interval
B. Absent tendon reflexes
C. Chovsteks sign
D. Serum $Mg^{2+} < 2.6$ mmol/L

66. All are true about critical limb ischemia *except:*
A. Dependent rubor B. Night pains
C. Paresthesias D. Claudication

67. Secondary prevention trials for lipid are all *except:*
A. 4S B. LIPID
C. WOSCOPS D. CARE

68. All are true about Kawasaki disease *except:*
A. Coronary aneurysm in 2%
B. Pericarditis may occur
C. Steroids not effective
D. Rare in India

69. All are seen in eosinophilic myocarditis *except:*
A. Myocarditis
B. Thrombosis
C. Endocardial fibro elastosis
D. MR

70. All are true about single lacunar infarct *except:*
A. Hemiparesis B. Binswanger disease
C. Ataxic stroke D. Sensory stroke

71. All are causes of diastolic dysfunction *except:*
A. DM B. Hypertension
C. Epicardial CAD D. LA dilatation

72. Least common cardiac manifestation of HIV:
A. Kaposi's
B. Primary lymphoma
C. Angiosarcoma
D. Secondary lymphoma

73. In all countries, death due to stroke is higher than MI *except:*
A. China B. Japan
C. India D. Africa

74. Viability of myocardium in ischemic cardiomyopathy can be assessed by all *except:*
A. $Thallium^{201}$ rest redistribution
B. Tc Sestamibi SPECT
C. High dose dobutamine echo
D. PET with myocardial metabolism

75. Romhilt Estes criteria score of 3 points suggestive of LVH are all *except:*
A. R in V_5 or $V_6 > 3$ mV
B. S in V_1 or $V_2 > 3$ mV
C. PTF in $V_1 > 4$ mV-msec
D. R in any limb lead > 1.1 mV

59 C 60 D 61 B 62 D 63 C 64 D 65 B 66 D 67 C 68 A 69 C 70 B 71 D
72 D 73 C 74 C 75 D

76. All are true about acromegaly *except:*
A. CHF
B. Hypertension
C. Sudden cardiac death
D. CHB

77. Which of the following is not seen in obesity?
A. Eccentric LVH
B. Increased filling pressure
C. Increased cardiac output
D. Conduction defects

78. Brugada syndrome: all are true *except:*
A. β-blockers decrease mortality
B. SCD in sleep
C. Procainamide unmasks ST elevation in V_1
D. Genetic abnormality SCN5a

79. Contrast echo most commonly used agent is:
A. Iopamol B. Microbubbles
C. Iohexol D. Gadolinium

80. Thermodilution method of cardiac output useful in:
A. VSD B. TR
C. TOF D. Low cardiac output

81. All are true about Coronary sinus *except:*
A. Saturation 30%
B. Can be used for pacing
C. Absence of CS is incompatible with life
D. LSVC may open into it

82. Sub arachnoid haemorrhage (SAH)–LQTs drugs not given:
A. Isoprenaline B. Pacing
C. β-blockers D. Magnesium

83. True about anaphylaxis are all *except:*
A. Can occur after 1 year of treatment
B. Epinephrine 2.5 ml (1:1000)
C. Cardiac arrest without respiratory arrest
D. Histamine, cysteine, leukotrienes may be responsible

84. Edema with low uric acid seen in:
A. Lead nephropathy B. CHF
C. PPH D. Liver disease

85. Braunwald classification of USA in a patient with rest angina in last 48 hours:
A. Class I B. Class II
C. Class III D. Class IV

86. Friedwald formula most useful in:
A. Type I hypercholesterolemia
B. Type II hypercholesterolemia
C. Type III hypercholesterolemia
D. Type IV hypercholesterolemia

87. Cardiac tamponade with absent paradoxus is seen in all *except:*
A. AR B. ASD
C. IPPV D. TB pericarditis

88. Coronary calcification best diagnosed by:
A. Helical CT B. EBCT
C. Cinefluoroscopy D. MRI

89. Triangle of Koch's contains:
A. SA node B. AV node
C. Bundle of HIS D. Purkinje fiber

90. Cardiac metabolism: all are true *except:*
A. Energy provided by anaerobic metabolism is 1%
B. Resting cardiac O_2 consumption is 2ml/100gm/min
C. 60% by Fats normally
D. >50% by triglycerides

76 D 77 D 78 A 79 B 80 A 81 C 82 A 83 B 84 D 85 C 86 B 87 D 88 B
89 B 90 A

AIIMS 2003 (June)

1. Latest Jones modification for rheumatic fever:
A. 1992 B. 2002
C. 1944 D. 1998

2. Systolic murmur grading by:
A. Frossman B. Paul wood
C. Levine D. Gruentzig

3. IE is diagnosed by which criteria:
A. Duke B. Jones
C. WHO D. None of the above

4. AICD; secondary prevention trial is:
A. MADIT 2 B. AVID
C. CIDS D. CASH

5. All are extracted from fungus *except:*
A. PnG B. Lovastatin
C. Cephalosporin D. Warfarin

6. Myopathy due to lovastatin is exacerbated by all *except:*
A. Erythromycin B. Rifampicin
C. Ketoconazole D. Cyclosporin

7. Pulmonary arterial wedge angiogram is done in:
A. MS B. ASD
C. PAH D. PDA

8. VEGF inhibitors are all *except:*
A. FGF
B. IL-8
C. TNF
D. Von Hippel gene

9. 2 D echo of fetus is useful in all *except:*
A. HLH
B. Atrial Flutter
C. Small VSD
D. Diaphragmatic hernia

10. Hypophosphatemia is caused by all *except:*
A. Alcohol withdrawal
B. DKA (recovering)s
C. Severe respiratory acidosis
D. Hyperalimentation

11. Magnesium therapy is useful in all *except:*
A. Renal tubular acidosis
B. MI
C. Hypokalemia
D. Tetany

12. All of the following suggest positive predictive value to diagnose infective endocarditis *except:*
A. Anemia
B. ↑ESR
C. Leucocytosis
D. Circulating immune complexes

13. All are used in enterococcal endocarditis *except:*
A. Ceftriaxone B. Ampicillin
C. Tiecoplanin D. Gentamycin

1 A 2 C 3 A 4 A 5 D 6 B 7 C 8 D 9 C 10 C 11 A 12 C 13 A

14. All are true about bicuspid AV *except:*
A. Commonest congenital cardiac lesion
B. IE prophylaxis necessary
C. Ascending aorta marked dilatation is seen
D. Can cause AR

15. AR with AV block is seen in all *except:*
A. Seronegative spondyloarthopathy
B. Senile calcification AS
C. RSOV
D. Takayasu aortitis

16. Mitral annular calcification is seen in all *except:*
A. Juvenile MS
B. HOCM
C. Hyperparathyroidism
D. Marfans syndrome

17. NIDDM least common in:
A. Chinese B. African Americans
C. Scandinavians D. Pacific islanders

18. Metabolic syndrome has all of the following features *except:*
A. ↓HDL
B. HT
C. ↑TG
D. Abnormal postprandial blood sugar

19. All is seen in diabetic dyslipidemia *except:*
A. Increased LDL
B. ↓HDL
C. ↑TG
D. Small dense LDL

20. 5-6mm ↓ in BP ↓es stroke by:
A. 24% B. 42%
C. 14% D. 58%

21. Annual stroke risk in symptomatic carotid stenosis at 1 year:
A. 15% B. 3%
C. 2% D. 7%

22. Mortality in acute MI is:
A. 10% B. 30%
C. 15% D. 4%

23. Bolus dose of heparin in MI:
A. 60 U/kg B. 30 U/kg
C. 70 U/kg D. 40 U/kg

24. Dose of IV amiodarone in resistant VF/pulseless VT:
A. IV 300 mg over 5 min
B. IV 300 mg bolus
C. IV 150 mg over 10 min
D. IV 150 mg bolus

25. All are true about digitalis toxicity *except:*
A. Bidirectional VT is typical of digitalis toxicity
B. PAT is not a reentrant tachycardia
C. Ectopics in children and bradycardia in adults
D. Depression in elderly in therapeutic disease

26. Normal HV interval:
A. 35-55 msec B. 15-25 msec
C. 20-40 msec D. 55-75 msec

27. ↓ LDL is seen in all *except:*
A. Anorexia nervosa
B. Abetalipoproteinaemia
C. HIV
D. Hemataologic malignancy with splenomegaly

28. Least nephrotoxic dye is:
A. Urograffin
B. Iohexol
C. Iopamidol
D. Idoxanol

29. Advantage of Tc99 over thallium are all *except:*
A. Better image
B. Rest ischemia imaging
C. Acute MI imaging
D. First Pass metabolism

14 C 15 D 16 A 17 C 18 D 19 A 20 B 21 D 22 B 23 A 24 D 25 C 26 A
27 A 28 D 29 B

30. Ciprofloxacin induced QT prolongation treated by all *except:*
A. Isoproterenol
B. β blocker
C. Pacing
D. Electrolytic imbalance correction

31. In sleep most common cause of sudden cardiac death is:
A. Brugada syndrome
B. Long QT syndrome
C. ARVD
D. HOCM

32. Sertraline causes:
A. Long QT
B. Bradycardia
C. VPC
D. Orthostatic hypotension

33. Orthostatic hypotension with postpradial hypotension: treatment of choice are all *except:*
A. Midodrine B. Octreotide
C. Brufen with meals D. Dopamine

34. Modified Jones criteria; what is not included:
A. Poly arthrtitis
B. Echo for carditis
C. ↑ASLO
D. Subcutaneous nodules

35. All of the following are features of carditis in acute rheumatic fever *except:*
A. Cardiomegaly
B. Subcutaneous nodules
C. Arthritis
D. ↑ASLO

36. All seen in acute rheumatic fever *except:*
A. Annular dilatation
B. Nodules over leaflet
C. Commissural fusion
D. MVP

37. Rapid Y descent is seen in all *except:*
A. Cardiac tamponade
B. TR
C. CCP
D. CCF

38. Commonest cause of holosystolic murmur of TR in India is:
A. Carcinoid B. COPD
C. RV infarct D. Rt sided EMF

39. All are seen in carcinoid *except:*
A. Hypotension
B. Pulmonary artery hypertension
C. Coronary spasm
D. TR

40. True about amyloidosis is all *except:*
A. Echo speckled appearance
B. AA is secondary amyloidosis
C. Digoxin sensitivity
D. Orthostatic hypotension

41. All are true about cardiac sarcoidosis *except:*
A. 5% incidence
B. AV block
C. ↑ ACE activity in 2/3rds
D. Restrictive cardiomyopathy can occur

42. Adolescent in swimming pool getting syncope: first investigation to do is:
A. TTE B. HUTT
C. ECG D. EPS

43. E : A > 3 : 1 with decrease deceleration time is seen in:
A. CCP B. Ac ischemia
C. MR (acute) D. Atrial fibrillation

44. Retinal artery occlusion is seen in all *except:*
A. Anti cardiolipin anitbody
B. Takayasu arteritis
C. Hypertensive encephalopathy
D. Giant cell arteritis

30 B 31 A 32 B 33 D 34 B 35 D 36 C 37 A 38 B 39 B 40 B 41 A 42 C
43 A 44 B

45. Least common site of intracranial haemorrhage:
A. Putamen
B. Globus pallidus
C. Cerebellum
D. Frontal lobe

46. Syncope is seen in all *except:*
A. Carotid arterial stenosis
B. Migraine
C. Pulmonary embolism
D. Internal bleed

47. Optimal BP according to JNC 7:
A. <80 mm Hg
B. 81-85 mm Hg
C. 85-90 mm Hg
D. None of the above

48. All are seen in electrical injury *except:*
A. ECG may mimic Hyperkalemia changes
B. Death may be due to apnea before cardiac arrest
C. Fixed dilated pupils indicates irreversible brain damage
D. Can cause MI

49. Cardiac trauma causes all *except:*
A. ASD
B. TR
C. Sudden death
D. MI

50. HIV–IE due to all *except:*
A. Staph aureus
B. Pseudomonas
C. Candida
D. Tubercle bacilli

51. Acute endocarditis is caused by all *except:*
A. β haemolytic streptococci
B. Coxiella
C. Staph aureus
D. Pneuomococus

52. Chronic aspirin use protects against all *except:*
A. Alzheimer's disease
B. Colorectal Carcinoma
C. MI in women
D. Diabetic retinopathy

53. All can be seen in Down's syndrome *except:*
A. Alzheimer's disease
B. Hypothyroidism
C. Duodenal atresia
D. TGA

54. All are true about amiodarone induced hypothyroidism *except:*
A. Due to iodine content of amiodarone
B. More common in iodine deficient person
C. ↑ TSH
D. L-thyroxine is useful

55. All are seen in CCF in infants *except:*
A. Raised JVP
B. Resp distress
C. Cardiomegaly
D. Hepatomegaly

56. Cardiac index 1.7 L/min/m^2, Oxygen saturation 92; Diagnosis is:
A. MI
B. TOF
C. Pulmonary embolism
D. ILD

57. TMT is not indicated in all *except:*
A. LVH
B. ST↓ more than 1 mm at rest
C. MI of 7 days
D. Routine screening of asymptomatic patients

58. P ligand binding peroxisome activity is seen in all *except:*
A. HLA antigen
B. Clofibrate
C. Linoleic acid
D. Rosiglitazone

59. Right aortic arch is least common in
A. TOF
B. Truncus arteriosus
C. VSD with Pulmonary atresia
D. TGA

60. Pulmonary artery ligation is not done in:
A. Multiple VSD
B. Single VSD with no PS
C. Ebstein's with no PS
D. TA with PAH

45 C 46 A 47 A 48 C 49 A 50 D 51 A 52 C 53 D 54 B 55 A 56 A 57 C
58 D 59 D 60 C

61. In TAPVC Lt innominate is present in:
A. 11% B. 36%
C. 16% D. 25%

62. Closure not needed in:
A. Small VSD B. ECD
C. Small PDA D. AP window

63. NO synthesis is done by all *except:*
A. Phosphodiesterase 3
B. L-Arginine
C. Nitric oxide synthase
D. Citrulline

64. All are true about cilastozol *except:*
A. ↓ HDL
B. ↑ Claudication distance
C. PDE III inhibitor
D. Inhibits platelets

65. Von Willibrand factor clearing metalloproteinase activity is decrease in:
A. TTP B. HVS
C. DIC D. Haemophilia

66. All are true about SVG graft intervention *except:*
A. ↑ Periprocedural MI than native plaque
B. GBIIb/IIIa inhibitors decrease the incidence of distal embolism
C. ↑ No reflow incidence
D. Distal protection devices has been proved to decrease adverse outcome

67. Vulnerable plaque has all the features *except:*
A. ↑ Lipid core
B. Thin fibrous cap
C. ↑ Polymorphonuclear infiltration
D. HLD DR + macrophage

68. All are true about warfarin in mechanical prosthesis *except:*
A. Loading dose not required
B. INR 2-3 in mechanical valve at mitral position
C. Skin necrosis with protein C deficiency
D. Reversal with vitamin K

69. Dicrotic pulse is seen in all *except:*
A. Fever
B. Cardiac tamponade
C. Hypovolemia
D. Hypertension HF

70. Paradoxical septal motion all *except:*
A. TR B. Septal infarct
C. PDA D. Post CABG

71. Accelerated atherosclerosis in post transplant heart is caused by all *except:*
A. Mycophenolate mofetil
B. CMV infection
C. Chronic rejection
D. ↑ Lipids

72. All can be seen in TMT of DCMP *except:*
A. HR > 85% of predicted
B. Arterial saturation 90%
C. Low anaerobic threshold
D. MVO_2 <14

73. Tumor causing conduction abnormality in infants:
A. Fibroma
B. Myxoma
C. Rhabdomyoma
D. Mesothelioma

74. Minor criteria of CHF are all *except:*
A. Weight gain
B. ↓ Vital capacity
C. + Hepatojugular reflux
D. Tachycardia > 120/min

75. All are seen in myxoma *except:*
A. Clubbing B. Hypoalbuminemia
C. ↑ ESR D. Polycythemia

---

61 B 62 A 63 D 64 A 65 A 66 B 67 C 68 B 69 D 70 C 71 A 72 B 73 D 74 A 75 B

76. Cholesterol is found in all *except:*
A. Coconut B. Fish
C. Red meat D. Milk products

77. Drugs showing decreased mortality in CHF are all *except:*
A. Bucindolol B. Metoprolol
C. Bisoprolol D. Carvedilol

78. Contraindication of r-tPA according to NIND trial are all *except:*
A. Recent MI
B. History of seizure at presentation
C. Symptoms < 3 hours
D. Resolving neurologic deficit

79. Rotablator chips are coated with:
A. Diamond B. Platinum
C. Steel D. Gold

80. High risk factors for SCD in HOCM are all *except:*
A. Adult onset
B. ↓BP response in TMT
C. Septal thickness >30 mm
D. Family history of SCD

81. Normal routine investigation initially done in hypertension are all *except:*
A. Echo B. Cholesterol
C. K^+ D. ECG

82. In CHF all ↑ *except:*
A. ANP
B. BNP
C. Effective arterial volume
D. Endothelin

83. All are seen in obesity *except:*
A. ↑ LVEDV
B. ↑ Blood pressure
C. ↑ Cardiac output
D. Concentric LVH

84. Predisposing condition for aortic dissection are all *except:*
A. Syphilis B. Marfan's syndrome
C. Pregnancy D. Bicuspid AV

85. Thiamine deficiency is seen in all *except:*
A. Alcoholism B. Food fadist
C. Pregnancy D. CHF on diuretics

86. MVP murmur is accentuated by all *except:*
A. Amylnitrate B. Valsalva
C. Standing D. Isometric exercise

87. ASD with cyanosis is seen in all *except:*
A. HT
B. Single atrium
C. Unroofed coronary sinus
D. Severe PS

88. Pulmonary hypertension is seen with all *except:*
A. Acidosis B. Hypoxia
C. Hypocarbia D. Left to right shunt

89. Ischemic heart tissue metabolises:
A. FFA B. Lactate
C. Sucrose D. Glucose

90. ↓ SVR is seen in all *except:*
A. Exercise B. Cor Pulmonale
C. Hypothyroidism D. Beriberi

76 A 77 A 78 C 79 A 80 A 81 A 82 C 83 D 84 A 85 C 86 D 87 A 88 C
89 D 90 C

AIIMS 2002 (December)

1. **The presence of cyanosis with a continuous murmur is seen in all of the following *except:***
   A. Sinus of valsalva aneurysm which has ruptured
   B. VSD with pulmonary atresia
   C. Pulmonary AV fistula
   D. TAPVC

2. **All of the following are seen in acute aortic regurgitation *except:***
   A. Pulses alternans
   B. Pulses bisferians
   C. Absence of S4
   D. Presence of "a" wave in aortic pressure tracing

3. **The middle cardiac vein is situation in the:**
   A. Anterior interventricular sulcus
   B. Posterior interventricular sulcus
   C. Anterior atrioventricular groove
   D. Posterior atrioventricular groove

4. **Reverse pulsus paradoxus is seen in all the following *except:***
   A. Hypertrophic Cardiomyopathy
   B. Positive pressure ventilation
   C. Isorhythmic dissociation
   D. Diaphragmatic palsy

5. **The presence of a low volume pulse following a premature ventricular contraction is seen in:**
   A. Left ventricular failure
   B. Atrial fibrillation
   C. Hypertrophic
   D. Cardiomyopathy

6. **Low volume pulse is seen in all the following *except:***
   A. Elderly
   B. Mitral stenosis
   C. Hypovolumia
   D. AS

7. **Kussmaul's sign is seen in all of the following *except:***
   A. Constrictive pericarditis
   B. Acute pulmonary thromboembolism
   C. Right ventricular infarction
   D. Cardiac tamponade

8. **Early systolic murmur is seen with all the following *except:***
   A. Tricuspid regurgitation
   B. Papillary muscle dysfunction
   C. Small VSD
   D. Aortic stenosis

9. **Poor progression of R wave is not seen in which of the following condition:**
   A. LBBB
   B. Chronic obstructive pulmonary disease
   C. Left pneumothorax
   D. Cardiac tamponade

1 A 2 B 3 B 4 D 5 C 6 A 7 D 8 D 9 D

10. All the following are true regarding U wave *except:*
A. Increased amplitude can be caused by drugs
B. Best seen in inferior leads
C. Inversion in precordial leads is pathological
D. May be caused by depolarization of Purkinje fibers

11. Which of the following is an absolute contra indication for exercise stress testing:
A. Myocardial infarction 1 week back
B. Unstable angina with recent rest pain
C. Peripheral vascular disease
D. Aortic stenosis

12. Which of the following is not an echocardiographic finding in normal individuals?
A. AR B. MR
C. PR D. TR

13. E:A ratio is increased in all of the following *except:*
A. Severe diastolic dysfunction
B. CCP
C. MS
D. Advanced DCM

14. In PET, decreased uptake of N and FDG implies:
A. Acute myocardial infarction
B. Ischemia
C. Chronic scarred tissue
D. Hibernating myocardium

15. All of the following are used in pharmacological stress testing *except:*
A. Dipyridamole
B. Adenosine
C. Theophylline
D. Dobutamine

16. The resting coronary sinus oxygen saturation is:
A. 30% B. 65%
C. 70% D. 85%

17. Thermodilution for cardiac output is unreliable in all of the following *except:*
A. Low Pulmonary output
B. VSD
C. Pulmonary regurgitation
D. Tricuspid regurgitation

18. Endothelium derived relaxing factor is derived from:
A. Guanosine
B. Endothelin
C. L-Arginine
D. Leukotriene

19. All the following are true regarding fast action potential in cardiac muscle *except:*
A. -40 to -70 mV
B. Increased speed of depolarization
C. Inhibited by tetrodoxin
D. Mediated by sodium channel

20. D2 dopaminergic stimulation cause all of the following *except:*
A. Decreased prolactin secretion
B. Vomiting
C. Renal vasodilatation
D. Decrease sympathetic

21. Adenosine causes all of the following *except:*
A. Coronary spasm
B. Chest pain
C. Bronchospasm
D. Pulmonary vasodilatation

22. All of the following can be seen in ventricular failure *except:*
A. Pulmonary artery saturation <80%
B. Increased lung thallium uptake
C. Positive hepatojugular reflux
D. Increased JVP

10 B 11 B 12 A 13 C 14 C 15 C 16 A 17 B 18 C 19 A 20 C 21 A 22 A

23. **All the following are features of apoptosis *except:***
A. Step ladder pattern in electron microscopy
B. Polymorphonuclear infiltrate
C. Rapid cell loss
D. Precipitated by hypoxia

24. **Digoxin toxcity is associated with all of the following *except:***
A. Bidirectional ventricular tachycardia
B. Atrial flutter
C. Supraventricular tachycardia with AV block
D. Hyperkalemia with massive overdose

25. **Digoxin level is increased by all the following *except:***
A. Omeprazole
B. Rifampicin
C. Amiodarone
D. Verapamil

26. **Which of the following is not an indication for transplantation in a patient with dilated cardiomyopathy?**
A. Pulmonary resistance = 5 units
B. Ejection fraction = 10%
C. O_2 uptake = 15 ml/kg/min
D. NYHA class III

27. **Myocardial oxygen consumption is dependent on all the following *except:***
A. Heart rate
B. Wall stress
C. Myocardial mass
D. External work

28. **All the following are synthesized in myocardium *except:***
A. Fatty acyl CoA
B. Myosin
C. Carnitine
D. Lactate

29. **The presence of pulmonary edema with a normal pulmonary capillary wedge pressure is seen with all of the following *except:***
A. Adult respiratory distress syndrome
B. After cardial surgery
C. Renal artery stenosis
D. Narcotic overdose

30. **The relationship between resistance of a vessel and its radius is given by which of the following:**
A. Bernouilli's equation
B. Poiseulli's law
C. Laplace's law
D. Gorlins equation

31. **Tachycardia associated with exercise is seen with all the following *except:***
A. Brugada syndrome
B. Romano Ward syndrome
C. CAD
D. RVOT obstruction

32. **The use of calcium gluconate is indicated in all of the following conditions *except:***
A. Hypocalcemia
B. Calcium channel blocker overdose
C. Routinely 1 minute after cardiac arrest
D. Electromechanical dissociation

33. **Vasovagal syncope may be caused by all of the following *except:***
A. Anemia
B. Pain
C. Prolonged standing
D. Chronic beta blocker therapy

34. **Polymorphic ventricular tachycardia is caused by all of the following *except:***
A. Old myocardial infarction
B. Ischemia
C. Sub arachnoid hemorrhage
D. Hypokalemia

23 B 24 B 25 B 26 C 27 D 28 C 29 C 30 B 31 A 32 C 33 D 34 A

35. Reentry can give rise to all of the following *except:*
A. Monomorphic ventricular tachycardia
B. Atrial flutter
C. Trsades de pointes
D. Junctional tachycardia with reciprocation

36. Permanent pacemaker is indicated in an asymptomatic patient in the presence of all of the following *except:*
A. Sinus pause > 3 seconds
B. Trifascicular block after MI
C. Bundle branch block with Mobitz II
D. Sick sinus syndrome

37. All of the following drugs cause prolonged QT *except:*
A. Erythromycin B. Mexiletine
C. Terfenadine D. Cisapride

38. Hypertension in Indian children is most commonly due to:
A. Fibromuscular dysplasia
B. Fibrointimal hyperplasia
C. Takayasu's arteritis
D. Thromboembolism

39. All of the following can be used as the first drug in hypertension *except:*
A. ACE inhibitor
B. Calcium channel blocker
C. Diuretic
D. Alpha blocker

40. Which of the following is the treatment of choice for pheochromocytoma with hypertension:
A. Esmolol B. Phentolamine
C. Methyldopa D. Reserpine

41. Hypertriglyceridemia is characterized by all of the following *except:*
A. Increased VLDL
B. Decreased HDL
C. Increased Chylomicrons
D. Decreased hepatic lipase

42. Which of the following drug is contra indicated in severe hypertriglyceridemia:
A. Statins
B. Fibric acid derivatives
C. Cholesytramine
D. Probucol

43. All of the following predisposes to thrombosis *except:*
A. Factor V Leiden
B. Homocysteinemia
C. Protein S deficiency
D. Bernard Soulier syndrome

44. In the emergency treatment of hypertension, all the following drugs are used intravenously *except:*
A. Fenoldapam B. Nifedipine
C. Urapidil D. Enalapril

45. Which of the following is not a lipid trial:
A. 4S B. CARE
C. WOSCOPS D. AVID

46. All of the following are contra-indicated in non QMI *except:*
A. Long acting dihydropyridine calcium channel blockers
B. Early PTCA
C. rtPA
D. Intracoronary thrombolysis

47. Decreased restenosis after PTCA is seen with the use of:
A. ACE inhibitor
B. Rapamycin
C. Heparin
D. Paclitaxel

48. All the following are poor prognostic factors in unstable angina *except:*
A. Recent onset chest pain
B. Prolonged chest pain
C. Trop T >0.41 ng/ml
D. Pulmonary edema

35 C 36 D 37 B 38 C 39 D 40 B 41 D 42 C 43 D 44 B 45 D 46 B 47 B 48 A

49. Coronary vasoconstriction is normally produced by all of the following *except:*
A. Thromboxanbe A2
B. Serotonin
C. Acetyl choline
D. No epinephrine

50. Recurrent ischemia after thrombolysis is due to:
A. Lipoprotein (a)
B. Antibody to thrombolytics
C. Fibrinopeptide-a
D. Hypertriglyceridemia

51. Troponin T is preferred over CPK in the diagnosis of myocardial infarction in all the following conditions *except:*
A. Small infarct
B. Post cardiac surgery
C. Re-infarction after 4 days
D. Bed side diagnosis of MI

52. All of the following predispose to atherosclerosis *except:*
A. Von willebrand disease
B. SLE
C. Type V hyperlipidemia
D. Nephrotic syndrome

53. Angioscopy after unstable angina is most likely to show:
A. Plaque without thrombosis
B. Mural thrombus with partial recanalization
C. Non occluding mural thrombus
D. Occluding thrombus

54. Poor prognosis in hypertrophic cardiomyopathy is indicated by all of the following *except:*
A. Gradient >100 mmHg
B. Septal thickness >25 mm
C. Family history of sudden cardiac death
D. Ventricular tacycardia on Holter monitoring

55. In the treatment of pericardial tamponade all of the following may be used *except:*
A. Frusemide
B. Intravenous saline
C. Isoproterenol
D. Atropine

56. All of the following are true regarding cardiac, amyloidosis *except:*
A. Congestive failure is uncommon in senile amyloidosis
B. Patient may be sensitive to nifedipine
C. High positivity may be present with the use of technetium pyrophosphate
D. Low voltage in limb leads and normal voltage in chest leads

57. Cyanotic spell in tetralogy of Fallot is precipitated by all the following *except:*
A. Anemia
B. Infection
C. Hypertension
D. Crying

58. Which of the following surgeries in neonates has a good long term prognosis:
A. Arterial switch
B. Senning's operation
C. Fontan
D. Cardiac transpant

59. Congestive failure in fetus is caused by all the following *except:*
A. Hypoplastic left heart
B. Anemia
C. Ebstein's anomaly
D. Complete heart block

60. Fontan operation is indicated for all of the following *except:*
A. Tricuspid atresia
B. Pulmonary stenosis with intact septum with HLH
C. Tetralogy of Fallot
D. Univentricular heart

61. All of the following can be seen in acute rheumatic carditis *except:*
A. Nodules on valve
B. Mitral valve prolapse
C. Annular dilatation
D. Paradoxical movement of posterior mitral leaflet

49 C 50 C 51 C 52 C 53 C 54 A 55 A 56 A 57 C 58 A 59 A 60 C 61 D

62. All of the following are high risk lesions for infective endocarditis *except:*
A. Ventricular septal defect
B. Blalock Taussig shunt
C. PDA
D. Eisenmenger

63. The most common cardiac tumor in a child is:
A. Fibroma B. Sarcoma
C. Rhabdomyoma D. Myxoma

64. Hematogenous spread of candida is least common to which of the following organs:
A. Retina B. Heart
C. Kidney D. Spleen

65. Osler's node is most common in infective endocarditis due to which of the following?
A. Staph aureus
B. Chronic candida
C. Pseudomonas
D. Libman Sach's endocarditis

66. Early prosthetic valve endocarditis is most commonly due to which of the following oganisms:
A. Staph. aureus B. Pseudomonas
C. HACEK D. Strep.Viridans

67. All the following predispose to pulmonary embolism *except:*
A. Obesity B. Sickle cell anemia
C. Progesterone D. Malignancy

68. Pulmonary embolism presents as all of the following *except:*
A. Bronchiectasis B. Syncope
C. Fever D. Paradoxical embolus

69. Pulmonary hypertension is seen with all the following *except:*
A. Toxic oil syndrome
B. Sickle cell anemia
C. Scleroderma
D. Argemone mexicana poisoning

70. Bosentan is an antagonist of:
A. Norepinephrine B. Angiotensin
C. Endothelin D. Acetylcholine

71. Di George syndrome is associated with chromosome:
A. 11q 13 B. 13 p 11.4
C. 17 D. 22

72. Noonan syndrome is associated with all of the following *except:*
A. Autosomal dominant inheritance
B. Hypertrophiccardiomyopathy
C. Cryptorchidism
D. Infertility (in females)

73. All of the following may occur in renal artery stenosis *except:*
A. Hypokalemia
B. Proteinuria
C. Loss of corticomedullary differentiation
D. Increase in urea after ACE inhibitor therapy

74. Which of the following disease is decreasing in incidence in India:
A. CAD
B. Endomyocardial fibrosis
C. Diabetes
D. Amyloidosis

75. All of the following are seen in malignant carcinoid *except:*
A. Labile hypertension
B. Coronary spasm
C. High cardiac output
D. Pulmonary arterial hypertension

76. Irradiation in childhood is associated with which of the following malignancies:
A. Lung B. Breast
C. Thyroid D. Melanoma

62 D 63 C 64 B 65 A 66 A 67 C 68 A 69 D 70 C 71 A 72 D 73 C 74 B
75 D 76 C

77. **The most common cause of metabolic alkalosis in a patient on the ventilator is:**
A. Hyperventilation
B. Extracellular volume depletion
C. External bicarbonate administration
D. Hyperkalemia

78. **Transudative pleural effusion is seen in all of the following *except:***
A. Pulmonary thromboembolism
B. Parapneumonic effusion
C. Renal artery stenosis
D. Cirrhosis

79. **Thiamine deficiency occurs due to following *except:***
A. Homocysteinemia
B. Food faddist
C. Alcohol
D. Congestive failure on diuretics

80. **Which of the following is the most common nosocomial infection:**
A. Urinary tract infection
B. Pneumonia
C. Skin infection
D. Infection at surgical site

81. **A patient has pH 7.05, HCO_3 – 5 mEq/Lt wt 50 kg base excess of 30. For correction how much HCO_3 has to be given in the next half hour:**
A. 250 mEq
B. 350 mEq
C. 600 mEq
D. 850 mEq

82. **All of the following are features of hypernatremia due to extrarenal mechanism *except:***
A. Neurological symptoms
B. Increased thirst
C. Free water loss
D. Dilute urine

83. **Intrapulmonary right to left shunt occurs in all of the following *except:***
A. Cirrhosis
B. Pneumonia
C. Osler Rendu Weber syndrome
D. Eisenmenger syndrome

84. **A pH 7.51, pCO_2 22 mmHg, PO_2 300 mmHg and SaO_2 60% seen in which of the following conditions:**
A. Carbon monoxide poisoning
B. Mechanical ventilation
C. Voluntary hyperventilation
D. Technical error

85. **All the following may be seen in hypomagnesemia *except:***
A. Prolonged QT interval
B. Chvostek's sign
C. Decreased tendon reflexes
D. Mg level of 1 mEq/L

86. **Decreased DLco is associated with all of the following *except:***
A. Goodpasture syndrome
B. Primary pulmonary hypertension
C. Interstitial lung disease
D. Emphysema

87. **Which of the following does not cause hyperventilation:**
A. Heart failure
B. Cirrhosis
C. Progesterone
D. Metabolic alkalosis

88. **The oxygen content of plasma while breathing room air is:**
A. 0.03 ml/dL
B. 3 ml/dL
C. 1.34 ml/dL
D. 19.4 ml/dL

77 B 78 B 79 A 80 A 81 A 82 C 83 D 84 D 85 C 86 A 87 D 88 A

89. INR as a method of standardization of PT is due to:

A. Indexes PT to normal value
B. Repeated PT measurements
C. Standardizes for thromboplastin activity
D. Internal normalization

90. PDA develop from:

A. Distal left sixth aortic arch
B. Left fourth arch
C. LVH fifth arch
D. Dorsal aorta

89 C 90 A

AIIMS 2002 (July)

1. Clubbing and cyanosis with normally split S2 is heard in:
A. Methemoglobinemia
B. Pulmonary A-V fistula
C. TAPVC
D. Cyanide toxicity

2. HTN may present as any of the following *except:*
A. Dizziness B. Migraine
C. Impotence D. Nocturia

3. Accessory pathway is not blocked by:
A. Digoxin B. Amiodarone
C. Quinidine D. Sotalol

4. Treatment of choice for torsades de pointes in a patient of SAH with long QT is:
A. Metoprolol B. Overdrive pacing
C. Mg D. DC shock

5. Secondary hyper aldosteronism not seen in:
A. Conn's syndrome B. Pregnancy
C. Portal hypertension D. CHF

6. CPK is not raised in:
A. Hypothyroidism B. Muscular dystrophy
C. Cerebral infarct D. Carnitine deficiency

7. ACE inhibitors do not cause:
A. Increased renin
B. Increased vasopressin
C. Decreased aldosterone
D. Decreased GFR

8. Syncope not found in:
A. Takayasu arteritis
B. Severe carotid stenosis
C. Basilar migraine
D. Hyperventilation

9. Square wave response on Valsalva is not seen in:
A. ASD B. MS
C. CHF D. PAH

10. Apex is obliterated in:
A. Endomyocardial fibrosis
B. Amyloidosis
C. Sarcoidosis
D. Hyper eosinophic syndrome

11. All are true about amyloidosis *except:*
A. Heart transplant is a treatment
B. Liver transplant is a treatment
C. Nifedipine can be used
D. CHF

12. All are true about apoptosis *except:*
A. Inflammatory exudate
B. Reperfusion is a cause
C. Cellular death
D. DNA fragmentation

1 B 2 B 3 A 4 A 5 A 6 D 7 B 8 B 9 D 10 A 11 C 12 A

13. CHF in fetus is seen in all *except:*
A. Ebstein B. Fetal anemia
C. Congenital CHB D. TGA

14. Haemoptysis is not seen in:
A. TOF B. Valvular PS
C. Eisenmenger D. Bronchial adenoma

15. PET scan mismatch is seen in:
A. Infarcted transmural myocardium
B. Isch. Viable myocardium
C. Scarred myocardium
D. Can be found in normal myocardium

16. ST elevation in V1 is seen in all *except:*
A. Pulmonary embolism
B. Brugada syndrome
C. Septal infarct
D. Pericarditis

17. AS with velocity 4m/sec; Gradient is:
A. 34 B. 64
C. 4 D. 100

18. DM–BP in JNC VI:
A. 135/85 B. 130/80
C. 120/75 D. 120/70

19. Not a coronary vasoconstrictor:
A. Adenosine B. Serotonin
C. Nor adrenaline D. Dopamine

20. Endothelium does not produce:
A. Fibrinogen B. vWF
C. Bradykinin D. Endothelin

21. Endothelial testing can be done using:
A. Acetyl choline B. Adrenaline
C. Atropine D. Serotonin

22. Worst prognosis:
A. Idiopathic DCMP
B. HIV related DCMP
C. Doxorubicin DCMP
D. Ischemic Cardiomyopathy

23. Refractory hypotension with adrenal insufficiency is seen with all *except:*
A. TB B. Meningococcus
C. Pseudomonas D. AIDS

24. Salmonella infection is seen in all *except:*
A. Elderly with aortic aneurysm
B. Asplenic patient
C. Sickle cell anaemia
D. IE

25. NO (inhaled) is useful in:
A. Persistent PPH of new born
B. Subarachnoid haemorrhage with HT
C. Hypertensive encephalopathy
D. Corpulmonale

26. Chronic AF with heart rate 60:
A. Digitalis toxicity
B. Hyperkalemia
C. Congenital heart block
D. Hypocalcemia

27. Warfarin effect decreased by:
A. Barbiturate
B. Erythromycin
C. Omeprazole
D. Griseofulvin

28. Tall R in V1is seen in all *except:*
A. Friedrichs ataxia
B. TOF
C. Muscular dystrophy
D. WPW type B

29. All are true about cardiac failure *except:*
A. Decrease A-V O2 difference
B. Decreased oxygen availability
C. Cyanosis
D. Extra pyramidal symptoms

13 D 14 B 15 B 16 A 17 B 18 A 19 A 20 C 21 A 22 B 23 C 24 B 25 A
26 A 27 A 28 A 29 A

30. Most common lipid disorder is:
A. Familial combined hyperlipidemia
B. Dysbeta lipoproteinemia
C. Polygenic hypercholesterolemia
D. Apo B deficiency

31. Dicrotic pulse not seen in:
A. HTN
B. Fever
C. Cardiac tamponade
D. Hypovolemic shock

32. Decreased in instent restenosis is seen with:
A. Sirolimous
B. Azathioprine
C. Heparin
D. Cyclosporin

33. Postural hypotension with tachycardia:
A. Bleeding peptic ulcer
B. Diabetic neuropathy
C. Vasovagal syncope
D. Autonomic insufficiency

34. All are true about polycythemia vera *except:*
A. Increased erythropoietin
B. Pruritus
C. Budd chiari syndrome
D. Peptic ulcer

35. Phospholamban:
A. Increased calcium in sarcoplasmic reticulum
B. Calcium regulatory protein
C. Decreased in heart failure
D. Responsible for contraction

36. Cardiac output by thermodilution is not affected in:
A. VSD
B. TR
C. PR
D. Low CO

37. Increased anion Gap acidosis is seen with all *except:*
A. RTA
B. Diarrhoea with shock
C. DKA
D. Acute renal failure

38. DC shock is effective in:
A. Atrial flutter with varying block
B. Digitalis toxicity
C. Torsades
D. Ventricular para systole

39. Clubbing is seen in all *except:*
A. NHL
B. Sarcoidosis
C. ILD
D. Crohn's disease

40. GPIIb/IIIa deficiency occurs in:
A. Bernard Soulier syndrome
B. Glanzman thrombasthenia
C. Scot's syndrome
D. Giant platelets

41. Treatment modality for AF include all *except:*
A. Maze operation
B. Ross operation
C. Amiodarone
D. RFA

42. All are true about ventricular action potential as compared to nodal action potential *except:*
A. More negative transmembrane potential
B. Conduction velocity is less in node than myocardium
C. β blockade causes decreased potential
D. None of the above

43. Resuscitation is not effective in:
A. Asystole
B. Primary VF
C. Pulse less electrical activity
D. Digitalis toxicity

44. Maximum mortality after MI:
A. Primary VF
B. Secondary VF
C. Aneurysm
D. Mitral regurgitation

30 A 31 A 32 A 33 A 34 A 35 A 36 A 37 A 38 A 39 A 40 B 41 B 42 C 43 A 44 B

45. Markedly hypoxic patient with alveolar–arterial difference of < 12 mm Hg; most probable diagnosis is:
A. Pickwickian syndrome
B. Pneumonia
C. Pulmonary embolism
D. MI

46. PO_2-80, PCO_2-20, PH 7.2, diagnosis:
A. Anxiety hyperventilation
B. Pneumonia
C. Pulmonary edema
D. DKA

47. PO_2-80, PCO_2-12, PH 7.55, diagnosis is:
A. Anxiety hyperventilation
B. PTE
C. Pulmonary edema
D. ARDS

48. Catch 22 is not seen in:
A. Pulmonary atresia B. Ebstein anomaly
C. Tricuspid atresia D. TOF

49. TMT–maximum predictability for pretest probability of CAD is:
A. 10% B. 20%
C. 50% D. 80%

50. All of the following can be normal *except:*
A. QS in V1
B. ST depressed 3 m in lateral leads
C. RBBB
D. ST elevation

51. Syncope after old MI; probable finding is:
A. LAD
B. RBBB
C. Pathological Q wave
D. RVH

52. All are common in female *except:*
A. Alzhemier B. HTN
C. DM D. Marfan

53. All are true in female *except:*
A. Increased HDL in female
B. Decreased TG in female
C. Increase waist hip ratio in female
D. Increased unstable angina in female

54. Alcohol cardiovascular effect include all *except:*
A. Hypertension
B. Raised TG
C. Raised LDL
D. Decreased HDL

55. Gene therapy is most successful in:
A. Cystic fibrosis
B. Peripheral vascular disease
C. Familial hypercholesterolemia
D. Duchenne muscular dystrophy

56. HOCM defect is in:
A. Myosin B. Tropomyosin
C. Troponin C D. Actin

57. Asymptomatic pericardial effusions is seen in all *except:*
A. Myxedema B. Hypoalbuminemia
C. Tuberculosis D. Post MI

58. Treatment of increased QT interval includes all *except:*
A. Potassium supplementation
B. Sotalol
C. Nicorandil
D. β blockers

59. Confidence interval of estimate means:
A. $p = 0.05$ to $p = 0.005$
B. Reliability of estimate
C. Standardization of estimate
D. Range of estimate in a population

60. Kussmaul sign not seen in:
A. Cardiac tamponade B. CCP
C. RVF D. RCM

45 A 46 C 47 A 48 B 49 C 50 B 51 C 52 D 53 C 54 D 55 B 56 A 57 B
58 B 59 D 60 A

61. Teratogenic drugs are all *except:*
A. Folinic acid
B. Phenylalanine
C. Alcohol
D. Retinoic acid

62. Primary investigation of choice in post MI when patient has precordial thrill:
A. Angiography
B. Echocardiogarphy
C. Chest X-ray
D. Nuclear scan

63. Target after CABG is:
A. LDL <100 mg/dL
B. LDL <130 mg/dL
C. LDL <160 mg/dL
D. LDL <60 mg/dL

64. Not to be given after nitrates:
A. Sildenafil
B. CCB
C. β blockers
D. Adenosine

65. All are true about vancomycin *except:*
A. <10% nephrotoxicity
B. Most common complication red Man syndrome
C. Should not be given with gentamicin
D. Can be used against enterococcus

66. Poisseulli equation:
A. To measure coronary artery stenosis
B. Measure resistance of blood flow
C. Measure coronary flow reserve
D. Measure endothelial dysfunction

67. Unstable angina; not to be given is:
A. rtPA
B. Abciximab
C. Statins
D. Tirofiban

68. All are increased in CCF *except:*
A. TNF
B. NA
C. Adrenalin
D. Na^+

69. All are seen in obesity *except:*
A. ↑T4
B. HTN
C. ↓ HDL
D. ↓ Leptin

70. Pulmonary artery hypertension; parasite involved:
A. Schistosomiasis
B. Paragonimiasis
C. Fasciolopsis
D. Trypanosoma

71. Arterial thrombus not seen in:
A. Factor V leiden
B. PNH
C. Hyper homocystenemia
D. Antiphospholipid antibodies

72. Weight loss by drug is statistically seen by:
A. Paired t test
B. Chi square test
C. Pearsons test
D. Spearman's test

73. Acute pulmonary embolism with RV dysfunction with normal systolic blood pressure; treatment is:
A. Thrombolytic therapy
B. LMWH
C. Surgery
D. Warfarin

74. Increased atherosclerosis is caused by:
A. Carbon disulphide
B. Carbon monoxide
C. Benzene
D. Cocaine

75. Jone's criteria are not applicable in all *except:*
A. Rheumatic chorea
B. Chronic carditis
C. First attack of rheumatic fever
D. Recurrent carditis

76. Compliment level is decreased in all *except:*
A. Acute rheumatic fever
B. IE
C. SLE
D. Glomerulonephritis

77. Genes for long QT syndrome include all *except:*
A. SCN5-A
B. HERG
C. KVLQT1
D. CIN

61 A 62 B 63 A 64 A 65 C 66 B 67 A 68 D 69 D 70 A 71 A 72 A 73 A
74 A 75 C 76 A 77 D

78. Hypertensive bleed most common at:
A. Thalamus
B. Putamen
C. Cerebellum
D. Cortex

79. Senile amyloidosis:
A. Can cause heart failure
B. Leads to systolic dysfunction
C. Autonomic involvement does not occur
D. Is associated with Alzheimer's disease

80. Gs ligand protein is associated with all *except:*
A. Insulin
B. ACTH
C. Adenosine
D. NO

81. All are true about unstable angina *except:*
A. Increased coronary sinus lactate
B. rtPA has mortality benefit
C. Occurs more in males
D. Plaque rupture is the predominant mechanism

82. H-V interval is decrease by all *except:*
A. Amiodarone
B. Xylocaine
C. Mexiletine
D. None of the above

83. Beta-1 mediated actions is:
A. Cardiostimulation
B. Cardioinhibition
C. Vasodilatation
D. None of the above

84. PTCA has adverse prognosis with:
A. Diabetes Mellitus
B. Concentric lesion
C. Distal lesion
D. Proximal LAD stenosis

85. In angina pectoris, all may be seen *except:*
A. Pulmonary congestion
B. Increase LVEDP
C. Decrease coronary sinus lactate
D. LV wall motion abnormality

86. Asymptomatic large pericardial effusion is seen in:
A. Rheumatic fever
B. Myxoedema
C. Sarcoidosis
D. Hypoalbuminemia

87. hrombolytic therapy saves how many lives per 1000 patients treated:
A. 17
B. 170
C. 50
D. 250

88. Seventy year old man with bifascicular block posted for hernia repair; best advice would be:
A. TMT
B. Temporary pacing
C. Close observation during surgery
D. EPS

89. In SHOCK trial, 30 day mortality with medical management was:
A. 36%
B. 75%
C. 56%
D. 80%

90. All are normal findings in ECG *except:*
A. T inversion in V1-V3
B. Qs in V1
C. ST depression in V2-V4
D. ST elevation in V4-V6

78 B 79 A 80 A 81 B 82 A 83 A 84 A 85 C 86 B 87 A 88 C 89 C 90 C

AIIMS 2001 (December)

1. **Complement levels is decreased in all *except:***
   - **A.** Rheumatic fever
   - **B.** Post streptococcal Glomerulonephritis
   - **C.** IE
   - **D.** SLE

2. **Jones criteria is not applicable in all of these *except:***
   - **A.** Rheumatic chorea
   - **B.** Chronic carditis
   - **C.** First attack of rheumatic fever
   - **D.** Recurrent carditis

3. **Osborn wave is seen in all *except:***
   - **A.** Hypothermia
   - **B.** Brugada syndrome
   - **C.** Hypokalemia
   - **D.** Hypercalcemia

4. **Early systolic murmur is heard in all *except:***
   - **A.** Traumatic TR
   - **B.** Small muscular VSD
   - **C.** Mild rheumatic MR
   - **D.** Ebstein

5. **All are true about penicillin prophylaxis *except:***
   - **A.** Anaphylaxis is fatal
   - **B.** Anaphylaxis may occur later
   - **C.** Continuous prophylaxis may cure the valve lesion
   - **D.** Continuous prophylaxis is less effective in a child than adult

6. **Prophylaxis for IE is given in:**
   - **A.** Uretheral dilatation
   - **B.** Fibre optic bronchoscopy
   - **C.** Cesarian section
   - **D.** Coronary angiography

7. **Maximum risk for IE:**
   - **A.** AS
   - **B.** VSD + AR
   - **C.** MR
   - **D.** MVP

8. **Best prophylaxis for SCD is:**
   - **A.** AICD
   - **B.** β blocker
   - **C.** Calcium channel blocker
   - **D.** Coronary risk factor prevention

9. **SCD is seen in all *except:***
   - **A.** Eisenmenger
   - **B.** MVP
   - **C.** Non obstructive HCM
   - **D.** Long QT

10. **Serum ammonia increase in all *except:***
    - **A.** Hepatic encephalopathy
    - **B.** Renal failure
    - **C.** Reye syndrome
    - **D.** Carinitiine deficiency

11. **In CCF which of the following does not increase:**
    - **A.** TNF
    - **B.** NA
    - **C.** Adrenalin
    - **D.** Na^+

---

1 A **2** C **3** C **4** C **5** C **6** A **7** B **8** D **9** B **10** B **11** D

12. Heart failure with pre renal azotemia: All can be seen *except:*
A. Fractional renal Na^+ excretion < 1
B. Urine osmolality <350 mosm
C. Ur/plasma creatinine >40
D. BUN/Creatinine >20

13. New Born cyanotic with oligemic lung fields with no cardiomegaly:
A. TOF
B. TGA
C. Pulmonary Atresia
D. Ebstein's anomaly

14. Maximum life expectancy is seen after:
A. Cardiac transplantation
B. Fontan operation
C. Mechanical valve prosthesis
D. TOF (operated)

15. 3rd day MI with LLSB thrill–investigation of choice:
A. TTE B. TEE
C. Angio D. MRI

16. Cholesterol emboli–all are correct *except:*
A. Seen after Coronary Angiography
B. Seen after warfarin therapy
C. Livedo reticularis
D. Anticoagulant can clear it

17. Premature CAD is seen in all *except:*
A. Progeria
B. SLE
C. Marfan
D. Pseudoxanthoma elasticum

18. Least risk–in patient with USA is seen in:
A. Rest angina, resolved
B. Age >65 yrs
C. Trop T +ve
D. Class II new onset

19. PET scan–perfusion mismatch is seen in:
A. Viable myocardium (ischemic)
B. Pulmonary edema
C. Pulmonary embolism
D. Primary pulmonary hypertension

20. RFA-least effective in:
A. AVNRT B. Atrial flutter
C. Ischemic VT D. AVRT

21. Least energy of DC cardioversion required in:
A. Atrial flutter
B. VT
C. Sinus tachycardia
D. Mahaim's tachycardia

22. Pulmonary embolism with RV dysfunction on echo: what to do in 30 year female:
A. Thrombolysis B. LMWH
C. Warfarin D. Aspirin

23. AF–what is not to be done:
A. Maze operation B. Ross operation
C. Amiodarone D. RFA

24. Sickle cell trait is associated with:
A. Painless hematuria
B. Acute chest syndrome
C. Painful crisis
D. Bone infarcts

25. All can be seen in chronic fatigue syndrome *except:*
A. Headache
B. Chest pain
C. Sleep disturbances
D. Lymphadenopathy

26. After blood pressure cuff application and withdrawal murmur is increased in all *except:*
A. HOCM B. MR
C. AR D. VSD

12 B 13 C 14 D 15 A 16 D 17 C 18 A 19 A 20 C 21 B 22 A 23 B 24 A
25 B 26 A

27. CCP –echo findings include all *except:*
A. Mitral deceleration slope increased
B. Septal bounce
C. Inspiratory collapse of IVC
D. E > A

28. Long QT syndrome not associated with gene:
A. SCN5-A B. HERG
C. KVLQT1 D. CIN

29. Confidence interval of estimate means:
A. p = 0.05 to p = 0.0005
B. Range of true estimate in population
C. Reliability of estimates
D. Standardization of estimates

30. Kussmaul sign is not found in:
A. CCP B. Cardiac tamponade
C. RVMI D. Pulmonary embolism

31. T wave alternans is seen in all *except:*
A. Ischemia B. Long QT
C. Cardiac tamponade D. Pericarditis

32. All are true about SVC syndrome *except:*
A. Histoplasmosis may be a cause
B. Stent is a palliative
C. Radiotherapy in small cell lung cancer
D. CT is reliable for diagnosis

33. Rib notching is seen in all *except:*
A. Neurofibromatosis
B. CoA
C. BT-shunt (modified)
D. Intercostal AV fistula

34. O_2 requirement in heart failure is decreased by all *except:*
A. ACE inhibitor
B. β blocker
C. Digoxin
D. Glucose Insulin potassium

35. Cyanosis, clubbing with normal S2 is seen in:
A. Pulmonary AV fistula
B. Methemoglobinaemia
C. Cyanide toxicity
D. TAPVC

36. Vasovagal syncope is not seen with:
A. Fasting
B. Prolong standing
C. β blocker
D. Autonomic insufficiency

37. SVT in children is decreased by all *except:*
A. Adenosine
B. Ice pack on face
C. β blocker
D. Calcium channel blocker

38. Metabolic alkalosis is seen in all *except:*
A. Conns syndrome
B. Cushing syndrome
C. Barter syndrome
D. G-6 PD deficiency

39. SIADH is caused by:
A. Acetazolamide B. Lasix
C. Thiazide D. Triamterene

40. Edema is caused by all *except:*
A. Cyclosporin B. IL-2
C. Nifedpine D. Captopril

41. PVR is increased by all *except:*
A. Acidosis B. Alkalosis
C. Serotonin D. Heart failure

42. Chronic mountain inhabitant can present with all *except:*
A. Monges disease
B. Acute mountain sickness
C. PDA
D. PPH

27 C 28 D 29 B 30 B 31 D 32 C 33 C 34 D 35 A 36 C 37 D 38 D 39 C
40 D 41 B 42 B

43. Pregnancy is well tolerated in:
A. Aorto arteritis
B. Marfan syndrome >50 mm aortic root dilatation
C. Mechanical valves
D. PPH

44. MS with > 1.3 cm² in 7 month pregnancy treatment of choice:
A. Medical management
B. Balloon valvotomy
C. Close valvotomy
D. Follow up

45. Clopidogrel: all of the following are true *except:*
A. Permanent platelet inhibitor
B. Inhibits ADP induced platelet aggregation
C. Peak action within 4 hours
D. Thienopyridine derivative

46. All are true about amyloid heart disease *except:*
A. Heart transplant is the treatment
B. Liver transplant is the treatment
C. Diuretic can be given
D. Nifedipine can be given

47. Which of the following is a clinically significant manifestation cardiac manifestation of AIDS?
A. Pericardial effusion
B. Secondary lymphoma
C. DCM
D. IE

48. In children junctional tachycardia caused by all *except:*
A. Atrial myxoma B. Mesothelioma
C. Rhabdomyoma D. Fibroma

49. In obesity which does not occur:
A. Hyperinsulinemia
B. HTN
C. Decreased HDL
D. Decreased Leptin

50. Endothelium testing is done by:
A. Ach B. Arecholine
C. Adrenaline D. Atropine

51. Statin is not effective in:
A. Polygenic hypercholesterolemia
B. Homozygous hypercholesterolemia
C. Heterozygous hypercholesterolemia
D. Non familial hypercholesterolemia

52. To inhibit conduction through accessory pathway drug used:
A. Digoxin
B. Procainamide
C. Adenosine
D. Verapamil

53. DM with hypertension, BP to be decreased to:
A. 135/85 B. 100/60
C. 140/90 D. 120/75

54. Hypertensive bleed most common at:
A. Thalamus B. Putamen
C. Cerebellum D. Cortex

55. TMT: ST elevation is caused by all *except:*
A. Aneurysm
B. Coronary vasospasm
C. Ischemia
D. Hibernating myocardium

56. Coronary vasoconstriction is caused by all *except:*
A. Adenosine
B. Serotonin
C. Nor Adrenaline
D. Dopamine

57. Cocaine heart disease is characterized by:
A. Eosinophilia
B. Contraction band necrosis
C. Apoptosis
D. LV thrombus

43 A 44 D 45 C 46 D 47 C 48 A 49 D 50 A 51 B 52 B 53 A 54 B 55 D
56 A 57 B

58. Best Post MI predictor of mortality:
- **A.** VT on 7th day
- **B.** Ejection fraction < 30%
- **C.** VPC ³10 per hour
- **D.** Class II symptoms

59. In Shock study, mortality of medical management was:
- **A.** 56% **B.** 76%
- **C.** 80% **D.** 36%

60. Cardiogenic shock is best treated by:
- **A.** PTCA **B.** Thrombolysis
- **C.** CABG **D.** PTCA with stent

61. TMT is best predictor when pretest probability is:
- **A.** 10% **B.** 20%
- **C.** 50% **D.** 80%

62. Subarachnoid haemorrhage with QT prolongation treatment of choice:
- **A.** β blocker **B.** Magnesium
- **C.** Over drive pacing **D.** DC Shock

63. All are antioxidant *except:*
- **A.** Vit E
- **B.** High dose vitamin C
- **C.** Ginkobiloba
- **D.** Carvedilol

64. TR jet velocity of 4 m/s is seen in all *except:*
- **A.** PS **B.** PAH
- **C.** ASD **D.** TOF

65. HTN is not seen in:
- **A.** Sleep apnea syndrome
- **B.** Hypothyroidism
- **C.** Barter syndrome
- **D.** Lead poisoning

66. Diastolic dysfunction is not seen in:
- **A.** Athelete heart **B.** HOCM
- **C.** Acute Ischemia **D.** CHF

67. PO_2-80, PCO_2-20, PH 7.55, diagnosis is:
- **A.** Anxiety hyperventilation
- **B.** PTE
- **C.** Pulmonary edema
- **D.** DKA

68. Pulmonary arterial saturation of 88% is seen in all *except:*
- **A.** TAPVC
- **B.** PAPVC
- **C.** Low Cardiac output
- **D.** TGA

69. Erectile dysfunction occur with all *except:*
- **A.** NTG
- **B.** β blocker
- **C.** Lehriche's syndrome
- **D.** Spironolactone

70. Tc^{99} is better than Thallium in all *except:*
- **A.** Acute MI
- **B.** Better image quality
- **C.** First pass metabolism
- **D.** Delayed imaging

71. All are true about carotid endarterectomy *except:*
- **A.** Done in symptomatic hemiparesis
- **B.** High Gr. Stenosis
- **C.** Perioperative mortality 10%
- **D.** Concurrent with CABG

72. CHB is seen in all *except:*
- **A.** Diphtheria myocarditis
- **B.** Chagas disease
- **C.** Myocardial sarcoidosis
- **D.** Acute rheumatic fever

73. MVP is not seen in:
- **A.** RF
- **B.** Marfan
- **C.** ASD
- **D.** Endomyocardial fibrosis

58 B 59 A 60 A 61 C 62 A 63 B 64 D 65 C 66 A 67 A 68 C 69 A 70 A
71 C 72 D 73 D

74. All are true about rubella syndrome *except:*
A. Does not occur in India
B. Common in 1st trimester of pregnancy
C. PS
D. Vaccination is contraindicated during pregnancy

75. VT with left axis deviation is seen in:
A. Uhl's anomaly
B. Structurally normal heart
C. Post MI
D. Myocarditis

76. GPIIb/IIIa deficiency occurs in:
A. Bernard Soulier syndrome
B. Glanzman thrombesthenia
C. Scott's syndrome
D. Giant platelets

77. Asymptomatic male having aortic stenosis with 4m/s jet: treatment of choice is:
A. Conservative
B. AVR
C. BAV
D. Open valvotomy

78. Long QT, torsades de pointes treatment of choice is:
A. $MgSO_4$
B. β blocker
C. Amiodarone
D. Overdrive pacing

79. Left SVC draining into coronary sinus derived from which brachial arch:
A. Left Common cardinal vein
B. Vitelline duct
C. Superior cardinal vein
D. Inferior cardinal vein

80. Adhesion molecules are all *except:*
A. Integrin
B. VCAM, ICAM
C. Selectin
D. Metalloproteinase

81. Markedly hypoxic patient with alveolar arterial difference of < 12 mmHg: Most probable diagnosis is:
A. Pickwickian syndrome
B. Pneumonia
C. Pulmonary embolism
D. MI

82. Calcium acts through all *except:*
A. Purinergic receptor
B. Na^+–K^+ ATPase
C. Dihydropyridine receptor
D. Ryanodine receptor (SERCA)

83. Least lipid soluble beta blocker is:
A. Atenolol
B. Labetelol
C. Propanolol
D. Metaprolol

84. Echocardiographic features of HOCM are all *except:*
A. Atrial septal hypertrophy
B. RVH
C. Concentric LVH
D. LV contractile dysfunction (late)

85. A seventy year old patient with bifascicular (RBBB + LAHB) block posted for hernia should undergo:
A. Close observation during surgery
B. TMT
C. Temporary pacing
D. EPS

86. Cyanosis in TOF is directly related to:
A. VSD
B. RVOT obstruction
C. Aortic override
D. RV hypertrophy

87. Diabetic patient with BP of 180/120 mm Hg with peripheral vascular disease and small right kidney should be taken up for:
A. Captopril test
B. Doppler USG
C. Renal angiography with ballooning if needed
D. MRI

74 A 75 B 76 B 77 A 78 A 79 A 80 D 81 A 82 A 83 A 84 A 85 A 86 B
87 C

88. Which of the following is least common in isolated inferior wall MI:

A. Myocardial rupture
B. Septal rupture
C. LV thrombus
D. MR

89. Which of the following is not true regarding AF in a 70 year male with high risk for stroke:

A. LA = 5 mm
B. CCF
C. RHD
D. HTN

90. TEE is indicated in all *except:*

A. Periaortic abscess
B. Aortic atheroma
C. LV apical thrombus
D. Sinus venosus ASD

88 C 89 A 90 C

AIIMS 2001 (June)

1. **All are cause of LBBB *except:***
   A. WPW right sided pathway
   B. Lev disease
   C. Subendocardial MI
   D. Hyperkalemia

2. **Rib notching is seen in all *except:***
   A. Intercostal neurofibroma
   B. CoA
   C. Modified BT Shunt
   D. Intercostal AV fistula

3. **Normal ECG can present with all *except:***
   A. QS in VI
   B. ST↑ V_1-V_3
   C. ST↓ V_2-V_4
   D. T↓ V_1-V_3

4. **Bowdich staircase phenomenon is:**
   A. ↑ Contractility with↑ rate
   B. Post extrasystolic increase in gradient in HOCM
   C. Radius varies inversely with rate of flow
   D. Increased after load increase contractility

5. **All are seen in Catch syndrome *except:***
   A. Ebstein
   B. TA
   C. Interrupted aortic arch
   D. TAPVC

6. **Drugs used in ↑QT interval are all *except:***
   A. Nicorandil
   B. Sotalol
   C. Nadolol
   D. Oral K^+

7. **Best correlation of O_2 demand of myocardium is with:**
   A. LVES dimension
   B. HR
   C. Contractility
   D. Metabolic activity

8. **In a female patient with long sinus pause, TMT THR 160/min with syncope, PPI of choice is:**
   A. AAI
   B. DDD
   C. VVIR
   D. DDDR

9. **Cyanosis, clubbing and normal split S2 is seen in:**
   A. Pulmonary A-V fistula
   B. TAPVC
   C. Methemoglobinaemia
   D. Cyanide toxicity

10. **Continuous murmur with diastolic component louder than systolic component is seen in all *except:***
    A. PDA
    B. AV fistula
    C. RSOV
    D. Coronary AV fistula

11. **Acute AR is associated with all *except:***
    A. No LVS4
    B. No IE
    C. Short murmur
    D. Wide pulse pressure

1 C 2 C 3 C 4 A 5 A 6 B 7 B 8 A 9 A 10 A 11 D

12. Most common cause of AS in 10 year old in India:
A. Unicuspid aortic valve
B. RHD
C. BAV
D. Hyperparathyroidism

13. Normal PA pressure in PR is indicated by:
A. High frequency murmur
B. Single S2
C. Gap between S2 and murmur
D. Ejection click

14. Inhaled NO is effective in:
A. Vasopspasm after SAH
B. Persistent PAH in new born
C. Cor pulmonale
D. Nitrate resistance

15. Refractory hypotension–probably due to Addison's crisis is suspected in all *except:*
A. AIDS
B. TB
C. Meningococcus sepsis
D. Pseudomonas sepsis

16. Salmonella infection is associated with all *except:*
A. Infected aortic aneurysm in elderly
B. Diarrhoea in dairy worker
C. Osteomyelitis in sickle cell disease
D. In asplenic patients

17. Nicorandil causes:
A. ↓ QT interval B. ↑ QT interval
C. ↑ QRS interval D. ST elevation

18. Which of the following does not increase survival in CHF ?
A. ACEI B. Digoxin
C. Aldacton D. β blocker

19. VT is most probable cause of syncope in IHD if following is present:
A. LVH B. Pathological Q wave
C. RBBB D. Normal heart

20. DC cardioversion is not effective in all *except:*
A. Flutter with varying block
B. Chronic AF
C. Automatic atrial tachycardia
D. Non paroxysmal junctional tachycardia

21. Confidence interval of estimate means:
A. P = 0.05 to p = 0.0005
B. Reliability of estimate
C. Standardization of estimates
D. Range of estimates in a population

22. Thermodilution cannot be used in all *except:*
A. VSD
B. MR
C. PR
D. Low cardiac output

23. Hypertension and hypokalemia respond to steroid in case of:
A. Barter syndrome
B. Liddle syndrome
C. 11β hydroxylase deficiency
D. Reninoma

24. Kussmaul's sign is seen in all *except:*
A. CCP
B. Cardiac tamponade
C. Pulmonary embolism
D. RVMI

25. Exudative hypertensive retinopathy is most likely with:
A. Renal artery stenosis
B. Conn's syndrome
C. CVA
D. Malignant hypertension

26. Not used in cardiac tamponade:
A. Isoprenaline B. Lasix
C. Dobutamine D. Fluid

12 A 13 C 14 B 15 D 16 D 17 A 18 B 19 B 20 A 21 D 22 A 23 C 24 B
25 A 26 B

27. Causes of sudden visual loss in DM with HT are all *except:*
A. Hypertensive crisis
B. Optic neuropathy
C. Retinal detachment
D. Vitreous haemorrhage

28. Postural hypotension with tachycardia is consistent with:
A. Bleeding peptic ulcer
B. Shy drager
C. Diabetic neuropathy
D. Parkinsonism

29. Polycythemia vera is associated with all *except:*
A. Clubbing
B. ↓ Erythropoietin
C. Microcytic erythrocytosis
D. Thrombocytosis

30. Osborne wave is seen in all *except:*
A. Hypothermia B. Hyperthermia
C. Hypercalcemia D. Hyperkalemia

31. Increase anion gap is seen in all *except:*
A. DKA
B. RTA
C. Ethyl glycol poisoning
D. Renal failure

32. Phospholamban:
A. ↑ Ca uptake by sarcoplasmic reticulum
B. ↓ in Heart failure
C. ↓ Ca uptake by sarcoplasmic reticulum
D. ↑ Ca uptake by T tubules

33. All are G protein linked *except:*
A. Adenosine B. Dopamine
C. ACTH D. Insulin

34. Main abnormality in HOCM is:
A. Myosin B. Actin
C. Tropomyosin D. Mitochondrial

35. IE prophylaxis is indicated in:
A. Subaortic AS < 20 mm Hg obstruction
B. Non obstructive HCM
C. MVP without murmur
D. MVP with stroke

36. ↑ Diastolic BP from supine to standing is suggestive of:
A. Essential HTN
B. Gestational HTN
C. Renovascular HTN
D. Pheochroma cytoma

37. Secondary hyperaldosteronism is seen in all *except:*
A. Conn's syndrome
B. Cirrhosis
C. Pregnancy
D. Nephrotic syndrome

38. Which of the following is a cause of SIADH ?
A. Acetazolamide B. Frusemide
C. Aldactone D. Thiazide

39. PO2-85, PCO2 20, pH 7.2; the most likely diagnosis is:
A. DKA
B. Anxiety
C. Phenobarbitone overdose
D. Pulmonary oedema

40. ↑ PVR is seen with all *except:*
A. Hypercarbia B. Acidosis
C. Alkalosis D. Polycythemia

41. MVP is seen in all *except:*
A. RHD B. ASD
C. Marfan's syndrome D. HOCM

42. In a patient with thrill in left sternal border 3 day after MI; Investigation of choice:
A. TEE B. TTE
C. MRI D. Cath

27 B 28 A 29 A 30 B 31 B 32 A 33 D 34 A 35 A 36 A 37 A 38 D 39 D
40 C 41 A 42 B

43. Congenital CHB is associated with all *except:*
A. SSA positive mother
B. c-TGA
C. Visceral heterotaxy
D. Kartagener syndrome

44. CCF in foetus occurs with all *except:*
A. Anemia B. CHB
C. d-TGA D. Hypoglycemia

45. CPK ↑ is present in all *except:*
A. Angina pectoris B. Cerebral infarct
C. Hypothyroid D. i.m injections

46. Tall R in V1 is present in all *except:*
A. DMD B. Fredrichs ataxia
C. TOF D. WPW

47. LDL cholesterol target in post CABG patient is:
A. <100 mg% B. <130 mg%
C. <60 mg% D. <150 mg%

48. Alcohol causes all *except:*
A. ↑ BP B. Cardiotoxicity
C. ↓ HDL D. AF

49. In a patient with DM with HT with CVA with BP 220/130:
A. ↓ BP to 180/110 B. No treatment
C. Give Manitol D. Statins

50. Patient on long acting nitrate should not receive:
A. ACE-inhibitors B. Sildenafil
C. Diuretic D. Nicroandil

51. Pregnancy is not well tolerated in:
A. CoA B. MR
C. Mild PS D. ASD

52. GpIIb/IIIa inhibitor proved useful in:
A. High risk PTCA
B. STEMI
C. Chronic angina
D. Subendocardial infarct

53. GPIIb/III activity decreased in:
A. Glanzmann thrombasthenia
B. Bernard Souliar syndrome
C. Grey Platelet syndrome
D. Wiskot Aldrich syndrome

54. Palpable purpura is seen in all *except:*
A. Warfarin necrosis
B. ITP
C. Cholesterol embolism
D. HS purpura

55. Warfarin activity is increased by all *except:*
A. Rifampicin B. Cimetidine
C. Erythromycin D. Miconazole

56. Clinical pulmonary edema is seen with all *except:*
A. Narcotic overdose B. Post CABG
C. Hypoalbuminemia D. Mountain sickness

57. ↑ PA pressure is seen in:
A. Anaphylactic shock
B. Septic shock
C. Hypovolemia
D. MI

58. Ross operation is done for:
A. MR B. AR
C. TGA D. MS

59. Cyanide poisoning is associated with all *except:*
A. ↓ Mixed venous oxygen saturation
B. Lactic acidosis
C. Treatment with sodium nitrite and thiosulphate
D. ↓ A-V oxygen difference

60. IV therapy in HTN crisis comprises all *except:*
A. Urapidil B. Fenoldopam
C. Nifedipine D. Enalaprilat

43 D 44 C 45 A 46 B 47 A 48 C 49 A 50 B 51 A 52 A 53 A 54 B 55 A
56 C 57 D 58 B 59 A

61. LBBB with MI is diagnosed by all *except:*
A. Q in I, AVL V_4-V_6
B. Notching of upstroke in V_3-V_6
C. ST↑ 3 mm in V_1-V_3
D. Primary ST-T change V_4-V_6

62. Best prognostic indicator in MI is:
A. VT on holter
B. Left main disease
C. LV ejection fraction
D. AF

63. Hemoptysis is seen in all *except:*
A. TOF
B. Eisenmenger syndrome
C. Pulmonary valve stenosis
D. Bronchial adenoma

64. Most likely to be observed in cyanotic spell:
A. ↓ BP
B. Absent murmur
C. Normal PaO_2 with decrease oxygen saturation
D. Sitting position

65. Very likely to be abnormal in pulmonary embolism is:
A. Perfusion scan B. Chest X-ray
C. ABG D. Echo

66. All are true about amyloidosis *except:*
A. Senile amyloidosis does not cause CCF
B. Sensitive to digoxin
C. ↑ Uptake of Technitium^{99}
D. Low voltage EGG

67. Least common in AIDS hearts is:
A. Kaposi sarcoma B. IE
C. Myocarditis D. Atherosclerosis

68. All are autosomal recessive *except:*
A. Neurofibromatosis
B. Hemochromatis
C. Ellis Van Creveld syndrome
D. Wilson's disease

69. Most useful for preventing SCD:
A. ↓ risk factor for CAD
B. Advanced life support by layman
C. ICD
D. Amiodarone

70. All are true about ventricular action potential as compared to nodal action potential *except:*
A. More negative transmembrane potential
B. Conduction velocity is more in node
C. β blockade causes decreased potential
D. None of the above

71. HV interval ↓ by all *except:*
A. Amiodarone B. Verapamil
C. Adenosine D. Procainamide

72. Gene therapy is most successful in:
A. Cystic fibrosis
B. Peripheral vascular disease
C. Alzheimer
D. Atherosclerosis

73. Endothelium secretes all *except:*
A. Prostacyclin B. Thrombomodulin
C. VWF D. Fibrinogen

74. Atherosclerosis is increased by:
A. Benzene B. CS_2
C. Iron D. CO_2

75. Result of effective ACE- inhibitors are all *except:*
A. ↑ Bradykinin
B. ↑ Vasopressin
C. ↓ Aldosterone
D. ↑ Renin

76. Poiseulli's law states that:
A. Pressure develop across stenosis
B. ↑ contractility with ↑ rate
C. Post extrasystolic potentiation
D. Increased after load increase contractility

60 C 61 C 62 C 63 C 64 B 65 A 66 A 67 B 68 A 69 A 70 C 71 A 72 B
73 D 74 B 75 B 76 A

77. Consequences of disease in old but not merely due to ageing are all *except:*
A. DM
B. Anemia
C. Heart failure
D. Bacteremia

78. In cardiac transplant most useful matching is:
A. ABO compatibility
B. HLA compatibility
C. Rh compatibility
D. Minor blood group antigens

79. PAH caused by parasite:
A. Paragonimiasis
B. Schistosomiasis
C. Filariasis
D. Liver fluke

80. Statins are useful in all *except:*
A. Hypertension
B. Primary prevention of MI
C. Plaque stabilization
D. Endothelial dysfunction

81. Most common hyperlipidemia is:
A. Combined hyperlipidemia
B. Type IV hyperlipidemia
C. Familial hypercholesterolemia
D. Type I hyperlipidemia

82. ACE is found in:
A. Alveolar epithelium
B. Vascular Endothelium
C. Liver
D. Alveolar interstitium

83. All are seen in apoptosis *except:*
A. Inflammatory exudates
B. Rapid cell death
C. DNA breakdown
D. Occurs in organogenesis

84. Increased in CCF are all *except:*
A. ↑ Renin
B. ↑ Vasopressin
C. ↑ Aldosterone
D. ↑ Na

85. Which of the following prevents conduction through accessory pathway:
A. Digoxin
B. Procainamide
C. Adenosine
D. Verapamil

86. As compared to men, women have all *except:*
A. Higher BP
B. ↓ TG
C. ↓ HDL
D. ↑ Waist hip ratio

87. Endothelium testing is done by:
A. Acetylcholine
B. Arecholine
C. Adrenaline
D. Atropine

88. In obesity, which does not occur?
A. Hyperinsulinaemia
B. Hypertension
C. Decrease HDL
D. Decrease Leptin

89. All are echocardiographic findings of CCP *except:*
A. Mitral deceleration slope increased
B. Septal bounce
C. Inspiratory collapse of IVC
D. E > A

90. Radio frequency ablation is least effective in:
A. AVNRT
B. Atrial flutter
C. Ischemic VT
D. AVRT

77 D 78 A 79 B 80 A 81 A 82 B 83 A 84 D 85 B 86 D 87 A 88 D 89 C
90 C

AIIMS 2000 (December)

1. **Which of the following is a known teratogenic?**
   A. Folic acid B. Retinoic acid
   C. Acetic acid D. Ascorbic acid

2. **Hypocalcemia is associated with:**
   A. Di George syndrome
   B. William syndrome
   C. Rubella
   D. Vater syndrome

3. **Most common cause of aortic stenosis in a 10 year old in India:**
   A. Bicuspid B. Rheumatic
   C. Unicuspid D. Subvalvular

4. **Exercise induced VT is associated with all *except:***
   A. Romanoward
   B. Brugada syndrome
   C. RVOT VT
   D. CAD

5. **CHF in fetus can occur with all *except:***
   A. SVT B. Anemia
   C. Severe CoA D. CHB

6. **LV dysfunction in infant is seen with all *except:***
   A. TOF
   B. ALCAPA
   C. Endothelial fibroelastosis
   D. None of the above

7. **Regarding cerebral abscess in cyanotic heart disease, all are true *except:***
   A. IE
   B. Age > 4 years
   C. Iron deficiency is not seen
   D. Severe polycythemia

8. **Least common lesion associated with IE:**
   A. ASD B. VSD
   C. PDA D. Cyanotic CHD

9. **Device closure is done in all *except:***
   A. ASD (20 mm)
   B. PFO (R $\rightarrow$ L)
   C. Supracristal VSD 4 mm
   D. PDA 5 mm

10. **All are true about supracristal VSD *except:***
    A. AR B. PAH
    C. LV to RA shunt D. CHF

11. **AR is associated with all *except:***
    A. Perimembranous VSD
    B. Supracrsital VSD
    C. ASD
    D. RSOV

12. **O_2 step up at IVC and RA junction is seen in:**
    A. RSOV
    B. VSD
    C. PDA
    D. AP window

1 B 2 A 3 C 4 B 5 C 6 A 7 C 8 A 9 C 10 C 11 C 12 A

13. Normal split S2 is heard in all *except:*
A. Pulmonary AV fistula
B. Methemoglobinaemia
C. TAPVC
D. Anomalous drainage of systemic veins into LA

14. Continuous murmur is heard in all *except:*
A. RSOV rupture into LV
B. Vein of Galen aneurysm
C. AV Fistula
D. Small PDA

15. CoA collateral involve all *except:*
A. 1st intercostals artery
B. 3rd intercostals artery
C. Hypogastric artery
D. Inferior epigastric artery

16. In TOF VSD is defined as:
A. Small PMVSD
B. Large unrestricted VSD
C. Muscular VSD
D. Pulmonary valve marks the margin of VSD

17. All are true about right atrium *except:*
A. Elongated and crooked finger appearance of RA appendage
B. Crista terminalis
C. Anterior and right position
D. Valve around fossa ovalis

18. Exudative retinopathy is seen with:
A. Conn's disease
B. Takayasu type 1
C. CoA
D. Pheochromocytoma

19. Postural drop is seen with all *except:*
A. Pheochromocytoma
B. Diuretic therapy
C. Shy Dragger syndrome
D. HT (essential)

20. All cause acidosis with normal anion gap *except:*
A. DKA
B. Potassium sparing diuretics
C. Diarrhoea
D. Renal tubular acidosis

21. Tall R wave (>10 mm) in V1 is seen in all *except:*
A. TGA
B. WPW in Ebstein's anomaly (Type B)
C. Duchenne dystrophy
D. TOF

22. HV interval is ↑ by all *except:*
A. Amiodarone **B.** Propafenone
C. Xylocaine **D.** Quinidine

23. LBBB is seen with all *except:*
A. Digitalis
B. Hyperkalemia
C. Lev's disease
D. WPW syndrome

24. All are true about Prosthetic valve *except:*
A. IABP to be used in patient with valve dysfunction causing AR
B. Thromboembolism/valve thrombosis in MV > AV
C. Absent click indicates PV thrombosis
D. Conduction defect in AV prosthesis suggest paravalvular abscess

25. Post MI causes acute MR due to:
A. Papillary muscle scarring
B. PM dysfunction
C. Dilatation of annulus & LV dysfunction
D. Rupture chordae

26. Absent uptake of C-14 and FDG on PET scan is suggestive of:
A. Scarred myocardium
B. Hibernating myocardium
C. Ischaemia
D. Normal myocardium

13 C 14 A 15 A 16 B 17 A 18 D 19 D 20 A 21 B 22 C 23 A 24 A 25 B
26 A

27. AF is least associated with:
A. Hypothyroidism
B. Post CABG
C. Thoracotomy for Ca lung
D. Alcohol Bing occasional

28. Objective of CABG are all *except:*
A. ↓ Angina
B. ↓ Mortality
C. ↓ Symptom
D. Prevent native arterial atherosclerosis

29. All are true about CAD after transplant *except:*
A. Intimal hyperplasia
B. 50% in 5 years
C. ↑ lipid not a risk factor
D. Related to repeated transplant rejection

30. All are done before cardiac transplantation *except:*
A. HLA typing
B. ABO grouping
C. Lymphocyte cross maching
D. CMV status

31. VSD is inoperable if:
A. PVR > 10 woods unit
B. >5
C. >2.5
D. >7.5

32. Bronchogenic CA with poorest prognosis is:
A. Alveolar **B.** Adeno
C. Squamous **D.** Small cell

33. Bioprosthesis is favored over mechanical valve in all *except:*
A. Young women
B. Children
C. Elderly
D. Recurrent Prosthetic valve thrombosis

34. Penicillin anaphylaxis is seen in:
A. 0.2-0.9/10,000
B. 0.2-0.9/1000
C. 0.4/lakh
D. 2/1000

35. Trop T is favored over CPK in all *except:*
A. Bed side diagnosis of MI
B. 4th day after MI
C. Within 32 hours of MI
D. Post CABG

36. ACE-I cause all *except:*
A. Left ventricular hypertrophy
B. ↑ Renin
C. ↑ Bradykinin
D. ↓ GFR

37. All are seen with old age *except:*
A. ↓ Resting HR
B. ↑ SBP
C. ↑ Closing lung volume
D. ↓ GFR

38. In CHF survival is not increased by:
A. Digitalis **B.** ACEI
C. Diùretus **D.** β blocker

39. In Unstable angina drug not to be used:
A. Gp IIb/IIIa inhibitor
B. CABG
C. Front loaded rtPA
D. Heparin

40. Rupture of myocardium is common in MI with all *except:*
A. Elderly
B. Recurrent infarct
C. MassiveMI
D. No history of previous angina

41. High risk CABG include all *except:*
A. CSA
B. CCS class IV
C. Urgent operation
D. Associated peripheral vascular disease

27 A 28 D 29 C 30 A 31 A 32 D 33 B 34 A 35 C 36 A 37 C 38 A 39 C
40 B 41 A

42. All are cause of death in Eisenmengers syndrome *except:*
A. Hemoptysis
B. GA for non cardiac surgery
C. IE
D. Pregnancy

43. Pregnancy is least tolerated in all *except:*
A. MVP (asymptomatic)
B. CoA
C. Marfan
D. PPH

44. Recurrent pulmonary embolism is least likely with:
A. Normal ECG
B. Normal TEE
C. Normal pulmonary scan
D. Normal Chest X-ray

45. Recurrent PTE is associated with all *except:*
A. Eosinophilic pneumonia
B. Fever
C. PHT
D. Paradoxical embolism

46. Pseudomonas IE is not found in:
A. Drug abusers (i/v)
B. Carcinoma Colon
C. Burns
D. None of the above

47. IE in IV drug abuse, all can be seen *except:*
A. Staph aureus is most common organism
B. Pulmonary valve is commonly involved
C. Most common site is tricuspid valve
D. Candida is most common fungal agent

48. LV aneurysm; surgery is done in all *except:*
A. Aneurysmal LV on angiogram
B. Symptomatic angina
C. Recurrent VT
D. LV dysfunction

49. All are true about effect of Ticlopidine *except:*
A. Drug allergy
B. Thrombocytopenia
C. Neutropenia
D. Decrease Restenosis

50. CVA in elderly with BP 220/130 (ischemic) .... is ideal BP control:
A. 180/105 mmHg
B. 115/95 mmHg
C. 110/80 mmHg
D. 140/90 mm Hg

51. NTG worsens pain in:
A. HOCM
B. Unstable angina
C. Chronic stable angina
D. Ischemic cardiomyopathy

52. Square wave response on Valsalva is seen in all *except:*
A. ASD
B. CHF
C. Cardiac transplant
D. HOCM

53. Chronic AR with normal LV function; which of the following is not seen:
A. ↑ LVEDV
B. ↑ EPSS
C. Mitra valve flutter
D. Reverse flow in descending aorta

54. ↑ RA pressure with (n) PCWP:
A. RVMI B. MS
C. IE D. CHF

55. Non cardiogenic pulmonary oedema is not seen with:
A. Bilateral renal artery stenosis
B. Post cardiopul bypass
C. HAPE
D. Narcotic overdose

42 C 43 A 44 C 45 A 46 B 47 B 48 A 49 D 50 A 51 A 52 B 53 B 54 A
55 A

56. Drug not used in CAD with HTN is:
A. Diazoxide
B. Frusemide
C. Carvedilol
D. Slow release ditiazem

57. Drugs not used in pregnancy are all *except:*
A. Adenosine B. Na Nitroprusside
C. ACEI D. ARB

58. Side effect of adenosine are all *except:*
A. Bronchospasm B. SVT
C. Bradycardia D. Anginal chest pain

59. Cardiac tamponade can be ruled out if following is absent:
A. ↑ intrapericardial pressure
B. Hypotension
C. Pulsus paradoxus
D. Decrease heart sound

60. Kussumaul's sign is seen in all *except:*
A. Cardiac tamponade
B. RCMP
C. CCP
D. RVMI

61. Least likely in CCP:
A. Very high pulmonary artery pressure
B. Diastolic dip and plateau
C. Equalization of pressure
D. Square root sign

62. For Pericardial calcification, most sensitive is:
A. MRI B. CT
C. TEE D. CXR

63. PR in pulmonary hypertension-true is:
A. High frequency murmur
B. Kite shaped murmur
C. Occur late after P2
D. ↑ with inspiration

64. All are true about coronary artery anatomy *except:*
A. LAD arises from left main coronary artery
B. RCA runs in A-V groove
C. Obtuse marginals are branches of RCA
D. In 85% cases, PDA arises from RCA

65. All are true about familial atrial myxoma *except:*
A. Atypical site
B. More recurrence
C. Younger age group
D. Mostly arises from valve tisssue

66. Transsaturated fatty acid is:
A. Lauristic B. Myristic acid
C. Oleic D. Eladic aicd

67. All are true about cyanide poisoning *except:*
A. Lactic acidosis
B. ↑ oxygen content of mixed venous blood
C. Cherry red in colour
D. Treatment is IV sod nitrite + sod thiosulphate

68. PO_2 300 mm Hg, pH 7.2, O2 sat 60%, PCO_2 30 mm Hg, Base excess +1, diagnosis is:
A. Cyanide poisoning
B. CO poisoning
C. Ventilator disturbance
D. HAPE

69. pH 7.589, Base excess + 15, PO_2 35 mm Hg, O_2 saturation 80% PCO_2 45 mm Hg in a patient with pneumonia with COPD; Diagnosis is:
A. Technical error
B. Metabolic acidosis
C. Septicemia with shock
D. Hypoxemia with respiratory failure

70. BE–30, weight- 51 kg, HCO3–5 meq/L, PO2 80 mm Hg, amount of bicarbonate needed in first half hour is:
A. 375 B. 250
C. 50 D. 30

56 A 57 A 58 B 59 A 60 A 61 A 62 B 63 A 64 C 65 D 66 B 67 C 68 C
69 A 70 B

71. pH 7.2, HCO3–12 meq/L, PCO2 55 mm Hg, Diagnosis is:
A. Respiratory acidosis
B. Compensatory respiratory acidosis
C. Metabolic acidosis
D. Respiratory acidosis and metabolic acidosis

72. Most important determinant of oxygen consumption of heart is:
A. EDV B. ESV
C. HR D. Contractility

73. Myocardial O_2 consumption depends on all *except:*
A. Increase Age B. HR
C. Contractility D. Wall stress

74. Contraindication in cardiac tamponade:
A. NTG B. Isoprenaline
C. Dobutamine D. IV saline

75. Atherosclerosis is predisposed by all *except:*
A. VWD
B. SLE
C. Type V hyperlipidemia
D. Combined hyperlipidemia

76. Familial hypercholesterolemia is differentiated from combined hyperlipidemia by:
A. Tendon xanthoma
B. Arcus senilis
C. Tuberous xanthoma
D. Absence of pancarditis

77. TNF is active in all *except:*
A. CHF
B. Rheumatoid arthritis
C. Crohn's disease
D. Normal myocardial function

78. EDRF derived from:
A. L-arginine B. Guanosin
C. Homocystein D. Endothelium

79. All act through G protein ligand *except:*
A. Insulin B. Acetylcholine
C. Adenosine D. Dobutamine

80. All are associated with pulmonary hypertension *except:*
A. Schistosomiasis
B. Toxic oil syndrome
C. Argemone Mexicana oil
D. Primary systemic sclerosis

81. Patient with BP of 90 mmHg with ventricular septal defect with flow across defect of 4 m/s; true is:
A. N pulmonary pressure
B. Moderate PHT
C. Severe PHT
D. Reversed shunt

82. Hyponatremia is seen with all *except:*
A. Diabetes insipidus
B. Diuretics
C. CHF
D. Polyuric phase of ATN

83. Confidence interval of estimate means:
A. p = 0.05 to p = 0.0005
B. Reliability of estimates
C. Standardization of estimates
D. Range of estimates in population

84. Risk factors for HOCM and SCD are all *except:*
A. Family history
B. Age < 30 years
C. VT on Holter
D. Severity of obstruction

85. All are true about apoptosis *except:*
A. Rapid cell loss
B. Exudative inflammation
C. Ladder pattern DNA
D. Hypoxic injury

71 D 72 C 73 A 74 A 75 C 76 A 77 D 78 A 79 A 80 C 81 A 82 A 83 D 84 D 85 B

86. Ebstein's anomaly is associated with abnormality of:

A. Morphological right A-V valve
B. Morphological left A-V valve
C. Outflow tract of RV
D. Outflow tract of LV

87. Operation of choice in first week of TGA is:

A. Arterial switch
B. Atrial switch
C. Pulmonary artery banding
D. B-T shunt

88. Most diagnostic of acute rheumatic carditis is:

A. Aschoff nodules
B. Fibrinous pericarditis
C. Presence of fibroblasts
D. None of the above

89. Which of the following is seen in rheumatic fever in old age with increasing frequency:

A. Arthritis
B. Carditis
C. Chorea
D. Subcutaneous nodules

90. All are true about streptococcus pyogenes *except:*

A. Form mucoid colonies
B. Penicillin resistance is not reported
C. M-protein is the virulence factor
D. Tetracycline is bactericidal

86 A 87 A 88 A 89 A 90 D

AIIMS 2000 (June)

1. **Q wave in V_1 is seen in all *except:***
   A. Severe P.S
   B. Anteroseptal ml
   C. Endomyocardial fibrosis
   D. C-TGA

2. **Catheter data-PaO_2 85, PCO_2 20, pH 7.2; diagnosis is:**
   A. Pulmonary edema **B.** Ketoacidosis
   C. Sedative overdose **D.** Hysterical

3. **CHF in utero can occur in all *except:***
   A. Ebstein's anomaly **B.** D-TGA
   C. Anaemia **D.** PSVT

4. **Adverse prognostic factor in AMI:**
   A. Left main block
   B. VT on stress test
   C. Decreased ejection fraction
   D. ST depression

5 **A 40 year old with stage I Hypertension with LDL 180 mg%,treatment of choice:**
   A. Dietary therapy **B.** Aspirin
   C. Alpha blocker **D.** Diuretics

6. **All can be closed by catheter based procedure *except:***
   A. Ostium secundum ASD > 20 mm
   B. Sub aortic VSD > 5 mm
   C. Large PDA
   D. Patent foramen ovale with right to left shunt

7. **Anion gap is increased in all *except:***
   A. Ethylene glycol
   B. Ketoacidosis
   C. Renal failure
   D. RTA

8. **All are true about cyanide poisoning *except:***
   A. Increased mixed venous oxygen saturation
   B. Treated with nitrite and thiosulphate
   C. Bitter almond odour
   D. Lactic acidosis

9. **Myocardial oxygen uptake depends most on:**
   A. Heart rate
   B. End systolic volume
   C. Physical activity
   D. After load

10. **High output failure occurs in all *except:***
   A. Multiple myeloma
   B. Ruptured aneurysm of Galen
   C. Hemangioma of liver
   D. RSOV

11. **Endocarditis is least common in:**
   A. ASD **B.** Small VSD
   C. MVP **D.** PS

12. **Cardiac teratogenicity is seen with all *except:***
   A. Folinic acid **B.** Phenylalanine
   C. Alcohol **D.** Retinoic acid

1 C 2 A 3 B 4 C 5 A 6 B 7 D 8 C 9 A 10 B 11 A 12 A

13. In significant pulmonary embolism all can be seen *except:*
A. Normal perfusion scan
B. Normal ECG
C. Normal chest X-ray
D. Normal PaO_2

14. Pulsus bisferians is best seen in:
A. Carotid B. Brachial
C. Femoral D. Radial

15. Poiseulli's law:
A. To measure coronary artery stenosis
B. Measure resistance of blood flow
C. Measure coronary flow reserve
D. Measure endothelial dysfunction

16. Normal pulmonary capillary wedge pressure with pulmonary edema is seen in:
A. Glomerulonephritis
B. Narcotic overdose
C. MR
D. HT

17. PCWP to LVEDP gradient is present in:
A. LA myxoma B. AR
C. CCF D. CCP

18. Not required to monitor in amiodarone therapy:
A. Serum levels B. LFT
C. TFT D. ECG

19. All prolong QT *except:*
A. Digoxin B. Amiodarone
C. Class Ia D. Hypocalcemia

20. Early thrombolysis has favorable effect in all *except:*
A. Immediate cardiac rupture (1 day)
B. Long term prognosis
C. Complex arrhythmias
D. Decreasing the size of infarct

21. CHB is seen in all *except:*
A. Diphtheria
B. Lyme's disease
C. Maternal lupus
D. Kearns Sayre syndrome

22. Nitric oxide is indicated in:
A. Vasospasm of Subarachnoid haemorrhage
B. Pulmonary artery hypertension in infants
C. Heart failure
D. Atherosclerosis

23. Most oxygen consumption per 100 gm of tissue:
A. Heart B. Kidney
C. Carotid body D. Lung

24. Adenosine can cause all *except:*
A. Chest pain B. Bronchospasm
C. Premature VPC D. Coronary spasm

25. True about adenosine are all *except:*
A. Can be reversed with atropine
B. Act through c-AMP dependent calcium channels
C. Open potassium channels
D. Causes transient AF

26. All acts through G protein *except:*
A. ACTH B. Adenosine
C. Insulin D. Dopamine

27. Inevitable consequences of aging are all *except:*
A. ↓ GFR
B. ↓ Heart rate
C. ↑ Blood pressure
D. ↑ Lung closing volume

28. About digitalis toxicity, all are true *except:*
A. AF with fixed heart rate
B. Hyperkalaemia never occurs with toxicity
C. Occurs at digitalis levels > 4 ng/dL
D. Cardioversion never attempted

13 A 14 A 15 B 16 B 17 A 18 A 19 A 20 A 21 C 22 B 23 C 24 D 25 B
26 C 27 D 28 B

29. LVOT gradient 60 mm Hg, EF 40%, asymptomatic AS–treatment of choice:
A. Observation B. Open valvotomy
C. AVR D. Balloon valvotomy

30. Investigation of choice for CCP:
A. TTE B. TEE
C. CT D. Thallium

31. Barkers hypothesis:
A. High CAD with low birthweight
B. High CAD with obesity
C. High CAD with HT
D. High CAD with dyslipidemia

32. Indications of surgery in IE are all *except:*
A. Late PVE
B. Persistent fever
C. Aortic root abscess
D. Unstable prosthesis

33. Staphylococcal infection is treated by all *except:*
A. Rifampicin B. Teicoplanin
C. Imipenem D. Cefuroxime

34. Drugs used in acute rheumatic pharyngitis are all *except:*
A. Oral penicillin V B. Amoxycillin
C. Cefadroxil D. Doxycycline

35. All help in differentiating VT from SVT *except:*
A. Hypotension
B. AV dissociation
C. Absent R wave V1-V6
D. Past history of AMI

36. Old AMI with EF 35% with VPCs: treatment of choice:
A. β-blockers B. AICD
C. CCB D. Digoxin

37. Which is not an indicator of heart transplant?
A. Oxygen consumption > 14 ml/min
B. Class III symptoms
C. EF <10%
D. PVR <5 W

38. All are seen in Noonan syndrome *except:*
A. COA
B. HOCM
C. Normal karyotype
D. Undescended testis

39. Hyperhomocystinemia drug of choice:
A. Folic acid B. Carnitine
C. Vitamin E D. Vit. B 12

40. HDL most effectively increased by:
A. Atorvastatin
B. Niacin
C. Fibrates
D. Pravastatin

41. LBBB pattern is seen in all *except:*
A. Bradyarrhythmia associated block
B. Post AMI
C. Hypokalemia
D. Lev's disease

42. All are indicated in USA *except:*
A. rtPA B. Heparin
C. Clopidogrel D. β blocker

43. All are true about hibernating myocardium *except:*
A. Associated with normal coronaries
B. Associated with decreased flow
C. Reversible condition
D. SPECT can be used to assess viability

44. Thallium scan is suggestive of LV dysfunction by:
A. Cold spot
B. Large defects
C. Redistribution
D. Increased lung uptake

---

29 C 30 C 31 A 32 A 33 D 34 D 35 A 36 A 37 A 38 A 39 A 40 B 41 C
42 A 43 A 44 D

45. All are true about renin-angiotensin system *except:*
A. Angiotensinogen is the precursor of ACE and is produced by the liver
B. ACE acts by inhibition of bradykinin pathway
C. ACE is produced by the lung
D. AT2 receptor is antithrombotic

46. Which of the following is associated with CAD?
A. SLE
B. Biliary cirrhosis
C. Type V hyperlipidemia
D. Marfan's syndrome

47. All are true about ventricular action potential compared to nodal action potential *except:*
A. More negative transmembrane potential
B. Conduction velocity is less in myocardium
C. Beta blockade causes decrease potential
D. None of the above

48. Confidence interval of estimate means:
A. p = 0.05 to p = 0.0005
B. Reliability of estimate
C. Standardization of estimate
D. Range of estimate in a population

49. In a patient of ischemic stroke with BP 210/130; it should be lowered down to:
A. 180/110
B. 140/90
C. No immediate intervention
D. Give heparin

50. Hypocalcemia in neonates is indicated by:
A. QTc >0.36 sec B. QTa >0.19 sec
C. QTc > 0.32 sec D. None of the above

51. Posterior papillary muscle is supplied by:
A. LAD B. PDA
C. Diagonals D. Septals

52. Kussmaul sign is seen in all *except:*
A. Cardiac tamponade
B. CCP
C. RVF
D. RCM

53. Seventy year old male with mild CHF with transient AF, treatment of choice is:
A. Oral anticoagulants
B. Dispirin
C. Dispirin + ticlopidine
D. Digoxin

54. Pulsus paradoxus is seen in all *except:*
A. Positive pressure ventilation
B. Cardiac tamponade
C. Bronchial asthma
D. Superior vena cava syndrome

55. CI 1.8, PCWP 10 with AMI; treatment of choice is:
A. IV fluids
B. Inotropes
C. ACE inhibitors
D. β blockers

56. All are true about beta blockers in CCF *except:*
A. Useful in both ischemic and non ischemic DCM
B. 85% population tolerate carefully titrated dose
C. Carvedilol have been successfully tried
D. Beneficial effect primarily by changes in sudden cardiac death

57. True about phospholamban is:
A. Increase calcium in sarcoplasmic reticulum
B. Calcium regulatory protein
C. Binds calcium in mitochondria
D. Binds calcium to troponin

58. All are used in hypertensive emergency *except:*
A. Urapidil
B. Fenoldopam
C. Enalaprilat
D. Nifedipine

45 A 46 A 47 C 48 D 49 A 50 B 51 B 52 A 53 A 54 A 55 A 56 D 57 A 58 D

59. Cyanosis with clubbing with normal S2 most likely diagnosis:
A. TAPVC
B. Methimoglobinemia
C. Pulmonary AV fistula
D. Cyanide poisoning

60. All are contraindicated in HOCM *except:*
A. Disopyramide
B. Digoxin
C. Diuretics
D. Milrinone

61. Gene therapy most successful:
A. Cystic fibrosis
B. Thalassaemia
C. Sickle cell anaemia
D. Duchenne muscular dystrophy

62. All are produced by genetic engineering *except:*
A. Fraxiparine B. Fab
C. Hirudin D. rtPA

63. Worst prognosis–pregnancy with:
A. MVP
B. Mild to moderate MR
C. COA
D. ASD

64. All statements are true *except:*
A. 1% decrease in S. cholesterol decreases mortality by 2%
B. Statins are HMG CoA inhibitors
C. HDL-C increases with exercise
D. Cereals and pulses have low cholesterol

65. According to JNC VI, 40 year old male with stage I hypertension with LDL cholesterol-180 mg%; treatment of choice is:
A. ACE-Inhibitors
B. Diuretics
C. Life style modification
D. α blocker

66. Dex-Fenfluramine causes all *except:*
A. Cardiomyopathy
B. AR
C. MR
D. Pulmonary hypertension

67. Vasogenic syncope occurs with all *except:*
A. Prolonged standing
B. β blockers
C. Increased sympathetic activity
D. Increased parasympathetic activity

68. Cardiac output by thermodilution is not affected in:
A. VSD B. TR
C. PR D. Low cardiac output

69. All are seen in acute AR *except:*
A. Wide pulse pressure
B. LVF
C. S3
D. S4

70. Most common cause of AS in a child of 10 years in India:
A. RHD
B. Congenital bicuspid
C. Congenital unicuspid
D. IE

71. All is true about amyloidosis *except:*
A. Senile amyloidosis is not associated with CCF
B. Digoxin sensitivity is increased
C. Decreased QRS amplitude in all precardial leads
D. RCM may be present

72. All are cardiac manifestation of AIDS *except:*
A. Staph endocarditis
B. Pericardial Kaposi sarcoma
C. Dilated cardiomyopathy
D. Coronary atherosclerosis

59 C **60** A **61** A **62** A **63** C **64** A **65** C **66** A **67** B **68** A **69** A **70** C **71** A **72** A

73. L-R shunt in ASD increased in:
A. PAH B. RVF
C. HTN D. MR

74. Tachycardia with postural hypotension is seen in:
A. Bleeding peptic ulcer
B. Vasovagal syncope
C. Shy Dragar syndrome
D. Diabetic neuropathy

75. Exudative retinopathy seen in:
A. CoA
B. Renal artery stenosis
C. Crohn's disease
D. Takayasu type 2

76. Primordial prevention is applicable to:
A. Persons with no risk factors
B. Persons with risk factors and disease
C. Community with low incidence of disease
D. Prevention in first degree relatives

77. In management of AMI; all are used *except:*
A. IV lidocaine
B. Primary PTCA
C. Aspirin
D. ACE-inhibitors

78. In athlete's heart all are seen *except:*
A. Ejection systolic murmur
B. Mobitz blocks
C. Early diastolic murmur
D. S3

79. Most saturated fatty acid:
A. Linoleic acid B. Linolenic acid
C. Myristic acid D. Eladic acid

80. All are true about salmonella *except:*
A. Can cause end arteritis in COA
B. Common cause of dairy workers diarrhoea
C. Osteomyelitis in sickle cell anemia
D. Infection in splenectomized patient

81. Ductal dependent circulation are all *except:*
A. CoA
B. Pulmonary atresia with intact IVS
C. HLHS
D. TGA

82. All are true about apoptosis *except:*
A. Inflammatory exudate
B. Seen in reperfusion
C. Spontaneous cellular death
D. Ladder pattern of DNA degeneration

83. All are true about pulmonary embolism *except:*
A. Paradoxical embolism may be seen
B. Spontaneous pneumothorax may occur
C. Hypotension
D. Raised SGOT

84. Drugs contraindicated in tamponade:
A. Diuretics B. Inotropes
C. I/v fluids D. Isoprenaline

85. Square wave sign in valsalva seen in all *except:*
A. HOCM
B. ASD
C. CCF
D. Autonomic neuropathy

86. Earliest sign of hyperkalemia is:
A. Tall/tented T waves
B. Widening of QRS
C. Decrease of P wave amplitude
D. CHB

87. Drug that is both an arteriolar and venodilator:
A. Nitroprusside B. Hydralazine
C. Nitrates D. Nifedipine

88. Amiodarone can cause all *except:*
A. Decrease ERP
B. Symptomatic bradycardia
C. Torsades de Pointes
D. Exacerbation of CHF

73 D 74 A 75 B 76 A 77 A 78 C 79 C 80 D 81 A 82 A 83 B 84 A 85 A
86 A 87 A 88 A

89. Tall R waves in V1 are seen in all *except:*
A. Duchenne's dystrophy
B. Freidrich's ataxia
C. TOF
D. WPW type A

90. Exercise induced VT is seen in:
A. Ventricular aneurysm
B. Prolonged QT syndrome (genetic)
C. WPW syndrome
D. Ebstein's anomaly

89 B 90 B

AIIMS 1999 (December)

1. **AVERT trial used:**
   A. Simvastatin B. Atorvastatin
   C. Lovastatin D. Cerivastatin

2. **Cardioselective β blockers are all *except:***
   A. Celiprolol B. Metoprolol
   C. Carvedilol D. Sotalol

3. **Syndrome X has the following features *except:***
   A. Typical angina B. Thallium normal
   C. Abnormal ECG D. Abnormal CAG

4. **Asymmetric septal hypertrophy is seen in all *except:***
   A. Post MI B. AS
   C. HOCM D. PAH

5. **Myocardial hypertrophy is mediated by all *except:***
   A. VEGF B. TGFB
   C. AII D. ANP

6. **Conduction defects are most commonly with:**
   A. AR B. AS
   C. MR D. MS

7. **Most common valve lesion in acute rheumatic fever is:**
   A. MR B. MS
   C. MS + MR D. AR

8. **Coronary vasodilator among the following is:**
   A. Vasopressin B. ANP
   C. Prazosin D. Adenosine

9. **Primordial prevention means:**
   A. Prevention in persons with no risk factor
   B. Prevention in communities with risk factor
   C. Prevention in persons with only risk factors for disease
   D. Antenatal prevention measures

10. **Pulses paradoxus is seen in all *except:***
    A. COPD B. IPPV
    C. CCP D. Cardiac tamponade

11. **In DCMP most commonly seen abnormality is:**
    A. LBBB
    B. RBBB
    C. Thallium perfusion defects
    D. Dysautonomia

12. **In HIV all are seen with increased frequency *except:***
    A. Myocarditis
    B. Staph. endocarditis
    C. Kaposi's sarcoma
    D. Tubercular pericardial effusion

13. **Most sensitive sign of C. tamponade is:**
    A. RA diastolic collapse
    B. RV diastolic collapse
    C. Pulsus paradoxus
    D. Low voltage ECG

1 B 2 C 3 D 4 A 5 D 6 B 7 A 8 D 9 A 10 B 11 A 12 B 13 A

14. Normal pericardial fluid:
A. 0-5 ml B. 15-50 ml
C. 5-15 ml D. >50 ml

15. Acute pulmonary embolism is characterised by all *except:*
A. Hemoptysis in few patients with pulmonary infarction
B. PASP >65 mmHg
C. ECG/CXR may be normal
D. PO_2 may be normal

16. pH 7.2, PO2–85 mm Hg, PCO2–22 mm Hg is suggestive of:
A. Pulmonary edema
B. Anxiety hyperventilation
C. Diabetic ketoacidosis
D. Barbiturates

17. In broad complex tachycardia; drug of choice can be:
A. Flecainide B. Esmolol
C. Adenosine D. Lignocaine

18. PAH develops early with:
A. c-TGA B. Noonans
C. Down's D. Rubella

19. CVA in Cyanotic congenital heart disease is most common with:
A. Polycythemia
B. Fe deficiency anaemia
C. Paradoxical embolization
D. Hypoxemia

20. Lowest risk of IE is with:
A. ASD B. MVP
C. PDA D. TOF

21. In congenital heart disease true is:
A. (Plump) moon facies with supravalvular AS
B. Turner's -ASD
C. Noonan's syndrome–peripheral PS
D. King syndrome–VSD

22. With cyanosis, all are true *except:*
A. At reduce Hb = 0.5 gm%
B. Polycythemia causes peripheral cyanosis
C. Bluish discolouration of skin
D. Associated with Right to left shunt

23. All bad in pregnancy *except:*
A. MVP
B. Coarctation
C. Marfans
D. Eisenmenger's

24. TOC in Eissenmenger's:
A. Heart transplant
B. Lung transplant
C. B/L lung transplant
D. Heart lung transplant

25. Dp/dt is decreased (in dissection) by:
A. Propranolol B. Diuretics
C. Nitroprusside D. Digoxin

26. Septation defects are all *except:*
A. DORV B. APW
C. TGA D. PDA

27. HDL ↑es maximum with:
A. Statins B. Resins
C. Probucol D. Niacin

28. Most potent LDL reducer is:
A. Fluvastatin B. Lovastatin
C. Simvastatin D. Atorvastatin

29. All are true regarding atherosclerosis *except:*
A. LDL receptor is present in smooth muscle
B. LDL causes smooth muscle proliferation
C. Endothelium produces prostacyclin
D. Prostacyclin is thrombo resistant

30. Gene therapy vectors are all *except:*
A. Adenovirus B. Retrovirus
C. Epstein bar virus D. CMV

14 B 15 B 16 A 17 C 18 C 19 B 20 A 21 C 22 A 23 A 24 D 25 A 26 D
27 D 28 D 29 B 30 D

31. Angiogenic factors include all *except:*
A. GM-CSF B. EDGF
C. FGF D. VEGF

32. Hibernating myocardium is assessed by all *except:*
A. Thallium B. Stress Echo
C. ECG D. PET

33. Contrast echo used for all *except:*
A. L → R shunt B. R → L shunt
C. Regurgitant lesions D. Stenotic lesions

34. Severity of AS by doppler is:
A. Overestimated B. Underestimated
C. Same D. Variable

35. Balloon angioplasty for coarctation is best suited for:
A. Adults B. Infants
C. Restenosis D. Preductal coarctation

36. For bicuspid AV; all are true *except:*
A. IE Prophylaxis required because of high risk
B. Coarctation also seen
C. Irregular and eccentric closure line
D. Can be both congenital and acquired

37. In pacing all are true *except:*
A. Pseudofusion means sensing problem
B. Fusion is a normal phenomenon
C. Epicardial pacing shows RBBB
D. DDD pacing is better than single chamber pacing

38. CPK is increased in all *except:*
A. Hypothyroidism B. DMD
C. Stroke D. Limb amputation

39. Best test for detecting viable myocardium is:
A. Thallium B. PET
C. ECG D. Contrast echo

40. 60 year old man with typical angina; the probability of CAD is:
A. 50% B. 60%
C. 90% D. 99%

41. Reversible ischemia is seen with all *except:*
A. Stress thallium B. Holter
C. TMT D. Angiography

42. PTCA is done in all *except:*
A. TVD
B. Unprotected left main disease
C. Diabetes mellitus with DVD
D. Instent Restenosis

43. True about radio activity are all *except:*
A. Radioactive stents decrease restenosis/smooth muscle proliferation
B. Iridium wire for restenosis with beta radiation
C. β radiation has low penetration
D. Phosphorus emits β radiation

44. All are examples of low pressure TR *except:*
A. Ebsteins
B. Trauma
C. EMF
D. Pulmonary embolism

45. Streptokinase is contraindicated in all *except:*
A. SAH
B. Active peptic ulcer
C. Prosthetic valve thrombosis
D. Streptokinase 1 year back

46. True about ASD are all *except:*
A. Ostium secundum shows RAD
B. Ostium primum shows RAD
C. MR seen with AV canal defect
D. In lutembacher's syndrome- ASD is present

47. Pulmonary edema with normal PCWP seen in:
A. HAPE B. MS
C. DCMP D. AMI

31 A 32 C 33 D 34 A 35 C 36 D 37 A 38 D 39 B 40 C 41 D 42 B 43 B
44 D 45 C 46 B 47 A

48. Situs solitus with dextrocardia is seen with:
A. AV canal defect B. d-TGA
C. TOF D. CoA

49. Patient with C.I.–1.6L/min/m^2 with PCWP = 10, Treatment of choice is:
A. DOPA B. IABP
C. IV fluids D. PTCA

50. IABP is contraindicated in:
A. VSD B. AR
C. MR D. C. shock

51. All are true about restrictive CMP *except:*
A. Max filling is in late diastole
B. Amyloidosis detected by endomyocardial biopsy
C. AF is common conduction defect
D. PASP > 45 is not uncommon

52. True about TAPVC are all *except:*
A. Obstruction decreases cyanosis and increases failure
B. Supracardiac TAPVC is seldom obstructive
C. Supracardiac TAPVC shows snowman appearance
D. TAPVC is associated with continuous murmur

53. All of the following statements are true *except:*
A. c-TGA associated with CHB
B. Cyanosis is seen in PDA
C. Continuous murmur of AV fistula can be confused with PDA
D. A-V canal defect can be associated with compete heart block

54. Lowest PO2 at catheterization is seen in:
A. Pulmonary veins
B. Coronary sinus
C. SVC
D. Pulmonary artery

55. NTG increases chest pain in:
A. TVD B. CHF
C. HOCM D. Pericarditis

56. Barkers hypothesis states:
A. Low birth weight infants have high probability of CAD
B. Low birth weight infants have low probability of CAD
C. Increased EDV increases QRS amplitude in ECG
D. Decrease EDV decreases QRS amplitude in ECG

57. In congestive heart failure all are true *except:*
A. ↓ A-VO2 difference
B. Oliguria
C. Hypotension
D. ↓ C.O.

58. CHF in 1st week of life is least likely in:
A. VSD B. PDA
C. Coarctation D. TGA

59. Commonest cyanotic congenital H.D is:
A. TGA B. VSD
C. TOF D. TAPVC

60. Wide fixed split S2 is seen in:
A. TAPVC
B. PAPVC
C. Straight back syndrome
D. MVP

61. Commonest cardiovascular problem in India:
A. HT B. CAD
C. RHD D. Stroke

62. Anatomic relationship between aorta and pulmonary artery:
A. Aorta is left anterior to PA
B. Aorta is right and anterior to PA
C. Aorta is left and posterior to PA
D. Aorta is right and posterior to PA

48 A 49 C 50 B 51 A 52 A 53 B 54 B 55 C 56 A 57 A 58 A 59 C 60 A
61 A 62 D

63. Syndrome X means:
A. Angina at rest
B. Microvascular angina
C. Associated with diabetes mellitus
D. Respond to nitrates

64. Genes for HOCM are located on all chromosomes *except:*
A. Chromosome 1 B. Chromosome 3
C. Chromosome 7 D. Chromosome 10

65. Rheumatic fever criteria which has ↑ed sensitivity in Indian context:
A. Polyarthralgia B. Carditis
C. Chorea D. Nodules

66. In constrictive pericarditis all are seen *except:*
A. Calcification
B. Systolic dysfunction
C. Pericardial thickness > 4 mm
D. Best diagnosed with TTE

67. True about SLE are all *except:*
A. CHB
B. Pericarditis is most common cardiac problem
C. Libman-Sach's endocarditis is seen
D. Acute myocarditis is frequently present

68. True about Coarctation of aorta is all *except:*
A. Bilateral symmetrical Rib notching
B. E sign on Chest X-ray
C. Associated with bicuspid aortic valve
D. Diagnosis cannot be established by Chest X-ray P-A film

69. Warfarin levels are increased by all *except:*
A. Amiodarone B. Metronidazole
C. Clofibrate D. Sucralfate

70. Cardiac tamponade is most likely to be associated with:
A. Hypothyroidism
B. Bronchogenic Ca
C. c-TGA
D. Rheumatic fever

71. True about acute MR are all *except:*
A. Increased P2
B. S3 present
C. Cardiomegaly
D. Systolic murmur heard

72. Homocysteine levels are decrease by all *except:*
A. Folic acid B. Vitamin B12
C. Niacin D. Pantothenic acid

73. True about hepato-jugular reflux are all *except:*
A. Sustained epigastric compression for 30 secs
B. Sustained rise of JVP ≥ 3 mm
C. Can be seen with increase PCWP
D. Seen in CHF

74. Side effects of ticlopidine are all *except:*
A. TTP B. Diarrhoea
C. Neutropenia D. Headache

75. True about hirudin are all *except:*
A. Direct antithrombin
B. Insensitive to platelet factor IV
C. Frequent APTT monitoring is not required
D. Low risk of intracranial haemorrhage

76. Best projection for Left main coronary artery is:
A. A-P caudal B. Lateral
C. LAO caudal D. LAO cranial

77. True about constrictive pericarditis are all *except:*
A. Tuberculosis is most common cause in India
B. Square root sign is present
C. Volume expansion is detrimental
D. Kussmaul sign is present

78. Fontan surgery is contraindicated in:
A. Tricuspid atresia
B. Hypoplastic left heart syndrome
C. Univentricular heart
D. TOF

63 B 64 D 65 A 66 B 67 D 68 B 69 D 70 B 71 C 72 D 73 A 74 D 75 C
76 A 77 C 78 D

79. Cong CHB is seen in:
A. cTGA
B. ASD (Ostium primum type)
C. VSD
D. CoA

80. True about tricuspid atresia are all *except:*
A. Lateral tunnel Fontans
B. Damus-Stansel kayes procedure done
C. In ECG - RAD + RAE + LVH
D. Associated with juxtaposition of atrial appendages

81. All are true about amyloidosis *except:*
A. Most common presentation is RCMP
B. Hypertension is common
C. Right sided Heart failure
D. Thickened interatrial septa

82. Most frequent arrhythmia in structurally normal heart is:
A. VPCS **B.** AF
C. Sinus arrhythmia **D.** Parasystole

83. Spurious hypertension may be seen with all *except:*
A. Small cuff **B.** Obesity
C. Anxiety **D.** Auscultatory gap

84. In SVT what is usually effective:
A. Morro's reflex
B. Bainbridge reflex
C. Divers reflex
D. Thump version

85. 10 mmHg difference in (pulse) pressure in a case of pulmonary stenosis after a VPC means:
A. CHF **B.** Intact IVS
C. VSD **D.** Infundibular P.S

86. Apical obliteration is seen in:
A. Amyloidosis
B. Sarcoidosis
C. EMF
D. Haemochromatosis

87. In MI with shock; which is effective in reducing mortality?
A. IABP **B.** PTCA
C. Thrombolysis **D.** CABG

88. ↑ HV interval is seen with:
A. β-blocker **B.** Digoxin
C. Amiodarone **D.** Diltiazem

89. Effective in reducing restenosis after PTCA is:
A. Aspirin **B.** Clopidogrel
C. Stent **D.** Rota

90. Severity of MR assessed by all *except:*
A. MDM
B. Split S2
C. Loud systolic murmur
D. Echocardiography

79 A 80 C 81 B 82 C 83 D 84 C 85 B 86 C 87 B 88 C 89 C 90 C

AIIMS 1999 (June)

1. Which of the following is a feature of a Normotensive TR:
A. High frequency murmur
B. Normal flow
C. Late systolic murmur
D. Early systolic murmur

2. All of the following are continuous murmurs *except:*
A. Cervical venous hum
B. Br collaterals
C. Ruptured sinus of valsalva
D. Unruptured sinus of valsalva

3. All of the following are ECG changes of myocarditis *except:*
A. CHB
B. Sinus Tachycardia
C. LBBB
D. Increased QRS voltage

4. In all of the following, serum creatinine increases abruptly with the use of ACE inhibitors *except:*
A. Hypovolemia **B.** Hypotension
C. NIDDM **D.** Diuretics

5. Atrial infarction in acute MI shows:
A. PR segment Elevation
B. PR interval change
C. Inverted T wave
D. U wave

6. Which of the following is true about TMT:
A. Positive in 5-10% of all asymptomatic patients
B. More sensitive than thallium in detecting viability
C. Can be performed in patients with LBBB
D. None of the above

7. Which of the following is true about strongly positive TMT:
A. Hypotensive response
B. Greater than 85% of predicted heart rate in Ist stage.
C. St depression in V3-V6
D. None of the above

8. Best treatment for Eisenmengers syndrome is:
A. Heart transplantation
B. Heart-lung transplantation
C. Bilateral lung transplantation
D. None of the above

9. Pregnancy is contraindicated in which of the following:
A. Eisenmengers syndrome
B. TOF
C. MVP
D. CoA

10. Viable myocardium is best shown by:
A. SPECT **B.** MRI
C. CT Scan **D.** PET

1 D 2 D 3 D 4 C 5 A 6 A 7 A 8 B 9 A 10 D

11. Contraindication of IABP is:
A. Ac AR B. VSD
C. MR D. ASD

12. True about cardiac output measurement is all *except:*
A. Thermodilution method for low cardiac output state
B. Fick's method suitable for low cardiac output
C. Cardiac output can be measured by catheterization study
D. None of the above

13. Aorta arises from:
A. Lt and Post to PA B. Lt and Ant to PA
C. Rt and Post to PA D. Rt and Ant to PA

14. Which of the following is not a X-ray finding in coarctation of aorta in a one year old child?
A. 3 sign B. Normal heart size
C. E sign D. None of the above

15. Which of the following is not a contraindication for BMV:
A. Subvalvular Fibrosis
B. MS with PAH
C. LA clot
D. Pregnancy

16. High risk Balloon pulmonary valvotomy is:
A. PS with cyanosis B. PS with CHF
C. Peripheral PS D. None of the above

17. Which of the following is not true about clubbing:
A. Infective endocarditis leads to clubbing in 4-6 weeks
B. Central cyanosis leads to clubbing in 3-4 weeks
C. Can occur in normal people
D. Aortic aneurysm can cause clubbing

18. Which of the following is used for treatment of hyperhomocystenemia:
A. Folic acid B. Ascorbic acid
C. Vit K D. Vit A

19. All of the following is true for Indian patients with MS *except:*
A. Younger age
B. Increased incidence of calcification
C. History of RF in only 50%
D. Associated TV disease

20. All of the following occur in CHF *except:*
A. Increased Pulse pressure
B. Low BP
C. Oedema
D. Raised JVP

21. Normal PCPW with pulmonary oedema can occur in:
A. High altitude pulmonary edema
B. MS
C. Cortriatriatum
D. Severe AS

22. Nitroglycerine is used in CHF to:
A. Decrease afterload
B. Decrease CO
C. Coronary vasodilation
D. Decrease Preload

23. Which of the following is an Angiotensin II receptor antagonist:
A. Enalapril B. Labetelol
C. Losartan D. Nicorandil

24. Drug that does not cross placental barrier:
A. Verapamil B. Heparin
C. Hydralazine D. ACE inhibitors

25. Murmur of MR in acute MI is due to all *except:*
A. Papillary muscle dysfunction
B. Valvular rupture
C. PM rupture
D. LV dilatation

---

11 A 12 A 13 C 14 C 15 B 16 B 17 B 18 A 19 B 20 A 21 A 22 D 23 C
24 B 25 B

26. Drug that blocks K^+ channel is:
A. Digoxin B. Amiodarone
C. Sotalol D. Verapamil

27. Drug of choice in wide QRS tachycardia; PSVT with aberration is:
A. Lidocaine
B. Flecainide
C. Adenosine
D. Esmolol

28. Chronic effort angina is characterized by all *except:*
A. Pain on exertion
B. ST segment depression on ECG
C. Pain lasting for 30-40 mts
D. Pain ppted by emotional or mental stress

29. Most common cause of syncope is:
A. Vasovagal
B. Drug induced
C. Stokes Adams syndrome
D. None of the above

30. According to specific activity scale, patient with class III CVS disability can perform activities requiring:
A. 9 mets B. 7 mets
C. 5 mets D. 2 mets

31. Pulsus Bisferians is best palpable in:
A. Carotid B. Brachial
C. Radial D. Femoral

32. All are signs of Hyperkinetic pulse *except:*
A. Mullers sign B. Hills sign
C. Duroziez sign D. Parvus pulse

33. Wise splitting of S2 is seen in all *except:*
A. LV paced beat
B. RBBB
C. Acute pulmonary thromboembolism
D. PS

34. Reversed splitting of S2 is seen with all *except:*
A. LBBB
B. Idiopathic dilatation of pulmonary artery
C. Angina pectoris
D. Severe aortic stenosis

35. MDM at apex is seen with all *except:*
A. ASD B. VSD
C. MR D. Ac rheumatic activity

36. Fontan's operation is done for:
A. TOF B. TGA
C. VSD D. Tricuspid atresia

37. LAD in ASD is seen with:
A. Ostium primum ASD
B. Ostium secundum ASD
C. AV canal defects
D. None of the above

38. Arrhythmia seen in HOCM patient after septal myomectomy is:
A. AF B. VT
C. CHB D. Atrial flutter

39. Which of the following is a cause of MI at 8 weeks of age:
A. Hyperlipidemia
B. Hypertension
C. AS
D. Anomalous origin of LA from PA

40. Congenital CHB is associated with:
A. Corrected TGA
B. Uncorrected TGA
C. Coarctation of Aorta
D. PDA

41. Chronic CP develops in all *except:*
A. Tuberculosis
B. SLE
C. Ac Rheumatic fever
D. Viral

26 B 27 C 28 C 29 A 30 D 31 A 32 D 33 C 34 B 35 A 36 D 37 A 38 C
39 D 40 A 41 C

42. Defects due to septation are seen in all *except:*
A. TOF
B. Truncus Arteriosus
C. DORV
D. PDA

43. RAD is seen all *except:*
A. Tricuspid atresia
B. Mitral atresia
C. Severe PS
D. Pulmonary hypertension

44. Infective endocarditis is common in all *except:*
A. VSD
B. PDA
C. TOF
D. ASD

45. Reversed differential cyanosis is seen in :
A. PDA
B. TOF
C. TGA with PDA reversal
D. Eisenmengers syndrome

46. PCPW = 30 mm: Diagnosis may be all *except:*
A. PS
B. MS
C. MR
D. Peripheral Pulmonary artery stenosis

47. IE occurs most commonly in:
A. MS
B. AS
C. PS
D. VSD

48. LPSH is seen in all *except:*
A. Eisenmengers ASD
B. Eisenmengers VSD
C. MS + PAH
D. PPH

49. Drug used in HOT trial were:
A. Felodipin + aspirin
B. Ticlopidine + aspirin
C. Warfarin + Clonidine
D. Aspirin

50. ACE inhibitors given in pregnancy can cause all *except:*
A. Polyhydramnios
B. Fetal HTN
C. Fetal malformation
D. None of the above

51. Anti-Hypertensive drug that does not increase lipids is:
A. Prazosin
B. Atenelol
C. Diuretics
D. Beta blockers

52. Highly lipid soluble Beta blocker that can cause CNS side effects is:
A. Sotalol
B. Esmolol
C. Labetelol
D. Propanalol

53. ACEI are contraindicated in patients with:
A. B/L Renal artery stenosis
B. CHF
C. DM
D. Unilateral renal artery stenosis with hypertension

54. Drug of choice in prolonged QT syndrome is:
A. Propanalol
B. Lidocaine
C. Mexiletine
D. Verapamil

55. Treatment of choice in an asymptomatic adult with VPC's is:
A. No drug treatment
B. Propranolol
C. Calcium channel blockers
D. None of the above

56. Primordial prevention means:
A. No risk factors; no disease
B. Risk factors +; no disease
C. Proper treatment of the existing disorder
D. None of the above

57. Pregnancy is contraindicated in all *except:*
A. TOF
B. Eisenmenger
C. MVP
D. CoA

42 D 43 A 44 D 45 C 46 A 47 D 48 B 49 A 50 A 51 A 52 D 53 A 54 A
55 A 56 A 57 C

58. Ductus dependant circulations are all *except:*
A. CoA
B. TGA
C. HLHS
D. Pulmonary atresia with intact IVS

59. Severity of TOF depends on:
A. VSD B. PS
C. ASD D. Overriding of aorta

60. Pulmonary hypertension can be caused by:
A. Paragonimiasis B. Filariasis
C. Schistosomiasis D. E Coli

61. Pulmonary thromboembolism is best diagnosed by:
A. Pulmonary Angiography
B. Chest X-ray
C. Perfusion scan
D. Echocardiography

62. Cardiac tamponade develops earliest in:
A. Bronchogenic Carcinoma
B. DCM
C. Hypothyroidism
D. Tuberculosis

63. CABG is best done in which of the following condition:
A. TVD with LV dysfunction
B. TVD with normal LV function
C. DVD with normal LV function
D. SVD with LV dysfunction

64. Calcium channel blockers are best for:
A. DCMP B. Silent MI
C. Acute MI D. Non Q MI

65. Non surgical pericardiotomy window is indicated in which of the following:
A. Pyogenic
B. Recurrent neoplasms
C. Tubercular
D. None of the above

66. Contraindication to STK therapy is:
A. DVT
B. STK administration within previous 3 weeks
C. Ac MI
D. Mestruation

67. Treatment of asymptomatic severe AS in a 50 year old man is:
A. AVR
B. Aortic valvotomy
C. Medical treatment
D. BAV

68. Drug to be stopped 1 week prior to CABG is:
A. Beta blockers
B. CCB
C. ACE I
D. Aspirin

69. Congenital CHB is seen in:
A. SLE B. PAN
C. AS D. Sarcoidosis

70. Ideal treatment of a one year old child with TOF is:
A. Total surgical correction
B. BT shunt
C. Medical management
D. Balloon Valvuloplasty

71. Indication for Fontan's operation are all *except:*
A. Tricuspid atresia
B. Single ventricle with PS
C. TGA with VSD with PS
D. Pulmonary atresia

72. Drug of choice in a patient with unstable angina with VPC is:
A. Beta blocker
B. Calcium channel blocker
C. Aspirin
D. Statins

58 A 59 B 60 C 61 A 62 A 63 A 64 D 65 B 66 B 67 A 68 D 69 A 70 A
71 C 72 A

73. Which of the following statements is correct?
- **A.** Asymptomatic adult patient with BT shunt should not undergo surgery
- **B.** Patient with pink TOF should not undergo surgery
- **C.** Total surgical correction in TOF should be performed as early as possible
- **D.** None of the above

74. Sexual dysfunction is not caused by:
- **A.** Verapamil
- **B.** Metoprolol
- **C.** Propranolol
- **D.** Alpha blocker

75. Pulmonary artery systolic pressure is 80 mm Hg, PADP = 70 mm Hg, Mean = 50 mm Hg; Diagnosis is:
- **A.** Peripheral pulmonary artery stenosis
- **B.** PPH
- **C.** MS with PAH
- **D.** None of the above

76. Precapillary hypertension is seen in:
- **A.** Left atrial myxoma
- **B.** Cortriatriatum
- **C.** MS
- **D.** PPH

77. Contrast Echo is useful to detect:
- **A.** Left to right shunt
- **B.** Right to left shunt
- **C.** AP window
- **D.** None of the above

78. Which of the following disease is seen exclusively in equatorial regions?
- **A.** Chagas disease
- **B.** Endomyocardial fibrosis
- **C.** Aortoarteritis
- **D.** Rheumatic fever

79. Patient with sick sinus syndrome and a history of syncope presented with arrhythmia. Best line of management would be:
- **A.** Antiarrhythmics without EPS
- **B.** AICD
- **C.** EPS followed by pacemaker implantation/AICD
- **D.** None of the above

80. All are true about loop diuretics *except:*
- **A.** Have bioavailability of 80-90%
- **B.** Causes sodium loss and hyponatremia
- **C.** Acts on loop of Henle
- **D.** None of the above

81. All can produce continuous murmur *except:*
- **A.** Venous hum
- **B.** Mammary souffle
- **C.** PDA
- **D.** Pulmonary artery stenosis

82. Increase incidence of CAD in overseas Indians is because of:
- **A.** Social deprivation
- **B.** Disturbed eating habits
- **C.** Glucose intolerance
- **D.** Increase smoking

83. PCWP can be measured to diagnose all *except:*
- **A.** Pulmonary veno-occlusive disease
- **B.** Peripheral pulmonary artery disease
- **C.** Pulmonary venous hypertension
- **D.** Cortriatriatum

84. Class IV symptomatic patient, according to specific activity scale cannot perform exercise workload of:
- **A.** ≤ 2 mets
- **B.** 4-5 mets
- **C.** ≤ 7 mets
- **D.** ≥ 9 mets

85. All can be seen in pheochromocytoma *except:*
- **A.** Perspiration
- **B.** Palpitation
- **C.** Pigmentation
- **D.** Pallor

86. Chances of haemoptysis is more after closure of PDA by:
- **A.** Umbrella device
- **B.** Coil
- **C.** Amplatzer device
- **D.** Surgical ligation

73 C 74 D 75 D 76 D 77 B 78 B 79 C 80 A 81 D 82 C 83 B 84 A 85 C 86 B

87. Late complication of balloon dilatation of coarctation of aorta is:
A. Aortic aneurysm
B. Aortic dissection
C. Aortic regurgitation
D. None of the above

88. Patient presented with HR of 220/min with no visible P wave. Previous ECG is not suggestive of preexcitation syndrome with rs in V1 Tachycardia in first 6 beats showing QRS alternans pattern. Most probable diagnosis is:
A. AVNRT
B. AVRT
C. Mahaim tract tachycardia
D. AVRT with accessory pathway

89. RV systolic pressure is more than LV systolic pressure in:
A. PS with intact IVS
B. TOF
C. TOF with pulmonary atresia
D. MR

90. RA pressure = 4 mm Hg, TR velocity jet is 4 m/sec. RVSP is:
A. 64 mm Hg
B. 68 mm Hg
C. 50 mm Hg
D. 58 mm Hg

87 A 88 A 89 A 90 B

AIIMS 1998 (June)

1. ECG in myocarditis; all are true *except:*

A. CHB B. Sinus Tachycardia
C. LBBB D. ↑ QRS Voltage

2. Management of VSD (Swiss Cheese) with CHF in infants despite medical Rx is:

A. Vasodilator
B. Heart lung transplantation
C. Patch closure
D. Pulmonary artery banding

3. Oxygen saturation at PA wedge position is:

A. 70% B. 40%
C. 95% D. 60%

4. Wide fixed S2 is heard in:

A. TAPVC B. PAPVC
C. TOF D. dTGA

5. Common site of interventricular septal rupture following myocardial infarction is:

A. Distal IVS B. Mid IVS
C. Proximal IVS D. Same

6. Confidence interval of estimate means:

A. P = 0.05 to p = 0.0005
B. Reliability of estimate
C. Standardization of estimate
D. Range of estimates in a population

7. Dp/Dt in aortic dissection is decreased by:

A. Propranolol B. Nitroprusside
C. Nitroglycerine D. None of the above

8. TMT with TVD with LMCA involvement will show:

A. Hypotension
B. Maximum predicted heart rate in stage I
C. Intraventricular conduction defects
D. ST depression > 3 mm

9. Arrhythmia depending on triggering activity is:

A. VPCs B. Torsades De Pointes
C. WPW D. AF

10. CAST Trial; True is:

A. Premature termination of trial
B. Compares antiarrhythmic with AICD
C. Shows significant decrease in mortality
D. None of the above

11. Class IV symptomatic patient is able to perform how much work according to specific activity scale:

A. 1 met B. 2 met
C. 4 me D. 5 met

12. All are true about clubbing *except:*

A. Occur within a year after central cyanosis
B. Can occur with Methemoglobinemia
C. Occurs within weeks after IE
D. Can occur with ulcerative colitis

1 D 2 D 3 C 4 A 5 A 6 D 7 A 8 A 9 B 10 A 11 A 12 A

13. Continuous Murmur is heard in all *except:*
A. Unruptured sinus of Valsalva
B. PDA
C. Peripheral pulmonary artery stenosis
D. TAPVC

14. Severity of AR is indicated by all *except:*
A. Loudness of murmur
B. Cardiomegaly
C. S3
D. Flow reversal in descending aorta

15. Normal coronary flow is:
A. 60-9 0ml/100 gm/min
B. 90-120 ml/100 gm/min
C. 0-60 ml/100gm/min
D. 120-150ml/100 gm/min

16. Stress test of choice in a patient with CAD and asthma is:
A. Dobutamine B. Dipyridamole
C. Adenosine D. Dopamine

17. LV dysfunction of recent onset in a 8 year old child is due to:
A. MS
B. HTN with RAS
C. Valvular moderate AS
D. ALCAPA

18. Congenital CHB is associated with:
A. cTGA B. ECD
C. TGA D. TOF

19. TGA repair by arterial switch is associated with all *except:*
A. Post operative arrhythmias are common
B. Conduction disturbances
C. Coronary ostial stenosis can occur
D. Infundibular stenosis can occur in long term

20. Peak occurrence of AMI is at:
A. Midnight to 6 AM B. 6 AM to 12 noon
C. 12 noon to 6 PM D. 6 PM to 12 AM

21. SVT with aberration and VT is differentiated by:
A. rSr' in V1
B. Monomorphic R in V1
C. Fusion beats
D. Rr' in V1

22. Indication of surgery in prosthetic valve endocarditis are all *except:*
A. Persistent fever
B. Late PV endocarditis
C. Aortic Root Abscess
D. Recurrent embolism

23. Na Nitroprusside is indicated in all *except:*
A. Eclampsia
B. Hypertensive encephalopathy
C. Dissection of aorta
D. None of the above

24. Pregnancy with adverse outcomes is seen in all *except:*
A. MVP
B. Coarctation
C. TOF
D. Eissenmenger's syndrome

25. Commonest cause of syncope is:
A. Postural
B. Vasovagal
C. Degenerative heart disease
D. Drug induced

26. PAH due to parasitic disease is caused by:
A. Paragonimiasis B. Schistosomiasis
C. Filariasis D. None of the above

27. All are antioxidants *except:*
A. Pantothenic acid B. Beta carotene
C. α-tocopherol D. Vitamin E

28. Treatment of hyperhomocystenemia is:
A. Folic acid B. Vitamin B12
C. Vitamin A D. Vitamin C

---

13 A 14 A 15 A 16 A 17 B 18 A 19 A 20 B 21 A 22 B 23 A 24 A 25 B
26 B 27 A 28 A

29. **Class III antiarrhythmic agents blocks:**
A. K^+ channels B. Na^+ channels
C. Ca^{++} channels D. Cl^- channels

30. **Which of the following is not required to monitor amiodarone toxicity:**
A. Thyroid function test
B. ECG
C. LFT
D. Serum levels

31. **Valvular AS versus subvalvular AS is differentiated by:**
A. Ejection click
B. Aortic root dilatation
C. Radiating murmur to carotid
D. Presence of AR

32. **CABG is best in:**
A. TVD with good LV function
B. TVD with LV dysfunction
C. DVD with good LV function
D. SVD with LV dysfunction

33. **All cause QT prolongation *except:***
A. Hyperkalemia B. Hypocalcemia
C. Hypokalemia D. Quinidine

34. **CI is 1.8 and PCWP is 10; Best treatment modality is:**
A. Inotropes B. i/v fluids
C. IABP D. NTG

35. **Cardiogenic shock in hospital; survival is maximum with:**
A. Angioplasty
B. IABP
C. Medical management
D. None of the above

36. **Drug that does not cross placenta is:**
A. Procainamide B. Quinidine
C. Propranolol D. Heparin

37. **High output is present in all *except:***
A. Thyrotoxicosis B. Pregnancy
C. Beriberi D. Anemia

38. **HTN with BPH; treatment of choice is:**
A. Prazosin
B. Beta blocker
C. ACE-Inhibitor
D. Calcium channel clocker

39. **CHF is characterized by all *except:***
A. ↓ A-VO2 difference
B. ↓ CO
C. ↑ ventricular filling pressure
D. Oliguria

40. **Apex is obliterated on Echo in:**
A. EMF B. Amyloidosis
C. Sarcoidosis D. HOCM

41. **ASH is seen in all *except:***
A. AS B. HOCM
C. Posterior wall MI D. PAH

42. **Catheterization data of a patient is RAP-19 mm Hg, RVEDP-20 mm Hg, LVEDP-20 mm Hg, LAP-19 mm Hg; Diagnosis is:**
A. Restrictive CMP
B. CCP
C. Pericardial effusion
D. Cardiac tamponade

43. **Fontan's operation is done for:**
A. TOF with PS
B. Single ventricle with PS
C. Tricuspid atresia with pulmonary stenosis
D. TGA

44. **Thrombolytic therapy in pulmonary embolism is given for:**
A. Preventing recurrent embolic episodes
B. Prevention of pulmonary infarction
C. Open occluded pulmonary artery
D. All of above

29 A 30 D 31 A 32 B 33 A 34 B 35 A 36 D 37 B 38 A 39 A
40 A 41 C 42 B 43 C 44 D

45. Bisferians pulse is best palpated in:
A. Brachial artery B. Carotid artery
C. Radial artery D. Femoral artery

46. All are true about cholesterol *except:*
A. 1 mg/dl decrease in total cholesterol leads to decrease in mortality by 2%
B. 1 mg/dl increase in HDL-C decreases CAD risk by 2% in male
C. Exercise increases HDL-C
D. Moderate alcohol consumption increases HDL-C

47. Isolated VPC that is asymptomatic is best managed by:
A. No drugs B. Amiodarone
C. i/v xylocaine D. Propranolol

48. Which index of LV contractility is not affected by afterload or preload:
A. Dp/dt
B. Velocity of myocardial fiber circumferential shortening
C. End systolic wall stress ratio
D. None of the above

49. ↑ Incidence in overseas Indians of CAD is because of:
A. Hyperlipidemia
B. Carbohydrate intolerance
C. Social deprivation
D. Smoking

50. EF is overestimated in:
A. AR B. MR
C. AS D. MS

51. ↑ L-R shunt in ASD is seen in:
A. MR B. MS
C. Anemia D. TR

52. Cyanotic spell can present with:
A. Absent murmur B. Hypotension
C. S2 wide split D. Normal SO_2

53. Mitral regurgitation can occur in MI by all of the following *except:*
A. Papillary muscle dysfunction
B. Rupture of papillary muscle
C. LV dilatation
D. Perforation of mitral valve

54. Diastolic murmur at apex are heard in all *except:*
A. ASD B. MR
C. VSD D. Ac Rheumatic fever

55. Severity of MR is related to all *except:*
A. Diastolic murmur
B. Cardiomegaly
C. Loudness of murmur
D. Wide split S_2

56. ACE inhibitors is not very useful in treatment of hypertension in:
A. Blacks
B. Reno vascular hypertension
C. Diabetes
D. CHF

57. In athletes, all are true *except:*
A. Presence of S3
B. Early Diastolic murmur
C. Intermittent mobitz block
D. ESM Grade II

58. Chest pain is aggravated with NTG in:
A. HOCM
B. Subendocardial Ischemia
C. Chronic stable angina
D. Hypertension

59. Cardiac Tamponade is most likely in:
A. Bronchogenic carcinoma
B. Acute rheumatic fever
C. Sarcoidosis
D. Tuberculosis

45 B 46 A 47 A 48 C 49 B 50 B 51 A 52 A 53 D 54 A 55 C 56 A 57 B
58 A 59 A

60. AF with HR of 60/mt is seen with:
A. Digitalis toxicity
B. Hypertension
C. Beta blockers
D. None of the above

61. ↑ QT interval is seen with all *except:*
A. Hypokalemia B. Hyperkalemia
C. Hypocalcaemia D. Quinidine

62. Congenital long QT interval; Treatment of choice is:
A. Beta Blocker B. Phenytoin
C. Sotalol D. Amiodarone

63. HOCM murmur increases with all *except:*
A. Valsalva
B. Leg raising
C. Isoprenanline
D. Post extra systolic beat

64. Pulmonary edema with normal PCWP is seen with:
A. High altitude pulmonary edema
B. MS
C. Cortriatriatum
D. Severe AS

65. Normotensive TR is seen with all *except:*
A. Pulmonary embolism
B. Ebsteins anomaly
C. Trauma
D. IE

66. Magnitude of cyanosis in TOF is decided by:
A. PS B. Override of aorta
C. VSD D. None of the above

67. Emergency TPI in acute MI is indicated in:
A. LBBB
B. New Wenckebach Type II A-V block
C. RBBB
D. RBBB + LAHB with first degree A-V block

68. Pacemaker of choice in a 65 year old lady with frequent long sinus pauses with HR on TMT around 180/min with narrow QRS complexes is:
A. AAI B. DDD
C. VDD D. VVI

69. Poor R wave progression is seen in all *except:*
A. RVMI B. RVH
C. RBBB D. None of the above

70. Normal resting heart uses:
A. FFA B. Glucose
C. Amino acids D. None of the above

71. Nonsynchronized DC shock is for:
A. VF
B. A flutter
C. A Fibrillation
D. Ventricular tachycardia

72. Arrhythmia least likely in structural normal heart is:
A. PSVT B. A Flutter
C. VT with LBBB D. VPCS

73. In treatment of unstable angina all are used *except:*
A. Thrombolytic therapy
B. Beta blockers
C. NTG
D. Aspirin

74. In pheochromocytoma; all are seen *except:*
A. Pallor B. Palpitation
C. Pigmentation D. Perspiration

75. A young female presented with pCO2-22, pO2-144, and pH of 7.55; Diagnosis is:
A. Pulmonary edema
B. Anxiety neurosis
C. Diuretic overdose
D. Pneumonia

60 A 61 B 62 A 63 B 64 A 65 A 66 A 67 D 68 A 69 C 70 A 71 A 72 B
73 A 74 C 75 B

76. Continuous murmur is seen in all *except:*
A. Peripheral Pulmonary artery stenosis
B. AP window
C. RSOV to RA
D. Pulmonary A-V fistula

77. Reversed split S2 is not seen with:
A. LBBB B. HOCM
C. RV Ectopics D. MVP

78. A 65 year male with intermittent AF; treatment may include all *except:*
A. Coronary angiography
B. Anticoagulation
C. Amiodarone
D. EPS

79. PSVT with aberrancy versus VT; most likely to differentiate between them is:
A. Adenosine
B. Calcium channel blockers
C. Beta blockers
D. Quinolones

80. All of the following are true about bisferian's pulse *except:*
A. Seen in severe AR with or without AS
B. DCMP with congestive heart failure
C. Seen in MVP
D. Seen in HOCM

81. VSD with Eisenmengers; treatment is:
A. Heart-lung transplantation
B. Heart Transplantation
C. Bilateral lung transplantation
D. Single lung transplantation

82. RF ablation is least successful in:
A. Accessory pathway
B. AF
C. AVNRT
D. VT

83. HUTT test is for:
A. LV dysfunction
B. Vasovagal syncope
C. Arrhythmia assessment
D. None of the above

84. In isotonic exercise in normal population, true is:
A. ↓ LVEDV B. ↑ LVEDV
C. Remains same D. None of the above

85. True about TMT is:
A. Highly sensitive
B. Affected by population being treated
C. Diagnostic in asymptomatic young patient
D. None of the above

86. Contraindicated in Prinzmetal angina is:
A. Beta-blocker
B. Calcium channel blocker
C. NTG
D. α blocker

87. Eisenmenger syndrome develops earliest in:
A. VSD B. PDA
C. ASD D. A-P window

88. Gynaecomastia is caused by:
A. Amiloride B. Spironolactone
C. Frusemide D. Thaizaides

89. Pulmonary artery saturation of 60% is in favor of:
A. Large left to right shunt
B. CHF
C. Distal pulmonary artery stenosis
D. TAPVC

90. Cardiotoxic effects of hyperkalemia is increased by:
A. Alkalosis B. Hypocalcemia
C. Hypercalcemia D. None of the above

76 B 77 D 78 A 79 A 80 B 81 A 82 B 83 B 84 B 85 B 86 A 87 D 88 B
89 B 90 B

AIIMS 1997 (December)

1. Following is not an echo finding in MS:
A. Decreased EF slope
B. Increased LA size
C. Paradoxical PML motion
D. P ½ <50

2. Treatment of cyanotic spell include all *except:*
A. Morphine B. Digoxin
C. Propranolol D. Ketamine

3. All are features of heart failure in infancy *except:*
A. Tachycardia B. Gallop
C. Cardiomegaly D. Pedal edema

4. Following is least likely to be found in cyanotic spell:
A. Normal PO_2
B. Decreased murmur
C. Hypertension
D. Loss of consciousness

5. All are seen as cardiac effects in HIV *except:*
A. Myocarditis
B. Kaposi's sarcoma (primary)
C. Pericardial effusion
D. CAD

6. Prostaglandin infusion is indicated in all *except:*
A. Coarctation of the aorta
B. Tricuspid atresia
C. Pulmonary atresia
D. HLHS

7. RAD on EKG is not associated with:
A. ASD B. VSD
C. Tricuspid atresia D. Pulmonary atresa

8. HV interval is not prolonged by all *except:*
A. Digoxin B. Verapamil
C. Propranolol D. Amiodarone

9. Commonest cardiovascular problem in India:
A. Hypertension B. CAD
C. RHD D. DCMP

10. Obliterated RV and LV apex on echo is seen in:
A. Carcinoid syndrome
B. Amyloidosis
C. Endomyocardial fibrosis
D. Cardiac tamponade

11. If mean PCWP is 30 mmHg then possible PA pressure are:

	PASP	*PADP*	*Mean PAP*
A.	40	30	20
B.	60	30	40
C.	60	30	20
D.	40	30	15

12. Atrial situs is best determined by:
A. Left bronchus
B. An air bubble in stomach
C. Right liver
D. Left atrium

1 D 2 B 3 D 4 A 5 B 6 A 7 C 8 D 9 A 10 C 11 B 12 A

13. Commonest valvular lesion (isolated or combined) is:
A. MS B. MR
C. MS + MR D. MS + AR

14. Commonest valvular lesions associated with conduction defect is:
A. MS B. MR
C. AS D. AR

15. Which of the following determine the level of R → L shunt maximum in TOF?
A. Degree of aortic over ride
B. Size of VSD
C. Degree of RVH
D. Degree of infundibular stenosis

16. L → R shunt in ASD will increase with:
A. PAH B. MR
C. RV dysfunction D. Anemia

17. Best investigation for detection of myocardial viability:
A. PET scan B. Adenosine echo
C. Stress thallium D. TMT

18. Best investigation for RVMI is:
A. TMT B. Stress thallium
C. Stress MUGA D. CART

19. Type III anti arrhythmic agent block:
A. Fast Na channel B. Slow Na channel
C. K channel D. Cl^- receptors

20. Best drug to differentiate SVT and VT:
A. Procainamide B. Verapamil
C. Digitalis D. Adenosine

21. All are seen in CHF *except:*
A. Decreased cardiac output
B. Decreased AV O_2 difference
C. Increased LV filling pressure
D. LVS3

22. Nitrates help in CHF by mainly:
A. Decreasing preload
B. Decreasing afterload
C. Increasing contractility
D. Decreasing heart rate

23. All are seen in isometric exercise *except:*
A. Increased heart rate B. Increase CO
C. Decrease PVR D. Increase PVR

24. Murmur of HOCM will be increased in all *except:*
A. Valsalva II
B. Isometric exercise
C. Straight leg raising
D. Standing

25. A patient of CHF with mean RA pressure 20 mm Hg, RVEDP 20 mm Hg, PCWP 20 mm Hg, LVEDP 19 mm Hg; most common diagnosis is:
A. Restrictive cardiopathy
B. Constrictive pericarditis
C. Cardiac tamponade
D. RVMI

26. Pulsus paradoxus is seen in all *except:*
A. COAD
B. Positive pressure ventilation
C. Constrictive pericarditis
D. Cardiac tamponade

27. Following interventions will decrease BP *except:*
A. ↓ Sodium intake to 2 gm/day
B. Exercise
C. Decreased calorie intake
D. Decreased alcohol intake

28. Asymmetric septal hypertrophy is seen in all *except:*
A. HOCM
B. Pulmonary arterial hypertension
C. Aortic stenosis
D. Posterior wall MI

13 C 14 C 15 D 16 B 17 A 18 C 19 C 20 D 21 B 22 A 23 C 24 C 25 B
26 B 27 C 28 D

29. Infective endocarditis is unlikely in:
A. ASD B. VSD
C. PDA D. TOF

30. Normally aorta arises:
A. Rt and posterior to PA
B. Rt and anterior to PA
C. Lt and posterior to PA
D. Lt and anterior to PA

31. For streptococci to be effective to cause Rheumatic fever, which of the following is necessary?
A. Throat infection
B. Localization in some tissue
C. Group D streptococci
D. None of the above

32. Primordial prevention is aimed at:
A. Persons with no risk factors
B. Prevention in first degree relatives
C. Persons with risk factors and disease
D. None of the above

33. HT in pregnancy useful treatment is:
A. Hydralazine B. Sodium nitroprusside
C. Captopril D. Diuretics

34. Most successful intervention to decease restenosis after PTCA:
A. Stent B. Brachytherapy
C. Statin D. Aspirin

35. RF ablation is most successful in:
A. WPW syndrome
B. AVNRT slow pathway
C. AVNRT fast pathway
D. AVRT

36. Young male with one day h/o palpitation; all are possible *except:*
A. Mahaim fiber mediated tachycardia
B. AVNRT
C. ARVD
D. Anxiety

37. Best treatment for asymptomatic patient with VPCs and structurally normal heart:
A. No treatment B. Flecainide
C. Amiodarone D. β blocker

38. Most sensitive echo sign of cardiac tamponade:
A. RA diastolic collapse
B. RV diastolic collapse
C. Pseudohypertrophy of the heart
D. Massive pericardial effusion

39. Which of the following is not usually seen with structurally normal heart:
A. VPC
B. Ventricular tachycardia
C. Atrial flutter
D. APC's

40. All are cardiac teratogen *except:*
A. Alcohol B. Warfarin
C. Lithium D. Retinoic acid

41. All are antioxidant *except:*
A. α tocopherol
B. Vitamin C
C. β carotene
D. Pantothenic acid

42. MI in a neonate; probable cause is:
A. Familial hyperlipidemia
B. Coronary AV fistula
C. Coronary artery from pulmonary artery
D. Coronary arterial spasm

43. Best treatment for cardiogenic shock in acute MI:
A. Thrombolysis B. PTCA
C. IABP D. Inotropic support

44. Bisferians pulse is best felt at:
A. Carotid B. Brachial artery
C. Popliteal D. Femoral

---

29 A 30 A 31 A 32 A 33 A 34 A 35 B 36 A 37 A 38 A 39 A 40 C 41 D
42 C 43 B 44 A

45. Wide fixed S2 is not seen in:
A. TAPVC
B. PAPVC
C. ASD
D. Massive pulmonary embolism

46. Chronic AF with HR of 60/min diagnosis is:
A. SA nodal dysfunction
B. Digoxin toxicity
C. Presence of accessory pathway
D. None of the above

47. Cardiac rupture in AMI usually occurs at:
A. First week B. 2nd week
C. 3rd week D. 4th week

48. Pathology of unstable angina is best diagnosed by:
A. Echo
B. Thallium stress test
C. EBCT
D. Coronary angioscopy

49. Best treatment for AMI with Cardiac index 1.8 L/min/m^2 and mean PCWP 10 is:
A. IABP B. Inotropic support
C. Diuretic D. Fluid

50. Significant MR is associated with all *except:*
A. Wide S2
B. MDM
C. Loudness of murmur
D. Cardiomegaly

51. Treatment of choice for congenital long QT syndrome:
A. β blocker B. Phenytoin
C. Sotalol D. Amiodarone

52. Pregnancy may be complicated in which of the following ?
A. Marfan syndrome B. AR
C. MR D. ASD

53. A patient with hypertension, DM, B/L renal artery stenosis should not receive:
A. Aspirin B. Thiazide
C. β blocker D. Enalapril

54. LAA clot is best diagnosed by:
A. TTE B. TEE
C. CT D. Angiocardiography

55. Following valvular lesion is most common in carcinoid syndrome:
A. MS B. MS + TR
C. TR + PS D. TS + PS

56. Pulmonary artery wedge pressure is more than LA pressure in:
A. Cortriatriatum B. LA myxoma
C. MS D. MR

57. STK is contraindicated in:
A. Prosthetic valve thrombosis
B. Acute Pulmonary embolism
C. DVT
D. Thrombolysis with STK in last 3 weeks

58. Normotensive TR is seen in all *except:*
A. Ebstein anomaly
B. Carcinoid syndrome
C. Acute Pulmonary embolism
D. Infective endocarditis

59. Cardiac tamponade can occur most likely in:
A. Bronchogenic carcinoma
B. Hypothyroidism
C. Tuberculosis
D. Idiopathic pericarditis

60. Contrast echo is used to detect:
A. L → R shunt
B. R → L shunt
C. Coronary blood flow
D. None of the above

45 D 46 B 47 A 48 D 49 D 50 C 51 A 52 A 53 D 54 B 55 C 56 A 57 D
58 C 59 A 60 B

61. **Pulmonary arterial saturation of 60% indicates:**
A. CHF B. MI
C. CCP D. EMF

62. **Site for mixed venous saturation sample for determination of cardiac output by Fick's method is:**
A. RA B. RV
C. Pulmonary artery D. Pulmonary vein

63. **Maximum desaturation is found at:**
A. SVC B. IVC
C. Coronary sinus D. Mid RA

64. **Treatment of choice for Eisenmenger's VSD:**
A. PA banding
B. Heart lung transplantation
C. Cardiac transplantation
D. Simple VSD closure

65. **MAT is commonly associated with:**
A. CAD B. COAD
C. HOCM D. CHF

66. **Osler nodes are best seen at:**
A. Pulp of the finger B. Thenar eminence
C. Palm D. Sole

67. **A patient with PO2 85 mm Hg, PCWP 20 mm Hg, pH 7.2; most likely diagnosis is:**
A. DKA B. Pulmonary edema
C. Sedative overdose D. None of the above

68. **Pulmonary edema with normal PCWP is seen in:**
A. High altitude pulmonary oedema
B. MS
C. Cortriatriatum
D. AS

69. **Best investigation for LV muscle mass is:**
A. MRI B. CT
C. Echo D. Angiography

70. **Commonest side effect of ACE inhibitors is:**
A. Cough
B. Nephropathy
C. Hypotension
D. Altered taste sensation

71. **PTCA is contraindicated in:**
A. TVD
B. Total coronary occlusion
C. Proximal LMC stenosis
D. Proximal LAD stenosis

72. **Drug used to reduce dp/dt in dissection of aorta is:**
A. Nitroprusside B. Hydralazine
C. Labetalol D. Frusemide

73. **IABP is contraindicated in:**
A. Acute MI with cardiogenic shock
B. Acute MR
C. Acute AR
D. Acute VSD

74. **Antihypertensive of choice in patient with HT and prostatic hypertrophy:**
A. Prazosin B. Amlodipine
C. Enalapril D. Atenolol

75. **Best investigation to diagnose neurocardiogenic syncope is:**
A. Holtar B. EPS
C. Stress echo D. HUTT

76. **Manoeuvre helpful in supraventricular tachycardia is:**
A. Diving reflex
B. Merie reflex
C. Bezold jarish reflex
D. Bainbridge reflex

77. **Peak time for acute MI is:**
A. 6 AM to 12 PM B. 12 PM to 6 PM
C. 12 AM to 6 AM D. 6 PM to 12 AM

---

61 A **62** C **63** C **64** B **65** B **66** A **67** B **68** A **69** A **70** A **71** C **72** C **73** C
74 A **75** D **76** A **77** A

78. BP difference of 5 mm Hg between between upper limbs is seen in:
A. Supravalvular AS B. Subvalvular AS
C. Valvular AS D. None of the above

79. Which finding on TMT is indicator of severe TVD/LM disease:
A. Hypotension
B. 85% MHR in stage I
C. Intraventricular conduction disturbances
D. ST depressant more than 3 mm

80. Overestimation of LV function by LVEF is seen in:
A. AR B. MR
C. AS D. MS

81. Thrombolytic treatment in pulmonary embolism is given for:
A. Prevention of further embolic episode
B. To prevent pulmonary infarction
C. To open the occluded pulmonary flow
D. All of the above

82. Parasite responsible for pulmonary arterial hypertension:
A. Trypanosomiasis B. Paragonimiasis
C. Schistosomiasis D. Filariasis

83. All are true about decreased in lipid *except:*
A. 1 mg% decrease in the total cholesterol leads to decrease in mortality by 2%
B. Decrease in HDL increases the risk of CAD
C. Regular exercise increases HDL
D. Moderate alcohol intake increases HDL-C

84. NTG increases the pain in:
A. HOCM
B. Variant angina
C. Intramyocardial bridging
D. MI

85. Commonest cause of syncope:
A. AV block B. Vasovagal
C. VT D. ARVD

86. In Athletes heart all are seen *except:*
A. Intermittent mobitz ype I
B. Grade II ESM
C. S3
D. Early diastolic murmur

87. Cardiotoxic effect of hyperkalemia is increased by:
A. Alkalosis B. Increased calcium
C. Decreased calcium D. None of the above

88. Child with valvular vs subvalvular AS is differentiated by:
A. Murmur radiation
B. Ejection click
C. Post stenotic dilatation
D. Presence of S4

89. Emergency TPI in acute MI is indicated in:
A. LBBB
B. RBBB
C. New wenckbach type II
D. RBBB + LAHB + 1st degree heart block

90. Randomized trials comparing CABG vs. medical treatment shows that CABG increases the survival in:
A. TVD with decreased EF
B. TVD with normal EF
C. DVD with normal EF
D. DVD with decreased EF

78 A 79 A 80 B 81 D 82 C 83 A 84 A 85 B 86 D 87 C 88 B 89 D 90 A

AIIMS 1997 (June)

1. **Infrequent in infant CHF is:**
   A. Sweating
   B. Ankle oedema
   C. Growth retardation
   D. Hepatomegaly

2. **Cyanosis in first week is seen in all *except:***
   A. Persistent fetal circulation
   B. PAPVC
   C. TGA
   D. TAPVC

3. **Common in rubella:**
   A. PDA B. ASD
   C. PS D. VSD

4. **Drug with cardiac teratogenic effect are all *except:***
   A. Warfarin B. Alcohol
   C. Retinoic acid D. Lithium

5. **Cause of AMI in child are all *except:***
   A. Pompes
   B. Hereditary hypercholesterolemia
   C. Homocystinuria
   D. Kawasaki

6. **AMI at 8 weeks in a child; diagnosis is:**
   A. ALCAPA
   B. ARCAPA
   C. Kawasaki's disease
   D. Glycogen storage disorder

7. **CHF in utero is seen in all *except:***
   A. TGA B. Anemia
   C. Ebsteins D. PSVT

8. **In cyanotic spell all can be given *except:***
   A. Phenylephrine B. Digitalis
   C. Lasix D. Aminophylline

9. **All can be seen in cardiac involvement in AIDS *except:***
   A. Kaposi's sarcoma
   B. Myocarditis
   C. Staph IE
   D. Tubercular pericardial effusion

10. **Sudden cardiac death: all are true *except:***
    A. 10% due to MVP
    B. IHD is an important cause
    C. AICD can be used in survivors
    D. >10 VPC/minute is an imp indicator of SCD

11. **PO_2 85, pCO_2 20, pH 7.2 is seen in:**
    A. DKA
    B. Pulmonary Edema
    C. Phenargan overdose
    D. Anxiety

12. **Constant ejection click is seen in all *except:***
    A. PS
    B. Tetrology of Fallot's
    C. Pulmonary hypertension
    D. Idiopathic dilatation of PA

---

1 B 2 B 3 A 4 D 5 A 6 A 7 A 8 B 9 C 10 A 11 B 12 A

13. All are true about TGA *except:*
A. Arterial switch at 2-3 weeks
B. Increased arrhythmias after arterial switch
C. Associated with situs ambiguous
D. Cyanosis present since birth

14. All are true about PSVT in an infant *except:*
A. I/v verapamil is drug of choice
B. RFA should not be used first
C. Bypass tract incidence is 40%
D. None of the above

15. Pregnancy is well tolerated in:
A. MVP B. Marfan's syndrome
C. CoA D. Eisenmengers

16. Treatment of Eisenmengers complex is:
A. Heart lung transplantation
B. Heart transplantation
C. Bilateral lung transplantation
D. Single lung transplantation

17. Infant with AS; Treatment of choice is:
A. Valvotomy B. Replacement
C. Medical treatment D. None of the above

18. Paradoxical split of S2 is seen in all *except:*
A. DCMP B. VSD
C. PDA D. AS

19. Cyanotic spell is characterized by:
A. Absent murmur B. Splitting of S2
C. Loud P2 D. None of the above

20. MS with TS with AF is characterized by:
A. Delayed y descent
B. Prominent 'a' wave
C. Pulmonary hypertension
D. Variable S1

21. Common cause of Congenital heart block is:
A. Coarctation of aorta
B. VSD
C. Corrected TGA
D. TA

22. 8 year old child with recent onset LV dysfunction is most probably due to:
A. Moderate AS
B. MS
C. Systemic HTN with RAS
D. TOF

23. Ventricularization of atrial pressure is seen in:
A. Acute MR B. MS
C. AR D. VSD

24. Embolism can occur with all *except:*
A. CART
B. Balloon Valvotomy
C. Swan Ganz Catheter
D. None of the above

25. IABP is contraindicated in:
A. Acute AR B. AS
C. Cardiogenic shock D. MR

26. Primordial prevention is:
A. Prevention in first degree relative
B. No risk factors; no disease
C. Treatment of existing risk factors in population
D. None of the above

27. Apical obstruction is seen in:
A. EMF B. Amyloidosis
C. Sarcoidosis D. CCP

28. Pulmonary HTN is caused by:
A. Trypanosomiasis B. Filariasis
C. Schistosomiasis D. None of the above

29. Aortic dissection is seen in all *except:*
A. Coarctation of aorta
B. Syphilis
C. Behcet's syndrome
D. BAV

13 B 14 A 15 A 16 A 17 A 18 B 19 A 20 A 21 C 22 C 23 A 24 C 25 A
26 B 27 A 28 C 29 B

30. LA Myxoma can cause all *except:*
A. Embolization
B. Clubbing
C. Fever
D. Anemia

31. Protective HDL is:
A. HDL1
B. HDL2
C. HDL3
D. HDL4

32. Drug that reduces HDL is:
A. Simvastatin
B. Vitamin C
C. Probucol
D. Nicotinic acid

33. Regression of atherosclerosis is by all *except:*
A. Statins
B. Nitrates
C. Calcium channel blockers
D. ACE-inhibitors

34. Drugs that increase HDL significantly is:
A. Niacin
B. Probucol
C. Lovastatin
D. None of the above

35. Treatment of choice in unstable angina is:
A. Intravenous heparin
B. i/v heparin + aspirin
C. i/v heparin + aspirin + anticoagulants
D. Thrombolytics + antianginals

36. Maximum decrease in mortality in AMI is seen with:
A. Aspirin + Thrombolytic therapy + Beta blocker
B. Aspirin + beta blocker
C. TLT with heparin
D. Beta blocker with heparin

37. Definition of Primary PTCA is:
A. Angioplasty performed directly as first line of reperfusion therapy in AMI
B. Angioplasty performed in failed thrombolysis
C. Angioplasty performed within first week of MI
D. None of the above

38. PTCA is contraindicated in:
A. Unprotected left main stenosis
B. LAD stenosis
C. Severe Triple vessel disease
D. SVD with LV dysfunction

39. RF ablation is least successful in which of the following?
A. Atrial fibrillation
B. Atrial flutter
C. WPW
D. AVNRT

40. Reduction in mortality with CABG is seen in:
A. TVD only
B. TVD with LV dysfunction
C. DVD with normal LV function
D. SVD with LV dysfunction

41. H-V interval is increased by:
A. Digoxin
B. Verapamil
C. Adenosine
D. Amiodarone

42. Absolute indication of stopping amiodarone is:
A. Worsening CHF
B. Pulmonary toxicity
C. Hypothyroidism
D. Corneal toxicity

43. Which of the following is contraindicated in early MI ?
A. Calcium channel blocker
B. ACE inhibitors
C. Beta blockers
D. Diuretics

44. EDRF is:
A. NO
B. NO_2
C. N
D. None of the above

45. True statement regarding cholesterol is:
A. 1% decrease in cholesterol decreases CAD risk by 1-2%
B. All nuts are very rich in cholesterol
C. LDL cholesterol is significantly decreased by Niacin therapy
D. Daily exercise decreases HDL cholesterol

30 B 31 B 32 C 33 B 34 A 35 B 36 A 37 A 38 A 39 A 40 B 41 D 42 B
43 A 44 A 45 A

46. Old MI with HT; Drug of choice is:
A. Diuretics B. Beta blockers
C. ACE inhibitors D. Alpha blockers

47. Drug of choice in pregnancy with HTN is:
A. Alpha methyldopa
B. Calcium channel blockers
C. ACE inhibitors
D. Beta blockers

48. Commonest side effect of ACE inhibitors is:
A. Cough B. Hypotension
C. Rash D. None of the above

49. In CHF, mortality benefit is seen with:
A. Beta blockers B. ACE inhibitors
C. Diuretics D. All of the above

50. Digitalis toxicity,all may be seen *except:*
A. AF with FVR
B. AF with junctional rhythm
C. PAT with block
D. VPC's

51. AF with heart rate of 50-60/min is most commonly seen in:
A. Digitalis toxicity B. AMI
C. COPD D. Beta blockers

52. CI < 1.8, PCPW 10; Treatment of choice is:
A. Intravenous fluids B. Inotropes
C. IABP D. NTG

53. Cardiogenic shock; treatment of choice is:
A. Primary PTCA B. CABG
C. STK D. Abciximab

54. VPC's with structurally normal heart; treatment of choice is:
A. No treatment B. Beta blockers
C. Amiodarone D. Lignocaine

55. Not associated with structurally normal heart is:
A. A Flutter B. VT with LBBB
C. PSVT D. VPC's

56. Investigation of choice for neurocardiogenic syncope is:
A. HUTT B. EPS
C. EEG D. ECG

57. TPI in Acute MI is indicated in:
A. AWMI with alternating bundle branch block
B. IWMI with A-V block
C. AWMI with prolonged PR interval
D. IWMI with RVMI

58. Treatment of choice for congenital long QT syndrome is:
A. Beta blocker
B. Alpha blocker
C. Inotropes
D. Class IB antiarrhythmics

59. QT interval is increased in all *except:*
A. JLN syndrome
B. Hyperkalemia
C. Romano Ward syndrome
D. Amiodarone

60. Which of the following statement is true about CAST trial:
A. Withdrawn early because of increased mortality
B. Shows significant decrease in mortality
C. Compares antiarrhythmic drugs with AICD
D. None of the above

61. Decreased restenosis is best seen with:
A. Stents
B. Radiation
C. Thrombolytic therapy
D. ACE-inhibitors

62. HCM murmur is increased by all *except:*
A. Passive leg raising B. NTG
C. Valsalva maneuver D. Standing

---

46 B 47 A 48 A 49 D 50 A 51 A 52 A 53 A 54 A 55 A 56 A 57 A 58 A
59 B 60 A 61 A 62 A

63. Nitrates aggravate angina in:
A. HOCM
B. Chronic stable angina
C. Unstable angina
D. DCMP

64. ASH is seen in all *except:*
A. PWMI
B. Pulm HTN
C. AS
D. HOCM

65. Paradoxical septal motion is seen in all *except:*
A. ASD
B. RV volume overload with ASD
C. TR
D. LV Volume overload

66. Myocarditis with CHF. Treatment of choice is:
A. ACE inhibitors
B. Prednisolone
C. Azathioprine
D. Diuretics

67. Best modality for testing viability of myocardium is:
A. PET
B. Exercise testing
C. Doppler echo
D. Thallium

68. Coronary calcification is best seen with :
A. Chest X-ray
B. CT scan
C. Fluoroscopy
D. MRI

69. Pulsus paradoxus is seen in all *except:*
A. IPPV
B. Constrictive pericarditis
C. Cardiac tamponade
D. COPD

70. In RA myxoma, all can be seen *except:*
A. TR
B. Pulmonary embolism
C. Tumor plop
D. Clubbing

71. Thrombolytic therapy is not used in which of the following:
A. Unstable angina
B. STEMI
C. Prosthetic valve thrombosis
D. None of the above

72. U wave inversion in TMT is specific for:
A. LAD territory ischemia
B. RCA territory ischemia
C. Global ischemia
D. Is a nonspecific finding

73. Isometric exercise can cause all *except:*
A. Decrease PVR
B. Increase force of contraction
C. Increase PVR
D. None of the above

74. All are true about CHF *except:*
A. Decrease A-V O2 difference
B. Increase serum norepinephrine
C. ACE inhibitors are useful in treatment
D. Oxygen hemoglobin dissociation curve is shifted to right

75. HAPE; true is all *except:*
A. Increase PCWP
B. Increase capillary constriction
C. Normal left atrial pressure
D. Pulmonary hypertension

76. Sodabicarb is not used in routine CPR due to:
A. Respiratory alkalosis
B. Hyperkalemia
C. Hypercalcemia
D. Respiratory acidosis

77. Calcium is not routinely used in CPR because of:
A. Intracellular accumulation causing uncoupling of oxidative phosphorylation
B. Promotion of hypokalemia
C. Promotion of acidosis
D. Promotion of alkalosis

63 A 64 A 65 D 66 A 67 A 68 B 69 A 70 D 71 A 72 A 73 A 74 A 75 A
76 D 77 A

78. Detection of CAD in patient with LBBB is done by:
A. TMT
B. Stress Echocardiography
C. CART
D. Thallium

79. Suprasystemic RV pressure is seen in:
A. PS with intact septum
B. Eissenmengers complex
C. TOF
D. TA with VSD with PS

80. BPH with HT; treatment of choice is:
A. Prazosin B. Beta blockers
C. ACE-inhibitors D. Diuretics

81. Confidence interval of estimate means:
A. P = 0.05 to p = 0.0005
B. Reliability of estimate
C. Standardization of estimates
D. Range of estimates in a population

82. TEE is used in all *except:*
A. LAA clot
B. Constrictive pericarditis
C. Poor echo window
D. Descending aorta dissection

83. BP is overestimated in all *except:*
A. Obesity B. Auscultatory gap
C. Small cuff D. Atherosclerosis

84. Cannon wave is seen in all *except:*
A. TS
B. CHB with pace maker (DDDR)
C. Junctional rhythm
D. AVNRT

85. ASD with increase left to right shunt is seen in:
A. MR B. Volume overload
C. PAH D. None of the above

86. Commonest cardiac disease in INDIA is:
A. RHD B. HTN
C. CAD D. Cardiomyopathy

87. Multifocal atrial tachycardia is most commonly associated with:
A. COAD B. CAD
C. HTN D. DCMP

88. LAD is seen in:
A. Secundum ASD with MVP
B. Primum ASD
C. Sinus venosus ASD
D. None of the above

89. Cyanosis with increased pulmonary blood flow is seen in:
A. Truncus arteriosus
B. Tricuspid atresia
C. RSOV
D. PDA reversal

90. All are true about Eisenmenger's syndrome *except:*
A. Syncope
B. Hemoptysis
C. History of squatting
D. History of respiratory tract infections

78 D 79 A 80 A 81 D 82 B 83 B 84 B 85 A 86 B 87 A 88 B 89 A 90 C

AIIMS 1996

1. **Drug that is both an arteriolar and venodilator:**
   A. Nitroprusside B. Hydralazine
   C. Nitrates D. Nifedepine

2. **Earliest sign of Hyperkalemia is:**
   A. Tall T/tented T
   B. Widening of QRS
   C. P wave amplitude decrease
   D. Complete heart block

3. **Which lipoprotein rises most in obesity:**
   A. HDL B. VLDL
   C. LDL D. Chylomicron

4. **In Barlow's syndrome, the drug that is to be avoided is:**
   A. Nitrates B. Beta blocker
   C. Aspirin D. Phenytoin

5. **Pulmonary vasodilators are all *except:***
   A. Dopamine B. Nitrates
   C. Nifedepin D. Isoproterenol

6. **LAD is found in which of the following CHD:**
   A. Eisenmengers
   B. Multiple VSD's
   C. VSD with Right to Left shunt
   D. VSD with PS

7. **Bioprosthetic valve is indicated in:**
   A. Child 5 years old
   B. 15 years old boy
   C. Pregnant women
   D. 70 year old male

8. **Plexogenic changes are seen in all *except:***
   A. PPH
   B. Pulomonary embolism
   C. Eisenmengers
   D. Left to Rt shunt

9. **Dose of propanalol in a child of TOF with cyanotic spells is:**
   A. 0.1 mg/kg
   B. 0.2-0.3 mg/kg
   C. 0.01-0.05 mg/kg
   D. 1 mg/kg

10. **BMV is absolutely contraindicated in:**
    A. Restenotic MS
    B. Calcific MS
    C. Pregnant MS
    D. Severe symptomatic MS

11. **Presence of gradient after BPV indicates:**
    A. Failed procedure
    B. Restenosis
    C. Infundibular stenosis
    D. None of the above

12. **Cyanotic spells are precipitated by all *except:***
    A. Fever B. Sleep
    C. Acidosis D. Digoxin

1 A 2 A 3 D 4 A 5 A 6 B 7 D 8 B 9 A 10 B 11 C 12 B

13. Five days old male baby asymptomatic small PDA: treatment of choice:
A. Surgery B. Balloon
C. Nothing D. IE prophylaxis

14. Thromboembolic episodes are least common in:
A. Lone AF B. HT with AF
C. RHD with AF D. DCM with AF

15. Cholesterol crystals in pericardial fluid are seen in:
A. Tubercular B. Ischemic
C. Traumatic D. Hypothyroidism

16. Continuous Murmur is least likely to occur in which of the following?
A. AP window B. RSOV
C. PDA D. Coronary AV fistula

17. All of the following can occur because of chest trauma *except:*
A. VSD B. MR
C. Coronary occlusion D. Aneurysm

18. Treatment of choice for Torsades de pointes syndrome is:
A. Overdrive pacing B. I/V magnesium
C. I/V Cordarone D. DC shock

19. Coronary artery origin can be best seen in which view:
A. PLAX view
B. Parasternal short axis view
C. Apical four chamber view
D. Apical two chamber view

20. Which of the following antihypertensives is not used in pregnancy:
A. Diuretics B. Beta Blockers
C. Hydralazine D. Methyl Dopa

21. Fetal echocardiogram is done at what gestational age:
A. 14 wks B. 16 wks
C. 20 wks D. 24 wks

22. Which of the following is not teratogenic:
A. Labetalol B. Lithium
C. Phenytoin D. Alcohol

23. Commonest complication of ACE inhibitor therapy:
A. Hyperkalemia
B. Angioedema
C. Renal impairment
D. Cough

24. Which of the following drug causes gynaecomastia:
A. Amiloride B. Frusemide
C. Thiazdes D. Spironolactone

25. Which pace maker is preferred in patients with HOCM and CHB:
A. VVI B. VVIR
C. DDD D. AAI

26. Murmur of HOCM decreases with:
A. Squatting
B. Standing
C. Amylnitrate
D. Strain phase of Valsalva

27. Prominent 'x' descent is seen with:
A. Tricuspid stenosis
B. Cardiac tamponade
C. Constrictive pericarditis
D. Pericardial effusion

28. Earliest peaking of which enzyme occurs in MI:
A. CPK MB B. LDH
C. SGOT D. Myoglobin

29. Myocardial rupture following MI occurs after:
A. 2-3 hrs B. 2-3 days
C. 2-3 wks D. 2-3 months

13 D 14 A 15 D 16 A 17 B 18 A 19 B 20 A 21 B 22 A 23 D 24 D 25 C
26 A 27 B 28 D 29 B

30. Treatment of choice for Dressler's syndrome is:
A. Aspirin B. NSAIDS
C. Corticosteroids D. Heparin

31. Angioplasty done within 3-4 hrs following acute MI without thrombolytic therapy is known as:
A. Primary PTCA
B. Rescue PTCA
C. Immediate PTCA
D. Deferred PTCA

32. Q waves might disappear after 6-12 months in how many cases of MI:
A. 2-3 % B. 20-30%
C. 10% D. 40%

33. Which of the following antilipid agents that lowers HDL has antioxidant therapy:
A. Probucol B. Nicotinic acid
C. Lovastatin D. Gemfibrozil

34. EDRF is actually what:
A. Interleukin B. TNF
C. NO D. Interferon

35. In patients of unstable angina, best therapy besides antianginals is:
A. I/V heparin and disprin
B. S/C heparin
C. I/V heparin
D. Disprin

36. Reliable sign of pericardial tamponade is:
A. Swinging heart in failure
B. Late diastolic RVOT collapse
C. Early diastolic RVOT collapse
D. Early diastolic RA collapse

37. Drug that is best used for producing vasospasm is:
A. Ergometrine B. Adenosine
C. Verapamil D. Isoprenaline

38. Drug that is contraindicated in prinzmetal angina is:
A. Nitrates
B. Calcium channel blockers
C. Disprin
D. Beta blockers

39. Hyperdynamic pulse in a one day old child could be because of:
A. PDA
B. Hypoxemia
C. Reverse coarctation
D. Systemic A-V Fistula

40. All of the following would be differential of wide QRS tachycardia *except:*
A. Preexcitation WPW syndrome with orthodromic conduction
B. Supraventricular tachycardia with previous existing a-v bundle branch block
C. Fascicular tachycardia
D. Association of M chain fibers

41. TEE is useful for diagnosing all *except:*
A. Pulmonary artery compliance
B. Assessing prosthetic valve vegetation
C. Aortic atheroma
D. Assess ascending aorta

42. Treatment of prosthetic valve thrombosis is:
A. I/V thrombolytic therapy
B. I/V heparin
C. Surgery
D. Oral anticoagulants

43. Evidence of atrial infarction on ECG is:
A. PR prolongation B. Raised PR
C. Prolonged QT D. Broad QRS

44. What happens to LVED volume at max isotonic exercise:
A. Increases B. Decreases
C. No change D. Varies with age

30 A 31 A 32 B 33 A 34 C 35 A 36 C 37 A 38 D 39 D 40 A 41 A 42 A
43 B 44 A

45. All are complication of modified BT shunt *except:*

A. Ipsilateral limb shortening
B. CCF
C. IE
D. Shunt blockage

46. Color Doppler is most useful in:

A. Large ASD **B.** Large VSD
C. Right to left shunt **D.** LV to RA shunt

47. Which of the following condition does not affect stress ECG:

A. Partial atrial degeneration
B. Multiple ectopics with normal ECG
C. RBBB with intermittent WPW
D. Severe LVH

48. Best treatment for patient of WPW syndrome is:

A. RFA therapy **B.** Cordarone
C. Surgery **D.** Digoxin

49. Best investigation for vasogenic syncope is:

A. HUTT **B.** Holter
C. Treadmill test **D.** SAECG

50. Following is the relation between pulmonary vascular resistance and systemic vascular resistance:

A. 1/8 of SVR **B.** 1/6 of SVR
C. 1/10 of SVR **D.** ¼ Of SVR

51. ROSS operation is:

A. Shift of aortic valve with homograft of pulmonary valve
B. Shift of aortic valve with xenograft of pulmonary valve
C. Shift of aortic valve with heterograft of pulmonary valve
D. None of the above

52. Brockenbrough Braunwald sign in HOCM is:

A. Post extrasystolic increase in gradient
B. Post extrasystolic decrease in pulse pressure
C. Post extrasystolic increase in murmur
D. Post extrasystolic increase in MR

53. Indication of pacemaker in sick sinus syndrome is:

A. Corrected sinus node recovery time > 525 msec
B. AF
C. Bradyarrhythmia
D. Pacing does not improve survival

54. Management of choice in an old patient with significant severe AS is:

A. Valvotomy
B. Medical therapy
C. Surgery with valve replacement
D. Any of the above

55. In balloon valvotomy, valve size increases due to:

A. Valve rupture
B. Opening up of adhesions at commissure
C. Breaking of cusps
D. Papillary muscle rupture

56. In a 4 year old child systolic murmur heard best at left axilla. On evaluation it reveals peripheral pulmonary stenosis. Patient should be taken for:

A. Surgery
B. Balloon angioplasty
C. Left as it is and reassured
D. None of the above

57. Best treatment that can be given at the earliest to a ACS is:

A. Intracoronary thrombolysis
B. Reteplase
C. PTCA
D. PTCA with stenting

45 A 46 D 47 B 48 A 49 A 50 C 51 A 52 B 53 A 54 C 55 B 56 C 57 D

58. All of the following are true for PE *except:*
A. Atrial arrhythmias
B. S1Q3T3 pattern in 15-25% cases
C. Nonspecific ST-T changes
D. PSVT

59. All of the following will have some histological changes in myocardium *except:*
A. Amyloidosis
B. Allograft rejection
C. DCMP
D. Doxorubicin induced cardiomyopathy

60. Balloon atrial septostomy is not needed in:
A. Fallot's tetrology
B. TGA
C. Tricuspid atresia
D. DORV

61. MR in patients with ostium primum ASD is due to:
A. Cleft in mitral valve leaflets
B. Mitral valve prolapse
C. Rheumatic
D. Infective endocarditis

62. In a patient of acute rheumatic fever, the commonest murmur is:
A. MR
B. AR
C. MS
D. AS

63. Increased morbidity and mortality during pregnancy is seen in all *except:*
A. Eisenmengers syndrome
B. PPH
C. TOF
D. MVP

64. Phasic ejection click is present in:
A. PS
B. AS
C. HOCM
D. MS

65. Eisenmengers syndrome develops early in:
A. ASD
B. VSD
C. Aortopulmonary window
D. PDA

66. Increase morbidity in pregnancy is seen with all *except:*
A. PPH
B. TOF
C. Eisenmengers
D. Coarctation of aorta

67. First dose effect of postural hypotension is seen with:
A. Methyldopa
B. Hydralazine
C. Prazosin
D. Beta blocker

68. Cholesterol increases in all *except:*
A. CRF
B. Common bile duct obstruction
C. Pregnancy
D. None of the above

69. Continuous murmur is present in all *except:*
A. RSOV
B. Pulmonary atresia
C. TAPVC
D. VSD with AR

70. Commonest accessory pathway for WPW is:
A. Left posteroseptal
B. Right free wall
C. Left free wall
D. Left anteroseptal

71. Quincke's pulse in AR is seen in:
A. Nail bed
B. Retina
C. Uvula
D. Forehead

72. Least affected valve in rheumatic heart disease is:
A. Tricuspid valve
B. Pulmonary valve
C. Mitral valve
D. Aortic valve

73. Polysplenia is associated with:
A. Right isomerism
B. Left isomerism
C. Dextrocardia
D. Mesocardia

58 D 59 C 60 A 61 A 62 A 63 D 64 A 65 C 66 D 67 C 68 C 69 D 70 C
71 A 72 B 73 B

74. Prosthetic valve dysfunction is best evaluated by:
A. TEE B. TTE
C. Chest X-ray D. CT scan

75. Giant T wave inversion is seen in:
A. Apical HOCM B. DCMP
C. RCMP D. None of the above

76. Prolonged PR interval is seen in:
A. Ostium secundum ASD
B. Muscular VSD
C. Ebstein's anomaly
D. Multiple VSD

77. Proximal RCA with 85 % stenosis, treatment of choice is:
A. Bypass surgery
B. PTCA without stent
C. Medical management
D. PTCA with stent

78. Following MI, aspirin should be given for:
A. 6 months B. 1 year
C. 3 years D. Life long

79. Treatment of choice for ventricular fibrillation:
A. Non-synchronized DC shock
B. Synchronized DC shock
C. I/V amiodarone
D. I/V xylocaine

80. Dose of rtPA is:
A. 25 mg B. 50 mg
C. 75 mg D. 100 mg

81. Hypertension with hypokalemia is seen in:
A. Conn's syndrome
B. CRF
C. Interstitial nephritis
D. Anuric phase of acute renal failure

82. In 1st week of life which cannot be detected:
A. Large VSD B. PS
C. AS D. TOF

83. Dobutamine vs. dopamine: true is:
A. Less vasoconstriction
B. More vasoconstrictive
C. Increase in heart rate
D. Decrease in heart rate

84. Advantage of TEE:
A. LAA thrombus B. LV apical thrombus
C. ASD D. Post MI VSD

85. ECG machine was invented by:
A. Waller B. Einthoven
C. Levine D. Harvey

86. Oxygen saturation at PA wedge position is:
A. 70% B. 40%
C. 95% D. 60%

87. Arrhythmia depending on triggering activity is:
A. VPCs B. Torsades De Pointes
C. WPW D. AF

88. VSD with Eissenmengers; treatment is:
A. Heart-lung transplantation
B. Heart Transplantation
C. Bilateral lung transplantation
D. Single lung transplantation

89. In athletes, all are true *except:*
A. Presence of S3
B. Early Diastolic murmur
C. Intermittent mobitz block
D. ESM Grade II

90. Na Nitroprusside is indicated in all *except:*
A. Eclampsia
B. Hypertensive encephalopathy
C. Dissection of aorta
D. None of the above

---

74 A 75 A 76 A 77 D 78 D 79 A 80 D 81 A 82 A 83 A 84 A 85 B 86 C
87 B 88 A 89 B 90 A

AIIMS 1995

1. Bounding pulses in a 2days old neonate is due to:

A. PDA
B. Systemic AV fistula
C. Hypoxia
D. Reverse Coarctation

2. IABP is contraindicated in:

A. Acute AR
B. Acute MR
C. Aortic dissection
D. AS

3. After acute MI being thrombolysed, what is the next line of therapy i.e. next step in asymptomatic patient:

A. Conservative therapy
B. Angiography ± revascularization
C. CABG
D. None of the above

4. Acute MI with Cardiogenic shock, the choice of therapy is:

A. IABP
B. PTCA
C. Thrombolysis
D. Inotropic drugs

5. Normal coronaries in acute MI are seen in how many cases:

A. <5%
B. 6-10%
C. 10-20%
D. None of the above

6. In a patient of bronchial asthma, stress echo is done by :

A. Adenosine
B. Dipyridamole
C. Dobutamine
D. None of the above

7. PTCA in acute MI without thrombolytic therapy is:

A. Primary PTCA
B. Deferred PTCA
C. Sequential PTCA
D. Rescue PTCA

8. 95% CI for a disease indicates:

A. Statistical significance
B. No statistical significance
C. Successful primary prevention
D. None of the above

9. Primordial prevention is for:

A. Persons with no risk factors
B. Person with risk factors
C. Prevention in first degree relatives
D. None of the above

10. Prevalence of a disease commonly affects:

A. Sensitivity
B. Specificity
C. + ve predictive value
D. – ve predictive value

11. All are correct about AS *except:*

A. Aortic ejection click is widely heard
B. Murmur is heard at the apex in the elderly
C. Rheumatic is the most common cause of AS in children
D. Valve replacement if gradient >75 mm of Hg in children.

1 B 2 A 3 A 4 B 5 A 6 C 7 A 8 A 9 A 10 C 11 C

12. Digitalis causes all *except:*
A. Blurring of vision
B. Yellow vision
C. Nephropathy, neuralgia
D. Nausea, vomiting. Anorexia

13. Digitalis toxicity is enhanced by all *except:*
A. Cor pulmonale B. CCP
C. Hypothyroidism D. Hyperthyroidism

14. In a patient with bilateral renal artery stenosis, drug contraindicated is:
A. ACE-I
B. Beta blockers
C. Calcium channel blockers
D. Diuretics

15. In CHF, all are increased *except:*
A. Renin B. Catecholamines
C. Vasopressin D. Sodium

16. Maximum O_2 consumption at rest and with maximum execise is:
A. 100/600 B. 200/1200
C. 200/600 D. 100/1200

17. JVP event occurring before QRS in ECG is:
A. Wave "a" B. Wave "c"
C. Descent "x" D. Wave "v"

18. Eisenmengers is seen earliest in:
A. AP window B. VSD
C. PDA D. ASD

19. Digoxin was discovered by:
A. William Wethering
B. Duckett Jones
C. Sones
D. Andrew Gruentzig

20. High output failure is likely in all of the following *except:*
A. Anemia B. Thyrotoxicosis
C. Pregnancy D. Beriberi

21. Treatment of hypertension prevents all *except:*
A. CAD B. CRF
C. CVA D. Heart failure

22. Mortality is highest with:
A. Supracardiac TAPVC
B. Infradiaphragmatic TAPVC
C. Intracardiac TAPVC
D. None of the above

23. Commonest cause of Cyanotic CHD after 1 month is:
A. VSD B. ASD
C. TOF D. Ebstein's anomaly

24. CHF is seen earliest in:
A. Hypoplastic Left heart syndrome
B. Myocarditis
C. Coronary arterial fistula
D. CoA

25. BT shunt is:
A. Subclavian artery to pulmonary artery
B. Descending aorta to pulmonary artery
C. Ascending aorta to pulmonary artery
D. None of the above

26. Worst proarrhythmic drug is:
A. Amiodarone B. Verapamil
C. Phenytoin D. Lidocaine

27. Least proarrhythmic drug among following is:
A. Amiodarone B. Flecainide
C. Phenytoin D. Quinidine

28. Treatment of choice in wide QRS tachycardia is:
A. Adenosine B. Procainamide
C. Verapamil D. Diltiazem

29. BP difference of 5 mm Hg between both upper limbs is seen with all *except:*
A. CoA
B. Subclavian artery from descending aorta
C. Supravalvular AS
D. Subaortic AS

---

12 C 13 B 14 A 15 D 16 B 17 A 18 A 19 A 20 C 21 A 22 B 23 C 24 A
25 A 26 A 27 C 28 B 29 D

30. Systolic thrill in ASD is suggestive of:
A. Large shunt
B. PS
C. Ostium primum ASD
D. Endocardial cushion defect

31. Predictor of prognosis within 12 hours after MI is:
A. Thallium scanning
B. Successful thrombolysis
C. CPK decrease
D. Angina

32. Low voltage DC shock is most successful in:
A. AF
B. Atrial flutter
C. PAT
D. Ventricular tachycardia

33. Post MI cardiac index is 1.8 L/min/m^2, CVP is 6; treatment of choice is:
A. i/v fluids B. NTG
C. Inotropes D. Beta blockers

34. Continuous murmur is heard in all *except:*
A. Lutembacher's syndrome
B. PS with PFO
C. Supracardiac TAPVC
D. PDA

35. Ideal management of ↑ PR, AH of 180 msec and HV of 100 msec and LBBB is:
A. AAI B. VVI
C. DDD D. None of the above

36. Pseudoinfarct pattern is seen in all *except:*
A. WPW Type A B. COPD
C. HOCM D. LVH

37. Vascular complications are maximum with:
A. SBP B. DBP
C. Mean BP D. None of the above

38. Intracoronary stenting is advantageous in all of the following forms *except:*
A. Decrease rate of restenosis < 25%
B. Prevents abrupt vessel closure
C. Decrease incidence of subacute thrombosis
D. None of the above

39. In resting membrane, permeability is decreased to all *except:*
A. Na B. Cl
C. K D. H_2O

40. Which reflex is used to terminate PSVT:
A. Diving refles B. Maries reflex
C. Bainbridge reflex D. Bezold Jarisch relex

41. LV enlargement is seen in:
A. VSD B. ASD
C. RSOV to RA D. PS

42. All of the following are true statements about RSOV *except:*
A. Occur in < 10 years age commonly
B. Supracristal VSD associated with rupture of Rt sided sinus of valsalva aneurysm
C. Noncoronary cusps generally ruptures into RA
D. Rupture of left coronary sinus is very rare

43. LAHB is confused with:
A. ASMI B. IWMI
C. Anterolateral MI D. Posterior wall MI

44. Least oxygen saturation is seen in:
A. RA B. RV
C. PA D. Coronary sinus

45. Best method of absorbing alveolar gas is:
A. IPPV
B. SIMV
C. 100% O_2 inhalation
D. None of the above

46. Which drugs worsens angina in HOCM:
A. Nitrates B. ACE #
C. Beta Blockers D. Aspirin

30 B 31 D 32 B 33 A 34 B 35 C 36 A 37 A 38 C 39 C 40 A 41 C 42 A
43 B 44 D 45 A 46 A

47. In CHF, nitrate is useful by:
A. Decreasing preload
B. Increase preload
C. Increasing heart rate
D. Increasing cardiac output

48. Idioventricular rhythm of 90/mt requires which of the following treatment:
A. No treatment B. I/v lignocaine
C. I/v procainamide D. Pacemaker

49. VT with increase QT require:
A. I/v propanalol B. Quinidine
C. Verapamil D. Mexiletine

50. Which of the following is not true about CPR:
A. Massage 80-100/minute
B. Sternal compression 3-5 cm
C. Lungs inflated 10-12/minute
D. Two breaths after 5 compressions with 2 rescuers

51. Treatment of choice for multiple VSD' s with CHF when medical treatment fails is:
A. Patch closure
B. Pulmonary artery banding
C. Fontan's operation
D. None of the above

52. Reversed split is seen in all *except:*
A. LBBB B. AS
C. PDA D. WPW Type A

53. Right sided aortic arch is commonly associated with:
A. Truncus arteriosus B. VSD
C. D-TGA D. Coarctation of aorta

54. HF in 3-6 months of life is seen in:
A. Primary endocardial fibroelastosis
B. VSD
C. ASD
D. Pulmonary atresia

55. Al are seen in acute AR *except:*
A. Hill's sign B. EDM
C. LVS4 D. Soft S1

56. Best drug for secondary prophylaxis after MI is:
A. Nitrates B. Beta Blockers
C. Aspirin D. Statins

57. Asymmetric septal hypertrophy is seen in all *except:*
A. HOCM B. AS
C. PS D. Post wall MI

58. RA pressure 8 mm Hg, TR jet 4m/sec RVSP is:
A. 72 mm Hg B. 80 mm Hg
C. 84 mm Hg D. 64 mm Hg

59. Predominant venous dilator is:
A. NTG B. Hydralazine
C. ACE inhibitor D. None of the above

60. Dp/Dt decrease is achieved by which drug in aortic dissection:
A. Propanolol
B. Calcium channel blocker
C. NTG
D. Na Nitraprusside

61. CASS trial shows significant mortality benefit in:
A. TVD with LV dysfunction
B. DVD with LV dysfunction
C. TVD with normal LV function
D. DVD with proximal LAD involvement

62. Pacemaker battery is made of:
A. Lithium B. Nickel cadmium
C. Gold D. Diamond

63. Pacemaker of choice in sick sinus syndrome with intact A-V nodal conduction is:
A. AAIR B. DDDR
C. VDDD D. VVVI

47 A 48 A 49 D 50 D 51 B 52 D 53 A 54 A 55 A 56 C 57 D 58 A 59 A
60 A 61 A 62 A 63 A

64. Treatment of choice in neurocardiogenic syncope is:
A. Beta blocker
B. DDDR
C. Disopyramide
D. Quinidine

65. Cyanosis may be seen in all of the following *except:*
A. Severe PS
B. TAPVC
C. Common Atrium
D. ASD

66. Cause of CHF in fetus can be:
A. Large VSD
B. PDA
C. Ostium primum ASD
D. Hypoplastic left heart syndrome

67. Fetal echocardiography cannot detect:
A. CHB
B. TGA
C. PDA
D. Hypoplastic left heart syndrome

68. Paradoxical septal motion is seen in:
A. HOCM
B. RV Volume overload
C. ASD
D. PDA

69. Gradient of AS in presence of PDA is:
A. Overestimated
B. Underestimated
C. No effect
D. None of the above

70. RV systolic pressure is more than LV systolic pressure in:
A. Eisenmenger syndrome
B. TOF
C. PS with Intact IVS
D. PDA with bidirectional shunt

71. In a patient of ASD with MS, PCWP is 15 mm Hg, RA pressure will be:
A. 5 mm Hg
B. 15 mm Hg
C. 20 mm Hg
D. 10 mm Hg

72. Nonionic dye used in coronary angiography has following benefits over ionic dye *except:*
A. Less allergy
B. Less arrhythmias
C. Less incidence of renal dysfunction
D. Decrease incidence of coronary thrombosis

73. Continuous wave doppler signal will be useful in all *except:*
A. RSOV
B. PDA
C. Coronary AV fistula
D. None of the above

74. Which of the following statement is false about myocardial bridging ?
A. Seen in 25% of patients with coronary artery disease
B. Generally seen in LAD territory
C. Can mimic acute coronary syndrome
D. Rarely seen in RCA territory

75. A2-OS gap is decreased in all *except:*
A. Severe MS
B. Subvalvular fusion
C. Aortic regurgitation
D. Calcification of valves

76. Delayed closure of TV in echocardiography is seen in:
A. Ebstein's anomaly
B. RA myxoma
C. TS
D. TR

77. Treatment of choice of acute occlusion during PTCA is:
A. Intracoronary stenting
B. Atherectomy
C. Thrombolysis
D. i/v heparin

64 A 65 D 66 D 67 C 68 B 69 A 70 C 71 B 72 D 73 D 74 A 75 C 76 A 77 A

78. Prominent y descent in JVP is seen in:
A. Constrictive pericarditis
B. Cardiac tamponade
C. PS
D. MS

79. Equalization of diastolic pressure in all 4 chambers is seen in:
A. CCP B. Cardiac tamponade
C. ASD D. VSD

80. In ECG disappearance of Q waves in case of MI occurs in what percentage of patients in 2 years?
A. 20-30% B. 5-10%
C. 10-70% D. 30-40%

81. Following statements is true about probucol:
A. Drug of choice in familial hypercholesterolemia
B. No antioxidant effect
C. Increase LDL-C
D. Decrease HDL-C

82. Treatment of asymptomatic severe AS in old age is:
A. AVR
B. Balloon aortic valvuloplasty
C. Conservative management
D. Beta blockers

83. Treatment of choice for severe PS is:
A. Balloon pulmonary valvuloplasty
B. Pulmonary valve replacement
C. Ross procedure
D. Diuretics

84. Fontan's operation is done in:
A. Tricuspid atresia B. TOF
C. D-TGA D. C-TGA

85. Complication of modified BT shunt are all *except:*
A. Ipsilateral limb shortening
B. IE
C. Shunt blockage
D. CHF

86. Longest action potential duration is seen in:
A. SA node B. AV node
C. Atrial muscle D. Purkinje fibers

87. Atrial situs is best made out by:
A. Descending aorta B. Stomach bubble
C. Liver D. Left bronchus

88. Following is least commonly seen in Down's syndrome:
A. AV canal defect B. PDA
C. TOF D. TGA

89. Pulmonary oedema with normal pulmonary capillary wedge pressure is seen in:
A. HAPE B. MS
C. Cortriatriatum D. AS

90. Which mechanism is responsible for atrial flutter:
A. Reentry
B. Automaticity
C. Triggered activity
D. None of the above

78 A 79 A 80 A 81 D 82 A 83 A 84 A 85 A 86 D 87 D 88 D 89 A 90 A

AIIMS 1994

1. **All of the following can occur because of chest trauma *except:***
   A. VSD B. MR
   C. Coronary occlusion D. Aneurysm

2. **Digitalis was discovered by:**
   A. William Withering
   B. Andreas Gruntzig
   C. Duckett Jones
   D. William Sones

3. **Treatment of choice for Torsades de pointes syndrome is:**
   A. Overdrive pacing B. iv magnesium
   C. iv amiodarone D. DC shock

4. **Coronary artery origin can be best seen in which view:**
   A. PLAX
   B. Parasternal short axis view
   C. Apical 4 chamber view
   D. None of the above

5. **Which of the following drug was not used in CAST trial:**
   A. Flecainide B. Moricizine
   C. Amiodarone D. Encainide

6. **Which of the following antihypertensives is not used in pregnancy:**
   A. Diuretics B. Beta blockers
   C. Hydralazine D. Methyl dopa

7. **Fetal echocardiogram is done at which gestational age:**
   A. 14 weeks B. 16 weeks
   C. 20 weeks D. 24 weeks

8. **Which of the following is not teratogenic:**
   A. Labetalol B. Lithium
   C. Phenytoin fetal D. Retinoic acid

9. **Commonest complication of ACE inhibitor therapy:**
   A. Hyperkalemia B. Angioedema
   C. Renal impairment D. Cough

10. **Drug causing gynecomastia:**
    A. Amiloride B. Frusemide
    C. Thiazdes D. Spironolactone

11. **Which pace maker is preferred in patients with HOCM:**
    A. VVI B. VVIR
    C. DDD D. AAI

12. **Murmur of HOCM decreases with:**
    A. Squatting
    B. Standing
    C. Amylnitrate
    D. Strain phase of valsalva

13. **Prominent × descent is seen with:**
    A. TS B. Cardiac tamponade
    C. CCP D. RCMP

1 D 2 A 3 B 4 B 5 C 6 A 7 B 8 A 9 D 10 D 11 C 12 A 13 B

14. Severity of MS is affected in what way by presence of AR by p ½ method:
A. Overestimated B. Underestimated
C. No effect D. None of the above

15. MVA calculated by p ½ is ......:
A. Inversely proportional
B. Directly proportional
C. Inverse to square
D. None of the above

16. Acute MI with normal coronaries at 4-6 hours interval is seen in:
A. Less than 5% B. 6-10%
C. 10-20% D. Greater than 20%

17. Earliest peaking of which enzyme occurs in MI:
A. CPK MB B. LDH
C. SGOT D. Myoglobin

18. Post myocardial infarction rupture occurs after:
A. 2-3 hrs B. 2-3 days
C. 2-3 weeks D. 2-3 months

19. Treatment of choice for Dressler syndrome is:
A. Aspirin B. NSAIDS
C. Paracetamol D. Heparin

20. Angioplasty done within 3-4 hours following acute MI without thrombolytic therapy is known as:
A. Primary PTCA B. Rescue PTCA
C. Immediate PTCA D. Deferred PTCA

21. Q waves might disappear after 2-3 years in how many cases of MI:
A. 2-3% B. 20-30%
C. None D. 10%

22. Lisinopril is used in which trial:
A. ISIS-4 B. GISSI-3
C. SAVE D. AIRE

23. In GUSTO trial, which of the following is most suitable thrombolytic therapy:
A. STK + heparin
B. rtPA + front loaded heparin + maintenance heparin
C. rtPA + S/c heparin
D. None of the above

24. Which of the following antilipid agents that lowers HDL has antioxidant property:
A. Probucol
B. Nicotinic acid
C. Lovastatin
D. Gemfibrozil

25. EDRF is actually what?
A. Interleukin B. TNF
C. NO D. Interferon

26. In patients of unstable angina, best therapy besides antianginals is:
A. IV heparin and disprin
B. s/c Heparin
C. IV heparin
D. Dispirin

27. Reliable sign of pericardial tamponade is:
A. Swinging heart in fluoroscopy
B. Right atrial diastolic collapse
C. RVOT diastolic collapse
D. Prominent × descent

28. In patients reaching after 3 hours of Ac MI, if CART is done then it will show spontaneous thrombolysis in:
A. 20-30% B. 10-15%
C. None D. 50%

29. Drug that is best used for producing vasospasm is:
A. Ergonovine B. Adenosine
C. Verapamil D. Dipyridamole

14 B 15 A 16 A 17 D 18 B 19 A 20 A 21 B 22 B 23 B 24 A 25 C 26 A
27 C 28 A 29 A

30. Drug that is contraindicated in prinzmetal angina is:
- **A.** Nitrates
- **B.** Calcium channel blockers
- **C.** Dispirn
- **D.** β blockers

31. pO_2 15mm, pCO_2 10 mm, pH 7.12 belongs to which of the following condition:
- **A.** TGA with large VSD
- **B.** Fallots with cyanotic spell
- **C.** Morphine overdose
- **D.** None of the above

32. Difference between non paroxysmal and paroxysmal junctional tachycardia is between:
- **A.** Rate
- **B.** A-V relationship
- **C.** Onset and offset
- **D.** None of the above

33. Hyperdynamic pulse in a one day old child could be because of:
- **A.** PDA
- **B.** CoA
- **C.** Reverse coarctation
- **D.** Systemic A-V Fistula

34. All of the following would be differential diagnosis of wide QRS tachycardia *except:*
- **A.** Preexcitation WPW syndrome with orthodromic conduction
- **B.** Supraventricular tachycardia with previous existing A-V bundle branch block
- **C.** Fascicular tachycardia
- **D.** Association of Mahaim fibres

35. Mahaim fibers terminate at:
- **A.** Anteroseptal region
- **B.** Posteroseptal region
- **C.** Bundle of HIS
- **D.** Upto A-V node

36. TEE is useful for diagnosing in all *except:*
- **A.** Pulmonary artery confluence
- **B.** Assessing prosthetic valve vegetation
- **C.** Aortic atheromas
- **D.** Assessing ascending aorta dissection

37. Treatment of thrombosis of prosthetic valves include:
- **A.** IV thrombolytic therapy
- **B.** IV heparin
- **C.** Surgery
- **D.** None of the above

38. Evidence of atrial infarction on ECG is:
- **A.** PR prolongation
- **B.** Raised PR segment
- **C.** Prolonged QT
- **D.** Q in II, III and aVF

39. Anti-platelet drugs are useful in angioplasty because they prevent:
- **A.** Long term reinfarction
- **B.** Subacute thrombosis
- **C.** Long term reocclusion
- **D.** Don't have any role

40. What happens to LVED vol at max isotonic exercise:
- **A.** Increases
- **B.** Decreases
- **C.** No change
- **D.** Varies with age

41. All are complication of modified BT shunt *except:*
- **A.** Shortening of limb
- **B.** IE
- **C.** Shunt blockage
- **D.** None of the above

42. Colour Doppler is most useful in:
- **A.** Large ASD
- **B.** Large VSD
- **C.** L-R shunt
- **D.** LV to RA shunt

43. Which of the following condition does not affect stress ECG:
- **A.** Presence of LBBB
- **B.** Multiple octopics with normal ECG
- **C.** RBBB with intermittent WPW
- **D.** None of the above

44. Best treatment for patient of WPW syndrome is:
- **A.** RFA therapy
- **B.** Amiodarone
- **C.** Surgery
- **D.** DC shock

---

30 D **31** B **32** C **33** D **34** A **35** D **36** A **37** A **38** B **39** B **40** A **41** A **42** D
43 B **44** A

45. Best investigation for vasovagal syncope is:
A. Holter test B. Treadmill test
C. Dobutamine test D. HUTT

46. Chances of embolisation are least common in:
A. Lone AF
B. Hypertension with AF
C. Rheumatic heart disease with AF
D. Dilated cardiomyopathy with AF

47. Following is the relation between pulmonary vascular resistance and systemic vascular resistance:
A. 1/8 of SVR B. 1/6 of SVR
C. 1/10 of SVR D. 1/4 of SVR

48. ROSS operation is:
A. Shift of aortic valve with homograft of pulmonary valve
B. Shift of aortic valve with xenograft of pulmonary valve
C. Shift of pulmonary valve with homograft of aortic valve
D. None of the above

49. Brokenbrough braunwald sign in HOCM is:
A. Post extrasystolic increase in gradient
B. Post extrasystolic decrease or normal pulse pressure
C. Post extrasystolic decrease in murmur
D. None of the above

50. Indication of pacemaker in sick sinus syndrome is:
A. Corrected SNRT > 525 msec
B. AF.
C. Bradyarrhythmias
D. Pacing does not improve survival

51. Highest concentration of oxygen is present in:
A. Hepaticveins
B. Coronary sinus
C. Popliteal vein
D. Superior mesenteric vein

52. Management of choice in a 64 year old asymptomatic male with severe AS is:
A. Valvotomy B. Medical therapy
C. AVR D. None of the above

53. In balloon valvotomy, valve size increases due to:
A. Valve rupture
B. Opening up of adhesions of commissure
C. Breaking of cusps
D. Papillary muscle rupture

54. In a 4 year old child systolic murmur was heard best at axilla. On evaluation it revealed peripheral pulmonary artery stenosis. Next line of management is:
A. Patient should be subjected to surgery
B. Balloon angioplasty
C. Left as it is and reassured
D. None of the above

55. Best treatment that can be given at the earliest to acute coronary syndrome is:
A. Intracoronary thrombolysis
B. i/v heparin
C. PTCA
D. PTCA with stenting

56. Myocardial infarction in a 4 year old child could be due to:
A. Anomalous origin of left coronary artery from pulmonary artery
B. Homozygous familial hypercholesterolemia
C. Combined hyperlipidemia
D. Trauma

57. Following are possible causes of childhood hypertension *except:*
A. Coarctation of aorta
B. William's syndrome
C. Subaortic stenosis
D. Renal artery stenosis

45 D 46 A 47 C 48 A 49 B 50 A 51 A 52 C 53 B 54 C 55 D 56 B 57 C

58. **All of the following are true for pulmonary embolism *except:***
A. Atrial arrhythmias
B. S1Q3T3 pattern in 25% cases
C. Non specific ST-T changes
D. PSVT

59. **All of the following will have some characteristic histological changes in myocardium *except:***
A. Amyloidosis
B. Doxorubicin toxicity
C. DCMP
D. Transplant rejection

60. **Balloon atrial septostomy is not needed in:**
A. Fallot's tetrology
B. TGA
C. Tricuspid atresia
D. Pulmonary atresia

61. **Normal HV interval is:**
A. 100-135 ms B. 75-100 ms
C. 55-75 ms D. 35-55 ms

62. **MR in patients with ostium primum ASD is due to:**
A. Cleft in mitral valve leaflets
B. Mitral valve prolapse
C. Rheumatic
D. None of the above

63. **In a patient of acute rheumatic fever, the commonest murmur is that of:**
A. MR
B. AR
C. MS
D. AS

64. **Increased morbidity and mortality during pregnancy is seen in all *except:***
A. Eisenmengers syndrome
B. TGA with VSD
C. Coarctation of aorta
D. TOF

65. **What is the blood supply to heart at maximum work:**
A. 300 ml/100gm B. 200 ml/100gm
C. 420 ml/100gm D. 100 ml/100gm

66. **Sphygmomanometer was discovered by:**
A. Rivorocci B. William Withering
C. Duckett Jones D. Andrews Gruentzig

67. **Phasic ejection click is present in:**
A. Pulmonary stenosis B. Aortic stenosis
C. Tricuspid stenosis D. Mitral stenosis

68. **In a patient of right sided aortic arch, PDA will be on:**
A. Right side
B. Left side
C. Side opposite to innominate artery
D. None of the above

69. **Eisenmenger syndrome develops early in:**
A. ASD
B. VSD
C. Aortopulmonary window
D. PDA

70. **Increase morbidity in pregnancy is seen with all *except:***
A. TGA
B. TOF
C. Eisenmengers
D. Coarctation of aorta

71. **First dose effect of postural hypotension is seen with:**
A. Methyldopa
B. Hydralazine
C. Prazosin
D. Calcium channel blockers

72. **Cholesterol increases in all *except:***
A. CRF B. CBD obstruction
C. Pregnancy D. Beta blockers

---

58 D 59 C 60 A 61 D 62 A 63 A 64 C 65 C 66 A 67 A 68 B 69 C 70 D
71 C 72 C

73. If after pulmonary balloon valvuloplasty the condition worsens then the cause could be:
A. Infundibular stenosis
B. Severe TR
C. Right to left shunt
D. Mild PR

74. CHF in infancy could be due to:
A. Coarctation of aorta
B. TGA
C. Ebsteins anomaly
D. Aortopulmonary window

75. MI in 8 weeks child could be due to:
A. Hyperaldosteronism
B. ALCAPA
C. Coronary artery dissection
D. ARCAPA

76. Cyanotic spell is precipitated by all *except:*
A. Digoxin B. Fever
C. Polycythemia D. Acidosis

77. Which of the following signifies a poor prognosis in aortic stenosis:
A. Angina B. Syncope
C. Heart failure D. None of the above

78. Spontaneous closure of VSD can occur upto what age ?
A. 2 years B. 4 years
C. 5 years D. 9 years

79. Systolic PAP-89 mm, Diastolic PAP-20 mm, Mean PAP-50 mm is seen in:
A. Valvular PS
B. Coarctation of aorta
C. Peripheral pulmonary artery stenosis
D. PAH

80. PAP can be calculated from:
A. TR B. PR jet
C. PS D. None of the above

81. PAH is seen earliest in:
A. ASD
B. VSD
C. PDA
D. Aorto pulmonary window

82. Continuous murmur is present in all *except:*
A. RSOV
B. Pulmonary atresia
C. TAPVC
D. VSD with AR

83. The commonest site of IE in PDA is:
A. Aortic valve
B. Pulmonary valve
C. Left pulmonary artery
D. Descending aorta

84. In a 52 year old male with a small PDA who is asymptomatic, treatment of choice is:
A. Surgical ligation
B. Device closure
C. IE prophylaxis
D. None of the above

85. Commonest accessory pathway for WPW is:
A. Anteroseptal
B. Posteroseptal
C. Left free wall
D. Right free wall

86. GISSI-I involves:
A. IV STK B. I/c STK
C. UK D. rtPA

87. All of the following drugs are useful in acute MI *except:*
A. Nifedipine B. Beta blocker
C. ACE inhibitor D. Aspirin

88. In a case of ASD, if thrill is found in left 2nd intercostal space, then there may be associated:
A. MS B. TR
C. MR D. PAH

73 A 74 B 75 B 76 C 77 C 78 D 79 C 80 A 81 D 82 D 83 C 84 A 85 C
86 A 87 A 88 A

89. In 10 year old child; most common cause of AS is:
- **A.** Unicuspid aortic valve
- **B.** Bicuspid aortic valve
- **C.** Tricuspid aortic valve
- **D.** Quadricuspid aortic valve

90. Survival into adulthood is seen in:
- **A.** Infracardiac TAPVC
- **B.** Ebsteins anomaly
- **C.** C-TGA
- **D.** Truncus arteriosus

89 A 90 C

AIIMS 1993

1. **ECG in myocarditis can show all *except:***
   A. CHB
   B. Sinus tachycardia
   C. LBBB
   D. ↑QRS amplitude

2. **Treatment of multiple VSD (swiss cheese) of infant with CHF is:**
   A. Primary closure
   B. Vasodilator
   C. Patch closure
   D. PA banding

3. **SPO_2 of PCWP sample is:**
   A. 70%
   B. 40%
   C. 98%
   D. 68%

4. **Wide fixed S2 is heard in:**
   A. TOF
   B. TAPVC
   C. PAPVC
   D. LBBB

5. **Incidence of VSD in AMI is maximum at:**
   A. 48 hours
   B. 2-4 days
   C. > 2 weeks
   D. > 4 weeks

6. **Dp/Dt in aortic dissection is decreased by:**
   A. Propranolol
   B. Calcium channel blockers
   C. ACE inhibitors
   D. α blockers

7. **TMT in TVD or LMCA stenosis can show:**
   A. Hypotension
   B. ST depression in V2-V4
   C. Q in II, III and aVF
   D. Inverted U in V1-V3

8. **Patient in class IV specific activity scale can perform:**
   A. 1 met
   B. 3 met
   C. 4 met
   D. 5 met

9. **All are true about clubbing *except:***
   A. Few weeks after IE
   B. Within 6 months of central cyanosis
   C. Can be seen in normal people
   D. Aortic aneurysm can produce clubbing

10. **Reverse splitting is heard in all *except:***
    A. MVP
    B. LBBB
    C. AS
    D. HOCM

11. **Continuous murmur is heard in all *except:***
    A. Unruptured sinus of valsalva
    B. RSOV
    C. PDA
    D. Coronary artery fistula

12. **Severity of AR is assessed by all *except:***
    A. Loudness of murmur
    B. Cardiomegaly
    C. length of murmur
    D. Positive Hill sign

13. **Normal coronary blood flow is:**
    A. 60-90 ml
    B. 90-120 ml
    C. 120-150 ml
    D. 150-190 ml

1 D 2 D 3 C 4 B 5 B 6 A 7 A 8 A 9 B 10 A 11 A 12 A 13 A

14. Stress test in patient with CAD with asthma can be performed using:
A. Dobutamine B. Dipyridamide
C. Adenosine D. None of the above

15. LV dysfunction of recent onset in 5 year old child with HTN is due to:
A. Renal artery stenosis
B. ALCAPA
C. RHD
D. Reverse Coarctation

16. Peak occurrence of AMI is between:
A. 6 AM to 12 noon B. 12 PM to 6 PM
C. 6 PM to 12 PM D. 12 PM to 6 AM

17. Drug of choice in differentiating SVT with aberrancy from VT is:
A. Adenosine
B. Amiodarone
C. Beta blocker
D. Calcium channel blocker

18. Indications of surgery in infective endocarditis are all *except:*
A. Persistent fever
B. A. root abscess
C. Late prosthetic valve endocarditis
D. Recurrent thrmboembolism

19. Success of CABG depends upon:
A. Number of vessels bypassed
B. State of LV function
C. Age of patient
D. Duration of angina

20. Adverse outcome in pregnancy is seen with all *except:*
A. MVP B. Coarctation
C. Eisenmenger D. TOF

21. Commonest cause of syncope:
A. Postural B. Vasovagal
C. Drugs D. None of the above

22. Pulmonary artery hypertension is caused by:
A. Paragonimiasis B. Schistosomiasis
C. Filariasis D. E Coli

23. All are antioxidants *except:*
A. Pantothenic acid B. Vitamin E
C. Vitamin C D. Vitamin A

24. Treatment of hyperhomocysteinemia is:
A. Folic acid B. Vit B12
C. Vit A D. Vit K

25. Class III antiarrhythmics acts through:
A. K^+ channels B. Cl^- channels
C. Na^+ channels D. Ca^{++} channels

26. Monitoring of amiodarone therapy requires all *except:*
A. Chest X-ray B. ECG
C. Serum level D. LFT

27. Valvular vs. subvalvular AS is differentiated by:
A. Ejection click
B. Aortic root dilatation
C. Soft A2
D. Ejection systolic murmur

28. CABG is better in:
A. TVD with good LV function
B. TVD with LV dysfunction
C. DVD with LV dysfunction
D. SVD with LV dysfunction

29. In hyperkalemia, cardiotoxicity is increased by:
A. Alkalosis
B. Hypocalcemia
C. Hyponatremia
D. None of the above

30. CI 1.8 L/min/m^2; PCWP 10 in a patient of MI. Treatment of choice is:
A. Inotropes B. IABP
C. IV fluids D. NTG

14 A 15 A 16 A 17 A 18 C 19 B 20 A 21 B 22 B 23 A 24 A 25 A 26 C
27 A 28 B 29 B 30 C

31. In cardiogenic shock; in hospital survival is improved by:
A. Angioplasty
B. IABP
C. Medical management
D. None of the above

32. Drug that does not cross placenta is:
A. Hydralazine B. Heparin
C. Quinidine D. Procainamide

33. Treatment of choice in BPH with hypertension is:
A. Prazosin
B. Beta blockers
C. Calcium channel blocker
D. Na nitroprusside

34. CHF is characterised by all *except:*
A. ↓ A-V O_2 difference
B. ↓ CO
C. ↑ LV filling pressure
D. Oliguria

35. Apical obliteration in echocardiography is seen in:
A. EMF B. Sarcoidosis
C. Amyloidosis D. HOCM

36. ASH is seen in all *except:*
A. AS B. HOCM
C. Post MI D. PAH

37. LVEDP = 20 mm Hg, RAP = 18 mm Hg, PCWP = 19 mm Hg, RVEDP = 20 mm Hg; Diagnosis is:
A. Restrictive CMP B. CCP
C. MI D. TAPVC

38. Fontan operation is done in:
A. TOF
B. Single ventricle with PS
C. TA with PS
D. TAPVC

39. STK in pulmonary embolism is given to:
A. Prevent recurrent embolic episodes
B. Open the occluded artery
C. Decrease the size of pulmonary infarction
D. All of the above

40. Bisferians pulse is best felt in:
A. Brachial artery
B. Carotid artery
C. Femoral artery
D. Radial artery

41. Regarding cholesterol; all are true *except:*
A. 1% decrease in HDL-C decreases the cardiac mortality by 2-3%
B. 1% increase in HDL-C decreases the CAD risk by 1-2%
C. Exercise increases HDL-C
D. Moderate alcohol intake increase HDL-C

42. Isolated VPC in a normal individual who is asymptomatic is best managed by:
A. No drugs
B. Beta blockers
C. Calcium channel blockers
D. Amiodarone

43. NTG is useful in CHF mainly by:
A. Decreasing preload
B. Decreasing Afterload
C. Decreasing cardiac output
D. Decreasing heart rate

44. ↑ Incidence of CAD in overseas Indians is because of:
A. Social deprivation
B. Carbohydrate intolerance
C. Alcoholism
D. Smoking

45. EF is overestimated in case of:
A. AR B. MS
C. MR D. AS

31 A 32 B 33 A 34 A 35 A 36 C 37 B 38 C 39 D 40 B 41 A 42 A 43 A
44 B 45 C

46. $\uparrow$ L $\rightarrow$ R shunt in ASD is seen with:
A. MR
B. AR
C. Anemia
D. PAH

47. All can be seen in cyanotic spells *except:*
A. Absent murmur
B. Hypotension
C. Normal splitting of second heart sound
D. Acidosis

48. Diastolic murmur at apex is heard in all *except:*
A. ASD
B. MR
C. VSD
D. Ac Rheumatic fever

49. Severity of MR is assessed by all *except:*
A. Cardiomegaly
B. Loudness of murmur
C. Wide splitting of S2
D. MDM

50. ACE inhibitor are not effective in:
A. Blacks
B. Renovascular HTN
C. Diabetic
D. LVH

51. In athletes all can be heard *except:*
A. S3
B. Early diastolic murmur
C. Ejection systolic murmur Gr.II
D. None of the above

52. Chest pain is aggravated with NTG in which of the following:
A. HOCM
B. Subendocardial ischaemia
C. Chronic stable angina
D. MI

53. Cardiac tamponade is most likely with:
A. Bronchogenic carcinoma
B. Acute rheumatic fever
C. Tuberculosis
D. Sarcoidosis

54. Atrial fibrillation with HR of 60/min indicates:
A. Digitalis toxicity
B. Beta blockers effect
C. Patient on amiodarone therapy
D. None of the above

55. $\uparrow$ QT is seen with all *except:*
A. Amiodarone
B. Quinidine
C. Flecainide
D. Xylocaine

56. Long QT interval is best treated by:
A. β blocker
B. Calcium channel blocker
C. Amiodarone
D. Quinidine

57. HOCM murmur increases with all *except:*
A. Valsalva II
B. Leg raising
C. Isoprenaline
D. Post extra systolic beat

58. Pulmonary oedema with normal PCWP is seen in:
A. MS
B. High altitude pulmonary oedema
C. Cortriatriatum
D. AS

59. Normotensive TR is seen in all *except:*
A. Pulmonary thromboembolism
B. Ebstein's anomaly
C. Trauma
D. Carcinoid

60. Severity of TOF is decided by:
A. Pulmonary stenosis
B. Override of aorta
C. VSD
D. ASD

46 A 47 C 48 A 49 B 50 A 51 B 52 A 53 A 54 A 55 D 56 A 57 B 58 B
59 A 60 A

61. Emergency TPI in MI is indicated in:
A. LBBB
B. First degree heart block
C. RBBB
D. Alternating bundle branch block

62. Pacemaker of choice in 65 year old lady with frequent long sinus pauses with maximum predicted heart rate of more than 95% on TMT is:
A. AAI B. DDD
C. VDD D. None of the above

63. Most common accessory pathway in WPW syndrome is:
A. Left Lateral pathway
B. Left Anteroseptal pathway
C. Left Posteroseptal pathway
D. Right free wall pathway

64. Non synchronized DC shock is used for:
A. VF B. A flutter
C. AF D. VT

65. Arrhythmia which is least likely to occur in a structurally normal heart is:
A. PSVT B. A flutter
C. VT with LBBB D. VPCS

66. In treatment of USA all are useful *except:*
A. Thrombolytic therapy
B. Beta blockers
C. Aspirin
D. Heparin

67. All can be seen in pheochromocytoma *except:*
A. Pallor B. Pigmentation
C. Palpitation D. Perspiration

68. PaO_2 = 85 mm Hg, P CO_2 = 20 mm Hg, pH-7.2; the likely diagnosis is:
A. Pulmonary oedema
B. Anxiety neurosis
C. Phenobarbiturate poisoning
D. DKA

69. Continuous murmur is heard in all *except:*
A. Peripheral PS B. AP Window
C. RSOV D. PDA

70. Normal coronaries in acute MI are seen in:
A. < 5% B. 6-10%
C. 10-20% D. 20-30%

71. Sixty year male with intermittent atrial fibrillation. All are indicated as treatment *except:*
A. PTCA
B. Anticoagulation
C. I c drugs
D. Amiodarone

72. Angiotensinogen is formed mainly by:
A. Lung B. Liver
C. Kidney D. Heart

73. Pulsus alternans is seen in all *except:*
A. SVT (recovering)
B. Severe AR with or without AS with normal LV function
C. Electrical alternans
D. LVF

74. VSD with Eissenmenger syndrome; best treatment is:
A. Heart lung transplantation
B. Heart transplantation
C. Bilateral lung transplantation
D. Unilateral Lung transplantation

75. R.F. ablation is successful in all *except:*
A. A.F B. AVNRT
C. A. flutter D. Accessory pathway

76. HUTT is useful in diagnosis of:
A. LV dysfunction
B. Vasovagal syncope
C. Myocardial viability
D. None of the above

61 D 62 A 63 A 64 A 65 B 66 A 67 B 68 A 69 B 70 A 71 A 72 B 73 B 74 A 75 A 76 B

77. Isotonic exercise will show:
A. LVEDV ↑ B. LVEDV ↓
C. Remains same D. None of the above

78. Snowman appearance on chest X-ray is characteristic of:
A. TAPVC B. PAPVC
C. ASD D. A-V septal defect

79. Contraindicated in prinzmetal angina:
A. β Blocker B. NTG
C. Ca^{++} blocker D. α Blocker

80. Weight of heart in adult man is:
A. 100 gm B. 250 gm
C. 350 gm D. 450 gm

81. Sail like sound is heard in:
A. Ebsteins anomaly
B. TR
C. RSOV
D. Bicuspid aortic valve

82. Reverse splitting is heard in all *except:*
A. LBBB B. HOCM
C. AS D. WPW type A

83. Balloon atrial septostomy is indicated in:
A. TGA B. TOF
C. C-TGA D. Tricuspid atresia

84. Amylnitrate in MVP will move murmur:
A. Close to S1 B. Away from S1
C. No effect D. None of the above

85. Equalisation of oxygen saturation of all 4 chambers indicates:
A. PAPVC B. TAPVC
C. ASD D. VSD

86. Reverse pulsus paradoxus is seen with:
A. IPPV B. COPD
C. Pregnancy D. Cardiac tamponade

87. Opening snap is heard in:
A. TS B. MS
C. ASD D. All of the above

88. Fetal heart will start beating by:
A. 3 weeks B. 6 weeks
C. 7 weeks D. 5 weeks

89. Incidence of tricuspid valve involvement in RHD is:
A. 10% B. 15%
C. 20-30% D. 50%

90. Balloon valvuloplasty is treatment of choice in:
A. PS B. TS
C. MS D. AS

77 A 78 A 79 A 80 C 81 A 82 D 83 A 84 A 85 B 86 A 87 D 88 A 89 C 90 A

SGPGI 2003 (December)

1. **Regarding cardiac transplant:**
   - **A.** Incomplete/complete RBBB very common
   - **B.** PR & QT prolonged
   - **C.** Transition zone shifted leftward
   - **D.** Supraventricular arrhythmias are often mild and self limited
   - **E.** Appearance of sudden AV block denotes rejection

2. **Bifid T wave in 12 lead ECG:**
   - **A.** Normally seen in 20% of children
   - **B.** In children best seen in V_1V_2
   - **C.** In adults best seen in V_5V_6
   - **D.** Always suggests ischemia
   - **E.** Suggests delayed RV repolarization

3. **Regarding T wave inversion in precordial leads in normal 12 lead ECG:**
   - **A.** Restricted to right precordial leads in children < 2 years
   - **B.** Common in elderly (female)
   - **C.** African Americans
   - **D.** Vagotonic patients
   - **E.** With ingestion of cold water

4. **Normal 12 lead ECG in 40 year male:**
   - **A.** Transition zone V_3V_4
   - **B.** RV forces overshadowed by LV forces and not represented
   - **C.** VAT is initial event of QRS to appears
   - **D.** VAT >0.06 secs
   - **E.** Atrial p wave activity improved by keeping both RA and LA leads over sternum

5. **U wave in 40 year old malesame direction as T wave:**
   - **A.** Taller in V_5V_6
   - **B.** Upto 10% of T wave amplitude
   - **C.** May be due to purkinje fibre repolarization
   - **D.** Tachycardia raises height of U waves
   - **E.** It may represent ventricular relaxation

6. **Atrial infarction:**
   - **A.** ≤10% of total MI
   - **B.** Isolated atrial infarction very rare
   - **C.** Ta depression may be associated with elevation in reciprocal leads
   - **D.** PR segment seen better with AV block
   - **E.** LA ruptures more commonly than RA rupture

7. **In acute MI additional ST elevation in 1st hour:**
   - **A.** Seen in >60% of reperfused patients
   - **B.** Infarct extension may be one of the cause
   - **C.** Persists with thrombolysis
   - **D.** Even after 30 days and 1 year, mortality same
   - **E.** Additional ST elevation comes down early with PTCA

8. **ECG in reperfusion:**
   - **A.** AIVR is good indicator
   - **B.** CPK higher peak early fall with reperfusion
   - **C.** Best indicator is settling ST segment
   - **D.** >50% ST elevation fall suggestive of good prognosis
   - **E.** Early settling ST segment–means decreased reinfarction

9. ECG in myocardial ischemia:

A. ST depression in V_5V_6 in IWMI is suggestive of RCA involvement
B. ST depression in aVF is suggestive of Px LCx lesion
C. ST depression is suggestive of subendocardial ischemia
D. ST elevation in $V_5V_6 > V_1V_2$ suggestive of LM disease
E. ST depression in V_1V_2 V_3 with elevation in II, V_4 R is suggestive of RCA in IWMI

10. LAE on ECG:

A. Proximal terminal force in V_1 >0.04 msec is more sensitive than proximal terminal force in V1 >1mm
B. Proximal terminal force V_1 >1mm more specific than $PTFV_1$ >0.04 sec
C. Duration between 2 peaks of P >0.04 sec is more sensitive for diagnosis than Morris index
D. Is characterised by shift of axis to the left
E. Shortening of PR segment

11. QT prolongation:

A. Hypokalemia and Hypocalcemia
B. Post tachycardia
C. Hypermagnesemia
D. SAH
E. Hypothermia

12. J Point shift:

A. Calcium channel blocker
B. Digoxin
C. Hypothermia
D. Ischemia
E. Tachycardia

13. In hepatic dysfunction, dose modification is required for:

A. Procainamide
B. Disopyramide
C. Amiodarone
D. Lidocaine
E. Ibutilide

14. Which drug acts on accessory pathway?

A. Adenosine
B. Procainamide
C. Digoxin
D. Quinidine
E. Disopyramide

15. Digoxin level:

A. Amiodarone increases its level
B. Verapamil increases its level
C. Dilzem decreases its level
D. Triamterene increases its level
E. Spironolactone decreases its level

16. Non peptide Gp IIb/IIIa inhibitors are:

A. Lamifiban
B. Eptifibatide
C. Tirofiban
D. Abciximab
E. Fradafiban

17. Antiplatelets with mechanism through ADP pathway:

A. Ridogrel
B. Ticlopidine
C. Aspirin
D. Abciximab
E. Tirofiban

18. Brain natriuretic peptide:

A. <20% of ANP
B. Normally secreted by normal LV
C. >100pg/ml suggestive of poor prognosis in CHF
D. No prognostic significance
E. Increased in RV dysfunction in cor pulmonale

19. Ventricle as necessary pathway in reentry:

A. AVNRT
B. AVRT
C. VT
D. AFib
E. Atrial flutter

20. Paradoxical split S_2 is heard in:

A. LV pacing
B. WPW type B
C. PDA
D. AR severe
E. PPH

21. Vectorcardiography:
A. Type A → ASD
B. Type C → COPD
C. Type A initially counterclockwise followed by clockwise right anterior
D. Type B mainly right and left posterior
E. Type C → counterclockwise right

22. Regarding rheumatic fever:
A. Endemic infection most common
B. All streptococcal strains may cause rheumatic fever
C. Persistent tonsilar infection is necessary
D. ASO titre specific
E. Genetic susceptibility seen

23. In Rheumatic fever:
A. Untreated arthritis last 2-3 months
B. Short P-R is a minor criteria
C. Carditis in 60% cases
D. Aschoff nodules pathognomonic
E. Chorea present in 3rd week

24. VSD with AR:
A. In 5-8% of the patients
B. AR will decrease left → Rt shunt
C. Subpulmonic VSD most common with AR
D. Perimembranous VSD → AR occurs because of lack of support of AV cusp
E. Commonly occurs by 5 years age

25. Obligatory mixture intracardiac shunting:
A. TAPVC
B. Complete TGA
C. Corrected TGA
D. Truncus arteriosus
E. Pulmonary atresia

26. Coronary anomalies:
A. Acquired in CoA
B. Congenital disease most commonly associated is TOF
C. Usually congenital in pulmonary atresia with intact VSD
D. Where coronary artery passes between aorta and pulmonary artery associated with CHD
E. When RCA passes between aorta and pulmonary artery not associated with CHD

27. In Acute coronary syndrome with mild coronary stenosis:
A. Less collaterals
B. Increased lipid content of plaque
C. More in numbers
D. Calcification
E. Increased collagen

28. According to NASPE pacemaker code:
A. 2nd letter suggestive of chamber sensed
B. 4th letter suggest antitachycardia pacing
C. 5th letter rate modulation
D. Programmability C for communicability
E. In antitachyarrhythmia, S suggests shock

29. Implanted permanent pacemaker:
A. Radiation may cause sensing dysfunction
B. Tip ectopy morphology same but not preceded by stimuli
C. Endless loop tachycardia always requires intact VA conduction
D. Atrial trial rhythm affected by DVI
E. Ventricular rhythm not affected by AT

30. Rate responsive pacemakers:
A. Accelerator sensor better than piezo electric
B. Transthoracic impudence is used for rate and respiratory volume
C. Arterial saturation better than mixed venous saturation
D. End of T wave used
E. Horizontal motion better than vertical motion

31. True about transmembrane potential of ventricular muscle cell:
A. RMP -80 to -90mV
B. Depolarisation upto + 30 mv
C. Vmax: 100-200v/sec
D. Propagation velocity 0.7 m/sec
E. Action potential amplitude 100-300 mv

32. True or False:
A. Calcium binds to trop I
B. Calcium binds to trop T
C. Tropomyosin inhibits actin myosin interaction
D. Myosin binds directed to Z line
E. CCB's acts on T type channels

33. True or False:

A. Calcium uptake during relaxation blocked by ryanodine
B. During relaxation calcium released by SERCA
C. β blocker inhibited by SERCA
D. Calsequestrin stores calcium
E. Calsequestrin degrades calcium

34. Atrial activity and ECG:

A. Vector of p wave 1st posterior and than anterior
B. Early activation of Right atrium septum
C. Atrial depolarisation and repolarization follow the same path
D. Ventricular depolarisation and repolarization occur in opposite direction
E. Prominent Ta mimick Q wave

35. True or False

A. Regular cannon in isorhythmic AV dissociation
B. Irregular cannon in AV junctional rhythm
C. 'a' may be absent in hyperkalemia
D. Single wave in TR
E. V wave prominent in Gerbode defect

36. Prominent y descent:

A. MR
B. RCM
C. CCP
D. Gerbode defect
E. LV aneurysm (Pseudo)

37. PCWP and LA pressure disparity is seen in:

A. MS
B. High pleural pressure
C. Catheter in dependent lung zone
D. Decreased ventricular compliance
E. Fluid overload

38. True or False about catheterization:

A. SV 55-70 ml/m^2
B. CI 2.6-4.2 L/min/m^2
C. AVO2 diff 3.5-4.0 ml/dL
D. Ventricularization of pressure by deep thrusting of catheter
E. Mean RA 0-8 mmHg

39. True/False about cardiac catheterization:

A. Fick's method is best in high CO
B. Angiography CO best for regurgitation
C. All valves areas determined by Gorlin's formula
D. L-R shunt detected by Cath upto Qp:Qs 1.1:1
E. SVR: 10-20 wood units

40. Echo in MS & MR:

A. Reduced EF slope specific
B. Doppler best non invasive technique for MR
C. Transthoracic better than Transesophageal for MR quantification
D. PISA for quantification of severity MR
E. Wilkins score used for BMV suitability

41. Reduced survival in DCMP:

A. Reduced Norepinephrine
B. Reduced Serum Na^+
C. Increased wall thickness
D. Reducing filling pressure
E. IVCD

42. Reversible defect T/F:

A. Seen only with thallium
B. PET for viable myocardium
C. Seen with reperfusion after acute MI
D. Indicates myocardial ischemia
E. 20% irreversible defects on thallium scan become reversible on PET

43. High risk:

A. Decreased NH_3 and No FDG uptake
B. Multiple defects in different vascular territories
C. Unable to do >3 mets
D. LV dilatation not seen
E. Exercise induced increased EDV and Increased ESV

44. Electrophysiologic study:

A. SNRT >1500 msec
B. AV internal 55-130
C. AV conduction from 1st deflection of HBE and Vent activity on HBE
D. HV interval from 1st deflection HBE to 1st deflection in surface ECG or ventricular depolarisation in HBE
E. In VT, HV interval less than normal sinus HV interval

45. Chronotropic incompetence:

A. Chronotropic incompetence suggestive of poor prognosis
B. Chronotropic index > 0.8 suggestive of poor prognosis
C. Chronotropic index: HR peak - HRrest/220 - age in years–HR rest
D. Digoxin may cause chronotropic incompetence
E. Unaffected by exercise protocol and exercise time

46. Myocardial involvement in pericarditis:

A. Antimyosin Indium antibody
B. Fibrinogen polymerisation test
C. Increased ADA in pericardial fluid
D. Exudative pericardial effusion
E. Raised myoglobin

47. Angiotensin II:

A. Mesangial contraction
B. Central (cerebral) dyspogesia
C. Afferent constriction
D. Decreased AVP
E. Myocyte hypertrophy

48. Trials ACE/ARB:

A. EUROPA with ramipril high risk patient
B. ELITE was with ARBS v/s ACE in LV dysfunction
C. CONSENSUS II with captopril with post MI patients
D. LIFE with lisinopril and losartan in HT patients
E. VALIANT: MI patients with normal LV function

49. Baroreceptor sensitivity:

A. Predicts ischemic ventricular response
B. <3 msec/mm Hg is a depressed response
C. Normal response: RR decrease with increased SBP
D. Post MI risk stratification
E. Post MI depression is associated with three fold increase in mortality

50. Exercise:

A. Initial increase in HR is because of vagal withdrawal
B. Supine position SV increase is because of increase in end diastolic volume
C. Standing position SV increase is because of decrease end systolic volume and increased end diastolic volume
D. Increase cardiac output after exercise upto 6 times of normal
E. Initial increase in stroke volume is due to increase in heart rate

51. Cardiopulmonary resuscitation: True/False:

A. 80-100/minute
B. Sternal compression of 3-5 cm
C. Breathing rate: 1 every 5 seconds
D. Two breath inhalations after every 5 compressions when 2 rescuers present
E. Sodium bicarbonate not preferred as it causes respiratory acidosis

52. Collagen vascular disease:

A. Polymyositis: conduction block
B. Scleroderma: pulmonary hypertension common
C. Low glucose effusion in Rh Arthritis
D. SLE: anti DSDNA maternal antibody responsible for CHB
E. Libman sach's vasculitis in ulcerative collitis

53. Hypertension:

A. Essential HT may be a cause in < 6 yrs
B. Bronchopulmonary dysplasia may be a cause in new born
C. Vascular renal and parenchymal disease is important cause beyond infancy
D. Most common cause in newborn is renal artery stenosis
E. CoA is an important cause in adolescence

54. Renal artery stenosis:

A. Aortoarteritis distal 2/3rd involved
B. Atherosclerosis >50% cases
C. Atherosclerosis affects proximal 1/3rd
D. Fibromuscular dysplasia in elderly females
E. Fibromuscular dysplasia proximal 2/3rd involved

55. Digoxin: chronic CHF in NSR:
- **A.** Improve symptoms and mortality
- **B.** Improves symptoms no effect mortality
- **C.** No effect on symptoms increased mortality
- **D.** Neurohormonal mechanism
- **E.** No effect on symptoms and mortality

56. RA desaturation more than RV:
- **A.** VSD
- **B.** LSVC–coronary sinus
- **C.** Unroofed coronary sinus
- **D.** Interrupted IVC
- **E.** SVC obstruction

57. Atrial switch operation:
- **A.** 20% atrial flutter
- **B.** <50% RV dysfunction
- **C.** Regurgitation of valve seen
- **D.** 80-90% survival at 20-30 years
- **E.** IVC and SVC obstruction goes unnoticed

58. Dystrophic calcification:
- **A.** Takes more than 6 months
- **B.** Increased acidotic environment at side
- **C.** CRF
- **D.** Posterolatral wall of LV with pseudoaneurysm
- **E.** Anterior wall of right ventricle following trauma

59. TMT in pre exitation:
- **A.** Sudden disappearance of delta wave implies shorter refractory period of antegrade pathway
- **B.** Type A WPW delta wave disappears more commonly than in type BWPW
- **C.** Delta wave disappearance with exercise is seen in 20-50%
- **D.** WPW syndrome does not compromise functional capacity
- **E.** Tachyarrhythmia's are common

60. Seen in normal person:
- **A.** RCA dominance >70%
- **B.** Sinus node artery from LCx upto 40%
- **C.** Conus artery supplies RV body
- **D.** LMCA absent
- **E.** Codominance in 7%

Answers

1 A T B T C F D F E F	2 A F B T C T D F E T	3 A T B T C T D T E T	4 A T B F C T D F E T	5 A T B F C T D T E T	6 A T B T C T D T E F	7 A F B T C T D F E T	8 A T B T C T D T E T	9 A F B F C T D F E T	10 A F B F C T D T E T
11 A T B T C F D T E T	12 A F B F C T D T E T	13 A F B T C T D T E T	14 A F B T C F D T E T	15 A T B T C F D T E F	16 A T B F C T D F E T	17 A F B T C F D F E F	18 A T B T C T D F E T	19 A F B T C T D F E F	20 A F B T C T D T E F
21 A F B T C T D F E T	22 A F B F C F D F E T	23 A F B F C F D T E F	24 A T B T C T D T E F	25 A T B T C F D F E T	26 A T B T C T D F E T	27 A T B T C T D F E F	28 A T B F C F D T E T	29 A T B T C T D T E T	30 A T B T C F D T E T
31 A T B T C T D F E F	32 A F B F C T D F E F	33 A F B F C F D T E F	34 A F B T C T D T E T	35 A T B T C T D T E T	36 A T B T C T D T E T	37 A F B F C F D F E F	38 A F B T C T D T E T	39 A F B F C T D F E T	40 A F B T C F D T E T
41 A F B T C F D F E F	42 A F B T C T D T E T	43 A F B T C T D F E F	44 A F B T C F D F E T	45 A F B F C T D T E T	46 A T B T C F D F E T	47 A T B T C F D F E T	48 A F B T C F D F E F	49 A T B T C F D T E T	50 A T B F C T D T E F
51 A T B T C T D F E T	52 A T B T C T D F E F	53 A F B T C T D T E T	54 A F B T C T D F E F	55 A F B T C F D T E F	56 A T B F C F D F E F	57 A T B T C T D T E T	58 A T B F C T D F E T	59 A F B T C T D T E T	60 A T B F C F D T E T

SGPGI 2003 (June)

1. Morphology of:
- **A.** LV-AV valve is inferior to RV-AV valves
- **B.** Multiple papillary muscles present in RV
- **C.** Moderators band is classical in RV than in LV
- **D.** Chordae of LV AV valves are attached to IVS
- **E.** Shape of RV is crescentric fine apical trabeculations

2. Sickle cell anemia is associated with:
- **A.** CMP
- **B.** Cor pulmonale
- **C.** Conduction defect
- **D.** Accelerated atherosclerosis
- **E.** Acute coronary event

3. Anti coagulants ↑sed effect due to:
- **A.** Barbiturates
- **B.** BDZ
- **C.** Phenylbutazone
- **D.** β blocker
- **E.** Amiodarone

4. Pregnancy is significantly contraindicated in which of the following:
- **A.** Eisenmengers syndrome
- **B.** Ebstein's anomaly
- **C.** Asymptomatic severe AS
- **D.** MVP with severe MR
- **E.** Marfan syndrome without AR & MR & aortic root dilatation of > 40 mmHg

5. Microvascular haemolytic anemia is seen in:
- **A.** Post CABG
- **B.** Free AR
- **C.** Prosthetic valve regurgitation
- **D.** Post aneurysmal repair
- **E.** RSOV

6. SLE features are:
- **A.** Coronary spasm
- **B.** Coronary arteritis
- **C.** Small contralateral heart
- **D.** Non-infective endocarditis
- **E.** Supraventricular tachycardia

7. Exercise and lipids are related as:
- **A.** ↓se LDL, ↓HDL, ↓TGS
- **B.** ↓se LDL, ↑se HDL
- **C.** ↓se LDL, ↓se TG
- **D.** No effect on LDL, ↓se TGS
- **E.** ↑se LDL, ↑se HDL

8. In TOF severity of cyanosis depends on:
- **A.** Site of VSD
- **B.** Severity of infundibular obstruction
- **C.** Presence of ASD
- **D.** Extent of Ao pulmonary collaterals
- **E.** Size of pulmonary artery

9. TAPVC:
- **A.** ¾ of infradiaphragmatic are obstructive
- **B.** Snowman's heart is diagnostic
- **C.** In figure of 8, the left side (upper) is formed by vertical vein
- **D.** Coronary sinus is obstructive type
- **E.** ASD in mandatory for survival

10. Vector cardiogram and RVH:
- **A.** Type A-ASD
- **B.** Type A is left & inferior with clockwise rotation
- **C.** Type B is right and posterior
- **D.** Type C is posterior & clockwise
- **E.** Type C is COPD

11. 4S study:
- **A.** ↓se in total mortality is directly correlated with ↓se in LDL-C
- **B.** ↓se in total mortality out of proportion to ↓se in LDL-C
- **C.** Mean cholesterol ↓se by 60%
- **D.** ↑se in non cardiac mortality
- **E.** ↓se TG and ↑se HDL

12. Cardiac tumors:
- **A.** Primary cardiac tumors 3.6%
- **B.** Rhabdomyomas are generally solitary
- **C.** Fibroelastomas are common at MV
- **D.** Mesotheliomas are common in females & cause SCD
- **E.** Cardiac fibroma cause SCD & arrhythmias conduction disturbances & obstructions

13. True/False:
- **A.** Atrial myxomas have hypoglobulinemia.
- **B.** 10% increase in globulins
- **C.** Raynaud's phenomenon 2.5-30%
- **D.** SCD 50%
- **E.** Rhabdomyoma are most common tumors in children

14. Secondary cardiomyopathy:
- **A.** Alcohol in the cause in 50% of secondary dilated CMP
- **B.** Diabetes has dilated CMP
- **C.** Peripartum CMP relieves completely in >50% of the patient
- **D.** Atrial flutter is major cardiac arrhythmia in alcoholic CM
- **E.** Holiday heart syndrome is associated with alcoholic CMP

15. CPK-MB:
- **A.** Carboxypeptidase converts MB-1 to MB-2
- **B.** ELISA is most sensitive and specific
- **C.** CK MB/CK activity > 71.5% is diagnostic
- **D.** MB Isoforms are elevated earlier
- **E.** Tongue & intestine are minor causes

16. True/False:
- **A.** Supravalvular AS Leopard syndrome
- **B.** Pulmonary dysplasia common in Lawwrence-Moon-Biedel syndrome
- **C.** Osler Weber Rendu–Right sided anomalies are common.
- **D.** Accelerated CAD-Progeria
- **E.** Di George syndrome-TOF

17. True/False:
- **A.** TAR-ASD
- **B.** Cornelia-de Lange syndrome-HCM
- **C.** Ellis van Creveld-Supravalvular AS
- **D.** Tuberous sclerosis–CMP & Myxomas
- **E.** Osler Weber Rendu–pulmonary AV fistula

18. Noonan syndrome:
- **A.** Malocclusion of tooth
- **B.** Undescended testes
- **C.** 50% has cardiac involvement
- **D.** Elfin facies
- **E.** Short stature

19. William Syndrome:
- **A.** Elfin facies
- **B.** Autosomal dominant
- **C.** Malocclusion of teeth
- **D.** Peripheral pulmonary artery stenosis
- **E.** Mental retardation

20. ACE inhibitor:
- **A.** Mechanism of action of angiotensin II is by type I receptor
- **B.** Tissue level of ACE are 6-7 times of circulating levels
- **C.** Nephropathy of DM1 and DM2 are prevented/ improved by
- **D.** Cough is due to histamine
- **E.** Proved to prevent coronary restenosis

21. True/False:
- **A.** When person breathes O_2 at >1 atm press HB-O_2 dissociation curve shift to right
- **B.** When 100% O_2 at ½ atm pressure PaO_2 is 700 mmHg
- **C.** 1 Atm pressure at sea level–760 mmHg
- **D.** O_2 dissolved in plasma is 0.003 ml/L
- **E.** Dissolve O_2 does not depend on Hb concentration

22. Post extrasystolic beat:
- **A.** Brokenbrough phenomenon present in valvular AS
- **B.** POST PVC–reduced filling ↑sed contractility of LV
- **C.** Long cycles–stroke volume ↑ses because of ↑se preload
- **D.** Short systole pre PVC ↓se afterload and ↑se contractility
- **E.** Post PVC–increase PS murmur

23. PTCA:
- **A.** Prevents MI
- **B.** Preserves hibernating myocardium
- **C.** Prolong survival always
- **D.** Prevent CHF
- **E.** Relieves severe angina pectoris

24. Apex phonocardiography:
- **A.** 'a' wave < 15 %
- **B.** E point denotes RV ejection
- **C.** After 'E' point there is gradual upstroke
- **D.** 'O' point coincides with mitral valve opening
- **E.** Helps in differentiating between different types of cardiac overload conditions

25. PET:
- **A.** Rb-Perfusion
- **B.** ^{15}O Perfusion
- **C.** FDG- Perfusion
- **D.** B-NH_3 Myocardial metabolism
- **E.** 20% non viable myocardium on thallium test is viable in PET

26. Proximal septal Notch:
- **A.** RBBB
- **B.** Severe TR
- **C.** Severe PR
- **D.** Congenital absence of pericardium
- **E.** Post CABG

27. Increased QT interval:
- **A.** Post tachycardia
- **B.** Subarachnoid hemorrhage
- **C.** Hypermagnesaemia
- **D.** Hypocalcemia
- **E.** Hypokalemia

28. Continuous murmur:
- **A.** ASD + MS
- **B.** VSD + AR
- **C.** Pulmonary atresia
- **D.** Severe coarctation of aorta
- **E.** Peripheral pulmonary artery stenosis

29. Cardiac transplantation:
- **A.** Severe DM–contraindicated
- **B.** End stage CAD contraindicated
- **C.** Age >50 yrs-CI
- **D.** Endomyocardial biopsy useful for detection of chronic rejection
- **E.** Accelerated atherosclerosis is commonly seen

30. CRF:
- **A.** Accelerate atherosclerosis
- **B.** Angina is singularly uncommon
- **C.** Clinically uremic pericarditis is diagnosed in 20% patient on chronic dialysis
- **D.** Can present as LV dysfunction without CAD
- **E.** Post transplant immunosuppression accelerate atherosclerosis

31. Acute MR:
- **A.** ↑se LVEDV
- **B.** ↑se LVESV
- **C.** ↓se EF
- **D.** LA pressure Normal
- **E.** LA compliance Normal

32. Re-entrant tachycardia:
- **A.** Atrial flutter
- **B.** Sinus tachycardia
- **C.** WPW associated tachycardia
- **D.** Post MI AIVR
- **E.** Prolonged QT

33. Delayed after depolarization depolarization:
A. Suppressed by CCB
B. Stimulated by catecholamines
C. Triggered activity
D. Increased automaticity
E. Prolonged cycle suppresses it

34. EMF:
A. Seen commonly in North India
B. Less common in cold climate
C. Subvalvular calcification is common
D. Severe AV regurgitation is uncommon
E. Surgery results are good

35. Cyanosis in 1st week:
A. TGA
B. TOF
C. ASD + PS
D. PA with intact vent septum
E. TAPVC

36. Cyanosis with normal heart:
A. Methemoglobinemia
B. Alveolar hypoventilation
C. Univentricular heart
D. ALCAPA
E. Anomalous systemic veins drainage to LA

37. Obligatory Intracardiac mixing:
A. TAPVC
B. Truncus arteriosus
C. Pul atresia
D. TGA
E. Corrected TGA

38. Coronary blood flow:
A. Coronary blood flow 70-90 ml/100 gm/min.
B. Myoc O_2 cons. At rest 15-20 ml/100 gm/min.
C. Coronary sinus O_2 saturation 5.5%
D. Coronary sinus O_2 content 5 ml/100 ml
E. Coronary sinus PO_2 18-20 mmHg

39. Sinus node:
A. Length 10-20 mm
B. Blood supply is by RCA in 70-80% of pts
C. Impulse originates from T cells
D. Posterior intraatrial bundles preferentially transmits from RA to LA
E. NE levels are 3-4 times more in atrial than ventricles

40. Renovascular hypertension:
A. More common in young males
B. Renin levels are high
C. In 40% of cases not responding to salt restriction
D. Salt sensitivity ↓se with age
E. High normal BP people may have low plasma volume

41. Pulsus paradoxus present in:
A. ASD
B. AR
C. PTE
D. Noneffusive constrictive pericarditis
E. Hypovolemic shock

42. Digoxin level:
A. Verapamil ↑ses
B. T4 has no effect
C. Quinidine ↑ses
D. Erythromycin ↑ses
E. Rifampicin ↓ses

43. Aneurysm:
A. Pseudoaneurysm of LV has narrow neck
B. Thoracic aneurysm operated only at size >6 cm
C. Operated if size ↑ses >0.5 m/yr.
D. Dissection progress usually proximally
E. Dissection most common in 1st trimester of pregnancy

44. Reactive hyperaemia:
A. Can occur even at occlusion of 200 msec
B. Maximal effect comes at 20 sec occlusion
C. Hypoxia, ↑se adenosine, ↑se NO, ↑se prostacyclin is responsible for it
D. Longer duration of occlusion results in ↑se duration
E. Depends on intracoronary pressure level

45. Cardiac troponins:

A. Prognostic level Trop I 1.5 and Trop T-0.1 ng/ml

B. Diagnostic level Trop I 0.1 and Trop T-0.01 ng/ml

C. Minor damage is suggested by ↑se trop T levels and normal CPK levels

D. Prognostic upper limit > 97.5%

E. In end stage renal disease: both are ↑sed

46. HUTT:

A. Optimum angle 60-80° for 20 to 45 min

B. >80° angle increases false positivity

C. Isoproterenol i/v high dose ↑se sensitivity

D. <40° angle ↓ses sensitivity

E. Sensitivity depend on population studies

47. True/False:

A. IL-1 causes hypotension, myocarditis

B. 5FU-CHF

C. Paclitaxel-arrhythmia

D. Cisplatin–Raynauds phenomenon

E. Doxorubicin-CMP

48. True/False:

A. On inspiration–TR & PR ↑ses

B. On expiration MS and MR ↑ses

C. Supravalvular gradient may occur in HOCM

D. Square wave response on valsalva in ASD and MS

E. Post extra systolic beat: PS increases

49. Post CABG ultra fast CT:

A. Proximal SVG occlusion easily visualized

B. I/V contrast is used

C. Does not visualize LIMA graft

D. Higher sensitivity and specificity for graft patency

E. Cannot distinguish fully patent and obstructed SVG

50. In A.S.:

A. Presence of anacrotic notch indicates significant AR

B. <10% of cases associated with AR

C. HF → survival for 2 years

D. Syncope–8-10 years survival

E. Angina is most common

51. True/False AS:

A. 50% are tricuspid < 15 years

B. Bicuspid valve causes severe obstruction in infancy

C. >65 years of age 40% are tricuspid

D. In rheumatoid involvement nodules thickening is present on commissure

E. As severity ↑ses murmur duration ↑ses

52. True/False:

A. In CCP no pericardial knock

B. In effuso-constrictive pericardial when pericardial fluid drained–still persistent ↑se in RA pressure–suggests SVC obstruction.

C. 80% filling in first half of diastole in RCMP

D. Systolic function is normal in RCMP

E. EMF–LV involvement in 20% cases

53. LMWH:

A. PF inhibition

B. Osteoporosis

C. Synthesized by UFH

D. Has significant role in platelet function

E. Can be given on OPD basis

54. True/False:

A. LV curve shift to left when ↓ses in LV complience

B. In cath peak to peak gradient is equal to gradient in ECHO

C. Transmitral gradient is more useful than viscoelastic properties of LV for LV filling

D. LVEDP is more useful for pulmonary congestion than mean LA pressure

E. LV tei is preload independent

55. Primary trial for SCD in amiodarone:

A. GESICA

B. Sword

C. CIDS

D. CHF-Stat

E. CAMIAT

56. SCD:
- **A.** RFA is useful in Rx of SCD
- **B.** CCB's are useful in post MI
- **C.** Mexiletine prevents primary VF
- **D.** β blockers are useful in long QT with ventricular arrhythmias
- **E.** MADIT-ICD is better than amiodarone

57. True/False:
- **A.** ↑se HR ↓ses ca entry into cell
- **B.** Relaxation requires more energy dependent Ca than contraction
- **C.** ↑se HR ↑se contractility all ↑se systolic duration (30-50%)
- **D.** Electrical activation mobilize Ca towards contract site
- **E.** Post PVC and PS↑

58. True/False:
- **A.** Diastolic movement of MV is normal in DCM
- **B.** LV elevated but RV Pr is never elevated in DCMP
- **C.** HOCM-dynamic obstruction
- **D.** Square root pattern of vent. Filling in HOCM
- **E.** Systolic functions are normal in RCM

59. Aortoarteritis:
- **A.** Inferior mesenteric artery spared
- **B.** Suprarenal aorta obstruction is MC presentation
- **C.** All three layers are involved
- **D.** Mixed lesions (stenosis/dilation) are usually present
- **E.** Retinopathy–25% of cases

60. Giant cell arteritis:
- **A.** Present in young, males & generally involve large artery
- **B.** Endarteritis is uncommon but arterial obstruction can occur
- **C.** Polymyalgia rheumatica in < 10% cases
- **D.** Rheumatic involvement of ascending aorta
- **E.** Atherosclerosis involves thoracic aorta in 25% of patients

Answers

1 A F B T C T D F E F	2 A T B T C F D F E T	3 A F B F C T D F E T	4 A T B F C T D F E T	5 A F B F C T D F E T	6 A F B T C T D T E T	7 A F B T C T D F E F	8 A F B T C F D T E F	9 A F B T C T D F E T	10 A F B T C T D F E T
11 A T B T C F D F E T	12 A F B F C T D T E T	13 A F B F C T D F E T	14 A F B F C T D F E T	15 A F B T C T D T E T	16 A F B F C F D T E T	17 A T B F C F D T E T	18 A F B T C T D F E T	19 A T B F C T D T E T	20 A T B F C T D F E F
21 A T B F C F D F E F	22 A F B F C T D F E T	23 A F B T C F D T E T	24 A T B T C F D F E T	25 A T B T C F D F E T	26 A T B T C T D T E T	27 A T B T C F D T E T	28 A T B F C T D T E T	29 A T B F C F D T E T	30 A T B T C F D T E T
31 A T B F C F D F E T	32 A T B F C T D F E F	33 A T B T C T D F E T	34 A F B T C F D F E F	35 A T B T C T D T E T	36 A T B T C F D F E T	37 A T B T C T D T E F	38 A T B F C F D T E T	39 A T B F C F D F E T	40 A F B T C F D F E T
41 A F B F C T D T E T	42 A T B F C T D T E T	43 A T B F C T D F E F	44 A F B T C T D F E F	45 A T B T C T D T E T	46 A T B T C T D T E T	47 A T B F C T D T E T	48 A T B T C F D T E T	49 A T B T C F D T E T	50 A F B F C T D F E T
51 A F B F C T D F E T	52 A F B F C T D T E F	53 A T B F C T D F E T	54 A T B F C F D T E T	55 A T B F C F D T E T	56 A T B F C F D T E T	57 A F B F C T D T E T	58 A F B F C T D F E T	59 A T B F C T D T E F	60 A F B T C T D F E F

SGPGI 2002 (December)

1. **Regarding atrioventricular valve:**
   A. Valves go along with ventricle
   B. Mitral valve has 3 papillary muscles
   C. TV is normally lower than MV
   D. TV chordae is attached to IVS
   E. MV is larger than TV

2. **Proarrhythmias:**
   A. Quinidine syncope is the first type described
   B. AV blocks may be seen
   C. Torsades de pointes because of after depolarisation and triggered activity
   D. Torsades de pointes more common in females
   E. Torsades de pointes is due to long-short R-R cycles

3. **Regarding sinus node and AV node:**
   A. Corrected SNRT normally <550 msec
   B. SA conduction time <150 msec
   C. AH <80 msec
   D. HV 35-55 msec
   E. PA <25 msec

4. **Heart rate variability:**
   A. Independent positive predictive marker SCD
   B. Reduced RR variability marker of recurrent infarction
   C. Reduced to 25% of normal after/for 2-3 wks post MI
   D. Time & frequency domain analysis both done
   E. Low Heart rate variability is a poor prognostic marker

5. **Exercise testing:**
   A. In consecutive 3 exercise testing the maximum exercise capacity occurs between 1 and 2
   B. Cooler temperature cause early ST-T changes
   C. In patient on digoxin absence of ST changes is a valid negative test
   D. Heparin increases exercise time
   E. Chronic smoking decreases ischemic threshold

6. **Pericardium and metabolism:**
   A. Occurrence of pericarditis is independent of etiology of renal failure
   B. In uremic pericarditis ECG changes of acute pericarditis generally not seen
   C. Uremic exudative pericarditis is rich in fibrin and inflammatory cells
   D. Occurs even with successful dialysis
   E. Can occur also in post transplant

7. **Normal cardiac cycle:**
   A. Isovolumic relaxation starts with AV closure
   B. Isovolumic contraction starts with MV opening
   C. Protoastolic phase follows aortic pressure tracing incisura
   D. MV closed in rapid ventricular filling phase
   E. Rapid ejection phase occurs after AoV opening

8. **First heart sound:**
   A. Paradoxical split RBBB
   B. LBBB single S1
   C. LGL–Loud S1
   D. Calcific MS (severe) Louder S1
   E. MVP S1 loud

9. Atrial myxoma:
- **A.** Tumor plop found in ventricular systole with soft S1
- **B.** Arises from post Lt wall
- **C.** MR & TR may occur
- **D.** Familial predisposition may be seen
- **E.** Histopathological examination of emboli may be diagnostic

10. RCMP:
- **A.** Marked systolic dysfunction with maximum diastolic filling during late phase
- **B.** Dip and plateau in atrial pressure tracing
- **C.** PA pressure usually >50 mm Hg
- **D.** EMB is highly diagnostic of cardiac amyloid
- **E.** Thrombosis common in EMF

11. Pacemakers:
- **A.** Hypotension, vertigo, syncope may occur in pacemaker syndrome
- **B.** Pacemaker syndrome most common seen in DDD pacemaker
- **C.** Intact ventriculo-atrial conduction necessary for pacemaker syndrome
- **D.** Skeletal muscle contraction causes reduced output of pulse generator battery with unipolar leads
- **E.** Hysteresis interval is escape interval that is different from pulse repetition cycle

12. Pulmonary vascular disease:
- **A.** In secondary pulmonary hypertension PCWP more than PA diastolic pressure
- **B.** For Ac Cor pulmonale to occur when >50% of pulmonary vascular bed is occluded
- **C.** Acute PTE in 24 hours 10-20% resolved
- **D.** RV enlargement on CXR most sensitive diagnosis PAH
- **E.** Perfusion lung scan differentiates primary from thrombotic PHT due to chronic pulmonary thomboembolism

13. Congenital MR is seen in:
- **A.** ALCAPA
- **B.** Parachute Mitral valve
- **C.** Endocardial cushion defect
- **D.** Pseudoxanthoma elasticum
- **E.** Ehler-Danlos syndrome

14. ALCAPA:
- **A.** Retrograde flow in LAD
- **B.** CHF in 1st month of life
- **C.** Large Q waves in inferior leads
- **D.** Continuous murmur is unusual
- **E.** LAD not arising from usual site from coronary sinus on angiography is diagnostic

15. Fetal circulation:
- **A.** Majority of IVC blood goes to LA through PFO
- **B.** RV cardiac output is 45% (contribution)
- **C.** IVC blood preferentially directed to descending aorta & SVC to ascending aorta
- **D.** Patent ductus functionally closes by 24 hrs
- **E.** Fetal pulmonary vasculature is highly reactive/ sensitive to change in O_2 conc.

16. Ductus dependent lesions:
- **A.** Tricuspid atresia
- **B.** Mitral atresia
- **C.** c-TGA
- **D.** Interrupted aortic arch
- **E.** TAPVC with restrictive ASD

17. Obligatory ASD must for survival:
- **A.** Pulmonary atresia with VSD
- **B.** Mitral atresia
- **C.** TGA
- **D.** Single ventricle with severe PS
- **E.** TAPVC

18. Cyanosis with ostium secundum ASD with normal PA pressure:
- **A.** LSVC to coronary sinus
- **B.** Raghlib syndrome
- **C.** PAPVC
- **D.** Multiple ASD at different sites
- **E.** Large Eustachian valve

19. Respiratory manoeuvres:
- **A.** ↑ed intensity of tricuspid OS with inspiration
- **B.** A2 moves less than P2 in splitting
- **C.** Presystolic murmur of Ebstein decrease with inspiration
- **D.** Hypertensive PR increases on inspiration
- **E.** Majority of murmur decrease with strain phase valsalva

20. Heparin:
- **A.** Molecular wt: LMWH 12,000-15,000
- **B.** Platelet inhibition minimal with LMWH
- **C.** Decrease factor IIa activity is minimal with LMWH
- **D.** UFH has predominant renal excretion
- **E.** Minimal protein binding with LMWH

21. Atherosclerotic plaque:
- **A.** Plaque disruption correlates with severity of stenosis on CAG
- **B.** NO acts directly on SM
- **C.** Transient improvement of endothelial dysfunction with NTG
- **D.** Even transient smoking causes endothelial dysfunction
- **E.** ↓ed endothelin levels in CHF

22. LV overload in valvular heart diseases:
- **A.** Acute MR produces increased stiffness
- **B.** Chronic compensated AR↓ stiffness (compliance↑)
- **C.** Compensated AS: Stiffness↑
- **D.** Stiffness inversely related to wall thickness
- **E.** Chambers volume ↓ed in compensated diagnosis

23. Balloon aortic valvulotomy in severe calcific AS is done in:
- **A.** Cardiogenic shock
- **B.** Ca breast with secondaries in lung
- **C.** Patient undergoing emergency urgent non cardiac surgery
- **D.** Moderate LV dysfunction without CHF
- **E.** If severity of AS is not assessable even after provocative testing

24. Relative indications of bioprosthetic valve over mechanical valve:
- **A.** Age =65 years
- **B.** CRF
- **C.** Pregnancy being contemplated
- **D.** IE (associated)
- **E.** Chronic AF

25. ACE inhibitors trials:
- **A.** AIRE
- **B.** Va-HeFT
- **C.** ISIS-1
- **D.** MADIT
- **E.** Consensus

26. Relative resistance of diuretics in CHF
- **A.** Decreased renal perfusion
- **B.** Combination of loop diuretic with thiazide
- **C.** Increased circulating catecholamines
- **D.** Concurrent use of indomethacin
- **E.** Hypomagnesaemia

27. Angiotensin II actions:
- **A.** Vasodilatation
- **B.** Kaliuresis
- **C.** Increased vasopressin
- **D.** Inhibits PAI 1
- **E.** Inhibits aldosterone

28. Inodilators:
- **A.** Dopamine
- **B.** Dobutamine
- **C.** Amrinone
- **D.** Enoximone
- **E.** Isoproterenol

29. Adenosine:
- **A.** Potassium channel blockers
- **B.** ½ life 60 sec
- **C.** Methyxanthines increases senstivity
- **D.** Dipyridamol ↑ses breakdown
- **E.** Useful in RVOT VT

30. Drugs that ↑ levels of warfarin:
- **A.** Phenytoin
- **B.** Pantoprazole
- **C.** Metronidazole
- **D.** Sulfinpyrazone
- **E.** Amiodarone

31. Which of the following fall in high risk category for developing IE?
- **A.** BT shunt
- **B.** MVP without MR
- **C.** CoA
- **D.** AICD
- **E.** Tricuspid valve disease

32. Situs solitus:
A. Right bronchus shorter
B. Right bronchus more horizontal
C. Right bronchus branches earlier
D. Left pulmonary artery lies below left bronchus
E. Right pulmonary artery lies above right bronchus

33. Latest modification of Jones Criteria:
A. Polyarthritis is a now minor criterion
B. Preceding streptococcal infection not an essential criteria
C. Arthralgia is a minor criteria
D. Erythema marginatum not seen in fair skinned
E. Useful only in 1st episode Rh Fever

34. HOCM:
A. LVOT gradient maximum in late systole
B. Post extrasystolic beat ↓ ventricular systolic pressure
C. Post extrasystolic pulse pressure ↓
D. Squatting ↓ LVOT gradient
E. Spike and dome pattern present during valsalva (strain phase) manoeuvre

35. Techniques for cardiac output measurement:
A. Douglas bag
B. Thermodilution
C. LV angiography
D. MUGA
E. Thallium scintigraphy

36. Open heart surgeries are:
A. BT shunt
B. Septectomy
C. PA banding
D. TMLR
E. Rastelli

37. In pregnancy:
A. Cardiac output ↑30-50 %
B. SVR ↓ max in 1st trimester
C. Blood volume ↑50%
D. Cardiac output ↑ in 3rd trimester because of increase in HR & SV
E. Cardiac output reaches maximum in 2nd trimester

38. Statin not used in which trials:
A. CARE
B. FATS
C. STAR
D. AVERT
E. CLAS-1

39. Acute PM rupture in acute IWMI:
A. Anterolateral papillary muscle dysfunction > posteromedial papillary muscle dysfunction
B. More common in small infarcts
C. Usually causes severe MR
D. Pulmonary edema common
E. Large 'v' wave on cath study diagnostic of acute PM rupture

40. Acute MI:
A. ↑ 2,3 DPG levels
B. ↓ P50
C. ↓ Reverse T3
D. ↓ DLCO
E. Decrease Insulin levels

41. CPK isoform:
A. ELISA more sensitive and specific than other methods
B. Tongue and intestine are minor contributors
C. CK-MB/C total >1.5% is more indicative of mass activity cardiac source than of musculoskeletal source.
D. Carboxypeptidase converts CPKMB-1 to MB-2
E. CPK-MB isoforms help in early diagnosis

42. True/False:
A. ↑HR ↑ contractility leads to Treppe
B. Post extrasystolic potentiation–Bowditch staircase phenomenon
C. Anrep: ↑ed AO pressure ↑ contractility
D. Laplace: Wall tension proportional to distending pressure
E. Concept of afterload preload mismatch is common in CHF

43. Pharmacotherapy of endothelial dysfunction:
A. Aspirin
B. ACEI
C. β blocker
D. HRT

E. GpIIb/IIIa inhibitor

44. Catheter RV 102/90 PA 90/48 mm Hg, mean 60 mm Hg, RA mean 12 mm Hg, PCWP 14 mm Hg, CI 2L/min/m^2:

A. Transvalvular gradient was 12 mm Hg
B. Patient has clinically significant pulmonary venous congestion
C. Patient is in gross CHF
D. Suggestive of primary pulmonary hypertension
E. PVR– 23 Wood index

45. Antiplatelets:

A. Clopidogrel reversible inhibitor
B. Low dose aspirin inhibits COX pathway for 7 days
C. Dipyridamole + aspirin is better in patients with prior CAD in large scale trials
D. Aspirin better than ACE-inhibitors after acute MI for secondary prevention
E. GpIIb/IIIa inhibitors useful in diabetic patients undergoing angioplasty

46. Echo finding of mitral stenosis are:

A. A reduced EF slope is diagnostic
B. Diastolic doming is best on M anode
C. Diastolic doming is diagnostic
D. Reduction of pressure to half of its peak correlates with valve orifice area
E. Pressure half time is not affected by presence of AR

47. Radionuclide angiography:

A. For a patient of LBBB pharmacological stress test + Radionuclide angiography is better than perfusion imaging
B. All coronary territory equally represented
C. Heparin administration may interfere with radionuclide angiography
D. Has high accuracy and reproducibility
E. Global and regional LV function can be assessed

48. Regional wall motion abnormality:

A. Hibernating-dyskinetic
B. Normal Blood flow -stunned
C. Abnormal calcium kinetics represents stunning
D. Hibernating myocardium has mild ↓BF
E. Stunned myocardium is associated with structural changes

49. MUGA (ERNA):

A. 1st Pass
B. Tc^{99} pertechnitium late
C. Respiratory gated
D. Pulmonary venous congestion detected
E. RV output better than echocardiography

50. Arch:

A. 1st Arch Maxillary a
B. 2nd Arch CCA
C. 5th Arch PA
D. 6th Arch PDA
E. Left 7th intersegmental artery–Left subclavian artery

51. Ventricular arrhythmias in non-ischemic CMP:

A. Amiodarone not useful
B. AICD useful in some cases
C. Torsades is most common arrhythmia
D. Class I_C are useful
E. Suppression of vent arrhythmia indicates good prognosis

52. True or false:

A. VSD is more common in IWMI than AWMI
B. PM involvement more distal than proximal
C. VSD is most common after 1st attack MI
D. Thrill more common in PMO v/s VSD
E. PMD more common in AWMI than IWMI

53. Athlete heart:

A. ↑LVEDV & LVESV↓
B. Junctional escape rhythm common
C. Exaggerated sinus arrhythmia common
D. ASH uncommon
E. Torsades common

54. CPR:

A. Chest compression 80/min
B. Respiration:Cardiac compression ratio is 1:10
C. Cardiac output is increased at least 1/3rd with CPR
D. Relaxation is equally important
E. Only cardiac massage without respiration is also

effective

55. Acute MI pericarditis:

A. Incidence <5%
B. Thrombolysis ↓ incidence
C. Indicates ↑ mortality
D. Acute pericarditis precludes use of anticoagulant
E. Related to infarct size

56. Mechanisms of b blockers in CHF:

A. Down regulation of b receptor
B. Protects heart from direct toxicity of catecholamines
C. Decreases NE synthesis in nerve terminals
D. Decreases NE release from noradrenergic nerve terminals
E. Inhibits renin-angiotensin system/aldosterone

57. Failing heart:

A. Down regulation of b receptors
B. Up regulation of a receptors
C. Concentration of $\beta 1$: $\beta 2$: α is 2:1:1
D. Elevated NE levels in cardiac veins
E. Plasma BNP: value >100 pg/mL diagnosed HF with a sensitivity, specificity, and predictive accuracy of 90, 76, and 83 percent

58. Primary prevention trials of lipids:

A. AFCAPS/TEXCAPS
B. Lipid
C. VAHIT
D. BIP
E. 4S

59. Genetic disease:

A. Neurofibromatosis-RAS
B. Tuberous sclerosis-PS
C. Noonan's–HOCM
D. Friedrichs-Rhabdomyosarcoma
E. TAR syndrome–ASD

60. PET:

A. Normal perfusion–normal or ↑ uptake in stunned myocardium
B. ↓ Perfusion–normal uptake in hibernating myocardium
C. ↓ Perfusion- ↓ uptake indicates scar
D. Mild or decrease blood flow may suggest fibrosis
E. ↓ Glucose uptake predicts improved contraction

Answers

1 A T B F C T D T E F	2 A T B T C T D T E T	3 A T B T C F D T E F	4 A F B F C T D T E T	5 A T B T C T D T E T	6 A T B T C F D T E T	7 A T B F C T D F E T	8 A F B T C T D F E T	9 A F B F C T D T E T	10 A F B F C T D F E T
11 A T B F C F D T E T	12 A F B F C T D F E F	13 A T B T C T D T E T	14 A T B F C F D F E F	15 A T B F C F D F E T	16 A T B T C F D T E T	17 A F B T C T D F E T	18 A F B T C F D F E T	19 A T B T C F D T E T	20 A F B T C T D T E T
21 A F B T C T D T E F	22 A T B T C T D F E F	23 A T B T C T D F E F	24 A T B F C T D F E F	25 A T B F C F D F E T	26 A T B F C T D T E F	27 A F B T C T D F E F	28 A F B T C T D F E F	29 A F B F C F D F E T	30 A F B T C T D T E T
31 A T B F C T D F E F	32 A T B F C T D F E F	33 A F B F C T D F E T	34 A T B F C T D T E T	35 A F B T C T D T E T	36 A F B T C F D F E T	37 A T B F C T D F E T	38 A F B T C T D F E T	39 A F B T C T D T E T	40 A T B F C F D T E T
41 A T B T C F D F E T	42 A T B F C T D T E T	43 A F B T C T D T E F	44 A F B F C T D T E F	45 A F B T C T D T E T	46 A F B F C T D T E F	47 A T B F C F D T E T	48 A T B T C T D T E F	49 A T B F C F D T E F	50 A T B F C F D T E T
51 A F B T C F D F E F	52 A F B T C T D F E F	53 A T B T C T D F E F	54 A T B F C T D T E F	55 A F B T C T D F E T	56 A F B T C F D T E T	57 A T B T C T D T E T	58 A T B F C F D F E F	59 A F B F C T D F E T	60 A T B T C T D F E F

SGPGI 2002 (June)

1. **Athletes heart:**
   - **A.** Paradoxical septal motion
   - **B.** ↑ RVEDP
   - **C.** ↑ LA size
   - **D.** 2nd degree type I AV block
   - **E.** Septal: PW thickness > 1.3:1

2. **SLE:**
   - **A.** Contracted small heart
   - **B.** Coronary artery spasm
   - **C.** Supraventricular tachycardia
   - **D.** Coronary arteritis
   - **E.** non infective endocarditis

3. **ACE inhibitors:**
   - **A.** Anti obesity
   - **B.** Anti thrombotic
   - **C.** Anti atherosclerotic
   - **D.** Anti insulin resistance
   - **E.** Most common side effect is cough

4. **Cyanotic with normal cardiac findings:**
   - **A.** ALCAPA
   - **B.** Alveolar hypoventilation
   - **C.** Methemoglobinaemia
   - **D.** Systemic venous return to left heart
   - **E.** Univentricular heart

5. **Obligatory intracardiac shunt are:**
   - **A.** Truncus arteriosis
   - **B.** c-TGA
   - **C.** Pulmonary atresia
   - **D.** TAPVC
   - **E.** d-TGA

6. **Degree of cyanosis in TOF depends on:**
   - **A.** Aortopulmonary collaterals
   - **B.** Presence of ASD
   - **C.** Size of VSD
   - **D.** RV outflow tract obstruction
   - **E.** Size of pulmonary arteries

7. **TAPVC:**
   - **A.** Presence of ASD necessary for survival
   - **B.** Coronary sinus variety often obstructive
   - **C.** 3/4th of infradiaphragmatic are obstructive
   - **D.** Snowman appearance is diagnostic
   - **E.** Upper part of figure of 8 formed by left vertical vein

8. **Exercise training:**
   - **A.** ↓ Parasympathetic tone
   - **B.** Mobitz type I Block
   - **C.** ↑ Oxygen consumption
   - **D.** Morphological P wave abnormality
   - **E.** ↓ ESV

9. **c-TGA:**
   - **A.** 95% situs solitus
   - **B.** 90% AV block
   - **C.** Lt A-V valve abnormality is commonest
   - **D.** Conduction abnormality due to inverted bundles
   - **E.** If asymptomatic normal survival (if no cardiac abnormality)

10. Acyanotic congenital heart disease:
- **A.** CoA presents with cerebral hemorrhage
- **B.** VSD associated with conduction block
- **C.** ASD commonest congenital abnormality
- **D.** I.E. prophylaxis is essence for PDA repair
- **E.** VSD with AR is common in age group of 5-9 years

11. Catecholamine receptor:
- **A.** α1 receptor block presynaptic receptors of NE
- **B.** α2 receptor mainly seen in post ganglionic and CNS
- **C.** Bronchioles contain β1 receptors
- **D.** β1 stimulation results in ↓ed AV node conduction
- **E.** Dopamine receptors D1 splanchnic vasodilator

12. Delayed after depolarization:
- **A.** Abnormal automaticity
- **B.** Abnormal triggered activity
- **C.** Abolished by catecholamine
- **D.** Abolished by calcium channel blocker
- **E.** Decreased by long cycles

13. Pregnancy:
- **A.** Cardiac output ↑ by 30-50%
- **B.** Blood volume ↑ by 50%
- **C.** PVR ↓ max in 1st trimester
- **D.** In 3rd trimester COP ↑ by ↑ HR and ↓ SVR
- **E.** Maximum diastolic BP decreased in second trimester

14. QT interval increased in:
- **A.** Hyperkalemia
- **B.** Hypocalcemia
- **C.** Hypermagnesaemia has no effect
- **D.** Hypothermia
- **E.** Mexiletine does not prolong QT interval

15. Primary prevention lipid trials are:
- **A.** 4S
- **B.** AFCAPS/Tex CAPS
- **C.** LIPIDS
- **D.** BIP
- **E.** Va-HIT

16. Intracoronary Ultrasonography is:
- **A.** Therapeutic and pathological dissection differentiation possible
- **B.** Detects thrombosis
- **C.** Quantify luminal diameter better than CAG
- **D.** Better detection of coronary vessel wall
- **E.** Pathology for coronary angioplasty

17. 4S trial:
- **A.** ↑ non cardiac mortality
- **B.** ↓ fatal, non fatal CV events directly related to LDL
- **C.** ↑ fatal non fatal cardio events out of proportion to ↓ LDL
- **D.** Cholesterol ↓ by 50%
- **E.** Also associated with ↑ HDL and ↓ TG

18. Pressure data: RA-12 mm Hg, RV 102/12mm Hg, PA-90/48 mm Hg, Mean–60 mm Hg, PCWP 14 mm Hg, CI 22/m^2/min:
- **A.** Transpulmonary gradient 12
- **B.** Patient in severe CHF
- **C.** PVR > 18 wood units
- **D.** Diagnosis PPH
- **E.** Patient having pulmonary venous congestion

19. Indication of Ao Valve replacement in patient of AR with Class II palpitation:
- **A.** LVEF <35%
- **B.** CT ratio > 50%
- **C.** LVESV >55 mi/m^2
- **D.** LVEDV >200 ml/m^2
- **E.** LVESD > 55 mm

20. **True or false:**
   A. Coronary Drug Project used nicotinic acid and showed no difference in coronary events in treated group
   B. Familial atherosclerosis treatment study (FATS) showed that angiographic evidence of atherosclerosis could be slowed, halted or even regressed in treatment group.
   C. The Helsinki Heart Study used gemfibrozil and showed that the treatment group had less fatal and non fatal coronary heart disease events
   D. US National Heart Lung and Blood Institute Type II coronary international study showed no difference in treatment and non Rx group for progression of atherosclerosis
   E. Lipid Research Clinics Coronary Primary Prevention Trial: used cholestyramine and found significant decrease in nonfatal MI and CAD death

21. **Endothelium and NO:**
   A. Normal endothelium inhibits proliferation of smooth muscle cells
   B. Experimental removal of endothelium allows initiation of mitogenic response of smooth muscle cells
   C. Smooth cells are relatively immature cells
   D. Cultured smooth cells exposed to Na Nitroprusside mimics NO
   E. NO plays a large role in control of vascular tone of large arteries

22. **Hemodynamic determinant of S3:**
   A. LA contractility
   B. LV diastolic compliance
   C. Thoracic architecture
   D. Rate of contraction of LV
   E. LV systolic volume

23. **Fatty streak:**
   A. Site same in children and old age
   B. Found in fetus
   C. Main content is oxidized cholesterol ester
   D. More in children than in adult
   E. T lymphocytes can be found

24. **In CHF drugs which prolong survival are:**
   A. Hydralazine with nitrate
   B. β blocker
   C. CCB
   D. Pimobendan
   E. Lanoxin

25. **Aortoarteritis:**
   A. Type IV most common in India
   B. Most common cause of secondary HT in India
   C. Retinopathy in 50%
   D. Spontaneous reactivity is common
   E. Mixed (Dilated and stenotic) lesions are commonest

26. **Stunning vs hibernating myocardium:**
   A. Inotropes improve contractility transiently
   B. ↑ Lactate in stunned myocardium
   C. ↓ Lactate in hibernating myocardium
   D. Normal flow in hibernating myocardium
   E. Normal flow ↓ FDG uptake in scar

27. **Branchial arches: derivatives are:**
   A. 1st arch-maxillary artery
   B. 2nd arch-Common carotid artery
   C. 6th arch-PDA
   D. 5th arch-pulmonary artery
   E. 7th arch-Intersegmental artery and left subclavian artery

28. **Right aortic arch commonly seen in:**
   A. Ebstein's anomaly
   B. Truncus arteriosus
   C. c-TGA
   D. Pulmonary atresia with VSD
   E. TOF

29. **Squatting effect:**
   A. ↑ RVS_3S_4
   B. ↑ LVS_3S_4
   C. ↑ MS murmur
   D. ↑ MR murmur
   E. ↑ VSD murmur

30. Post extrasystole:

A. ↑ed contractility because of ↑ preload after long pause
B. ↑ed contractility because of increased afterload
C. ↑ heart rate → ↑ Ca^{++}
D. Calcium electrically driven
E. Increased contractility with increase heart rate

31. Rubella–congenital heart disease:

A. Macrocephaly and retinal abnormality and VSD
B. Lithium associated with PS
C. Peripheral pulmonary stenosis can present as hemoptysis
D. Alcohol associated with VSD
E. Phenytoin ASD & PDA

32. Termination of pregnancy is indicated in:

A. Marfan with severe MR
B. All cases of cyanotic congenital heart disease
C. All cases of DCM
D. CoA
E. PPH

33. JVP:

A. Same wave pattern in jugular vein and RA
B. In AF, no 'a' wave and prominent Y descent
C. 'W' pattern in cardiac tamponade
D. Cannon 'a' wave in PA stenosis
E. Y descent corresponds to ventricular systole

34. cTrop T and cTrop I:

A. ↑ in end stage heart failure
B. Minor myocardial damage Trop T increased and CPKMB normal
C. cTrop T 0.1 ng/ml, c Trop I 1.5 ng/ml diagnostic
D. cTrop T 0.01 ng/ml Trop I 0.1 ng/ml prognostic
E. Cut off for diagnostic Trop T is > 97.5 percentile

35. Vectorcardiography and RVH:

A. Type A ASD
B. Type C COPD
C. Type A clockwise and anterior
D. Type B right and posterior
E. Type C clockwise and posterior

36. True/false:

A. Person breathes > 1 atm pressure Hb dissociation curve to right
B. At sea level partial Pr O_2 760 mmHg
C. Dissolved O_2 is independent of Hb
D. Dissolved O_2 is 0.3 m/Lt (of plasma)
E. 100% oxygen inhalation at ½ atm will increase PO_2 to 700

37. Regarding murmurs:

A. Inspiration–diastolic murmur of TS and PR accentuated
B. Expiration diastolic murmur of MS and systolic murmur of MR increases
C. Inspiration ↑ LV size and causes ↓ of MVP
D. Square root valsalva in ASD, MS
E. During VPC systolic murmur of PS ↓

38. Chemical toxicity:

A. Cobalt-RCM
B. Co → transient biventricular dysfunction
C. Methysergide → Right sided valvular lesion
D. Cocaine causes Acute MI
E. Phenothiazine: sudden cardiac death

39. Normal cardiac cycle:

A. Tricuspid valve opens before mitral valve
B. Aortic valve opens before pulmonary valve
C. Aortic valve closes before pulmonary valve
D. Tricuspid valve closes before mitral valve
E. RA mean pressure higher than mean PCWP

40. In CHD:

A. All cardiac congenital disorders associated with chromosomal abnormalities
B. Cardiac abnormality: 10 times more common in still birth than live birth
C. Extracardiac abnormalities in 25%
D. VSD is commonest at birth
E. Patients of hypoplastic left heart syndrome die at birth

41. Viable myocardium and PE:
- **A.** Normal blood flow and increased glucose uptake suggestive of stunned myocardium
- **B.** ↓ Blood flow, normal glucose s/o hibernating myocardium
- **C.** ↓ BF and ↓ glucose s/o scar
- **D.** Mild ↓se flow s/o tissue fibrosis
- **E.** ↓ Glucose uptake predicts improved contraction

42. Ankylosing spondylitis v/s rheumatoid arthritis:
- **A.** Corticosteroids regress lesions of ankylosing spondylitis
- **B.** Ankylosing spondylosis causes MR
- **C.** 30% pericarditis in RA
- **D.** RA causes MR by involving mitral leaflets
- **E.** Ankylosing spondylosis causes AR by involving aortic annulus

43. Situs solitus:
- **A.** Rt bronchus more wide than left
- **B.** Rt bronchus shorter than left
- **C.** Rt bronchus passes above right PA
- **D.** Lt bronchus passes below leftt PA
- **E.** Rt Bronchus divides early

44. Bioprosthetic valve over mechanical valve:
- **A.** Adolescence
- **B.** 70 year male with severe MR and LV dysfunction
- **C.** Hemodialysis
- **D.** Redosurgery of mechanical valve
- **E.** Thrombosis of mechanical valve

45. Indications of BMV in asymptomatic patient:
- **A.** Chest pain
- **B.** Episodes of pulmonary edema
- **C.** Thromboembolism
- **D.** Post CMV moderate MS
- **E.** Severe MS suitable for BMV

46. EPS:
- **A.** SNRT most commonly used for SN dysfunction
- **B.** Symptomatic CHB
- **C.** Infra HIS unpredictable course and requires permanent pacemaker implantation
- **D.** Asymptomatic SN dysfunction
- **E.** SN dysfunction commonly associated with AV nodal disease

47. PPH can present as:
- **A.** Hoarse of voice
- **B.** Syncope
- **C.** Pulmonary congestion
- **D.** Angina
- **E.** Cyanosis

48. Echo findings in diastolic dysfunction of LV:
- **A.** Posterior Ao root motion in diastole
- **B.** ↓ deceleration time
- **C.** ↑ isovolumetric relaxation time
- **D.** ↓ IVRT during pseudonormalization
- **E.** ↑ deceleration time during pseudonormalization

49. HCM:
- **A.** In asymptomatic patients drugs are beneficial
- **B.** Response to β-blockers and CCB predictable
- **C.** Diuretics ↓ dyspnea
- **D.** Disopyramide found better than amiodarone in large scale trials
- **E.** Nifedipine better tolerated than verapamil

50. Dangerous plaque:
- **A.** Covered with fibrous cap
- **B.** Rupture in mid line
- **C.** Usually occupies whole of vessel wall
- **D.** Atherosclerosis occurs in intima of vessel
- **E.** ↑ content of macrophage & ↓ smooth muscle cells

51. Digoxin serum levels:
- **A.** ↑se by Rifampicin
- **B.** ↑se by verapamil
- **C.** ↑ by cyclosporine
- **D.** ↓ ed by quinidine
- **E.** ↑ by Phenytoin

52. In Ac MI pericarditis:
- **A.** Acute pericarditis in 5%
- **B.** Not related to infarct size
- **C.** Does not r/o anticoagulant
- **D.** Prognosis/mortality not affected
- **E.** Thrombolysis ↑ pericarditis

53. Pulsus paradoxus seen in:
- **A.** ASD
- **B.** AR
- **C.** Pulmonary embolism
- **D.** Hypovolemic shock
- **E.** Constrictive pericarditis with effusion

54. In cardiac cycle:
- **A.** Protodiastole begins with incisura of Ao pressure tracing
- **B.** Isovolumic contraction begins with MV closure
- **C.** Isovolumic relaxation begins with AV closure
- **D.** LV systole begins with MV opening
- **E.** LV systole followed by slow RA filling

55. Cardiac tumors:
- **A.** Most common is lipoma
- **B.** Carney syndrome–endocrine under activity
- **C.** IL6 denotes active phase with stimulation of complement and clotting cascade
- **D.** Calcification in 40% myxomas
- **E.** Metastatic tumors are commonest

56. Pericarditis:
- **A.** Pericardial inflammation autopsy 30-40%
- **B.** Vascularity and fibrin deposition is low
- **C.** Pericardial friction rub presystolic component in 30% cases and is loudest
- **D.** ST segement axis varies from 30°-60°
- **E.** Pericardial pain ↑ by recumbency

57. Giant cell arteritis:
- **A.** More common in young and in large arteries
- **B.** Endarteritis not a feature of mural involvement
- **C.** Polymyalgia rheumatica <10%
- **D.** Leutic aneurysm involves ascending aorta
- **E.** In 25% involves thoracic aorta

58. Kawasaki disease:
- **A.** Coronary artery involvement < 3 days
- **B.** Death by MI/pericarditis/myocarditis by 3-4 weeks
- **C.** α1-antitrypsin is diagnostic
- **D.** Aneurysm of noncoronary medium arteries seen
- **E.** Pancarditis: late feature

59. Basic life support:
- **A.** Chest compression at 80 min
- **B.** Chest compression: ventilation 5:1
- **C.** 1/3rd cardiac output may be increased by proper CPR
- **D.** Relaxation important in chest compression
- **E.** CPR without respiration also effective

60. Endothelin True/False:
- **A.** Three receptors ET-A, ET-B, ET-C
- **B.** BT-123 is ET-B blocker
- **C.** ET-A in vascular smooth muscle
- **D.** ET-A responsible for smooth muscle contraction and vasoconstriction
- **E.** ET-B responsible for ↑ NO and vasodilatation

Answers

Q	A	B	C	D	E
1	F	F	F	T	T
2	F	F	T	T	T
3	F	T	T	F	T
4	F	T	T	T	F
5	T	F	T	T	T
6	T	F	F	T	F
7	T	F	F	T	T
8	F	T	T	T	T
9	F	F	T	T	F
10	F	T	F	T	T
11	F	F	F	F	T
12	F	T	F	T	T
13	T	T	F	F	T
14	F	T	T	T	T
15	F	T	F	F	F
16	T	T	T	T	F
17	F	T	F	F	T
18	T	F	T	T	F
19	T	F	T	T	T
20	T	T	T	F	T
21	T	T	F	T	F
22	F	T	T	F	T
23	T	F	F	F	T
24	T	T	F	F	F
25	F	F	T	T	T
26	F	F	F	F	F
27	T	F	T	F	T
28	F	T	F	T	F
29	T	F	T	T	T
30	T	F	T	T	T
31	F	F	T	T	T
32	T	T	F	F	T
33	T	F	F	F	F
34	T	T	T	T	T
35	T	T	T	F	F
36	T	F	F	F	F
37	T	T	F	T	T
38	T	T	T	T	T
39	T	F	T	F	F
40	T	T	T	T	T
41	T	T	T	F	F
42	F	T	F	F	T
43	T	T	T	T	T
44	F	T	F	T	F
45	T	T	T	F	T
46	T	F	T	F	T
47	T	T	F	T	F
48	T	T	F	T	F
49	T	T	T	T	F
50	F	F	T	T	T
51	F	T	T	F	T
52	F	F	T	F	F
53	F	F	T	T	T
54	T	T	T	T	F
55	F	F	T	T	T
56	F	F	F	T	T
57	F	F	F	T	T
58	F	T	F	T	F
59	F	F	F	T	T
60	T	F	T	T	T

SGPGI 2001

1. **Endothelium dysfunction–True/false:**
   A. Vasoconstriction due to endothelin
   B. Excess NO production
   C. Vasoconstriction due to acetylcholine
   D. Increased incidence of CAD
   E. Commonly associated with acute coronary events

2. S:
   A. Soft in acute AR
   B. Increased in WPW
   C. Pneumothorax with gastric dilatation decrease
   D. Ebstein's is associated with muffled sound
   E. Loud in mobile LA myxoma

3. **Amyl nitrate inhalation:**
   A. ↑ed MR murmur intensity
   B. ↓ed intensity of AS murmur
   C. MVP murmur decreases
   D. Increase murmur of HOCM
   E. Murmur of AR decreased

4. **Regarding murmur:**
   A. High pitched murmur indicates high gradient
   B. Short murmur indicate severe stenosis
   C. Late peaking indicates severe stenosis
   D. Perimembranous VSD can cause midsystolic murmur
   E. End Diastolic murmur in dysplastic pulmonary valve

5. **Mid diastolic murmur of MS:**
   A. ↑es in intensity with squatting
   B. Louder murmur indicates severe stenosis
   C. RV hypertrophy can cause silent MS
   D. TS decreases intensity of MS murmur
   E. Presystolic accentuation always absent with AF

6. **Cyanotic spells; management:**
   A. Morphine is the primary modality of treatment
   B. Knee chest position decreases cyanosis by cutting out venous return from legs
   C. Carotid baroreceptor play primary role
   D. Propranolol dose is 0.1 mg/kg
   E. Is seen in pulmonary atresia

7. **Fatty streaks:**
   A. Commonly seen in children
   B. Occur at same sites in both Young adults and old individuals
   C. Cholesterol esters founds
   D. T lymphocytes are also seen
   E. Seen in fetal life also

8. **TS:**
   A. Seen in 1/3rd of pathological specimens
   B. Invariably associated with MS in RHD
   C. Isolated TS more common than mixed lesions
   D. Early diastolic hepatic pulsation in TS
   E. RV heave felt

9. **TS:**
   A. Pedal edema occurs if RA pressure >10 mmHg
   B. Dyspnea & fatigue are common presentations
   C. Increases severity of MS
   D. Organic TS more common than TR
   E. Myxoma seen in LA only

10. **Myxoma:**
A. Seen in only RA
B. 90% are in LA
C. Endocrine manifestation in sporadic myxoma
D. Familial is common in sporadic myxoma
E. Carney's syndrome and familial myxoma

11. **EMF:**
A. Common in northern India
B. Less common in cold climates
C. AV regurgitation common
D. Subvalvular calcification common
E. Surgical results are good

12. **Cardiac amyloidosis:**
A. M mode can diagnose
B. RCM is common
C. Conduction abnormalities are uncommon
D. Diagnosed by rectal biopsy
E. Wide pulse pressure seen

13. **Pheochromocytoma should be suspected in presence of:**
A. Neurofibromatosis
B. Palpable abdominal mass
C. Orthostatic hypertension
D. Inappropriate hyponatremia
E. Pressure response to β blockers

14. **Coronary calcification:**
A. Signify significant stenosis
B. Identify with ultrafast CT
C. Made of calcium carbonate
D. Found in advanced atheromas
E. IVUS can detect calcification in adventitia

15. **Ultrafast CT/Cine CT:**
A. Help to detect occlusion of coronary artery
B. Help in detection of calcium even in distal coronary artery
C. Detects occlusion in saphenous venous graft
D. Requires less radiation
E. Detects occlusion best in venous graft than arterial

16. **Inotropic drugs:**
A. Dobutamine stimulate dopamine receptors
B. Norepinephrine more arrhythmogenic than Dopamine
C. Dopamine acts on α, β1 and β2 receptors
D. Isoproterenol acts on β and α receptors
E. Carvedilol acts on α, β1 and β2 receptors

17. **Digoxin:**
A. ↑ PR, ↑ A-H interval
B. ↑ AV conduction time
C. ↑ atrial RFP
D. ↑ atrial automaticity
E. Sympatholytic more than parasympathomimetic

18. **β blocker with vasodilator:**
A. Carteolol
B. Carvedilol
C. Bisoprolol
D. Celiprolol
E. Bucindolol

19. **Properties of plaque disruption:**
A. ↑ lipid content
B. ↓ smooth muscle cell
C. ↑ macrophage content
D. Decreased intraplaque temperature
E. Thin fibrous cap

20. **Chronic congestive heart failure:**
A. ↓ sympathetic activity
B. RAS activation
C. ↑ vasopressin
D. ↑ vasodilatation
E. ↑ aldosterone

21. **Endothelin:**
A. ↓ in AMI
B. ↑ BP
C. ↑ in CHF
D. Vasodilation
E. Stimulate cardiac hypertrophy

22. **Hyperhomocystinemia:**
A. ↑ in chronic renal failure
B. Treatment is Vitamin B-6, B-12 and folate
C. Premature atherosclerosis is associated
D. Recurrent venous thrombosis
E. Normal range is 5-15 mmol/L in fasting state

23. Lp (a):
- **A.** Does not indicate atherogenesis
- **B.** Small dense LDL is more atherogenic
- **C.** Lp(a) cannot be modified by diet
- **D.** HDL is formed by Apo (a) and Apo (b)
- **E.** Lipoprotein (a) is LDL with apoprotein 'a'

24. CHF management:
- **A.** Dynamic cardiomyoplasty increases survival
- **B.** SOLVD showed increase mortality with enalapril
- **C.** SAVE showed improve mortality with Captopril
- **D.** DCMP and CHF should be invariable anticoagulated
- **E.** Patient can be allowed to exercise till maximum symptoms

25. TOF with severe pulmonary stenosis (cyanotic):
- **A.** ↑RA pressure
- **B.** ↑ PA pressure (n)
- **C.** Equal pressures in RV and LV
- **D.** Arterial PO_2 is decreased
- **E.** LV may be normal

26. ASD with no pulmonary stenosis:
- **A.** Ostium primum always associated with cleft MV
- **B.** Increase LA pressure with Increase in pulmonary artery pressure
- **C.** Sinus venosus defect associated with anomalous pulmonary vein
- **D.** Ostium secundum associated with RBBB
- **E.** Ostium primum associated with LAD with LBBB

27. CABG indication:
- **A.** Double vessel disease with LV dysfunction
- **B.** Single vessels disease –Proximal LAD stenosis
- **C.** TVD with LV dysfunction
- **D.** LM disease
- **E.** TVD with normal LV function

28. In unstable angina:
- **A.** Unfractionated heparin is superior to LMWH
- **B.** LMWH heparin is superior to UFH
- **C.** LMWH given for prolonged period
- **D.** Dipyridamole equals aspirin in ischemic events
- **E.** Thrombolysis can be given

29. Unstable angina:
- **A.** 10% patient have normal coronaries
- **B.** 80% thrombus contained lesions
- **C.** Complicated plaque found
- **D.** 50% culprit lesions cannot be detected
- **E.** On initial presentation > 50% have TVD

30. PDA-Eisenmenger:
- **A.** ↓ LV systolic pressures
- **B.** LV pressure is normal
- **C.** ↑ RA pressure
- **D.** Diastolic murmur across shunt
- **E.** RV pressures suprasystemic

31. Ticlopidine:
- **A.** Irreversible ADP blockade
- **B.** Action start within 72 hours
- **C.** CAPRIE Trial: ticlopidine decreases mortality in embolic events
- **D.** Ticlopidine with clopidogrel has bone marrow toxicity
- **E.** Blocks GpIIb activation specific for ADP pathway

32. Baroreflex:
- **A.** ↑ Efferent sympathetics
- **B.** ↑ Efferent parasympathetic
- **C.** ↑ Baroreceptor activity in heart failure
- **D.** Digoxin improve baroreceptor activity
- **E.** Digoxin parasympathomimetic and sympatholytics

33. Severe MS + TS:
- **A.** ↑ LA pressure
- **B.** ↑ LV end diastolic volume
- **C.** Severe RVH and MS murmur silent
- **D.** Normal RVEDP
- **E.** 1/3rd cases of RHD have TS associated with MS

34. Severe AS + mild AR:
- **A.** Gradient across LA and LV
- **B.** LV end diastolic pressure ↑
- **C.** LV systolic pressure ↓
- **D.** Pulmonary capillary pressure↑
- **E.** In AS- Diastolic murmur of AR seen in < 10% cases

35. Severe chronic MS:
- **A.** Haemosiderosis
- **B.** LA not markedly enlarged
- **C.** RA pressure ↑
- **D.** No gradient across LA/LV
- **E.** Loudness of murmur indicates severity

36. Culture negative endocarditis:
- **A.** Q fever
- **B.** Bartonella
- **C.** Acinetobacter
- **D.** E Coli
- **E.** Brucella

37. Braunwald-Brokenbrough phenomenon:
- **A.** Occur in premature ventricular contraction
- **B.** Pulse pressure decreases
- **C.** LV systolic pressure increases
- **D.** Gradient increases
- **E.** Systolic aortic pressure decreases than control beat

38. Phosphocreatinine ATP ratio:
- **A.** Markers of bio energy
- **B.** ↓ratio suggest poor prognosis
- **C.** ↓ in cardiomyopathy
- **D.** Always < 1
- **E.** Predictor of DCMP

39. ASD:
- **A.** Ostium primum has LBBB
- **B.** Ostium secundum ASD has RAD with RBBB
- **C.** Sinus venosus ASD is usually associated with anomalous pulmonary venous drainage
- **D.** ↑ pulmonary capacitance
- **E.** Wide and fixed S2 can persist even after surgery

40. Situs solitus:
- **AS.** Horizontal right bronchus
- **B.** Right diaphragm is elevated > left diaphragm
- **C.** Right trilobed lung
- **D.** Aorta and IVC on one either of the spine
- **E.** Right pulmonary artery passes below right bronchus

41. Large ASD and VSD: hemodynamic pattern?
- **A.** O_2 does not increase a RV level
- **B.** Wide split S_2
- **C.** ↑ Pulmonary capacitance
- **D.** Pulmonary capillary pressure elevated
- **E.** O_2 step up in RA

42. In normal heart hemadynamics:
- **A.** LVEDP upto 18 mm Hg
- **B.** PCWP is 5-13 mm Hg
- **C.** Mean RA pressure is 0-12 mm Hg
- **D.** Small gradient between RV and PA
- **E.** PCWP and PAEDP are approximately same

43. In Cardiac tamponade:
- **A.** RA pressure always increased
- **B.** Always lead to constriction
- **C.** Hypovolemia collapse does not occur
- **D.** Pericardiocentesis is treatment of choice
- **E.** RA pressure > intrapericardial pressure

44. Idiopathic DCM:
- **A.** Myocyte atrophy
- **B.** Myocyte hypertrophy
- **C.** Lymphocyte infiltration at necrotic zones
- **D.** Increase interstitial connective tissue
- **E.** Histological changes in DCMP do not correlate with severity of illness

45. Pulmonary embolism:
- **A.** Ventilation defect ≥ 3 segmental perfusion defect ≥ 2 defect: does not signify pulmonary embolism
- **B.** Intrapulmonary urokinase in acute pulmonary embolism
- **C.** Chronic pulmonary embolism: pulmonary embolectomy is treatment of choice
- **D.** Ultrafast CT less sensitive in diagnosing pulmonary embolism than echo
- **E.** D-dimers more > 500 ng/ml is useful in establishing diagnosis

46. Square wave response on valsalva:
- **A.** HCM
- **B.** MS
- **C.** ASD
- **D.** CCF
- **E.** CCP

47. In JVP:
- **A.** Slow Y descent in TS
- **B.** 'a' wave due to RV contractility
- **C.** 'cv' wave of TR
- **D.** High venous pressure can be detected by examining dorsum of hand
- **E.** Kussmaul's sign in chronic RVF

48. Pulse:
- **A.** Pulsus bigeminus in carotids
- **B.** Reverse paradoxus in HOCM/IPPV
- **C.** Pulsus alternans is regularly irregular
- **D.** 'Coanda' effect in subvalvular AS
- **E.** Pulsus bigeminus is double beat pulse

49. Hangout interval:
- **A.** Depends on impedance of post capillary and aortic pressure
- **B.** ¾ inspiratory splitting due to ↑ pulmonary capacitance
- **C.** It is due to inspiratory ↑ in capacitance of pulmonary vessels
- **D.** Pulmonary capacitance more than aortic capacitance
- **E.** P2 hangout interval is increased in ASD

50. Functional class:
- **A.** CCS II- angina on walking or climbing upstairs rapidly
- **B.** CCS I–measured in blocks and flights
- **C.** Specific score activity is more sensitive than NYHA
- **D.** NYHA III cannot perform < 2 mets
- **E.** NYHA is a better predictor than CCS for specificity

51. True/False:
- **A.** 1 met = 3.5 ml/kg/min for 40 year male of 70 kg
- **B.** Bruce protocol stage I = 5 mets
- **C.** Class IV NYHA is 2 mets
- **D.** Strongly positive TMT, if patient cannot perform > 5 mets
- **E.** Strongly positive TMT when ST depression appears in stage I of Bruce protocol

52. Squatting:
- **A.** ↓ VSD murmur
- **B.** ↑ left sided S3/S4 but ↓ at Right S3-S4
- **C.** ↑ HOCM murmur
- **D.** ↑ MR murmur
- **E.** ↑ SVR

53. Antiphospholipid syndrome:
- **A.** Increase rate of arterial and venous thrombosis
- **B.** Thrombocytosis
- **C.** Increase abortion
- **D.** Livedo reticularis
- **E.** Valvular lesions more often Regurgitant

54. Severe MR with severe AR:
- **A.** LV grossly enlarged
- **B.** LV dysfunction at late stages
- **C.** LAP increases
- **D.** Brisk carotids
- **E.** LVESV provides useful overall index of myocardial function

55. Carotid baroreceptors at carotid sinus respond to increase arterial pressure by:
- **A.** Increase efferent sympathetic activity
- **B.** Decrease parasympathetic neuronal outflow
- **C.** Decrease in heart rate
- **D.** No effect on heart rate
- **E.** Increase release of renin from kidney

56. Valsalva phases:
- **A.** Bradycardia is seen in phase IV
- **B.** Abrupt decline in pressure in phase III
- **C.** Increase venous return in phase IV
- **D.** A2-P2 gap increase in phase II
- **E.** Valsalva phase I and III normal in CHF

57. Cardiac rupture:
- **A.** > 50% increase in mortality after MI in 1st week
- **B.** Seen in 1st infarction
- **C.** More common in females
- **D.** Commonly seen in 2nd week
- **E.** Associated with diffuse TVD

58. HRT:

A. Decrease Triglyceride levels
B. Increase LDL oxidation
C. Increase HDL
D. Decrease insulin requirement
E. Decrease in plasma level of LDL

59. Isometric exercise:

A. Increase PVR
B. Increase LV filling pressure
C. Increase heart size
D. Increase Cardiac output
E. Increase MR murmur

60. S1: True/False:

A. Paradoxical in RBBB
B. Lown Ganong Levine has loud S1
C. MVP has loud S1
D. Calcific MS has loud S1
E. LBBB has single S1

Answers

1 A T B F C T D T E T	2 A T B T C T D F E T	3 A F B F C T D T E T	4 A T B F C T D F E F	5 A T B F C T D T E F	6 A T B T C F D F E T	7 A T B T C T D T E T	8 A F B T C F D F E F	9 A F B T C F D F E F	10 A F B T C F D F E T
11 A F B T C T D F E F	12 A F B T C F D T E F	13 A T B T C F D T E T	14 A F B T C T D T E T	15 A T B T C T D F E T	16 A F B T C T D F E T	17 A T B T C T D T E F	18 A F B T C F D F E T	19 A T B T C T D F E T	20 A F B T C T D F E T
21 A F B T C T D F E T	22 A T B T C T D T E T	23 A F B T C T D F E T	24 A F B F C T D F E T	25 A F B F C T D T E T	26 A T B F C T D T E F	27 A T B F C T D T E T	28 A F B T C F D F E F	29 A F B F C T D F E F	30 A F B F C T D F E F
31 A T B T C T D T E T	32 A F B T C F D T E T	33 A T B F C F D T E T	34 A F B T C F D T E F	35 A T B F C T D F E F	36 A T B T C T D F E T	37 A T B T C T D T E T	38 A T B T C T D F E T	39 A F B T C T D T E T	40 A F B T C T D T E T
41 A F B T C T D F E T	42 A F B T C F D T E T	43 A F B T C F D T E F	44 A T B T C T D T E F	45 A F B F C T D F E T	46 A F B T C T D T E T	47 A T B F C T D T E T	48 A F B T C T D T E F	49 A T B T C T D T E T	50 A T B F C T D F E T
51 A T B T C T D T E T	52 A F B F C F D T E T	53 A T B F C T D T E T	54 A T B F C T D T E T	55 A F B F C T D F E F	56 A T B F C T D F E F	57 A T B T C T D F E F	58 A F B F C T D F E F	59 A T B F C F D T E T	60 A F B F C T D F E T

SGPGI 2000 (December)

1. **Endocardial prophylaxis is needed—True/False:**
   A. Biscuspid AV valve with AR
   B. Prior CABG
   C. VSD with shunt ratio <1.5
   D. BT shunt
   E. ICD

2. **True/False:**
   A. Anrep effect → ↑Aortic pressure–↑ contractility
   B. Laplace law → wall stress = pressure × radius/ 2 × wall thickness
   C. Treppe phenomenon → ↑ HR–↑ contractility
   D. Post extrasystolic potentiation of obstruction in HOCM
   E. Preload-afterload mismatch is seen in cases of congestive heart failure

3. **Familial hypertriglyceridemia:**
   A. ↑ 5 fold risk of CAD
   B. Occurs in 1% people
   C. Apo E_3 associated with ↑ cholesterol
   D. Apo E3 inhibit binding of IDL to hepatic receptor
   E. Xanthelesma strongly positive

4. **Variant angina: True/false:**
   A. Always at rest
   B. Associated with ventricular fibrillation/death
   C. Generalized tone ↑
   D. Ergometrine increases generalized tone of vessel
   E. Involves septal vessels

5. **Cardiac output can be measured by:**
   A. Ventriculography
   B. Dye dilution method
   C. MUGA
   D. Douglas BAG
   E. Thallium scintigraphy

6. **Which of the following is open cardiac surgery:**
   A. AS closure
   B. BT shunt
   C. Rastelli procedure
   D. Closure of PDA by wire
   E. VSD closure

7. **Surgical indication of IE:**
   A. Staphylococcus responding to R_x
   B. Fever > 10 days not responding to antibiotics
   C. Unstable prosthesis
   D. Fungal endocarditis
   E. Refractory heart failure

8. **True or false:**
   A. Sinus venosus ASD-Left atrial rhythm
   B. Sinus venosus ASD-Increased PR interval
   C. ASD secundum–RBBB due to increased distance
   D. ASD primum type may have CHB
   E. PR interval ↑ in all types of ASD

9. **Papillary muscle rupture:**
   A. Requires small infarct
   B. Anterior rupture common
   C. Pulmonary edema common
   D. Murmur is intense
   E. Thrill is common

10. RV infarction:
A. ECG not helpful
B. Always associated with IW MI
C. Rarely it can occur in isolated form
D. I/V fluids is R_x of choice
E. PA pressure ↑

11. In TOF:
A. Cyanosis occur after 2 years
B. Severity of pulmonary stenosis is inversely related to size of aortic root
C. Monoallelic disease
D. 50% associated with right sided aortic arch
E. P_2 is not recorded in phonocardiogram

12. Morphological right ventricle differentiated from left ventricle:
A. Have moderator band
B. Irregular papillary muscle
C. Tricuspud valve more apical than mitral
D. RV-fine trabeculations
E. Thebasian vein in RA/RV directly

13. Sarco tubular system:
A. Store energy for muscle contraction
B. Helps transmission from SA node to AV node
C. Has a role in relaxation
D. Calcium pumps plays the dominant role in calcium uptake during diastole
E. Related to sarcomere/tubular system

14. APSAC:
A. Highest molecular weight
B. Higher antigenicity than STK
C. Associated with hypotension
D. Fibrin specific
E. Given as a bolus dose

15. True/False:
A. Clopidogrel is reversible inhibitor
B. Dipyridamole ↑ survival in MI if given with aspirin
C. Aspirin in low dose prevents platelet action for 7 days
D. GpIIb/IIIa antagonist is mostly useful in Diabetic patients
E. Aspirin is better than ACE inhibitor in event prevention

16. Dangerous plaque:
A. Covered with thin fibrous cap
B. Rupture in mid line
C. Usually occupies whole of vessel wall
D. Atherosclerosis occurs in intima of vessel
E. ↑ content of macrophage & ↓ smooth muscle cells

17. Ejection sound:
A. A2-ejection click interval is 40 m.sec
B. Ejection sound heard rarely
C. Non aortic non pulmonary click heard in ventricular septal aneurysm
D. Pulmonary click diminished in inspiration
E. Aortic ejection sound best heard at apex

18. Auscultation of precordium:
A. Most cardiac sounds have frequency of <1000 Hz
B. Higher frequency heard over wide area
C. Smaller tube transmits low pitched sound
D. Double tube is good for low frequency
E. High frequency sounds attenuated by long tube

19. P_2:
A. In most adults in pulmonary area A_2 is louder than P_2
B. In TOF, P_2 is not recordable even on phonocardiogram
C. In mild PPH P_2 is louder than A_2 in aortic area
D. P2 single in patients of Eisenmenger's complex
E. In truncus arteriosus, P_2 is loud

20. For edema:
A. In Hypoproteinemia fast pitting edema disappears in <40 second
B. At least 4 kg of fluid required to produce edema
C. Slow edema → pitting that persist for > 1 minute
D. Ascites with increase intrabdominal pressure can cause slow oedema
E. Slow oedema is due to congestion

21. **EPS:**
A. In CHB, EPS is required
B. Infra hisian block has bad prognosis
C. SA node dysfunction is usually associated with AV node dysfunction
D. In SA node dysfunction, EPS is required
E. SNRT is a useful test

22. **True/false:**
A. LCA supplies AV node in 40%
B. LCA forms Circle of Vieussens for supply of AV node
C. SN artery arises from RCA in 50-60% cases
D. Dominant RCA in 85%
E. In 85-90% cases, AV node supplied by branch of RCA

23. **Loudness of S1:**
A. Increase in Ebstein anomaly
B. Decrease in pneumothorax
C. Increase in Type B WPW
D. Increase in Hiatus hernia
E. Increase in MVP

24. **Stress testing:**
A. Contraindication in uncontrolled diabetics
B. < 3 mets is present in persons with sedentary life style
C. 1 Met–2.5 ml/O_2/kg/min
D. After AMI > 3 MET at 10 weeks increases risk
E. Exercise is directly proportional to VO_2 Max

25. **Prognostic factor for DCM:**
A. Thickening of myocardium
B. Conduction abnormalities
C. ↑ Sympathetic activity
D. Hypoxic arrhythmia
E. ↓ Filling pressure

26. **Apoptosis**
A. Energy dependent
B. Common in end stage LVF
C. Anti apoptotic ↑ survival in CHF
D. Inflammatory exudate
E. β2 receptors via G_1 cause of apoptosis

27. **Angiogenesis:**
A. Effective in coronary as well as peripheral circulation
B. Effective after PTCA
C. VEGF is most potent
D. Is responsible for plaque stability
E. Angiostatin in endogenous inhibitor of angiogenesis

28. **Ultrafast CT:**
A. Helpful to detect occlusion of coronary artery
B. Helpful in detection of calcium even in distal coronary artery
C. Detects occlusion in saphenous venous graft
D. Requires less radiation
E. I/V contrast needed

29. **In Noonan sydrome:**
A. Dwarfism
B. Undescended testis
C. Malocclusion of teeth
D. Mental retardation
E. Pulmonary stenosis

30. **True/False:**
A. In multiple lentigenosis AS is common
B. Ellis van Creveld → webbing of nail bed is common
C. Di George syndrome TOF never occur
D. In Ellis van Creveld VSD is common
E. In Noonan's syndrome: dysplastic pulmonary valve is common

31. **True/False:**
A. Post extra systolic potentiation–Braunwald-Brockenbrough effect
B. Accelerated atherosclerosis is common in progeria
C. Takayasu is the most common cause of HTN in India
D. Takayasu's arteritis is also known as reversed coarctation
E. Type III Takayasu arteritis is most common in India

32. DCMP:
- **A.** Alcoholic CMP → commonest arrhythmia AF
- **B.** Alcoholics have > 50% of DCMP
- **C.** Diabetic CMP is dilated type
- **D.** Pure LV EMF accounts for 20% of all EMF
- **E.** Peripartum CMP associated with a type of myocarditis

33. Definative indication of stopping TMT:
- **A.** Chest pain
- **B.** ST ↓ >1 mm
- **C.** ST ↑ > 1 mm in non q leads
- **D.** ST ↑ > 2 mm in non q leads
- **E.** Decreasing heart rate

34. Oxygen saturation in RA > RV:
- **A.** Unroofed coronary sinus
- **B.** VSD
- **C.** Interrupted IVC
- **D.** LSVC → coronary sinus
- **E.** Gerbode defect

35. M-valve opening in T/F:
- **A.** Isovolumic contraction phase
- **B.** T.V closure before M.V.
- **C.** A_2 louder than P_2 in Aortic area
- **D.** A_2-P_2 closure depends on P_2
- **E.** A-V closure at beginning of isovolumic relaxation

36. Aortic stenosis:
- **A.** 10% have AR
- **B.** Commoner symptom in Angina
- **C.** Syncope develops in-3-10 yrs
- **D.** CHF in-2 yrs.
- **E.** Anacrotic notch indicates severe AR

37. True/False:
- **A.** Perimembranous VSD causes ESM
- **B.** High frequency murmur means high gradient
- **C.** Late systolic murmur → ↑ severity
- **D.** Length of murmur increases with increased severity
- **E.** AS murmur may be continuous

38. A_2–OS interval:
- **A.** ↑ by bradycardia
- **B.** ↑ by ↑ systolic blood pressure
- **C.** ↑ in severe AR
- **D.** Narrow interval → severity
- **E.** Calcification of valve ↓ A_2-OS interval

39. IE prophylaxis is needed in:
- **A.** Modified BT shunt
- **B.** AS with AR
- **C.** AICD
- **D.** Post CABG
- **E.** VSD > 1.5 mm

40. Aortoarteritis:
- **A.** Type IV is most common in India
- **B.** 50% have retinopathy
- **C.** Most common cause of secondary hypertension
- **D.** Mixed lesions are most common
- **E.** Relapses are common

41. Paradoxical S_2:
- **A.** Severe AR
- **B.** PDA
- **C.** PPH
- **D.** LV paced beat
- **E.** LBBB

42. In Pregnancy:
- **A.** Cardiac output increases by 30-50%
- **B.** Blood Volume ↑ by 50%
- **C.** ↑ in cardiac output during third trimester by increase in SV and increased heart rate
- **D.** Pulse pressure decreases maximum in 1st trimester
- **E.** SVR keeps falling till 20 week

43. ACE inhibitors:
- **A.** Acts on AT_1 receptors
- **B.** Histamine is responsible for cough
- **C.** Concentration increases by 6-7 times in tissue
- **D.** Decrease restenosis
- **E.** ↓ diabetic nephropathy in NIDDM/IDDM

44. True/False:
- A. Leopard syndrome → PS
- B. Tuberous sclerosis → cardiomyopathy
- C. Lung AV fistula → Osler weber Rendu
- D. Brachydactyly with PS/AS
- E. Interrupted aortic arch → Catch 22 syndrome

45. CPK-MB:
- A. CPKMB mass/CPK > 1.5 suggest MI
- B. Helps in early diagnosis Of MI
- C. Tongue & small intestine → minor contribution
- D. Carboxypeptidase converts MB1 to MB2
- E. More sensitive than troponin T & I for diagnosis of MI

46. Postextrasystole:
- A. ↑ preload → ↑ contractility
- B. ↓ afterload → ↓ contractility
- C. ↑ systolic time → ↑ contractility
- D. ↑ heart rate → ↑ C.O → ↑ contractility
- E. ↑ diastolic time → ↑ contractility

47. True/False:
- A. Mitral valve opens during Isovolumetric contraction
- B. Aortic valve closes at the beginning of IVRT
- C. Pulmonary valve opens before RV systole
- D. Tricuspid valve closes before M.V
- E. Pulmonary valve opens before aortic valve

48. EPS:
- A. Symptomatic infrahisian block → require permanent pacemaker
- B. SNRT is common parameter for sinus node dysfunction
- C. Asymptomatic sinus node dysfunction requires EPS
- D. SN dysfunction commonly associated with AV node dysfunction
- E. Symptomatic third degree heart block → EPS done

49. RA mean 12 mm Hg, RV 110/12 mm Hg, PA-60 mmHg, PCWP-12 mm Hg: diagnosis is:
- A. PPH
- B. Pulmonary odema with severe pulmonary congestion
- C. Severe CHF
- D. MS
- E. Trans pulmonary gradient present

50. Amyl Nitrite inhalation:
- A. ↑ MR murmur intensity
- B. ↓ intensity of AS murmur
- C. MVP murmur ↓
- D. ↑ murmur of HOCM
- E. In MVP; click becomes earlier

51. True/False:
- A. Trop I binds to Myosin
- B. Trop C binds to Calcium
- C. Trop T & I used in clinical practice
- D. Trop T levels are elevated for >4 day
- D. Trop T levels are elevated > 20 times in acute MI

52. True/False:
- A. Xanthelesma associated with lipid abnormalities in 50% patient
- B. Palmar xanthoma is seen in type III hyperlipidemia
- C. Tuberous xanthoma can be seen in type II hyperlipidemia
- D. Eruptive xanthoma can be seen in type II hyperlipidemia
- E. Tuboeruptive lesions can be seen in type IV hyperlipidemia

53. IDDM patient with good glycemic control:
- A. Still have ↑ atherosclerotic risk factor as compared to general population
- B. Have same risk of developing CAD as compared to general population
- C. Does not affect risk factor status
- D. Is associated with worse outcome after CABG
- E. Is associated with worse outcome after PTCA

54. HOCM:
- A. LVOT gradient maximum in late systole
- B. Post extrasystole beat ↓ ventricular systolic pressure
- C. Post extrasystole pulse pressure ↓
- D. Squatting ↓ LVOT gradient
- E. Spike & dome pattern present during valsalva

55. Digoxin:
A. ↑ AV conduction time
B. ↑ atrial refractory period
C. ↑ atrial automaticity
D. ↑ PR & AH interval
E. Parasympathomimetic effect move than sympatholytic

56. Normal response to exercise:
A. ↑ P wave amplitude
B. ↓ PR interval
C. ↓ R wave amplitude
D. Right axis deviation
E. J point depression & decreased T wave amplitude ↓

57. Body surface potential mapping applied to diagnosis of:
A. Old IWMI
B. localization of bypass tract in WPW
C. Recognition of ventricular hypertrophy
D. Estimation of size of M I
E. Congenital heart disease

58. Continuous murmur:
A. ASD + MS
B. VSD + AR
C. Pulmonary atresia
D. Severe coarctation of aorta
E. Peripheral pulmonary artery stenosis

59. LMWH:
A. Platelet factor inhibition
B. Osteoporosis
C. Synthesized from UFH
D. Has a significant role in platelet function & vascular integrity
E. Cannot be given on OPD basis

60. Chronic CHF:
A. ↓ sympathetic activation
B. RAS activation
C. ↑ Aldosterone
D. ↑ vasopressin
E. ↑ vasodilation

Answers

1 A T B F C T D T E F	2 A T B T C T D T E T	3 A F B T C F D F E F	4 A F B F C T D T E T	5 A T B T C T D T E T	6 A T B F C T D F E T	7 A F B T C T D T E T	8 A T B T C F D T E T	9 A T B F C T D F E F	10 A F B F C T D T E F
11 A F B F C T D F E T	12 A T B T C T D F E T	13 A F B F C T D T E T	14 A T B F C T D F E T	15 A F B F C T D T E T	16 A T B F C F D T E T	17 A T B T C T D T E T	18 A T B T C T D F E T	19 A T B F C T D T E F	20 A T B T C T D T E T
21 A F B T C T D T E T	22 A F B F C T D T E T	23 A T B T C T D F E T	24 A F B F C F D F E T	25 A F B T C F D T E F	26 A T B T C T D F E F	27 A T B T C T D T E T	28 A T B T C T D T E T	29 A T B T C F D T E T	30 A F B T C F D F E T
31 A F B T C F D T E T	32 A T B F C F D F E F	33 A F B F C T D T E F	34 A T B F C F D F E T	35 A F B F C T D T E F	36 A F B T C F D T E F	37 A F B T C T D T E F	38 A T B F C T D T E T	39 A T B T C F D F E T	40 A F B F C F D T E T
41 A T B T C F D F E T	42 A T B T C F D T E F	43 A F B F C F D F E T	44 A T B F C T D T E T	45 A F B T C T D F E F	46 A T B F C T D T E T	47 A F B T C F D F E T	48 A T B T C F D T E F	49 A F B F C F D F E T	50 A F B F C F D T E T
51 A F B T C T D T E T	52 A F B T C T D F E F	53 A T B F C F D F E T	54 A T B T C T D T E T	55 A T B F C T D T E T	56 A T B T C F D F E T	57 A T B T C F D T E F	58 A T B F C T D T E T	59 A T B F C T D F E F	60 A F B T C T D T E F

SGPGI 2000 (June)

1. **Atrial fibrillation in Acute MI:**
   - **A.** Commoner than flutter
   - **B.** Frequent with inferior than with anterior
   - **C.** Common after 24 hours
   - **D.** Common with LV failure
   - **E.** Does not adversely affect prognosis

2. **Platelet:**
   - **A.** ADP stimulate platelet activation
   - **B.** Ticlopidine inhibits cyclooxygenase pathway
   - **C.** Platelet adhesion through subendothelial VWF
   - **D.** PAF stimulate macrophages and PMN leucocytes
   - **E.** GbIIb/IIIa attach to platelet fibrinogen

3. **Post MI, Free wall rupture:**
   - **A.** Female > male
   - **B.** Common in second week
   - **C.** Occurs with diffuse disease
   - **D.** Occurs with 1st infarct
   - **E.** Occur in 25% of patients dying in hospital with MI

4. **Positive abdominal jugular reflex:**
   - **A.** Positive with increased PCWP
   - **B.** The venous pressure can be measured
   - **C.** 'a' wave with RV systole
   - **D.** TS: 'y'descent is gradual
   - **E.** Clue for acute heart failure

5. **Squatting effect:**
   - **A.** ↑ RVS_3S_4
   - **B.** ↑ LVS_3S_4
   - **C.** ↑ MS murmur
   - **D.** ↑ MR murmur
   - **E.** ↑ VSD murmur

6. **Regarding hangout interval:**
   - **A.** Pulmonary hangout interval is increased in ASD
   - **B.** Normal split S2–¾ of the split is caused by P2 delay
   - **C.** Hangout increases with increase capacitance and decreased resistance
   - **D.** Aortic hangout increases in Systemic HT
   - **E.** Pulmonary hangout interval > aortic hangout interval

7. **Square wave response:**
   - **A.** ASD
   - **B.** HOCM
   - **C.** CCP
   - **D.** MS
   - **E.** CHF

8. **Isometric exercise:**
   - **A.** Decreased cardiac output
   - **B.** ↓ Heart size
   - **C.** ↓ LVF
   - **D.** ↑ SVR
   - **E.** ↓ LVOT murmur in HOCM

9. **Valsalva:**
   - **A.** Phase IV-increase SVR
   - **B.** Phase II A2P2 increased
   - **C.** Phase III-BP decreased (sudden)
   - **D.** Phase IV-reflex bradycardia
   - **E.** Phase II-S3 S4 increased

10. **Arterial baroreflexes in hypertension:**
    - **A.** Inhibit efferent sympathetic outflow
    - **B.** Increased rennin release
    - **C.** Decreased heart rate
    - **D.** No effect on heart rate
    - **E.** Inhibit efferent para sympathetic outflow

11. Brockenbrough-Braunwald phenomenon:
A. Nonobstructed HCM
B. PVC
C. Pulse pressure decreased
D. LV pressure more than control beat
E. LVOT gradient higher in post ectopic beat

12. Vasodilator beta blockers:
A. Carvidalol
B. Bucindolol
C. Cartelol
D. Celiprolol
E. Bevantolol

13. Unstable angina:
A. Dipyridamole + aspirin is effective
B. Aspirin + heparin more effective than warfarin
C. Ticlopidine better than placebo
D. LMWH inferior to UFH
E. LMWH given for prolonged periods

14. TOF:
A. Arterial desaturation always despite minimal cyanosis
B. LVP = RVP
C. RAP ↑
D. PAP normal
E. LV could be normal

15. MS +TS:
A. RAP & LAP ↑
B. LVEDP ↑
C. RVEDP normal
D. Rt to Lt shunt due to increased RAP
E. O_2 saturation normal

16. Normal hemodynamics:
A. Mean PAP 6-12 mmHg
B. Mean PCP 5-13 mmHg
C. PCWP mean = PADP
D. Small gradient between pulmonary vein and pulmonary artery
E. LVEDP upto 18 mm

17. Heart with situs solitus:
A. Right bronchus horizontal
B. RPA below Right bronchus
C. Right diaphragm higher due to liver
D. IVC to left of spine
E. Aorta left half of spine

18. ASD with valvular PS:
A. Gradient across PV 60 mmHg
B. RVP increased in late stages
C. LAP increased 1-2 mm than RAP
D. Additional step up of oxygen at ventricular level
E. Asymptomatic course is benign

19. MS with PVH with PAH:
A. R-L shunt at atrial level
B. Pulmonary haemosiderosis
C. LA mildly increased in size
D. LVEDP may be increased
E. RAP increased

20. Infundibular PS with intact IVS:
A. RVP suprasystemic
B. Myocardial sinusoios seen
C. Cyanosis in late stages
D. RAP increased
E. No gradient across PV

21. ASD L → R Qp/Qs 2.5 : 1
A. O_2 step up at atrial level
B. PCWP could be increased
C. No systemic desaturation
D. S2 wide fixed split
E. Increased systolic pressure of RV

22. PDA with severe PAH causing Eisenmenger's:
A. Cyanosis arm > leg
B. RVP is suprasystemic
C. RAP normal
D. Diastolic shunt murmur
E. LV pressure is decreased

23. AR + MR
A. ↑ heart size
B. LAP severely elevated
C. RAP normal
D. Pulmonary edema occurs early
E. Generally well tolerated in pregnancy

24. Hyperhomocystenemia:
A. Increases in CRF
B. ↑ atherogenicity
C: Vit B complex given
D. Known to cause venous embolism
E. Associated with Pernicious anemia

25. Unstable angina and angiography:
A. 10% normal CAG
B. 80 % contain thrombus on CAG
C. Culprit lesion in 50% identified
D. Angioscopy sensitivity for thrombus
E. IVUS most specific to identify culprit lesion

26. Culture negative endocarditis:
A. Q fever
B. C burnetti
C. B Quintana
D. Ekinella
E. Acinetobacter

27. Idiopathic DCMP histology:
A. Myocyte hypertrophy
B. No myofilament loss
C. Myocyte atrophy
D. Normal extramural artery and capillary
E. Myocyte necrosis

28. DCMP with adrenergic system:
A. β1 receptor decreased
B. β2 receptor ↑
C. Inhibitory G1 ↓
D. β2 receptor uncoupling
E. Inotropic response to β agonist

29. Primary APLS:
A. Recurrent arterial thrombosis
B. Thrombocytosis
C. Recurrent abortion
D. Anticardiolipin antibodies are elevated
E. Lupus anticoagulant is elevated

30. Cardiac tamponade:
A. Atrial pressure always ↑
B. Pericardiocentesis required
C. Always leads to constriction
D. Intra pericardial pressure higher than atrial
E. ECG: electrical alternans

31. Coronary calcification:
A. EBCT helps in detection of coronary calcification
B. Plaque has $CaCO_3$ deposition related to Vit D3 intake
C. Degree of calcification relation to severity of CAD
D. Calcified medial sclerosis associated with increased risk of acute coronary syndrome
E. Coronary calcification seen usually in adventitia by IVUS

32. CABG in stable angina: improvement in survival is seen in:
A. Left main coronary
B. TVD with normal LV function
C. DVD with impaired LV function
D. SVD without LAD disease
E. SVI/DVD with LAD involvement

33. True/False:
A. NYHA III moderate limitation of physical activity
B. NYHA II mild limitation of physical activity
C. Stage III < 2 METS
D. NYHA better predictor of mortality than specific activity scale
E. CCS is for angina only

34. Exercise stress test in supine position:
A. 1 met 4.5 ml/kg/min
B. Delayed fall in systolic pressure is ominous
C. Stage 1 Bruce is 5 METS
D. Specific activity scale in stage III is less than 2 METS
E. Can be performed in severe aortic stenosis prior to surgery

35. True/false:
A. Pulsus Bisferians is best seen in carotids
B. Pulsus bigeminous is twice beating pulse
C. Coanda effect is seen in subvalvular AS
D. Pulsus alternans: regularly beating pulse
E. Reverse pulse paradoxus in HOCM

36. Exercise testing:

- **A.** Initially increased cardiac ouput due to increase in SVR
- **B.** Later on ↑ CO due to ↑ HR
- **C.** Diastolic BP normally falls
- **D.** Vaso constriction
- **E.** Pulmonary vasculature capable of accommodating six times increase in cardiac output

37. Lp(a):

- **A.** Level protects against atherosclerosis
- **B.** Homologous to plasminogen
- **C.** Decrease by niacin
- **D.** LDL more atherogenic than buoyant LDL
- **E.** Lipids contain core of lipoproteins surrounded by apoprotein and phospholipids.

38. ASD:

- **A.** Ostium primum–LAD + LBBB
- **B.** Ostium secundum: RAD with incomplete RBBB
- **C.** Sinus venosus with left upper pulmonary vein
- **D.** Ostium primum associated with invariably defective mitral valve
- **E.** Operation before 25 years is not beneficial

39. HRT in females:

- **A.** ↑ HDL level
- **B.** ↓ PAI–1 level
- **C.** ↓ TG
- **D.** ↑ LDL oxidation
- **E.** ↓ insulin requirement in DM

40. In CHF:

- **A.** ↑ epinephrine
- **B.** Activation of renin angiotensin axis
- **C.** ↑ vasopressin levels
- **D.** ↑ aldosterone levels
- **E.** ↑ endothelin

41. True/false:

- **A.** Dopamine act at DA receptor
- **B.** Isoproterenol acts at β2 receptor
- **C.** Dopamine acts at β1 receptor
- **D.** Dopamine does not act on β2
- **E.** Dopamine does not act on α2

42. Phosphocreatinine/ATP ratio:

- **A.** Is not a prognostic marker with CMP
- **B.** Is a prognostic marker with CMP
- **C.** Marker of mitochondrial energy reserve
- **D.** Ratio always less than 1
- **E.** Dynamic cardiomyoplasty decreases mortality

43. Regarding endothelin:

- **A.** Endothelium derived vasodilator
- **B.** Myocyte hypertrophy
- **C.** Decreased in AMI
- **D.** Increase in CHF
- **E.** Has a role in the management of CHF

44. True/false:

- **A.** Frank sterling mechanism related to fibre shortening in ventricular tension
- **B.** T tubules play role in initiation of contraction coupling
- **C.** Myocytes are not rich in mitochondria
- **D.** Increase heart rate and increased contractility-Treppe effect
- **E.** Increased aortic pressure leads to increased contractility: Anrep effect

45. Incidence of plaque rupture is related to:

- **A.** Degree of angiographic stenosis
- **B.** SMC content of plaque
- **C.** Macrophage content of plaque
- **D.** Intraplaque core lipids
- **E.** Increase in collagen content

46. CAPRIE trial:

- **A.** Ticlopidine and clopidogrel: both associated with neutropenia
- **B.** Ticlopidine better than aspirin in end points like stroke and MI
- **C.** Acts by binding ADP receptors to fibrinogen molecules
- **D.** Inclusion criteria included recent ischemic stroke, recent myocardial infarction (MI), or established peripheral arterial disease
- **E.** Inhibitory effect related to half life of drug

47. Treatment for thromboembolism:

A. In history of venous thromboembolism pulmonary embolectomy should be done
B. If 1 segmental and 3 subsegmental areas are involved in lung perfusion scan PT is doubtful.
C. Treatment of choice of acute PT is urokinase
D. Management of DVT of large vessel thrombectomy
E. Greenfield filter is commonly used for recurrent pulmonary thromboembolism

48. Cardiac output measurement:

A. Angiographic cardiac output measurements are preferred to Fick and thermodilution methods for calculation of stenotic valve areas in patients with severe aortic or mitral regurgitation
B. Variability of upto 10% in calculations of cardiac output by the Fick's method
C. When interpreting results of the indicator dilution method, the area under the curve is directly related to the cardiac output
D. Left to right shunts results in early recirculation on indicator dilution or thermodilution curves
E. Thermodilution cardiac outputs may cause a falsely elevated cardiac output value in low output states

49. Cardiac cycle:

A. The third heart sound corresponds to the rapid early diastolic filling of the ventricles
B. Prominent 'a' wave on the right or left atrial pressure tracing is typical of AF
C. The QRS complex on the ECG corresponds to the timing of isovolumic ventricular contraction
D. The 'v' wave on the right or left atrial pressure tracing occurs after the 'T' wave on the ECG
E. The mitral valve opens in diastole when the left atrial pressure falls below that of the left ventricle

50. Sudden cardiac death:

A. Is the first clinical manifestation of coronary artery disease in approximately 25% patients
B. LV dysfunction and ventricular ectopic activity after MI increase the risk of SCD
C. The most common mechanism of cardiac arrest is cardiac asystole
D. Onset of brain death occurs within 4-6 minutes of unattended ventricular fibrillation
E. The outcome of patients with bradycardiac/asystolic out of hospital cardiac arrest is worse than if VF is the initial arrhythmia

51. Pacemaker complications:

A. Acceptable rates of lead dislodgement are less than 1% for ventricular leads and less than 2-3% for atrial leads
B. In the presence of a wire fracture, the lead impedance is high
C. In the presence of an insulation break, the lead impedance is low
D. In the presence of lead dislodgement, the lead impedance is normal
E. Early infection after pacemaker implantation is most commonly caused by streptococci

52. Post MI LV aneurysm:

A. Usually due to total occlusion of the LAD
B. Usually range in size from 1-8 cm in diameter
C. Inferoposterior aneurysms are slightly more common than apical aneurysm
D. Similar mortality to those patients with MI with no LV aneurysm and similar LVEF
E. Persistent ST segment elevation in ECG indicates a large infarct but does not necessarily indicate an aneurysm

53. Cyanosis in cyanotic congenital heart disease:

A. Is due to levels of reduced hemoglobin in excess of 2 gm/dl
B. Peripheral cyanosis is due to increase oxygen extraction from normally saturated arterial blood
C. Is not affected by physical exertion
D. Differential cyanosis usually results from the presence of aortic coarctation and left to right shunting
E. Is sometimes improved by squatting posture

54. Cardiac amyloidosis:
- **A.** Restrictive cardiomyopathy
- **B.** Cardiac tamponade
- **C.** Orthostatic hypotension
- **D.** Systolic dysfunction
- **E.** Pericardial constriction

55. Increased LV preload is seen in the presence of:
- **A.** Sepsis
- **B.** Right ventricular failure
- **C.** Mitral regurgitation
- **D.** Dehydration
- **E.** Renal failure with oliguria

56. Syndrome X:
- **A.** May have abnormal nuclear scintigraphy
- **B.** Abnormal pain perception and increased sympathetic tone are potential causative mechanisms
- **C.** Aggressive modification of cardiac risk factors is not indicated
- **D.** Calcium channel blockers are useful
- **E.** Seen in 50-70% postmenopausal women

57. Syncope:
- **A.** Unidentifiable cause in upto 50% cases
- **B.** One year mortality in patients with syncope with unknown cause is 6%
- **C.** One year mortality in patients with syncope with noncardiac causes is < 15%
- **D.** One year mortality in patients with syncope with cardiac causes is 19-30%
- **E.** EPS in patients with unexplained syncope and structurally normal heart has diagnostic yield of 70%

58. TIMI risk score:
- **A.** Elevated cardiac markers
- **B.** Prior stenosis of coronary ≥ 75%
- **C.** ≥ 1 episode of angina within past 24 hours
- **D.** Prior use of aspirin and clopidogrel in past 24 hours
- **E.** ≥ 3 risk factors for CAD

59. Brugada criteria for ventricular tachycardia:
- **A.** Superior QRS axis
- **B.** Absence of RS complex in all precordial leads
- **C.** R to S interval > 100msec in 1 precordial
- **D.** Fusion beats
- **E.** QRS width > 0.14 sec

60. RV infarction:
- **A.** ST elevation of at least 0.1 mV in lead aVR is very sensitive and specific for diagnosis
- **B.** Kussmaul's sign is common
- **C.** Typical hemodynamic findings include a right atrial pressure > 75-80% of wedge pressure
- **D.** Intravenous NTG is relatively contraindicated
- **E.** Volume loading to achieve a right atrial pressure above 18 mm Hg is usually required to optimize hemodynamics and forward flow

Answers

Q	A	B	C	D	E
1	T	F	F	T	F
2	T	F	T	F	T
3	T	F	F	T	F
4	T	T	F	T	T
5	T	T	T	T	T
6	T	T	T	F	T
7	T	F	T	T	T
8	F	F	F	T	T
9	T	F	T	T	F
10	T	F	T	F	F
11	F	T	T	T	T
12	T	T	F	F	F
13	F	T	T	F	F
14	T	T	F	T	T
15	T	F	F	F	T
16	F	T	T	T	F
17	F	T	T	F	T
18	T	T	F	F	T
19	F	T	F	F	T
20	T	T	F	T	T
21	T	F	T	T	F
22	F	F	F	F	F
23	T	T	F	T	T
24	T	T	T	T	T
25	F	T	F	T	F
26	T	T	T	T	T
27	T	F	T	F	T
28	T	T	F	F	T
29	T	F	T	T	T
30	F	T	F	T	T
31	T	F	F	F	F
32	T	F	T	F	T
33	T	T	F	F	T
34	F	T	T	F	F
35	T	F	F	T	T
36	T	T	F	F	T
37	F	T	T	T	F
38	F	T	F	T	F
39	T	T	F	F	F
40	T	T	T	T	T
41	T	T	T	F	T
42	F	T	T	F	F
43	F	T	F	T	F
44	T	T	F	T	T
45	F	T	T	T	F
46	T	T	T	T	F
47	F	T	F	F	T
48	T	T	F	T	T
49	T	F	T	T	F
50	T	T	F	T	T
51	T	T	T	T	F
52	T	T	F	F	T
53	F	T	F	F	T
54	T	F	T	T	F
55	F	F	T	F	T
56	T	T	F	T	T
57	T	T	T	T	F
58	T	F	F	F	T
59	F	T	T	F	F
60	T	T	T	T	F

SGPGI 1999

1. **Autosomal dominant disorders are:**
   A. Holt Oram syndrome
   B. Noonan's syndrome
   C. Ellis van Crevald syndrome
   D. Turner syndrome
   E. Down syndrome

2. **Following drugs are safe in pregnancy:**
   A. Beta blocker
   B. Ca Channel blocker
   C. Na Nitroprusside
   D. Digoxin
   E. ACE inhibitor

3. **Following are true of ACE:**
   A. Convert angiotensinogen I to II
   B. Help in degradation of angiotensinogen
   C. Causes constriction of efferent renal arteriole
   D. Increase bradykinin level
   E. Increase norepinephrine level

4. **Following drugs have antiproliferative effect on ventricular hypertrophy:**
   A. ACEI
   B. Beta blocker
   C. Diuretics
   D. Alpha blocker
   E. Hydralazine

5. **Wide splitting of S2 is seen in:**
   A. RBBB
   B. Ac MR
   C. Ac PE
   D. PDA
   E. Hypertensive heart disease

6. **Mid diastolic murmur is heard in:**
   A. PR (normal PA pressure)
   B. MR
   C. VSD
   D. RSOV to LV
   E. CHB

7. **Following are true of syndrome X:**
   A. Increased HDL
   B. Decreased triglyceride
   C. Increase PAI-1
   D. Increase small dense LDL
   E. Normal buoyant LDL

8. **Peripheral pulmonary artery stenosis:**
   A. Has 3 anatomic types
   B. Type II has multiple peripheral stenoses
   C. Produce continuous murmur
   D. Murmur spread to whole of thorax
   E. Rubella is 2nd commonest cause of PPS

9. **Neurocardiogenic syncope:**
   A. Beta blocker is drug of choice
   B. Permanent pacing treatment of choice
   C. Caused by stimulation of ventricular mechano-receptors
   D. Cardio inhibitory response is inhibited by beta blockers
   E. Vasodepressor response is improved by beta blockers

10. **Following drug increase HV interval:**
   A. Procainamide
   B. Flecainide
   C. Digoxin
   D. Amiodarone
   E. Phenytoin

11. QT interval decrease in following conditions:
A. Hypercalcemia
B. Hypocalcemia
C. Hyperkalemia
D. Hypokalemia
E. Digoxin

12. Following drugs decrease lower esophageal sphincter tone:
A. ACEI
B. Nitrates
C. Beta blocker
D. Smoking
E. Fatty meal

13. Adenosine is used in following situation:
A. AVNRT
B. PAH
C. Ectopic atrial tachycardia
D. Angina
E. DCMP

14. Exercise is contraindicated in following:
A. Sev AR
B. Severe AS
C. HCM
D. PPH
E. CHB

15. Cardiac output in severe PS is dependent upon:
A. Severity of PS
B. RV function
C. ASD
D. PFO
E. Infundibular PS

16. Following are not consistent with TOF diagnosis?
A. RBBB
B. Absent RVH
C. RA enlargement
D. QRS axis > 150
E. QRS transition shifted to left

17. ASD repair in a 30 year age is helpful because:
A. Increased longevity
B. Decreased chances of PAH
C. Decrease Paradoxical embolization
D. Improves exercise capacity
E. Prevents CVA

18. Apex phonocardiography:
A. 'a' wave < 15 %
B. E point denotes RV ejection
C. After 'E' point there is gradual upstroke
D. 'O' point coincides with mitral valve opening
E. Helps in differentiating between different types of cardiac overload conditions

19. Ebstein's anomaly:
A. Box shaped heart
B. Multiple heart sounds
C. Type A WPW
D. Decrease pulmonary blood flow
E. Cyanosis can occur because of right to left shunt at atrial level

20. Radiotherapy is associated with:
A. Increase incidence of MR
B. AS
C. AR
D. Effusive pericarditis
E. Conduction defects

21. Signs of CCF in infant;
A. Tachypnea
B. Peripheral oedema
C. Orthopnoea
D. Cyanosis
E. Poor feeding

22. LV S3 is found in:
A. Tricuspid atresia with large collaterals
B. RSOV into RA
C. TAPVC
D. Acute MR
E. Acute AR

23. Mechanism of nitrate tolerance:
A. Decreased sulfhydryl group
B. Reflex increase in sympathetic tone
C. Increased renin
D. Decreased nitrate receptor
E. Plasma volume expansion

24. Straight back syndrome is associated with:
A. rsr' pattern
B. RAD
C. ECG usually abnormal
D. Otherwise LAD with RsR in lead V1
E. Non specific T changes

25. Difference between fetal and adult heart disease:
A. More non contractile pattern in fetal heart
B. Only one intracardiac shunt in fetus
C. Better diastolic relaxation with fetal myocyte of V1 type
D. PVR = SVR
E. Decrease parasympathetic stimuli

26. Vasodilator in CCF causes:
A. Increased HR
B. Increased CO
C. Increased ESV
D. Decrease PCWP
E. Reduction in mean BP

27. Endothelin is:
A. Vasoconstrictor
B. Dilator
C. Used in HT
D. Decreased in CHF
E. Absent myocardial hypertrophy

28. Parathyroid disease and heart:
A. Cardiac arrhythmia
B. Hypertrophy can be seen without even hypertension
C. Increase risk of CAD with chronic hypercalcemia
D. Calcium deposition mainly in endocardium
E. Most common ECG feature is short QT and 1/v conduction defects

29. Absolutely contra indication to thrombolytic therapy:
A. DBP 100
B. Pregnancy
C. Subclavian/internal jugular vein cannulation
D. Oral anticoagulant therapy
E. A-V malformation or tumor in spinal cord

30. Rapid weight reduction is associated with:
A. CHF
B. Cardiac atrophy
C. Decrease cardiac contractility
D. Increase QT interval
E. SCD

31. Sexual dysfunction is associated with:
A. Beta blockers
B. Occur in 50% of patients
C. Can be reduced by decreased dose
D. Does not occur with selective beta blockers
E. Improved by nitrates

32. Following are coronary dilators:
A. Nitrates
B. Beta blocker
C. Hypoxia
D. NO
E. Acetylcholine

33. About Lutembacher's syndrome:
A. MS is rheumatic in origin
B. Valvotomy is treatment of choice
C. Most common in females
D. Signs of MS predominate
E. Prominent 'a' wave in JVP

34. MVP is associated with:
A. Ehler Danlos syndrome
B. Polydactyly
C. Straight back syndrome
D. Pectus Excavatum
E. Thoracic lumbar scoliosis

35. About absent pulmonary valve syndrome; not seen is:
A. PR associated
B. PS
C. PDA
D. PFO
E. Hypoplastic pulmonary arteries

36. Serum homocysteine:
A. Very difficult to estimate
B. Decrease level associated with risk of CAD
C. Associated with vascular events
D. Seen in < 5% of patients with CAD
E. Increase incidence of stroke

37. **Regarding xanthomas:**
   A. Xanthelesma indicates CAD in > 50% cases
   B. Tuboeruptive in Type II
   C. Palmar in Type III
   D. Eruptive in Type II
   E. Palmar–type II homozygous hypercholesterolemia

38. **Regarding troponin:**
   A. TnI bind to myosin
   B. Tnc binds to calcium
   C. TnT 20 times the base level in ac MI
   D. Trop T and I are specific for myocardial injury
   E. Trop I remain elevated for 14 days

39. **Tricuspid anomaly associated with following drugs:**
   A. Lithium
   B. Alcohol
   C. Thalidomide
   D. Fenfluramine
   E. Hydralazine

40. **Flosequinan used as vasodilator is now banned because:**
   A. Other better drugs available
   B. Cause fatal arrhythmia
   C. Increase mortality
   D. Irreversible side effects
   E. Did not show any benefit

41. **Advantages of unfractionated heparin:**
   A. Inhibits clot bound thrombin
   B. Does not require monitoring
   C. Narrow therapeutic range
   D. Does not inhibit platelet aggregation
   E. Effect proportional to dosage

42. **All of the following lesions are ductus dependant:**
   A. Ebstein's anomaly with ASD
   B. ASD with TGA with normal IVS
   C. VSD with pulmonary atresia
   D. Pulmonary atresia with ASD with normal IVS
   E. Tricuspid atresia

43. **IDDM with CAD:**
   A. Incidence more than general population
   B. Incidence same as general population
   C. IDDM with good glycemic control is still a risk factor for high risk CABG and PTCA
   D. Glycemic control reduced risk factor
   E. CABG gives better results than multivessel PTCA

44. **Improvement in endothelial function by:**
   A. Decreased cholesterol
   B. Nitrate rich diet
   C. Exercise
   D. Increase Acetylcholine esterase orally
   E. Estrogens

45. **Pravastatin:**
   A. Dose 20 mg/day
   B. Decrease restenosis after PTCA
   C. Not effective in women
   D. Decrease strokes
   E. Decrease LDL by 25-30%

46. **Regarding DM and CAD:**
   A. CAD is 4 times more common in diabetic than non-diabetics
   B. Even if there is good glycemic control, still there is risk in PTCA
   C. Abciximab decrease restenosis more in DM
   D. Apple type of obesity
   E. Platelet aggregation is inhibited by aspirin in normal people but not in DM

47. **Isopotential body surface mapping:**
   A. Used to detect old MI
   B. Size and site of MI
   C. To detect pre excitation syndrome
   D. For diagnosis of CHD
   E. For detection of LVH

48. **Congenital HD is:**
   A. In monozygotic twins, only male affected
   B. Low incidence of CHD in monozygotic twins
   C. If mother has CHD, chances of child having CHD is more than if father is affected
   D. Increase risk by 10 times in sibling, if sibling has CHD
   E. Malformations are concordant or partially concordant in families

49. Congenital heart disease with decrease pulmonary blood flow?
- **A.** Pulmonary atresia
- **B.** Ebstein anomaly
- **C.** Rupture of sinus of valsalva
- **D.** Tricuspid atresia
- **E.** TAPVC

50. X-ray findings associated with MVP:
- **A.** Pectus excavation
- **B.** Loss of thoracic kyphosis
- **C.** Straight back syndrome
- **D.** Polydactyly
- **E.** RV enlargement

51. IE prophylaxis is done in?
- **A.** Bronchoscopy
- **B.** Prostate surgery
- **C.** GI surgery
- **D.** Oral ingestion of local anesthetic
- **E.** Prolonged cardiac catheterization

52. Digoxin levels are increased with:
- **A.** Verapamil
- **B.** Erythromycin
- **C.** Rifampicin
- **D.** Phenytoin
- **E.** Quinidine

53. Wide split S2 in:
- **A.** RBBB
- **B.** Acute MR
- **C.** PDA
- **D.** Hypertensive heart disease
- **E.** VSD

54. Pheochromocytoma; clinical clues are:
- **A.** Inappropriate hyponatraemia
- **B.** Pressure response to beta blockers
- **C.** Neurofibromatosis
- **D.** Orthostatic hypotension
- **E.** Abdominal lump

55. Apoptosis; True/False:
- **A.** Programmed cell death
- **B.** Does not require energy
- **C.** Seen in end stage heart failure
- **D.** Associated with cell swelling
- **E.** DNA fragmentation is seen

56. ASD; true/false:
- **A.** Ostium primum shows LBBB
- **B.** Ostium secundum shows RAD with incomplete RBBB
- **C.** Sinus venosus with left upper pulmonary vein in RA
- **D.** Operation before 25 years
- **E.** Ostium primum defects associated invariably with mitral valve disease

57. True/False:
- **A.** VSD is more common in IWMI than AWMI
- **B.** VSD is most common following 1st attack of MI
- **C.** Thrill is more common in MR as compared to VSD
- **D.** Papillary muscle dysfunction is more common in AWMI than IWMI
- **E.** Papillary muscle involvement is more distal than proximal

58. True/False:
- **A.** Heyde's syndrome is angiodysplasia of colon with congenital AS
- **B.** LAD is associated with PS with rubella
- **C.** Most common lesion in RHD is MS
- **D.** Septal tricuspid leaflet displacement in Ebsteins anomaly is > 8mm/m ^{2}
- **E.** Most common cardiovascular disease in India is MI

59. HRT in females:
- **A.** Increase HDL levels
- **B.** Decrease PAI-I levels
- **C.** Decrease Triglycerides
- **D.** Increase LDL-oxidation
- **E.** Decrease insulin requirement in diabetes

60. Square wave response in valsalva:
- **A.** ASD
- **B.** HOCM
- **C.** CCP
- **D.** MS
- **E.** CHF

Answers

1 A T B T C F D F E F	2 A T B T C F D T E F	3 A T B F C T D T E T	4 A T B T C T D T E F	5 A T B T C F D F E F	6 A T B T C T D F E T	7 A F B F C T D T E F	8 A F B F C T D T E F	9 A T B F C T D F E T	10 A T B T C F D T E F
11 A T B F C T D F E T	12 A F B T C T D T E F	13 A T B T C F D F E F	14 A F B T C T D T E F	15 A T B T C F D F E T	16 A F B T C F D T E T	17 A T B F C T D T E F	18 A T B F C F D T E T	19 A T B T C F D T E T	20 A T B T C T D T E T
21 A T B F C F D T E T	22 A T B T C F D T E T	23 A T B T C T D F E T	24 A T B T C F D F E T	25 A T B T C F D F E F	26 A T B T C F D T E T	27 A T B F C F D F E F	28 A T B T C T D T E T	29 A F B F C F D F E T	30 A F B T C T D T E T
31 A T B F C T D F E T	32 A T B F C T D T E F	33 A T B F C T D F E T	34 A T B T C T D T E T	35 A T B T C F D T E F	36 A F B F C T D T E T	37 A F B F C T D F E T	38 A T B T C T D T E T	39 A T B F C F D T E F	40 A T B T C T D F E T
41 A F B F C F D T E T	42 A F B F C T D T E F	43 A T B F C T D T E T	44 A T B F C T D F E T	45 A F B T C F D T E T	46 A T B T C T D T E F	47 A T B T C T D F E T	48 A F B T C T D F E T	49 A T B T C F D T E F	50 A T B F C T D T E F
51 A F B T C T D F E F	52 A T B T C F D F E T	53 A T B T C F D F E T	54 A F B T C T D T E T	55 A T B F C T D F E T	56 A F B T C F D F E T	57 A F B T C F D F E F	58 A T B T C F D T E F	59 A T B T C F D F E F	60 A T B F C T D T E T

SGPGI 1998 (December)

1. Calculate median from the following: 10, 9, 9, 8, 7, 6, 7:

A. 10 B. 9
C. 8 D. 7

2. Correlation co-efficient lies between:

A. 0-1
B. 1-2
C. -1 to +1
D. -2 to +2

3. PQLI: all are true *except:*

A. Infant mortality rate
B. Literacy rate
C. Per capita income
D. Mortality at 1 year of age

4. IUGR on USG is diagnosed best by monitoring:

A. Biparietal diameter
B. Abdominal circumference
C. Femur length
D. Head circumference: abdominal circumference ratio

5. Drug causing pulmonary fibrosis is:

A. Diuretics
B. ACE inhibitors
C. Beta blockers
D. Calcium channel blockers

6. Which of the following increases cholesterol?

A. Diuretics
B. Alcohol
C. Hypothyroidism
D. Diabetes mellitus

7. Dicrotic pulse: all are true *except:*

A. Hypovolemic shock
B. Rare for SBP <130
C. Can be seen normally
D. Typhoid

8. Combined oral contraceptive pills $\uparrow$ risk for all *except:*

A. Acute MI
B. Venous thrombosis
C. SAH
D. Stroke (Ischemic)

9. Young female, aspirin sensitive menorrhagia, bleeding, PT normal, aPPT increase, BT increase, platelets normal. Diagnosis is:

A. Von Willebrand disease
B. Hemophilia A
C. Factor VII deficiency
D. Christmas disease

10. Anion gap is not increased in:

A. Lactic acidosis
B. Renal failure
C. DKA
D. Diarrhoea

---

1 C 2 C 3 C 4 B 5 C 6 C 7 B 8 C 9 A 10 D

11. M_1-T_1 > 65 msec in:
A. MS
B. Ebstein
C. TS
D. Cortriatriatum

12. Splitting of S1 is seen in:
A. RBBB
B. LBBB
C. RV pacing
D. VSD

13. All are true for LA myxoma *except:*
A. Soft S1
B. MDM
C. Systolic mitral murmur
D. Tumor plop

14. Rheumatoid arthritis: which is true?
A. CVS manifestations before joint manifestation
B. CVS manifestations when nodules present in myocardium
C. Pericarditis is rare
D. Coronary arteritis is rare

15. 20 year old with coarctation following is unlikely to be seen:
A. Dissection of aorta
B. Infective endocarditis of aortic valve (bicuspid)
C. Subarachnoid hemorrhage
D. CHF

16. $PaSO_2$ > AoSO2 is seen in all *except:*
A. TGA
B. Mitral atresia
C. TAPVC
D. DORV with subpulmonic VSD

17. Adenosine success rate in SVT:
A. 95% success rate in 30 sec
B. 95% success rate in 2 min
C. 80% success rate in 5 min
D. 95% success rate in 1 min

18. Atrial arrhythmias which is not true:
A. Significant structural heart disease
B. CS massage usually converts atrial arrhythmia
C. PAT with block usually due to digoxin
D. Atrial arrhythmias can be treated by surgery

19. In diagnosis of sick sinus syndrome, which is not required?
A. Holter
B. SN Conduction time
C. SNRT
D. His purkinje studies

20. Fastest conduction velocity is seen in
A. SA node
B. AV node
C. Ventricular muscle
D. His purkinje system

21. S3 is heard in:
A. d-TGA
B. TA with large collaterals
C. TAPVC
D. c-TGA

22. Reversed splitting of S2 is seen in:
A. LBBB
B. RBBB
C. LV pacing
D. PS

23. DCMP: all are true *except:*
A. Embolism
B. Reverse splitting of S2
C. Late systolic murmur
D. S3

24. Endomyocardial biopsy is useful for diagnosis of:
A. Allograft rejection
B. Dilated cardiomyopathy
C. Amyloidosis
D. Fabry's disease

11 B 12 A 13 A 14 D 15 D 16 B 17 A 18 B 19 D 20 D 21 B 22 A 23 C 24 A

25. Murmur which decrease with isometric handgrip is:
- A. AS
- B. MR
- C. AR
- D. None of the above

26. SLE: all are true *except:*
- A. Arterial and venous thrombosis
- B. Pancarditis
- C. Decrease fertility
- D. Coronary arteritis

27. Drug causing SLE is:
- A. Procainamide
- B. Digoxin
- C. Amiodarone
- D. Beta blockers

28. Side effects of disopyramide include all *except:*
- A. Worsening of LV function in known LV dysfunction
- B. Anticholinergic effects
- C. Vagomimetic
- D. Hypotension

29. VT suspected in wide QRS tachycardia if:
- A. Variable pulses
- B. QRS < 0.12 sec
- C. Rate < 110 bpm
- D. rsr' in V1

30. Atrial flutter: which is not true?
- A. Always signifies significant heart disease
- B. Cannot be diagnosed on ECG if there is no flutter waves
- C. Difficult to control with drugs
- D. Mechanism is triggered activity

31. WPW syndrome which is true:
- A. Prolonged HV if AV nodal conduction is tested
- B. 2% incidence in asymptomatic population
- C. Left lateral pathways is most common
- D. Left posteroseptal pathway is rare

32. β receptors:
- A. Ahlquist discovered them (β1 & β2)
- B. Beta-2 is cardioselective
- C. Beta-1 is for lipolysis
- D. Bisoprolol is beta-2 selective

33. ANP: all are true *except:*
- A. Discovered in 1961
- B. Cause both Na and K^+ diuresis
- C. Inhibit rennin angiotensin system
- D. Secreted in atrium

34. JVP: which of the following is true?
- A. External jugular vein is of no significance
- B. Intermittent 'a' is prominent in CHB
- C. 'y' descent is due to ventricular systole in normal hearts
- D. Only 'v' is prominent in TR

35. Elderly HT: which is true?
- A. Isolated systolic hypertension is defined for patients more than 80 years
- B. ISH does not require any treatment
- C. ACE inhibitors are drugs of choice
- D. Diuretics and beta blockers are used as first line of therapy

36. Hypertension: all are true *except:*
- A. JNC criteria is applicable to persons more than 18 years
- B. Hypertension is defined when the blood pressure is > 140/90 mm Hg
- C. Ideal BP goal in diabetics is < 130/80 mmHg
- D. Methyldopa is the first line of therapy in hypertensive females

37. Atrial fibrillation: all are true *except:*
- A. Mortality is independent of cause
- B. Hypertension may be a cause of atrial fibrillation
- C. Most common in elderly
- D. Atrial fibrillation in myocardial infarction increases mortality

25 A 26 C 27 A 28 C 29 A 30 D 31 C 32 A 33 B 34 B 35 D 36 D 37 A

38. Cardioversion: which is true?
- A. Embolism risk increases with cardioversion of atrial fibrillation
- B. Atrial fibrillation can be cardioverted successfully with 10 joules
- C. Atrial flutter can always be reverted with drugs
- D. I/v bolus of 400mg amiodarone is needed for cardioversion of VT

39. In favour of CCP:
- A. Pulsus paradoxus
- B. PAH
- C. Equal RVEDP & LVEDP
- D. Early diastolic RV collapse

40. Restrictive CMP: which is true?
- A. Restrictive CMP is the commonest cause of death in amyloidosis
- B. Hypertrophy is never seen
- C. S3 is never heard
- D. Can be easily differentiated from CCP by clinical examination

41. Vaughan Williams classification: following is true?
- A. Amiodarone is potassium channel blocker
- B. Mexiletine is Class II agent
- C. All class I drugs are potassium channel blockers
- D. Digoxin is class IV drug

42. Sinus node dysfunction: all are true *except:*
- A. p wave is absent
- B. Sinus bradycardia-tachycardia can be one of the manifestation
- C. Atrial fibrillation is also one of the manifestation
- D. Digitalis can cause it

43. Multifocal atrial tachycardia: which is true?
- A. Usually occurs in the setting of chronic respiratory disease
- B. Regular p waves are seen
- C. Most common in young persons
- D. Diagnosed by at least two different morphologies of 'p' wave

44. Exercise test: which is true?
- A. Increasing ST segment depression increases the sensitivity and specificity
- B. Patient desire to stop is a relative contraindication of TMT
- C. Heparin decreases exercise duration
- D. Exercise time < 8 min is a high risk criteria

45. All are false about S2 *except:*
- A. Wide and fixed in ASD
- B. Wide in LBBB
- C. P2 is loud in TOF
- D. Expiration increases A2-P2 interval

46. Systolic click is heard in all *except:*
- A. Pulmonary hypertension
- B. HOCM
- C. AS
- D. MVP

47. Secondary hypertension is suspected in all *except:*
- A. BP 220/140
- B. ↑Renin levels
- C. Target organ damage
- D. Diastolic bruit over flank

48. A 30 year old male presents to emergency room with acute chest pain: Right arm BP is 180/110 mm Hg, Left arm BP is 110/70 mm Hg, early diastolic murmur in left Parasternal areas: diagnosis is:
- A. Acute MI
- B. Proximal ascending aorta dissection
- C. Aortic regurgitation
- D. Takayasu arteritis

49. Not shown to decrease mortality in LV dysfunction is:
- A. ACE-inhibitor
- B. Nitrate + Hydralazine
- C. Carvedilol
- D. Prazosin

38 A 39 C 40 A 41 A 42 A 43 A 44 A 45 A 46 B 47 C 48 B 49 D

50. Dressler's syndrome: which is true?
- **A.** 20% patients of MI
- **B.** Tamponade is rare
- **C.** Seen after 6 weeks of AMI
- **D.** NSAIDS is used for treatment

51. Pericarditis in MI:
- **A.** Indicates transmural infarction
- **B.** Not related to size of myocardial infarction
- **C.** Dressler's syndrome is usually seen after 3 months of MI
- **D.** Most common with inferior MI

52. Epinephrine is used in all *except:*
- **A.** Status asthmaticus
- **B.** Anaphylactic shock
- **C.** Acute MI
- **D.** Local anesthesia

53. Thrombolysis is used in all *except:*
- **A.** Prosthetic valve thrombosis
- **B.** Unstable angina
- **C.** Pulmonary embolism
- **D.** Deep vein thrombosis

54. True about thrombophlebitis in pregnancy:
- **A.** Superficial thrombophlebitis does not require anticoagulation
- **B.** Best initial investigation for DVT is angiography
- **C.** Pregnancy is an anticoagulant state
- **D.** Risk of pulmonary embolism increases 10 times in pregnancy

55. Heparin: which is true?
- **A.** Always necessary after thrombolysis
- **B.** Does not inhibits platelet aggregation
- **C.** Is inferior to LMWH in NSTEMI
- **D.** Bolus 60 U/kg in acute myocardial infarction

56. True about Infective endocarditis is:
- **A.** Staph aureus usually involves anatomically normal valves
- **B.** Staph aureus is commonest organism
- **C.** In drug addicts mixed flora is commonest
- **D.** All cases should be treated with antibiotics for 6 weeks

57. True about heart block:
- **A.** Asymptomatic third degree heart block always requires pacemaker
- **B.** PR interval is constant in Mobitz type II
- **C.** In congenital CHB, rate is < 30/min
- **D.** EPS should be done in all cases of CHB

58. Blunt trauma to heart: which is true?
- **A.** Commonest cause of death is acute MI
- **B.** Commonest coronary lesion is thrombosis
- **C.** Cardiac enzyme elevation helps in diagnosis
- **D.** Right atrium is the most common chamber involved

59. Atherosclerosis: which is false?
- **A.** Fatty streak consists of macrophages
- **B.** Vascular smooth muscle play important role
- **C.** Statin decrease atherosclerosis
- **D.** Premature atherosclerosis is not seen in progeria

60. Screening for primary prevention: which is tested?
- **A.** Total cholesterols
- **B.** LDL levels decide drug therapy requirement
- **C.** Total cholesterol: HDL ratio
- **D.** Tendon xanthomas

61. Prophylaxis for Rheumatic fever in established RHD is given for:
- **A.** 5 years
- **B.** 18 years
- **C.** Life long
- **D.** 2 year

62. Bisferian's pulse is seen in all *except:*
- **A.** Pure AR
- **B.** AS with AR
- **C.** HOCM
- **D.** Cardiac tamponade

50 B 51 A 52 C 53 B 54 A 55 D 56 A 57 B 58 C 59 D 60 A 61 C 62 D

63. Severity of AR is indicated by all *except:*
A. Bisferian's pulse
B. Signs of distal run off
C. Ejection systolic murmur
D. Murmur occupying > 50% of diastole

64. Acute MR: true are all *except:*
A. Small LV size
B. Pan systolic murmur
C. S3
D. Early systolic murmur

65. Examination of apex beat: all true *except:*
A. Tapping apex is due to high velocity of closure of mitral valve
B. LA impulse felt in right sternal border in severe MR
C. Sustained apex in aortic stenosis
D. Ill sustained apex in AR

66. True about S1:
A. Loud S1 always means MS
B. Split S1 in RBBB
C. Soft S1 in MVP
D. S1 is narrowly split in ASD

67. Long QT syndrome which is true:
A. Romano ward is AR
B. Long QT syndrome causes SCD in young adults
C. SCD is prevented by PPI
D. Normal QT interval > 0.42 sec

68. LAFB:
A. Causes right axis deviation on EKG
B. Acute appearance indicates poor prognosis in acute MI
C. Diagnosed by deep S in II, III, aVF and tall R in L_I AV_L
D. Least common block

69. Q waves: all are true *except:*
A. Always indicate old MI
B. Significant if >25% of succeeding R wave
C. Can be seen in normal person
D. 30% q waves disappear within 6-12 months after MI

70. A 65 year female undergone surgery for fracture femur, 2 days later she develops bilateral crepts, S3 audible, pedal oedema present, increased JVP, diagnosis is:
A. Cardiogenic shock
B. Hypervolemia
C. Fat embolism syndrome
D. Acute MR

71. All are indicators of CHF in infants *except:*
A. Sweating
B. Tachypnea
C. Tachycardia
D. Cough

72. Mean of a data is 20, Standard deviation is 2, 95% of data will lie between:
A. 20-22
B. 18-22
C. 16-24
D. 15-25

73. Digoxin level is increased by all *except:*
A. Quinidine
B. Verapamil
C. Cholestyramine
D. Amiodarone

74. Choose the best pair for SVT (without accessory pathway):
A. Convert with digoxin, maintain with adenosine
B. Convert with adenosine, maintain with digoxin
C. Convert with DC maintained with digoxin
D. Convert with adenosine, maintain with quinidine

75. Best variable to choose surgical treatment in MR:
A. ESV B. EDV
C. EDD D. LA/Ao

63 C 64 B 65 B 66 B 67 B 68 C 69 A 70 C 71 D 72 C 73 C 74 D 75 A

76. All are true about MI *except:*
A. 10% have normal ECG
B. IWMI usually associated with MR murmur
C. Free wall rupture is more common with anterior wall MI than IWMI
D. More common in females

77. Toxicity of digoxin is worsened with concomitant:
A. Hypokalemia
B. Hyponatremia
C. Hypocalcemia
D. Hyperkalemia

78. Commonest cause of CCP:
A. TB
B. Ischemia
C. Hemorrhage
D. Neoplastic

79. Maximum chances of fetal malfunction if taken prenatally:
A. Alcohol
B. Phenytoin
C. Lithium
D. Xylocaine

80. Cerebrovascular accidents: all are true about ECG changes *except:*
A. 15-20% patients show changes on ECG
B. ST-T changes are the only changes
C. Changes are functional and not due to organic heart disease
D. QT prolongation can occur

81. Drug causing cardiac necrosis:
A. Cyclophosphamide
B. Vincristine
C. Doxorubicin
D. Mycophenolate

82. All are components of syndrome X *except:*
A. HT
B. ↓Insulin levels
C. Hyperlipidemia
D. Increase triglycerides

83. Which is true?
A. Acidosis shifts the oxygen dissociation curve to right
B. Least oxygen saturation in RA
C. Increased temperature shifts the oxygen dissociation curve to left
D. None of the above

84. Drug useful in diastolic dysfunction:
A. Diltiazem
B. Verapamil
C. Adenosine
D. Diuretic

85. Infective endocarditis is most common in:
A. PS
B. MS
C. CAD
D. Floppy valve with regurgitation

86. Drug precipitating malignant hyperthermia in a susceptible patient:
A. Dantrolene
B. Succinylcholine
C. Bucindolol
D. Prazosin

87. ACE inhibitors should be started in myocardial infarction:
A. Within 24 hours
B. Within 48 hours
C. Within 72 hours
D. After one week

88. Drug of choice for Kala Azar is:
A. Pentamidine
B. Amphotericin B
C. Sodium stibogluconate
D. Penicillin

76 D 77 A 78 A 79 A 80 B 81 A 82 B 83 A 84 B 85 D 86 B 87 A 88 A

89. RVH is not seen in:
A. TOF
B. TGA
C. Tricuspid atresia
D. MS

90. True regarding digoxin is:
A. Absorbed in colon
B. Absorption decreased by cholestyramine and metoclopramide
C. Verapamil has no interaction with digoxin
D. Decrease mortality in CHF

91. Estrogen protect against all *except:*
A. Fatal & non fatal MI
B. Osteoporosis
C. Endothelial dysfunction
D. Lipoprotein (a)

92. To develop rheumatic heart disease. All are true *except:*
A. Immune reaction is important
B. Cross reactive with heart
C. Pharyngeal carrier state and invasion required
D. Duration of carrier state

93. Digoxin causes all *except:*
A. Increased refractory period of atrial and ventricular muscle
B. Never causes Mobitz type II block
C. Increased PR interval
D. Bidirectional VT is suggestive of digoxin toxicity

94. Thyrocardiac disease: all are true *except:*
A. Increase sensitivity of digoxin
B. MVP is common
C. Atrial fibrillation is commonest arrhythmia
D. Cardiomegaly can occur

95. Drug of choice for PSVT is:
A. Digoxin
B. Verapamil
C. Disopyramide
D. Adenosine

96. LVS3: all are true *except:*
A. Pulmonary embolism
B. VSD
C. MR
D. AR

97. All are complications of amiodarone *except:*
A. Thyroid disorder
B. Corneal deposits
C. Pulmonary toxicity
D. Diabetes Mellitus

98. Cyanosis with increased pulmonary blood flow is seen in all *except:*
A. TGA
B. Ebstein's anomaly
C. Univentricular heart
D. TAPVC

99. All are type A lesions *except:*
A. Ostial lesions
B. Concentric lesions
C. Noncalcified
D. Angulation less than 45 degrees

100. All are true about acute MR *except:*
A. Large LA
B. Normal heart size
C. Increased LA pressure
D. Increased PA pressure

89 C 90 B 91 A 92 D 93 A 94 A 95 D 96 A 97 D 98 B 99 A 100 A

Srichitra 2004

1. **Canon 'a' wave is found in:**
   A. TS
   B. PPH
   C. PS
   D. All of the above
   E. None of the above

2. **Tg > 600 mg%, HDL-C-40 mg%, Total cholesterol-200 mg%, LDL-C is:**
   A. 100 mg%
   B. 120 mg%
   C. 150 mg%
   D. Cannot be estimated

3. **TMT is used in all *except:***
   A. Diagnosis of unstable angina
   B. Post CABG
   C. Males with atypical symptoms
   D. Post MI with stent implantation

4. **Most specific in assessment of myocardial viability by stress echo is:**
   A. Increase in contractility with smaller doses and decrease in contractility at higher doses
   B. No change in smaller doses but increase contractility with higher doses
   C. Decrease in contractility in smaller doses and increase in higher doses
   D. None of the above

5. **Beta blocker not shown to be of benefit in CHF is:**
   A. Atenolol
   B. Metoprolol
   C. Bisoprolol
   D. Carvedilol

6. **Selective alpha-2 antagonist is:**
   A. Yohimbine
   B. Prazosin
   C. Clonidine
   D. Guanosine

7. **On doppler echocardiography-object moving away is seen with:**
   A. Decrease velocity, decrease frequency
   B. Velocity same, frequency increased
   C. Velocity same, frequency decreased
   D. Velocity increased, frequency decreased

8. **Valsalva maneuver in stage IV will show:**
   A. Increase BP, decrease HR
   B. Decrease BP, decrease HR
   C. Increase BP, Increase HR
   D. Decrease BP, Increase HR

9. **True about Korotokoff's sound is:**
   A. Stage IV-muffling
   B. Stage II-Tapping
   C. Stage III-Progressive decrease in velocity
   D. Stage I-Soft

1 E 2 D 3 A 4 A 5 A 6 A 7 C 8 A 9 A

10. Echo data in patient with CHF–LVID in diastole is 42 mm and systole is 36 mm. Diagnosis is:

A. Acute MR
B. CCP
C. RCMP
D. Cardiac tamponade

11. LVID (d)–36 mm, LVID (s)–24 mm, RVID-36 mm, LA= 2 cm, Aorta 2.4 cm: Diagnosis is:

A. Acute MR
B. PPH
C. CCP
D. Severe MS

12. False statement about heparin induced thrombocytopenia is:

A. Low incidence in LMWH
B. Type I associated with platelet factor 4
C. Continuous heparin may improve it
D. Occurs within few days

13. Factor Xa inhibitor is:

A. Ximalagatran
B. Argatroban
C. Fondaparinaux
D. Hirudin

14. Systolic and diastolic bruit indicates stenosis of around:

A. 80%
B. 50%
C. 20%
D. Total occlusion

15. False in pregnancy is:

A. Cardiac output increased by 40%
B. Blood volume increased by 30%
C. PDA with PAH is poorly tolerated
D. S3 is normal

16. HOCM is best described as:

A. Myocardial disease with asymmetrical hypertrophy
B. Myocardial disease with dynamic LVOT obstruction
C. Myocardial disease with ACE polymorphism
D. Myocardial disease with sarcomere protein abnormality

17. True about HOCM diagnosis is:

A. Decreased pulse pressure in post ectopic beat
B. Increased gradient in post ectopic beat
C. Increased pulse pressure in post ectopic beat
D. Decreased gradient in post ectopic beat

18. Which of the following statements is false:

A. Warfarin embryopathy is dose related
B. Patient of HOCM during labor and delivery requires IE prophylaxis
C. Peripartum CMP can be seen upto 6 months following delivery
D. BP > 140/90 mm Hg on two occasions for diagnosing preeclampsia

19. Right aortic arch with mirror image distribution of vessel is seen in:

A. TOF
B. Truncus arteriosus
C. D-TGA
D. VSD

20. True about anthracycline cardiotoxicity is all *except:*

A. Contraindicated in EF<30%
B. Chronic toxicity usually seen with dose > 550 mg/m^2
C. Commonest adverse effect of acute toxicity is nonspecific ST-T changes
D. Does not occur after 1 year of completion of treatment

21. Continuous murmur is heard in:

A. Truncus arteriosus
B. Peripheral PS
C. VSD with AR
D. TOF with absent pulmonary valve

10 A 11 B 12 B 13 C 14 A 15 B 16 D 17 A 18 B 19 B 20 D 21 B

22. Regarding S1: False is:
A. M1 before T1
B. Sail sound due to loud T1 in Ebstein's anomaly
C. LV pacing causes paradoxical split
D. Mitral obstruction causes reverse split

23. True about ASD is:
A. Atrial arrhythmias are more common in children
B. MVP is seen in more than 50% cases
C. Shunt depends on ventricular compliance
D. IE prophylaxis in adult

24. All are true about hyperkalemia *except:*
A. Tall T waves
B. Prominent U waves
C. Sine waves
D. ST-T inversion

25. True about troponin is:
A. Early release from cytoplasmic pool
B. Late release from contractile protein pool
C. Does not correlate with severity
D. Persist for 6-10 days
E. All of the above

26. CPK-MB is raised in:
A. Myocarditis
B. Pericarditis
C. Polymyositis
D. Post CABG
E. All of the above

27. BP response in near maximal exercise:
A. Increased diastolic pressure
B. Increased systolic pressure
C. Increased mean pressure
D. Increased pulse pressure

28. Coronary flow reserve: all are true *except:*
A. Velocity ratio < 2 is favorable for revascularization
B. FFR > 0.75 is suggestive of critical obstruction
C. Diastolic: Systolic ratio > 1.7
D. FFR requires both distal and proximal measurements

29. Rapid and regular pulse with altered volume suggest:
A. AF
B. AVNRT
C. PJRT
D. VT

30. All are true about ectopic atrial tachycardia *except:*
A. DC shock
B. AV nodal blocking drugs
C. RFA
D. None of the above
E. All of the above

31. Dilzem is used for:
A. Rhythm control
B. Rate control
C. To prevent VT
D. All of the above

32. Which is atherogenic virus?
A. H.Pylori
B. Chlamydia pneumonia
C. Mycoplasma
D. All of the above
E. None of the above

33. Contraindicated in pregnancy is:
A. Captopril
B. Methyl Dopa
C. Digoxin
D. Metoprolol

34. Conotruncal anomalies is seen with:
A. Retinoic acid
B. Lithium
C. Alcohol
D. Valproic acid

22 C 23 C 24 B 25 E 26 E 27 D 28 B 29 D 30 A 31 B 32 E 33 A 34 A

35. Remnants of sinus venosus are all *except:*
A. Right atrial appendage
B. Thebesian valve
C. Crista terminalis
D. Eustachian valve

36. Action potential phases: Dv/Dt change is maximum in:
A. Phase 4
B. Phase 3
C. Phase 2
D. Phase 1
E. Phase 0

37. True about HOCM is:
A. Isovolumic relaxation is decreased
B. Sudden death related to severity of obstruction
C. Apical cardiomyopathy has poor prognosis
D. Biventricular pacing is effective therapy

38. Oral hypoglycemic agent worsening CAD is:
A. Glibenclamide
B. Pioglitazone
C. Metformin
D. Glimepiride
E. None of the above

39. Following is not used in non ST elevation MI:
A. Thrombolytics
B. Beta blockers
C. Aspirin
D. Statins

40. False statement about Prinzmetal angina is:
A. Aspirin is drug of choice
B. Ergonovine is sensitive in detecting coronary vasospasm
C. Ergonovine has alpha adrenergic and 5-HT agonist activity
D. Alcohol may prevent spasm

41. Phosphodiesterase inhibitors are:
A. Dipyridamole
B. Cilastazole
C. Clopidogrel
D. A + C
E. A and B
F. None of the above

42. All are true about IE *except:*
A. Earliest manifestation is NBTE
B. Streptococcus viridans has best prognosis
C. Tricuspid involvement in drug abusers
D. Staph epidermidis is most common nosocomial infection

43. True about Staph epidermidis is:
A. Early prosthetic valve endocarditis
B. Drug abusers
C. Late PVE
D. Early infection after pacemaker implantation

44. All are true about HOCM *except:*
A. Normal ECG rules out diagnosis of HOCM
B. LVET prolonged
C. Extent of hypertrophy is a predictor of SCD
D. Alcohol ablation is as effective as surgical myectomy

45. Most common cardiac malignant tumor in adult is:
A. Angiosarcoma
B. Rhabdomyosarcoma
C. Teratocarcinoma
D. Mesothelioma

46. True about thrombolysis in acute MI is:
A. Not useful in 6-12 hours
B. Repeat thrombolysis is not beneficial
C. Not useful in more than 75 year old patient
D. None of the above

47. All are true about parasystole *except:*
A. Asynchronous discharge from different focus
B. Interectopic interval is multiple of basic interval
C. Entry block can be continuous or intermittent
D. Not altered by basic rhythm

35 A 36 E 37 A 38 A 39 A 40 A 41 E 42 D 43 A 44 A 45 A 46 D 47 C

48. **All are true about AV fistula *except:***
A. Bradycardia
B. Increase AV oxygen difference
C. Arterial desaturation
D. None of the above

49. **Rheumatoid arthritis: all are extraarticular manifestations *except:***
A. Raynaud's phenomenon
B. ILD
C. Osteoporosis
D. Hypersplenism
E. Felty's syndrome

50. **All are true about rheumatoid arthritis *except:***
A. Rheumatic nodule is seen in more than 50% cases
B. Vasculitis can involve any organ
C. Rheumatoid factor has prognostic significance
D. Methotrexate is a disease modifying drug

51. **Most common cause of nephrotic syndrome in adults is:**
A. Membranous
B. Focal and segmental glomerulosclerosis
C. Mesangiproliferative
D. Membranoproliferative

52. **All are true about membranoproliferative glomerulonephritis *except:***
A. Normal complement
B. Hypertension
C. Azotemia
D. Active sediments

53. **All are true about Wilson's disease *except:***
A. Normal serum ceruloplasmin rules out diagnosis
B. Urine ceruloplasmin > 200 is not pathognomonic
C. Serum copper low
D. Penicillamine is used for treatment

54. **All are true about MEN-I *except:***
A. Medullary carcinoma thyroid
B. Pancreatic tumor
C. Parathyroid tumor
D. Pituitary tumor

55. **All are true about Zollinger Ellison syndrome *except:***
A. Pancreatic body is the commonest site for gastrinoma
B. Watery diarrhoea may occur
C. Fasting gastrin level > 1000 pg/ml is diagnostic
D. Peptic ulcer-commonest site is duodenum
E. Part of MEN in 50% cases

56. **All are true about cystic fibrosis *except:***
A. Chromosome 10 involvement
B. Multiorgan involvement
C. > 25% reach adulthood
D. Autosomal recessive

57. **All are true about H. pylori *except:***
A. Spiral gram + organism
B. Found in > 90% cases of duodenal ulcer
C. Does not invade blood
D. Found in > 50% of normal population
E. Chronic/acute gastritis

58. **All are myeloproliferative *except:***
A. CML
B. Polycythemia vera
C. Essential thrombocytosis
D. Myeloid metaplasia
E. Hairy cell leukemia

59. **All are true about polycythemia vera *except:***
A. Increased erythropoietin
B. Increased RBC mass
C. Increased basophil
D. Pruritus after taking bath

60. **All are true about erythropoietin *except:***
A. Formed in spleen in fetus
B. 30 Kda protein
C. Secreted by kidney in adult
D. Secretion increased in hypoxia

48 D 49 A 50 A 51 A 52 A 53 A 54 A 55 A 56 A 57 A 58 E 59 A 60 A

61. Martel's sign is seen in:
A. Gout
B. Osteoarthritis
C. Psoriatic arthropathy
D. Rheumatoid arthritis

62. All are true about iron deficiency anemia *except:*
A. Decrease ferritin is earliest to occur
B. Fe containing enzymes affected the least
C. Microcytosis is invariably present
D. Hypocellular marrow

63. All are true about iron absorption *except:*
A. In duodenum and ileum
B. Mostly in ferric form from diet
C. Transferrin is iron transporting protein
D. Exact mechanism unknown
E. 10% of 10-20 mg absorbed

64. Leptin:
A. Increase growth hormone
B. Increase insulin sensitivity
C. Increase melatonin
D. Increased LH-FSH secretion

65. Triple test is used to assess all *except:*
A. HCG
B. Alpha fetoprotein
C. Estradiol
D. Prolactin

66. Most common joint involvement in Lyme's disease is:
A. Knee
B. Hip
C. Ankle
D. Elbow

67. Hypersensitivity reaction in fungal infection with erythema nodosum, erythema multiforme, and arthritis:
A. Histoplasmosis
B. Coccidioidomycosis
C. Blastomycosis
D. Candida

68. All are true about Polyglandular autoimmune syndrome *except:*
A. Mucocutaneous candidiasis Type I
B. Type I DM with Type II PGA
C. Hypoparathyroid only with type II
D. Type III causes diabetes insipidus

69. True about sickle cell trait are all *except:*
A. HbA-40%, HbS-60%
B. Splenic infarct may occur
C. Protected against plasmodium falciparum
D. Usually asymptomatic

70. All are true about G6PD deficiency *except:*
A. X linked
B. More than 400 variants
C. Aging in 120 days decrease G6PD by 50%
D. Normal type is A
E. Most common RBC enzyme deficiency disorder

71. Anti RNP antibody is found in:
A. MCTD
B. RA
C. SLE
D. PSS

72. All are true about MCTD *except:*
A. Progressive systemic sclerosis
B. SLE
C. Rheumatoid arthritis
D. Sjogren's syndrome
E. Polymyositis

73. Bullous myringitis is caused by:
A. Mycoplasma
B. EB virus
C. Chlamydia
D. HSV

61 A 62 C 63 A 64 D 65 D 66 A 67 A 68 C 69 A 70 D 71 A 72 D 73 A

74. Not a nucleoside reverse transcriptase inhibitor:
A. Nevirapine
B. Didanosine
C. Zidovudine
D. Zalcitabine

75. Suprarenal artery:
A. Superior from inferior phrenic
B. Middle from aorta
C. Inferior from renal
D. A and C
E. A and B
F. All are correct

76. All are true about eosinophilic pneumonia *except:*
A. Eosinophils < 500
B. Bronchial asthma
C. Infiltrates
D. Aspergillus fumigatus precipitin

77. Immunoglobulin with longest half life is:
A. IgG
B. IgA
C. IgM
D. IgE

78. True about multiple myeloma is:
A. Interleukin 6 drives proliferation
B. Osteoblastic proliferation
C. Bone pain at night
D. Radioisotope scan better than chest X-ray

79. Scarlet fever is caused by:
A. Group B streptococcus
B. Group A streptococcus
C. Group C streptococcus
D. Staphylococcus

80. All are true about asthma *except:*
A. Extrinsic asthma is caused by IgG
B. Infant male: female ratio is 2:1
C. Associated with urticaria
D. Food allergy may be associated

81. ECF concentration is more than ICF:
A. Cl^-
B. Mg^{2+}
C. PO_4
D. HCO_3^-
E. A and B
F. A and D

82. Normal anion gap acidosis is seen in all *except:*
A. Diarrhoea
B. Diabetic ketoacidosis
C. Renal tubular acidosis
D. None of the above

83. Which is not an acute phase reactant?
A. Serum AA
B. CRP
C. Fibrinogen
D. α-TNF

84. Which of the following is a normal value?
A. PCO_2 : 35-45 mm Hg
B. pH : 7.45-7.55
C. PaO_2 : 70 mm Hg
D. HCO_3^- : 16

85. Ethyl alcohol is used in:
A. Methanol poisoning
B. Ethylene glycol poisoning
C. Lithium
D. A and B
E. A and C
F. All of the above

86. True about renal cell carcinoma are all *except:*
A. Clear cell carcinoma is commonest
B. Most commonly seen in 20-30years
C. Smoking is strongly associated
D. Most common tumor of kidney

74 A 75 F 76 A 77 A 78 A 79 A 80 A 81 A 82 B 83 D 84 A 85 D 86 B

87. Glucagonoma from:
- A. Alpha cell
- B. Beta cell
- C. Delta cell
- D. Theta cell

88. True about ARDS is:
- A. Alveolocapillary membrane abnormality
- B. PCWP > 25 mm Hg
- C. Inhaled NO is a modality of treatment
- D. Ventilation in lateral position is most effective

89. All are true about jerks *except:*
- A. Triceps-C_5-C_6
- B. Jaw jerk-Pons
- C. Ankle jerk-$S_{1,2}$
- D. Knee jerk-L_3, L_4

90. True about hepatitis virus is all *except:*
- A. Hepatitis A-RNA
- B. Hepatitis B-DNA
- C. Hepatitis C-RNA
- D. Hepatitis D-DNA

91. All cause hypercalcemia *except:*
- A. Anticonvulsant therapy
- B. Lithium
- C. Sarcoidosis
- D. Vitamin D intoxication

92. Anorexia nervosa: psychiatric change is:
- A. Perfectionist
- B. Depression
- C. Bipolar
- D. Schizophrenic

93. Sustained VT:
- A. > 30 secs
- B. > 3 sec
- C. > 3 beats
- D. Syncope

94. NO donor is:
- A. Molsidomine
- B. Nicorandil
- C. Aplha-2 blocker
- D. Eternacept

95. Hepatorenal syndrome: true are all *except:*
- A. Associated with cirrhosis and ascites
- B. Kidney normal
- C. Kidney biopsy abnormal
- D. Treatment unsuccessful

96. Renin is decreased by:
- A. Salt loading
- B. Sudden standing
- C. Diuretics
- D. All of the above

97. Ann Arbor classification: Lymph node both above and below diaphragm:
- A. Stage I
- B. Stage II
- C. Stage III
- D. Stage IV

98. Amphotericin B is used in which of the other infections other than systemic fungal infection:
- A. Leishmaniasis
- B. Amoebiasis
- C. Pneumocystis carinii pneumonia
- D. None of the above

99. ACC/AHA recommendations: following MVR INR should be:
- A. 2.0-3.0
- B. 2.0-3.0 + aspirin 75 mg
- C. 2.0-3.0 + aspirin 150 mg
- D. 2.5-3.5

100. Preeclampsia: all are true *except:*
- A. In 5% pregnancy
- B. HELPP syndrome increase morbidity and mortality
- C. Multiple organ vascular events
- D. Risk factors extreme age, obesity, ACE gene polymorphism
- E. Predisposes to chronic epilepsy

87 A 88 A 89 A 90 D 91 A 92 A 93 A 94 A 95 C 96 A 97 C 98 A 99 D 100 E

Srichitra 2003

1. **Early systolic murmur is caused by all *except:***
   A. Gallavardin phenomenon
   B. Low pressure TR
   C. VSD
   D. MR

2. **All are true about common atrium *except:***
   A. Axis more than –30
   B. Clockwise rotation of QRS
   C. P wave left axis
   D. Incomplete RBBB

3. **In HOCM, NYHA class IV cath study, PCWP 28, LV pressure 120/90, Aortic pressure 120/86, no MR: treatment is:**
   A. Alcohol septal ablation
   B. Diuresis
   C. DDD pacing
   D. Septal myomectomy with MVR

4. **Mechanism of benefit of DDD pacing in HOCM:**
   A. Ventricular resynchronization
   B. Septal preexcitation
   C. AV synchronization
   D. Rhythm control

5. **VY descent in Wiggers cycle corresponds to:**
   A. End of early diastolic filling
   B. End of ejection
   C. End of isovolumetric relaxation
   D. Onset of isovolumetric relaxation

6. **Iso volumetric relaxation occurs between:**
   A. Mitral valve closure and AV opening
   B. Mitral opening and AV closure
   C. S3 and aortic valve closure
   D. S4 and aortic valve closure

7. **Most common site of opening in TAPVC:**
   A. Left innominate vein
   B. Coronary sinus
   C. Rt SVC
   D. Portal system

8. **In Takayasu's arteritis, most common artery involved is:**
   A. Carotid
   B. Renal
   C. Subclavian
   D. Coronary

9. **Myxoma arises most commonly from:**
   A. Interatrial septum
   B. Lt atrial appendage
   C. AV annulus
   D. Right atrial appendage

10. **Least beneficial in Unstable angina undergoing conservative management:**
    A. Tirofiban
    B. Aspirin
    C. Unfractionated heparin
    D. Abciximab

1 A 2 B 3 B 4 B 5 A 6 B 7 A 8 C 9 A 10 D

11. Apo B 100 is the only apolipoprotein for:
A. LDL
B. IDL
C. HDL
D. Chylomicron

12. LDL Cholesterol increases in:
A. PBC
B. Obesity
C. Diabetic
D. Alcohol

13. Contraindicated in CHF:
A. Insulin
B. Biguanides
C. Sulfonylurea
D. Thiazolindinediones

14. Not seen in ulcerative colitis:
A. Maximum incidence between age 20-40
B. Obesity
C. Tenderness of Lt iliac fossa
D. Diarrhoea

15. Commonest site of carcinoid:
A. Hindgut
B. Foregut
C. Midgut
D. Lung

16. Tendon of todaro is the continuation of:
A. Coronary sinus
B. Eustachian valve
C. Tricuspid annulus
D. Semilunar valve

17. Ductus venosus remnant:
A. Eustachian valve
B. Crista terminalis
C. Fossa ovalis
D. Crista supraventricularis

18. All are true about multiple myeloma *except:*
A. Secondary amyloidosis
B. Metastatic calcification
C. AVM of neck of femur
D. Decreased anion gap

19. Serum alkaline phosphatase is increased in all *except:*
A. Multiple myeloma
B. Cholestatic hepatitis
C. Paget's disease
D. Osteomalacia

20. Liddle's syndrome; true is:
A. HTN, hypokalemia, alkalosis
B. Spironolactone is drug of choice
C. Amiloride is ineffective
D. Increased aldosterone

21. Diuretic acting by inhibiting sodium channel in epithelial cells:
A. Amiloride
B. Frusemide
C. Thiazide
D. Acetazolamide

22. True about metalazone:
A. K^+ sparing
B. Act on thick ascending limb of Loop of Henley
C. Effective even in renal insufficiency
D. All of the above

23. Least likely to cause torsades:
A. Procainamide
B. Sotalol
C. Ibutilide
D. Flecainide

24. Which of the following decreases QT interval:
A. Digitalis
B. Hypokalemia
C. Hypomagnesemia
D. Hypocalcemia

11 A 12 A 13 D 14 B 15 D 16 B 17 A 18 D 19 A 20 A 21 A 22 A 23 D

25. **Autosomal dominant disorder is:**
A. Huntingtons chorea
B. Haemophilia
C. Night blindness
D. Fibrocystic disease

26. **Most common sensitive screening test for hemophilia:**
A. BT
B. CT
C. PT
D. CRT

27. **Most common Hb in adults:**
A. HbA
B. HbC
C. HbA_2
D. HbE

28. **False above thalassemia:**
A. HbH: Beta thalassemia
B. Thallessemia trait is heterozygote
C. Cause microcytic hypochromic anemia
D. Gene therapy may be effective

29. **Not an antioxidant:**
A. Vitamin C
B. β carotene
C. Vitamin E
D. Folic acid

30. **Not used in the treatment of homocystenemia:**
A. Vitamin B6
B. Vitamin B12
C. Folate
D. Ascorbic acid

31. **Catastrophic in APLS is:**
A. Recurrent miscarriage
B. Recurrent arterial or venous thrombosis
C. Microangiopathy involving >3 organs
D. Prolonged APTT

32. **False about RSOV:**
A. 1/3rd associated with VSD
B. Right sided drainage is most common
C. Non coronary sinus rupture commonly in R^
D. Continuous murmur

33. **True about long QT syndrome:**
A. Romano ward syndrome is autosomal recessive
B. Jarvel Lange Neilson is associated with deafness
C. Long RR cycle precipitates VT i congenital form
D. Calcium gluconate used in treatment

34. **45 year old male with > 2 hr chest pain with hypotension, ST elevation in II, III aVF and V_4R; treatment of choice:**
A. IABP
B. NTG/morphine
C. RV assist device
D. IV Fluid

35. **AMI > 96 hours; marker of choice:**
A. Myoglobin
B. Troponin
C. CPK-MB
D. LDH

36. **Which of the following disease states does not alter pharmacokinetics of cardiovascular drugs:**
A. AMI
B. Bronchial asthma
C. CLD
D. CRF

37. **True about COPD is:**
A. Expiratory reserve volume is decreased
B. TLC is decreased
C. FRC is decreased
D. VC is decreased

24 A 25 A 26 B 27 A 28 A 29 D 30 D 31 C 32 A 33 B 34 D 35 B 36 B
37 D

38. False about Hepatocellular carcinoma is:
A. Most common in Asians/Africans
B. Four times more common in males
C. Occur ½ decade earlier in male
D. HBV not HCV is causative

39. Salmonella; true are all *except:*
A. >500 subtypes are known
B. Cause enteric fever, food poisoning, and asymptomatic carrier state
C. Cause osteomylitis in sickle cell anaemia
D. Common cause of IE in HIV positive patients

40. Most sensitive test for diagnosis of enteric fever:
A. Blood culture
B. Buffy coat culture
C. Stool culture
D. Bone marrow culture

41. True about Pseudohypoparathyrodism:
A. Normal parathyroid histology
B. Decreased Calcitonin
C. Increased PTH
D. Hyper calcemia

42. True about calcitonin:
A. Secreted by Para follicular cells of parathyroid
B. Secreted by Para follicular cells of thymus
C. Increased serum calcium levels
D. Physiological antidote of PTH

43. Maintenance of sinus rhythm in AF patients:
A. Ibutilide
B. Dofetilide
C. Verapamil
D. Digoxin

44. Echocontrast in systemic vein reach LA after few cardiac cycle: diagnosis is:
A. Pulmonary AVF
B. Anomalous drainage of SVC into LA
C. Distal AP window
D. PDA

45. Which is antidopominergic:
A. Metoclopramide
B. Bromocryptin
C. Fenoldopam
D. A and B

46. Bromocriptine is used in all *except:*
A. Acromegaly
B. Cushing syndrome
C. Hyperprolactinemia
D. Parkinsonism

47. False about Conn syndrome:
A. Hyperkalemia
B. Increased activity of zona glomerulosa
C. Alkalosis
D. Oedema is absent

48. Which is false:
A. Norepinephrine has no β2 receptor agonist activity
B. Epinephrine has no β1 activity
C. Dobutamine has no dopominergic activity
D. Isoprenaline has no a activity

49. Carvedilol is:
A. Non selective β blocker with a blocking activity
B. Selective β blocker with a blocking activity
C. Non selective β blocker with direct vasodilator property
D. Selective β blocker with direct vasodilator property

50. Which of the following causes wide QRS complex tachycardia:
A. Orthodromic AVRT with bundle of Kent
B. AVRT with Mahaim bundle
C. Junctional re-entrant tachycardia
D. AVRT with concealed accessory pathway

38 D 39 A 40 D 41 A 42 D 43 B 44 A 45 A 46 B 47 A 48 B 49 A 50 B

51. In Ectropic atrial trachycardia, which is not given ?
A. DC cardioversion
B. β blocker
C. Amiodarone
D. CCB

52. Male with recurrent syncopal attack, EP shows RVOT–VT; Treatment of choice is:
A. RFA
B. ICD
C. Amiodarone
D. CCB

53. Most common in females is:
A. CoA
B. PDA
C. Biscuspid AV
D. AV canal defect

54. In utero death is least common in:
A. Congenital CHB
B. Ventricular tachycardia
C. TGA
D. Ebstein anomaly

55. Ventricular enlargemnt in new born:
A. Ebstein with TR
B. TGA with non restrictive VSD
C. Non restrictive VSD
D. TOF

56. Cyanosis occurs in neonates in:
A. Gerbode defect
B. Ostium primum ASD
C. Complete AV septal defect
D. Non restrictive VSD

57. Small cardiac vein runs in:
A. Lt AV groove
B. Rt AV groove
C. Ant int vent. groove
D. Post interventricular groove

58. Which is true:
A. RCA is dominant if it gives PDA and supplies posterior surface of LV
B. LCx is codominant if supplying posterior surface of Left ventricle
C. LCx is dominant if supplies posterior surface of LV and gives rise to PDA
D. All of the above

59. Which is false about Ca stomach:
A. Gastrectomy is only curative treatment
B. >70% ulcerative lesions occurs in pylorus
C. Always be investigated for screening cases of microcytic hypochromic anemia
D. Is an uncommon malignancy of GI tract

60. Zollinger Ellison Syndrome doesn't cause:
A. Watery diarrhoea
B. Peptic ulcers
C. Islet hyperplasia/adenoma
D. Increased secretion of pancreazymin

61. Which is true about sarcomere?
A. Distance between 2 M bands
B. Optimal length is 2.2 mm
C. Myosin is attached to Z line directly
D. Actin is thick filament

62. Athlete with ST and J elevation in mid precordial leads:
A. Early repolarization
B. HOCM
C. ALCAPA
D. Myopericarditis

63. Double product–Max range is:
A. 21-40,000
B. > 40000
C. 15-25,000
D. < 10,000

51 A 52 A 53 B 54 C 55 A 56 C 57 D 58 D 59 D 60 D 61 B 62 A 63 A

64. Which is false about V O_2 max:
A. Trainėd athelete can increase it by 4 folds
B. Value increases in females
C. Value decreases with age
D. Value less in females

65. Thrombocytosis is seen in all *except:*
A. CML
B. Hyposplenism
C. Kawasaki's disease
D. Idiopathic myelofibrosis

66. Osteoporosis is seen in all *except:*
A. Hypoparathyroidism
B. Cushings
C. Steroid
D. Alcohol

67. Radiation exposure is not seen in:
A. Chest X-ray
B. CT
C. MRI
D. Bronchoscopy

68. Pressure half time of mitral valve is 150 msec; MVA is:
A. 1 cm^2 B. 0.5
C. 1.5 D. 2.5

69. Thrombolytic with shortest t ½:
A. STK
B. t-PA
C. r-PA
D. Tenecteplase

70. Erectile dysfunction is seen with all *except:*
A. Thiazides
B. β blockers
C. Atorvastatin
D. Sickle cell anemia

71. Porphyria is not caused by:
A. OCP
B. Gabapentin
C. CBZ
D. Phenothiazine

72. Double switch procedure is done for:
A. c-TGA
B. Simple TGA
C. DORV
D. SV with PS

73. RV dependent coronary blood flow is seen in:
A. Hypoplastic left heart syndrome
B. Pulmonary artesia
C. Anamolous origin of LCA from pulmonary artery
D. TOF

74. EB virus causes all *except:*
A. Burkitts
B. Lymphoma in immunocompromised host
C. Adult T cell lymphoma leukemia
D. Hodgkins

75. True about infectious mononucleosis is all *except:*
A. Incubation period 7-10 days
B. Highly infectious
C. Common in adolescence
D. Caused by EBV

76. QRS –ve in AVR and AVL, QRS axis is:
A. +60 to +120
B. 120 to 180
C. +30 to +90
D. -30 to -90

77. Hypotension–pre renal azotemia can be differentiated from intrinsic renal azotemia by all *except:*
A. BUN/Cr >20:1
B. Ur Na <20
C. Ur. Cr/Sr. Cr <20:1
D. None of the above

64 B 65 B 66 A 67 C 68 C 69 B 70 C 71 D 72 A 73 A 74 C 75 B 76 B 77 C

78. True about malaria are all *except:*
- **A.** P vivax is more common in India
- **B.** P ovale is rarest
- **C.** P. Falciparum can cause increase mortality
- **D.** Chloroquin resistance is not seen in India

79. All are true about Entamoeba *except:*
- **A.** E. histolytica is most common sub groups
- **B.** Both trophozoite and cyst are infective
- **C.** Patient is afifbrile
- **D.** Amebic liver abscess should be treated with lumicidal and anti trophozite drugs

80. LGV is caused by:
- **A.** H. ducreyi
- **B.** Donovani granulomatis
- **C.** Ureaplasma urealytica
- **D.** Chlamydia

81. Acanthous nigricans should lead to search for:
- **A.** DM
- **B.** Visceral malignancy
- **C.** Hematological malignancy
- **D.** Congenital heart disease

82. All are true about Pancoast tumor *except:*
- **A.** Rib erosion
- **B.** Upper brachial plexus involvement
- **C.** Horner's syndrome
- **D.** Upper lobe opacity

83. Type 2 respiratory failure:
- **A.** Hypoxemia plus hypercapnia
- **B.** Only hypoxemia
- **C.** Cyanosis
- **D.** Chronic respiratory insufficiency

84. All are true about tetanus *except:*
- **A.** CSF pleocytosis
- **B.** Trismus
- **C.** Neck rigidity
- **D.** Normal mental status

85. Malignancy is associated with:
- **A.** Dermatomyositis
- **B.** Scleroderma
- **C.** SLE
- **D.** Rheumatoid Arthritis

86. Opoid agonist are:
- **A.** Methadone
- **B.** Naloxone
- **C.** Naltrexone
- **D.** All of the above

87. Smoking addiction–for nicotine withdrawal used is:
- **A.** Bupropion
- **B.** Clonidine
- **C.** Nicotine patch
- **D.** All of the above

88. Most common cause of HTN in young adult:
- **A.** Renal parenchymal disease
- **B.** Reno-vascular hypertension
- **C.** CoA
- **D.** Pheochromocytoma

89. Which of the following is not seen in acute pancreatitis?
- **A.** Hypotension
- **B.** Murphy's sign
- **C.** Gray Turner sign
- **D.** Cullen sign

90. For diagnosis of variant angina: drug used for provocative test is:
- **A.** Ergonovine
- **B.** Serotonin
- **C.** Dipyridamole
- **D.** Adenosine

91. True about delayed after depolarization:
- **A.** Mechanism for digitalis toxicity
- **B.** Precipitate by catecholamine excess
- **C.** Can be terminated by premature stimulation
- **D.** All of the above

---

78 D 79 B 80 B 81 B 82 B 83 A 84 A 85 A 86 A 87 D 88 A 89 B 90 A
91 D

92. Integrins are:
A. Related to platelet receptors
B. Related to oncogenesis
C. Assist in cell mobilisation
D. Increased gastric motility

93. Which of the following causes to and fro murmur?
A. VSD with AR
B. RSOV
C. Pulmonary artery hypertension with PR
D. PDA

94. Which of the following is ganglion blocker?
A. Reserprine
B. Clonidine
C. Trimethoprim
D. Atenelol

95. Anrep effect is:
A. Abrupt increase in aortic pressure lead to positive inotropic effect
B. Increase in heart rate increase the force of contraction
C. Wall stress is directly related to pressure and radius
D. None of the above

96. Tamm-Horsfall protein is:
A. Secreted by renal tubule
B. Found in urine in multiple myeloma
C. Increase in Type 2 renal tubular acidosis
D. Suggests glomerular damage

97. Increase LH secretion occurs in:
A. Testicular feminization syndrome
B. 5-alpha reductase deficiency
C. Turner's syndrome
D. Hyperprolactinemia

98. Which of the following is thrombogenic at endothelial level?
A. Activated protein C
B. Thrombomodulin
C. Antithrombin 3
D. Thrombospondin

99. Maximum action potential duration is seen in:
A. SA node
B. AV node
C. Ventricle
D. Purkinje cell

100. Maximum rate of rise of voltage is seen in which phase of action potential:
A. Phase 0
B. Phase 1
C. Phase 2
D. Phase 3

92 A 93 A 94 C 95 A 96 A 97 A 98 D 99 D 100 A

Srichitra 2002

1. Least amenable to treatment in NVE:
- **A.** Fungi
- **B.** Aerobic gram negative Bacteria
- **C.** Staph aureus
- **D.** Enterococci

2. HACEK includes:
- **A.** Cardiobacterium
- **B.** Acinitobacter
- **C.** E. coli
- **D.** Klebsiella

3. Janeway's lesion:
- **A.** Tender
- **B.** Nodular
- **C.** Most common in trunk
- **D.** Blanches on pressure

4. HACEK true is:
- **A.** Gram positive
- **B.** Anaerobes
- **C.** Nutritionally deficient
- **D.** As a group most common cause of endocarditis

5. True about mycotic aneurysm:
- **A.** Caused by fungi
- **B.** Always affect intracranial vessels
- **C.** Intervention required if>5mm
- **D.** Do not rupture if infection controlled

6. Most common congenital heart disease at birth:
- **A.** PDA
- **B.** VSD
- **C.** ASD
- **D.** TOF

7. Congenital heart disease is more common with:
- **A.** Situs inversus with dextrocardia
- **B.** Sintus solitus with levocardia
- **C.** Situs solitus with dextrocardia
- **D.** Kategener syndrome

8. Highest incidence of congenital heart disease in baby of mother with:
- **A.** Marfans syndrome
- **B.** ASD
- **C.** VSD
- **D.** TOF

9. Simple TGA true is:
- **A.** Ductal dependent circulation
- **B.** More than 90% mortality within a year after birth
- **C.** Should be operated as early as possible after birth
- **D.** None of the above

10. DORV true is:
- **A.** RVSP > LVSP if VSD is restrictive
- **B.** LVSP > RVSP if VSD is small and restrictive
- **C.** RVSP > aortic pressure if VSD is restrictive
- **D.** LVSP = PA pressure

1 A **2** A **3** D **4** C **5** C **6** B **7** C **8** A **9** B **10** A

11. Step down of pulmonary artery saturation in PDA:
- A. Eisenmenger PDA
- B. TOF with PDA
- C. TGA with PDA
- D. TAPVC with PDA
- E. AP Window

12. RVSP 120 mmHg, pulmonary artery 30 mmHg, diagnosis is:
- A. PS
- B. cTGA
- C. dTGA
- D. All of the above

13. Volume of all 4 chamber equal in:
- A. Gerbode's VSD
- B. Gassoul's VSD
- C. Membranous VSD
- D. Muscular VSD
- E. Sub pulmonic VSD

14. Holt Oram syndrome true is:
- A. Upper limb dysplasia
- B. ASD
- C. Chromosome 5q results in ASD and AV anomaly
- D. AV node abnormality
- E. All of the above

15. All are true about Di George syndrome *except:*
- A. Hypercalcemia
- B. Truncus arterioses
- C. IAA
- D. Thymic hypoplasia

16. Click at apex in child with LVOT obstruction suggestive of:
- A. Congenital valvular AS
- B. HOCM
- C. Supravalvular AS
- D. Sub valvular AS

17. Valsalva maneuver; true is:
- A. Index >1.6 suggestive of CHF
- B. Ph 1 & 3 response is normal in CHF
- C. Forced inspiration against closed glottis
- D. Decreased SBP, decreased DBP, decreased HR in phase 2

18. True about circulation time is all *except:*
- A. >25 sec is suggestive of CHF
- B. Last phase of dehydrochloric acid is facial flushing
- C. Helps to differentiate pulmonary and cardiac dyspnea
- D. In high output failure normal circulation time

19. In HOCM murmur is decreased by:
- A. Phenylephrine
- B. Valsalva strain phase
- C. Amylnitrite
- D. All of the above

20. Isometric exercise in comparison to isotonic exercise:
- A. Increased HR
- B. Increased CO
- C. Increased stroke volume
- D. Increased PVR

21. Isotonic exercise:
- A. 10 time increase in CO
- B. 10 time increase in SV
- C. 10 time increase in HR
- D. All of the above
- E. None of the above

22. Pulmonary hypertension is least common in:
- A. Systemic sclerosis
- B. CREST
- C. SLE
- D. RA

23. AR and aortic root dilatation not found in:
- A. Marfans syndrome
- B. Ehler-Danlos syndrome
- C. Pseudoxanthoma elasticum
- D. Osteogenesis imperfecta

11 C 12 A 13 A 14 E 15 A 16 A 17 B 18 B 19 A 20 D 21 E 22 D 23 C

24. True about ankylosing spondylitis are all *except:*
A. AR
B. MR
C. Ascending aorta aneurysm
D. Conduction defects

25. In 3 orthogonal leads PR is calculated by:
A. Shortest PR
B. Longest PR
C. Peak of P to peak of R in any lead
D. Beginning of p to QRS

26. Negative P terminal force which is significant is:
A. 1 mV and 40 msec
B. 1 mV and 20 msec
C. 0.1 mV and 40 msec
D. 0.1 mV and 20 msec

27. Tall R in aVR and aVF axis is:
A. 0 to 60º
B. 60 to 120º
C. 120º to 180º
D. –60 to –120º

28. QT interval shortens in:
A. Hypothermia
B. Hypokalemia
C. Hypocalcemia
D. Acidosis

29. Romhilt Estes criteria for LVH includes:
A. LAD
B. LAE
C. ST opposite to QRS
D. A and B
E. B and C
F. All of the above

30. PR interval includes:
A. AH and HV
B. PA and AH
C. PA and HV
D. None of the above

31. BP of 146/104 JNC VI:
A. Stage 2
B. Stage 1
C. Stage 3
D. Stage 4

32. According to BMI obesity is:
A. 25 kg/m^2
B. 30 kg/m^2
C. 35 kg/m^2
D. 40 kg/m^2

33. ARB is:
A. Losartan
B. Enalapril
C. Ramipril
D. Amlodipine

34. Omapatrilat is:
A. Vasopeptidase inhibitor
B. Prodrug of enalapril
C. ARB
D. Endothelin antagonist

35. Statin if given with following drugs causes rhabdomyolisis *except:*
A. Gemfibrozil
B. Itraconazol
C. Cholestyramine
D. Nicotinic acid

36. Least effective in dyslipidemia is:
A. Probucol
B. Gemfibrozil
C. Niacinamide
D. Cholestyramine

37. Cardioselective β blocker is:
A. Bisoprolol
B. Bucindolol
C. Carvidilol
D. All of the above

24 C 25 D 26 C 27 C 28 D 29 F 30 D 31 A 32 B 33 A 34 A 35 C 36 A 37 A

38. Dose reduction not required in reduced GFR:
A. Fosinopril
B. Lisinopril
C. Enalapril
D. Captopril

39. Atrial fibrillation–long term maintenance of sinus rhythm is not effective with:
A. Esmolol
B. Amiodarone
C. Quinidine
D. Flecanide

40. Hypertension, Hypokalemia, urine potassium >30 meq/L:
A. Diuresis
B. Primary aldosteronism
C. Renovascular HT
D. Licoric ingestion

41. Isolated diastolic dysfunction isolated as compared to systolic dysfunction:
A. Increased EDV
B. Increased ESV
C. Increased EF
D. None of the above

42. Beginning of LV systole characterized by:
A. Mitral closure, tricuspid closure, aortic closure, pulmonary opening
B. Mitral closure, tricuspid closure, pulmonary opening, aortic opening
C. Tricuspid closure, mitral closure, aorta opening, pulmonary closure
D. Tricuspid closure, mitral closure, pulmonary opening, aorta opening

43. Not true about pulsus alternans:
A. Indicates LV dysfunction
B. Always accompanied by electrical alternans
C. Can be started by standing
D. Can be initiated by VPC

44. For BP measurement least important is:
A. Arm cuff at heart level
B. Manometer at heart level
C. Arm cuff >80% arm circumference
D. Manometer should be vertical

45. Mitral diastolic and aortic systolic flow not equal in:
A. VSD
B. PDA
C. ASD
D. TOF/TGA

46. Gene defective in Marfans is:
A. Collagen
B. Fibrillin
C. Elastin
D. Cathepsin

47. Most sensitive non invasive test for pulmonary embolism:
A. Abnormal ventilation scan
B. Abnormal perfusion scan
C. Impedance plethysmography
D. Pulmonary arteriogram

48. ABG in pulmonary embolism:
A. Hypercapnia
B. Hypocapnia
C. Respiratory acidosis
D. Metabolic alkalosis

49. In Hot spot which is used:
A. Tc^{99} pyrophosphate
B. Tc^{99} Sistamibi
C. Tc^{99} teboroxine
D. Thallium

50. tPA differs from STK by all *except:*
A. Less allergic
B. Long plasma ½ life
C. Fibrin specific
D. Binds to plasminogen

38 A 39 A 40 B 41 D 42 B 43 B 44 B 45 A 46 B 47 B 48 B 49 A 50 B

51. Reinfarction in acute MI least useful:
A. CPK
B. CPKMB
C. Trop T
D. Myoglobin

52. Earliest enzyme to appear in Acute MI:
A. Myoglobin
B. Trop T
C. Trop I
D. CPKMB

53. UFH differs from LMWH:
A. Long ½ life
B. Binds to platelet factor 4 and platelets
C. More bleeding
D. All of the above

54. Natural anticoagulants are all *except:*
A. Protein C
B. Protein S
C. Antithrombin III
D. Fibrinogen
E. Plasminogen

55. Natural prothombotic is:
A. Thrombospondin
B. Thrombomodulin
C. PAI
D. Fibronectin

56. Least important risk factor for preeclampsia:
A. Nulliparity
B. Multiparity
C. Multi gestation
D. Age <15, >35 yrs

57. HT and stroke–risk factor for stroke means:
A. Casual relationship
B. Strong association
C. Controlling HT prevents stroke
D. All of the above

58. All cause pancytopenia *except:*
A. Chloramphenicol
B. Ticlopidine
C. Sulphonamide
D. Carbenicillin

59. LDL contains:
A. Apo B48
B. Apo B 100
C. Lp(a)
D. Apo(a)
E. Apo (e)

60. In circulatory shock, lactate level is:
A. 0.1 mmol/L
B. 1.5 mmol/L
C. 10 mmol/L
D. 20 mmol/L

61. In cardiogenic shock true are all are *except:*
A. Increased cardiac index
B. Increased PCWP
C. Increased RA pressure
D. Increased SVR
E. Increased HR

62. X linked recessive disease is characterized by:
A. Father to son transmission absent
B. Females recessive and dominance both important
C. Phenotypic manifestation of mutant gene in males
D. Father to daughter would become carrier
E. All of the above

63. All are true about Fredrich's ataxia *except:*
A. Dorsal root ganglia destroyed
B. Pupillary reflex normal
C. Autosomal dominant
D. ECG in most patients is abnormal

51 C 52 A 53 D 54 D 55 C 56 B 57 C 58 D 59 B 60 C 61 A 62 E 63 C

64. Tetany is aggravated by:
A. Hyperphosphataemia
B. Increased Hydrogen ions
C. Hypermagnesemia
D. Hypokalemia

65. Visual hallucinations seen with:
A. L dopa
B. β blockers
C. Tricyclic antidepressant
D. Phenothiazines
E. All of the above

66. Parasympathetic overactivity by:
A. Organophosphorous compounds
B. Cocaine
C. Hydrocarbons
D. All of the above

67. Eosophageal varices–GI bleeding drug of choice:
A. Octreotide
B. Vasopressin
C. Propanolol
D. NTG

68. Hepatic encephalopathy in cirrhosis is precipitated by all *except:*
A. Vomiting
B. Acidosis
C. GI bleed
D. Viral hepatitis
E. Pneumonia

69. P-ANCA is associated with:
A. Primary biliary cirrhosis
B. Sclerosing cholangitis
C. Viral hepatitis
D. All of the above

70. All are true about Chronic hepatitis *except:*
A. Hepatitis B
B. Hepatitis C
C. Hepatitis D
D. Hepatitis E

71. First to appear in Hepatitis B is:
A. HbsAg
B. HbeAg
C. HbcAg
D. Anti-HBc

72. Ranson criteria for acute pancreatitis include all *except:*
A. PaO_2 <8 Pa
B. RBS <7 mmol/L
C. LDH >600
D. Ca^{2+} <2 mmol/L

73. Least oxygen extraction in basal state by:
A. Liver
B. Heart
C. Kidney
D. Brain

74. Primary hemochromatosis is benign in:
A. Heart
B. Liver
C. Pancreas
D. Brain

75. PICA is a branch of:
A. Vertebral artery
B. Basilar artery
C. Anterior spinal artery
D. Posterior cerebral artery

76. Cell wall synthesis inhibitor is:
A. Sulpha drugs
B. Penicillin
C. Tetracyclin
D. Macrolides

77. Patient of penicillin allergy cannot be given all *except:*
A. Cephalosporins
B. Monobactams
C. Macrolides
D. Carbapenems

64 A 65 E 66 A 67 A 68 B 69 B 70 D 71 A 72 B 73 C 74 B 75 A 76 B 77 C

78. Renal osteodystrophy is caused by all *except:*
A. Hyper PO_4.
B. Washed out calcium and vit.D by dialysis
C. Decreased production of 1-25 dihydroxy Vit.D
D. Aluminium antacids
E. Metabolic acidosis

79. Which of the following can be measured by spirometer:
A. ERV
B. RV
C. TLC
D. FRC

80. Bronchospasm is not seen with:
A. Silica
B. Cotton dust
C. Pollen
D. Flax

81. All are true about H1 receptors *except:*
A. Blocked by terfinadine
B. Mediate pruritus
C. Secretes acids
D. Acts on vascular and non vascular smooth muscle cell

82. All may be seen in paraneoplastic *except:*
A. SIADH
B. Acromegaly
C. Hypocalcemia
D. Gynaecomastia

83. In Nephrotic syndrome thrombosis is due to:
A. Loss of coagulation factor
B. Less synthesis of anticoagulants
C. Hypercholesterolemia
D. Thrombocytosis and increased platelet activity
E. A and D
F. All of the above

84. Galactorrhea is due to:
A. Domperidone
B. Phenothiazines
C. M-dopa
D. Tricyclic antidepressants
E. All except A

85. Allelic heterogenicity is:
A. Same locus different mutation–identical phenotype
B. Mutation in different locus on same gene-different phenotype
C. Single mutation–different phenotype
D. All of the above

86. Half life of IgG:
A. 8 hrs
B. 14 days
C. 7 days
D. 21 days
E. 1 month

87. Skin pigmentation seen in:
A. Primary biliary cirrhosis
B. Vitamin B_{12} deficiency
C. Nelson disease
D. Gilbert disease

88. Cystic fibrosis most common extrapulmonary manifestation is:
A. Endocrine pancreatic deficiency
B. Exocrine pancreatic deficiency
C. Liver failure
D. Cardiac failure

89. All are true about gastrinoma *except:*
A. Rarely malignant
B. Most common in pancreas and duodenum
C. Diabetes in 40% cases
D. Asymptomatic in man

90. Which is more common in females than males?
A. Osteoporosis
B. Alzheimer's disease
C. DM 2
D. All of the above
E. None of the above

78 E 79 A 80 D 81 C 82 C 83 E 84 E 85 A 86 D 87 C 88 B 89 A 90 D

91. Filiariform larvae is:
A. Ascariasis
B. Trichuris trichuria
C. E.vermicularis
D. Necator and Stercoralis

92. Co-enzyme Q-10 deficiency can lead to all *except:*
A. Muscle weakness
B. Huntingtons chorea
C. Sometime antioxidant sometime pro-oxidant
D. Part of mitochondrial transfer chain from 2 to 11

93. Cardiac cachexia–factors responsible are:
A. Increased TNF
B. Increased noradrenaline
C. Increased renin
D. Increased ANP

94. Most common infection in neutropenic patients:
A. H. influenzae
B. S.aureus
C. S.Pneumonia
D. Aerobic gram –ve

95. Weaning from ventilator–all true *except:*
A. Tidal volume >5 ml/kg
B. Vital capacity > 10 ml/kg
C. PEEP >10 cm of water
D. Tidal volume >15 ml/kg

96. TB in HIV difficult to diagnose because of:
A. AFB negative
B. PPD negative
C. Atypical chest X-ray
D. All of the above
E. None of the above

97. Sick euthyroid syndrome characterized by:
A. Normal T3, normal T4, decreased TSH
B. Normal T3, normal T4, Normal TSH
C. Normal T3, decreased T4, increased TSH
D. Normal T4, decreased TSH

98. Best prognosis in Hodgkin's is of:
A. Lymphocytic predominant
B. Lymphocytic depletion
C. Nodular
D. Mixed

99. Valvular graft taken from human cadaver to human is:
A. Autograft
B. Allograft
C. Heterograft
D. None of the above

100. High altitude pulmonary odema–true is:
A. Increased pulmonary capillary wedge pressure
B. Normal pulmonary capillary wedge pressure
C. Decreased pulmonary capillary wedge pressure
D. Increased pulmonary artery pressure with normal pulmonary capillary wedge pressure

91 D 92 B 93 A 94 D 95 C 96 C 97 C 98 A 99 B 100 D

Srichitra 2001

1. **True statements:**
   A. Mitral closes before tricuspid valve
   B. Pulmonary open before aortic valve
   C. Aortic closes before pulmonary valve
   D. Tricuspid opens before mitral valve
   E. All of the above
   F. None of the above

Match the following:

2. **Na^+K^+2Cl transport**	A. Frusemide
3. **Na Cl**	B. Spironolactone
4. **Apical Na^+ channel**	C. Hydrochlorothiazide
	D. Acetazolamide
	E. Amiloride

Match the following:

5. **Minoxidil**	A. Pericardial effusion
6. **Cyclosporin**	B. Thromboembolism
7. **Estrogen**	C. Hypertension
8. **Doxorubicin**	D. Dilated cardiomyopathy
9. **Cisapride**	E. Torsades de pointes
	F. Hypertrophic cardiomyopathy

10. **High RV pressure is found in:**
    A. Ebstein
    B. Isolated EMF of RV
    C. Pulmonary atresia with intact IVS
    D. Uhl's anomaly

11. **Cyanotic congenital heart disease:**
    A. Coronary cameral fistula
    B. Left SVC draining into unroofed coronary sinus
    C. ALCAPA
    D. PAPVC
    E. Scimitar syndrome

12. **Dilated coronary sinus commonest cause is:**
    A. Obstructive IVC with azygous continuation
    B. Right SVC obstruction
    C. TAPVC draining into coronary sinus
    D. Persistent left SVC

13. **Ejection systolic murmur with delayed peak in pulmonary area:**
    A. Isolated valvular PS
    B. TOF with Severe obstruction
    C. Single ventricle with PS
    D. AS

14. **O_2 saturation 60% with PCO_2 36 mmHg and alveolar arterial gradient <10 diagnosis is:**
    A. High altitude
    B. COPD
    C. Right to left intracardiac shunt
    D. Hypoventilation

15. **Atrial rate equal to ventricular rate in:**
    A. AVRT
    B. Atrial tachycardia
    C. Bundle branch re-entry
    D. Atrial flutter with bypass tract

1 E 2 A 3 C 4 E 5 A 6 C 7 B 8 D 9 E 10 C 11 B 12 D 13 A 14 A 15 A

16. Regarding concealed AV bypass tract true is:
- **A.** Retrograde VA conduction does not occur
- **B.** Does not participate in AVRT
- **C.** Ventricular fibrillation will not occur if it develops AF
- **D.** All of the above
- **E.** None of the above

17. AF with bypass tract treatment of choice is:
- **A.** Verapamil
- **B.** Adenosine
- **C.** Flecainide
- **D.** Digitalis

18. Drug used to revert AF to normal sinus rhythm:
- **A.** Verapamil
- **B.** Moricizine
- **C.** Digoxin
- **D.** Mexiletine
- **E.** All of the above

19. Rate control needed before conversion of AF to sinus rhythm:
- **A.** Quinidine
- **B.** Procainamide
- **C.** Flecainide
- **D.** All of the above

20. 'p' wave on ST segment: least likely arrhythmia is:
- **A.** AVRT
- **B.** AVNRT
- **C.** Junctional tachycardia
- **D.** SA nodal reentry tachycardia

21. Veins draining to coronary sinus:
- **A.** Middle cardiac vein
- **B.** Anterior interventricular vein
- **C.** Vein of Marshall
- **D.** All of the above
- **E.** None of the above

22. Tissue perfusion is best measured by:
- **A.** HR × CO × AVO_2 difference
- **B.** HR × SV × AVO_2 difference
- **C.** HR × SV
- **D.** None of the above

23. Fibrinolytic which can be given in bolus:
- **A.** TNK-tPA
- **B.** Lanateplase
- **C.** Reteplase
- **D.** All of the above
- **E.** None of the above

24. Low molecular weight heparin in comparison to unfractionated heparin: true is:
- **A.** Better than UFH in NSTEMI
- **B.** Early onset of action
- **C.** aPTT is best to monitor the activity
- **D.** Enoxaparin is the most commonly used LMWH in clinical trials

25. 35 year old male, rhythm strips showing constant PR interval of 200 msec possible diagnosis is:
- **A.** Wenckbach AV block
- **B.** CHB
- **C.** First degree AV block
- **D.** Trifascicular block

26. Event farthest from QRS onset is:
- **A.** Z event of atrial pressure tracing
- **B.** Onset of rise of aortic pressure
- **C.** Onset of isovolumetric contraction
- **D.** Closure of mitral valve

27. Speed of blood flow in aorta:
- **A.** 0.6-1.2 m/s
- **B.** 1.2-2 m/s
- **C.** 2-2.5 m/s
- **D.** 0.3-0.6 m/s

16 E 17 C 18 B 19 D 20 D 21 D 22 B 23 D 24 D 25 C 26 A 27 D

28. O_2 saturation in pulmonary artery more than descending aorta in:
A. C-TGA
B. d-TGA
C. PDA with Eisenmengers
D. VSD with Eisenmengers

29. In which condition murmur intensity decreases with phenylephrine:
A. MR of MVP
B. Rheumatic MR
C. HOCM
D. VSD

30. Cardiac tamponade in comparison to CCP will show:
A. VY collapse
B. Kussmaul's sign
C. Pericardial knock
D. All of the above
E. None of the above

31. Wall stress is inversely proportional to:
A. Wall thickness
B. Radius
C. Pressure
D. All of the above
E. None of the above

32. Regarding HOCM true is:
A. 90% have resting gradient
B. All have ASH
C. All have SAM if there is LVOT obstruction
D. All have mutation for beta MHC

33. Which is a nitro vasodilator?
A. Nicorandil
B. Molsidomine
C. Vesnarinone
D. Pimobendan
E. None of the above

34. Acute aortic dissection with severe hypertension: treatment of choice:
A. Esmolol
B. Sodium nitroprusside
C. Hydralazine
D. Diazoxide

35. His bundle branch originates beneath:
A. Right coronary and non coronary cusp
B. Left and right coronary cusp
C. Left and non coronary cusp
D. Below non coronary cusp

36. Pulmonary AV fistula can cause all *except:*
A. Deep cyanosis
B. High output state
C. Equal appearance of contrast in RA and LA
D. None of the above

37. Murmur with non organic cardiac disease:
A. Austin Flint
B. Graham Steel
C. Carey Coomb's murmur
D. Still's murmur

38. Paradoxical splitting of S2 seen in:
A. WPW type A
B. RV apical pacing for CHB
C. Severe PS
D. None of the above

39. Which of the following is not a primary siti of carcinoid?
A. Bronchus
B. Appendix
C. Ileum
D. Liver

40. Carcinoid causes:
A. Paroxysmal HTN
B. Flushing
C. Bronchoconstriction
D. Diarrhoea
E. All of the above

28 B 29 C 30 E 31 A 32 C 33 B 34 B 35 A 36 C 37 D 38 B 39 D 40 E

41. Hypokalemia is seen in:
A. Liddle's syndrome
B. Bartter syndrome
C. Conn's syndrome
D. All of the a bove

42. Primary hyperaldosteronism: all true *except:*
A. Hypokalemia
B. Metabolic alkalosis
C. Hyperreninemia
D. Salt intake fails to increase urine osmolality

43. Isometric exercise in comparison to isotonic exercise causes:
A. Increased Heart rate
B. Increased cardiac output
C. Increased Stroke volume
D. Increased peripheral vascular resistance

44. Primary atrial septostomy in patient of d-TGA helps in:
A. Increased pulmonary blood flow
B. Increased aortic blood flow
C. Decreased LV overload
D. Bidirectional mixing of blood

45. Warfarin dose needs to be increased with:
A. Griseofulvin
B. Amiodarone
C. Quinidine
D. All of the above
E. None of the above

46. Inhibitor of cytochrome p-450:
A. Phenytoin
B. Barbiturate
C. Cimetidine
D. Rifampicin

47. QT interval is not increased with:
A. Acidosis
B. Hyperkalemia
C. Hypercalcemia
D. Digoxin
E. All of the above
F. None of the above

48. SA node is nearer to all *except:*
A. SVC
B. Cristae terminalis
C. Right atrial appendage
D. Tendon of Todaro

49. PR interval shortening is seen with:
A. Exercise
B. Short cycle atrial pacing
C. Both of the above
D. None of the above

50. Favorable lipid effect is seen with:
A. Alpha blocker
B. Ace inhibitor
C. ARB
D. Non selective beta blocker
E. None of the above

51. True about Korotokoff's sound is:
A. Stage IV-muffling
B. Stage II-Tapping
C. Stage III-Progressive decrease in velocity
D. Stage I-Soft

52. In standard ECG, V6 is positioned in:
A. 5th space mid axillary line
B. 5th space posterior axillary line
C. 6th space mid axillary line
D. At the level of V4–mid axillary line

53. Haemophiliac father with heterozygous mother. Son's chance of having haemophilia:
A. 25%
B. 50%
C. 75%
D. 100%

41 D 42 C 43 D 44 D 45 A 46 C 47 E 48 D 49 C 50 A 51 A 52 A 53 B

54. Following are minor criteria of rheumatic fever:
A. Erythema multiforme
B. Rising ASO titre
C. Positive streptococcal throat culture
D. Rapid streptococcal antigen test
E. All of the above
F. None of the above

55. Regarding rheumatic subcutaneous nodules: true is:
A. Tender
B. Fixed to underlying bone
C. Commonly associated with carditis
D. Seen in 50% cases of rheumatic fever

56. Adenosine antagonist:
A. Theophylline
B. Disopyramide
C. Dipyridamole
D. Verapamil

57. Primary biliary cirrhosis is characterized by:
A. Antimitochondrial antibody positive in 95% cases
B. Hypercholesterolemia
C. Increased alkaline phosphatase
D. All of the above

58. All are seen in nephrotic syndrome *except:*
A. Hypercholesterolemia
B. Hypocalcemia
C. Hypofibrinogenaemia
D. Hypogammaglobulinaemia
E. Renal vein thrombosis

59. Lenticular cataract is seen in all *except:*
A. Neurofibromatosis
B. Homocysteinemia
C. Myotonic dystrophy
D. Galactosemia

60. pH 7.45, bicarbonate increased, PCO_2 increased:
A. Respiratory acidosis with metabolic compensation
B. Respiratory alkalosis with metabolic compensation
C. Metabolic acidosis with respiratory compensation
D. Metabolic alkalosis with respiratory compensation

61. H. pylori; true statement are all *except:*
A. Gram positive
B. Can be diagnosed on culture
C. Commonly associated with gastric ulcer
D. Urease producing

62. Bilateral cortical necrosis of kidneys seen with:
A. Scleroderma
B. Sickle cell disease
C. Septic abortion
D. Hepato renal syndrome

63. Flow of fluid in a vessel depends mostly on:
A. Fluid viscosity
B. Fluid density
C. Vessel diameter
D. Velocity

64. As per WHO, ORS solution contain all *except:*
A. Sodium
B. Potassium
C. Chloride
D. Citrate
E. Bicarbonate

65. All decrease seizure threshold *except:*
A. Ciprofloxacin
B. Acetazolamide
C. Metoclopramide
D. Lithium

54 F 55 C 56 A 57 D 58 C 59 B 60 D 61 A 62 C 63 C 64 D 65 B

66. Metoclopramide causes all *except:*
A. Delayed gastric emptying
B. Dystonia
C. Decreased prolactin release
D. Act on CTZ
E. Equipotent to domperidone

67. PUO for weeks can be due to all *except:*
A. Renal cell carcinoma
B. Bronchogenic carcinoma
C. Lymphoma
D. Leukemia

68. Werthin-Finkeldey cells in measles are:
A. T4
B. T8
C. Fibroblast
D. Histiocytic giant cell

69. Paget's disease: all true *except:*
A. Hypercalcemia
B. Increased calcitonin
C. Increased acid phosphatase
D. Autosomal dominant
E. Hypoparathyroidism

70. Rheumatoid arthritis causes all *except:*
A. Neuropathy
B. Retinopathy
C. Splenomegaly
D. Atlanto-axial dislocation

71. Anaphylaxis is mediated by:
A. IgE
B. IgA
C. IgG
D. IgM
E. Immune complex

72. Commonest cause of immunodeficiency is:
A. IgA deficiency
B. Di George's syndrome
C. Job syndrome
D. Common variable immunodeficiency

73. Sildenafil: all statements are true *except:*
A. Act by inhibiting phosphodiesterase-5
B. Nitrates contraindicated
C. Increased cyclic AMP level
D. Treatment of choice for primary erectile dysfunction in males
E. Act through potassium channels

74. Clozapine causes:
A. Aplastic anemia
B. Thrombocytopenia
C. Megaloblastic anemia
D. Agranulocytosis

75. Hepatorenal syndrome: true are all *except:*
A. Associated with cirrhosis and ascites
B. Kidney normal
C. Kidney biopsy abnormal
D. Treatment unsuccessful

76. Not true about anaphylaxis:
A. Mediated by IgA
B. Angioedema and urticaria occurs
C. Mediated by IgE
D. None of the above

77. Which of the following has faeco-oral route:
A. Hepatitis B
B. Hepatitis C
C. Hepatitis E
D. Non-A, Non-B

78. Regarding hepatitis E: true statement is:
A. Transmission same as hepatitis B
B. Commonly leads to cirrhosis
C. High incidence of mortality in pregnancy
D. Transmitted through blood

79. Hypokalemia is seen in all *except:*
A. Leukemia
B. Hyperosmolality
C. Renal tubular acidosis
D. Diuretic used

66 A 67 B 68 D 69 A 70 B 71 A 72 A 73 E 74 D 75 C 76 A 77 C 78 C 79 A

80. Acidosis with increased anion gap is seen in all *except:*
A. Renal tubular acidosis
B. Lactic acidosis
C. Salicylate poisoning
D. Diabetic ketoacidosis
E. CRF

81. Regarding ATT: all are true *except:*
A. Streptomycin is useful in TBM
B. Pyrazinamide causes hyperuricaemia
C. Ethambutol causes optic neuritis
D. Rifampicin acts through DNA dependent RNA polymerase

82. With hypocalcemia chance of tetany is increased by:
A. Increased blood phosphate
B. Decreased potassium
C. Increased magnesium
D. Increased hydrogen ion

83. Delayed excretion of contrast in unilateral kidney can be due to:
A. Polycystic kidney
B. Hypoplastic kidney
C. CRF
D. Renal artery stenosis

84. All are associated with diabetes *except:*
A. Somogyi effect
B. Dawn's phenomenon
C. Myotonic dystrophica
D. Kalmann syndrome
E. Lipoidosis en sibre

85. Hyper segmented macrophage with decreased myelin synthesis is seen in:
A. SSPE
B. Multiple sclerosis
C. Cerebral lipoidosis
D. Krabbe's disease

86. In an old man, PSA is 35 ng/ml (normal 4ng/ml): next stage of screening:
A. Skeletal X-ray
B. CT
C. MRI
D. $Tech^{99}$ bone scan
E. TRUS guided biopsy

87. Child hood autism: true statement is:
A. Developmental pervasive behavioral disorder
B. No neurological defect
C. Starts after 5 years of age
D. Boys are commonly affected

88. Treatment with Vitamin B12 in subacute combined degeneration of spinal cord: earliest evidence of response to treatment:
A. Improvement in sense of vibration
B. Improvement in sense of position
C. Increase in reticulocyte count
D. Decrease in hyper segmented neutrophils

89. All are markers of decreased survival in acute pancreatitis *except:*
A. LDH> 400 IU/Lt
B. AST > 250 IU/Lt
C. RBS <200 mg%
D. PO_2 <60 mm Hg

90. Following are endocrinal pancreatic tumors *except:*
A. Gastrinoma
B. Glucagonoma
C. Somatostatinoma
D. Carcinoid

91. Which causes obstructive pulmonary disease?
A. Cystic fibrosis
B. Primary alveolar fibrosis
C. Kyphoscoliosis
D. None of the above

80 A 81 A 82 A 83 D 84 D 85 D 86 E 87 D 88 A 89 C 90 D 91 A

92. 42 year old female with SLE, scleroderma and polymyositis like syndrome diagnostic test is:
A. Anti DNA
B. Anti RNP
C. Anti SS DNA
D. Anti Ro

93. Which of the following indicates total lung capacity?
A. Residual volume + ERV + Forced inspiratory capacity
B. Residual volume + vital capacity
C. FRC + inspirtory capacity
D. All of the above
E. None of the above

94. Neostigmine reverses the action of all *except:*
A. Pancuronium
B. Succinyl choline
C. Vancuronium
D. Tubocurarine

95. Hangout interval means:
A. Cross over point of ventricular and arterial pressure
B. Cross over point of ventricular and atrial pressure
C. Cross over point of atrial and arterial pressure
D. Cross over point of interatrial pressures

96. Coronary filling occurs mostly in:
A. Systole
B. Diastole
C. RCA-Systole LCA-diastole
D. LCA-systole RCA-diastole

97. In enduring athletes, which is true?
A. 20 times increase in CO
B. 6 times increase in Stroke volume
C. PO_2 increase by 10%
D. CO_2 decrease by 20%

98. Drug induced thrombocytopenia: all are true *except:*
A. 80% diagnosed by recent test
B. Sudden improvement on stoppage of drug
C. Increased megakaryocytes
D. Caused by Binge alcohol drinking
E. Complement mediated

99. Sustained VT:
A. > 30 secs
B. > 3 sec
C. > 3 beats
D. Syncope

100. Which is not an acute phase reactant?
A. Serum AA
B. CRP
C. Fibrinogen
D. α-TNF

92 B 93 D 94 D 95 A 96 B 97 B 98 A 99 A 100 D

BHU 2004

1. **What is the normal coronary blood flow?**
   A. 60-90 ml/min/100 gm
   B. 0-60 ml/min/100 gm
   C. 90-120 ml/min/100 gm
   D. 120-150 ml/min/100 gm

2. **In 1998, nobel prize was given for discovery of:**
   A. NO
   B. Sub lingual nitrate
   C. Sildenafil
   D. EDRF

3. **Maximum stress of cardiac systole is on which valve:**
   A. Aortic valve
   B. Tricuspid valve
   C. Mitral valve
   D. Pulmonary valve

4. **Age group in 4S trial was:**
   A. 35-70 years
   B. 40-70 years
   C. 40-80 years
   D. 45-75 years

5. **Ramipril in HOPE: the dosing pattern was:**
   A. 1.25 mg–7 days, 2.5 mg–14 days, 10 mg–long
   B. 1.25 mg–14 days, 2.5 mg–21 days, 10 mg for long
   C. 2.5 mg for 7 days, 5 mg–21 days, 10 mg–long
   D. 5 mg for 7 days, 10 mg–21 days, 15 mg–long

6. **Lipid tetrad index of 15,000 falls in which category?**
   A. Low
   B. High
   C. Borderline
   D. Moderate

7. **NCEP guidelines: cholesterol measurement should be done at:**
   A. 20 years
   B. 30 years
   C. 40 years
   D. 50 years

8. **Maximum decrease in triglycerides is by:**
   A. Statins
   B. Fibrates + niacin
   C. Statins + fibrates
   D. Statin + niacin

9. **Normal PR interval is:**
   A. < 100 msecs
   B. 120-160 msecs
   C. 160-200 msecs
   D. > 200 msecs

10. **Not true about Lp(a) is:**
    A. 10 times more atherogenic than LDL
    B. Premature CAD occurs
    C. Expressed after 5 years of age
    D. Homologous to plasminogen

1 A 2 A 3 C 4 A 5 C 6 B 7 A 8 B 9 B 10 C

11. Increase in homocysteine is by all *except:*
A. Folate antagonists
B. Increase LDL cholesterol oxidation
C. Premature atherosclerosis
D. Increase EDRF

12. High Lp(a) levels is treated by:
A. Niacin
B. Fibrates
C. Statins
D. ACE-inhibitors

13. Most powerful antioxidant is:
A. Vitamin E
B. Beta carotene
C. Vitamin C
D. Carvedilol

14. Congenital absence of pericardium was discovered by:
A. Dexter
B. Galen
C. Harvey
D. Columbus

15. First successful heart transplant was carried out at:
A. AIIMS
B. Escorts
C. Madras
D. Apollo

16. Eisenmenger's VSD is best treated by:
A. VSD closure
B. Heart transplantation
C. Heart-lung transplantation
D. Lung transplantation

17. Mortality in severe AS is:
A. 10%
B. 20%
C. 40%
D. 50%

18. In a patient with aortic valve area of 0.6 cm^2, the continuous wave Doppler velocity will be:
A. 2-3 m/sec
B. 3-4 m/sec
C. 4-5 m/sec
D. > 5 m/sec

19. Successful balloon septostomy in TGA with intact IVS reduces transeptal gradient by:
A. < 2 mm Hg
B. < 3 mm Hg
C. < 4 mm Hg
D. < 5 mm Hg

20. TGA with PS: true is:
A. VSD is always present
B. Systemic to pulmonary shunt effectively decreases cyanosis
C. Stenosis is usually valvular
D. Following correction, mitral valve is damaged and there is AV conduction defects

21. Serotonin helps in differentiating which of the following murmurs:
A. AS and PS
B. Graham Steel and AR
C. MS and TS
D. AS and IHSS

22. Most common paroxysmal narrow complex tachycardia is:
A. AVNRT
B. AVRT
C. SNRT
D. Ectopic atrial tachycardia

23. Effective platelet inhibition for GbIIb/IIIa inhibitors requires what percentage of receptor blockage?
A. < 50%
B. 50-80%
C. > 80%
D. 100%

11 D 12 A 13 A 14 D 15 A 16 C 17 D 18 D 19 A 20 B 21 B 22 A 23 C

24. **Echo on AR: all are seen *except:***
A. Fluttering (diastolic) of AML
B. Fluttering of IVS of LV
C. Fluttering of PML
D. Fluttering of PW

25. **All are causes of ASH *except:***
A. AS
B. PWMI
C. PAH
D. IHSS

26. **High output heart failure is seen in all *except:***
A. Anemia
B. Thyrotoxicosis
C. Beriberi
D. Pregnancy

27. **M1-T1 interval is:**
A. 20-30 msec
B. 40-60 msec
C. 60-90 msec
D. 90-120 msec

28. **Oxygen saturation of ascending aorta in fetus is:**
A. 46-48%
B. 36-38%
C. 26-28%
D. 16-18%

29. **Umbilical venous oxygen saturation is:**
A. 40-55%
B. 62-68%
C. 30-35%
D. None of the above

30. **Which of the following agents is a noncompetitive, high-affinity blocker of the GP IIb/IIIa integrin?**
A. Abciximab
B. Enoxaparin
C. Eptifibatide
D. Tirofiban

31. **ICD prevents SCD in:**
A. 54%
B. 74%
C. 64%
D. 94%

32. **Drug used in EPISTENT was:**
A. Abciximab
B. Eptifibatide
C. Hirudin
D. Tirofiban

33. **TIMI-14 trail used:**
A. Hirudin
B. Abciximab
C. TNK-tPA
D. Intracoronary radiation

34. **US carvedilol was prematurely terminated due to decrease in mortality by:**
A. 35%
B. 65%
C. 54%
D. 75%

35. **Rapamycin true about action of:**
A. Inhibit elastic recoil
B. Inhibit late remodeling
C. Inhibit neointimal proliferation
D. Inhibit thrombus formation

36. **Following DCA: incidence of restenosis at 1 year is:**
A. 35%
B. 30%
C. 40%
D. 60%

37. **Slew rate is important in:**
A. Pacemaker
B. IHSS
C. Alternative name of sinus bradycardia
D. Cardiac tamponade

---

24 C 25 B 26 D 27 A 28 C 29 C 30 A 31 A 32 A 33 C 34 B 35 C 36 A
37 A

38. Reverse splitting of S2 occurs in all *except:*
A. LBBB
B. RV ectopic
C. HOCM
D. MVP

39. Thirty year female with RA pressure-22 mm Hg, LA-23 mm Hg, PA-40/20 mm Hg, RVEDP-26 mm Hg, LVEDP-28 mm Hg, Aorta-110/70 mm Hg, RA shows small a and v waves: Diagnosis is:
A. Hemochromatosis
B. EMF
C. CCP
D. Severe MS

40. Persistent Kerley B lines after successful BMV are seen in:
A. Mild MR
B. Mild AR
C. Haemosiderosis
D. Increase pulmonary venous pressure

41. Poor outcome in Takayasu arteritis is with:
A. HLA A-10
B. HLA Bw-52
C. HLA DR-W12
D. HLA B5

42. Gene involved in DCMP is:
A. Dystrophin
B. Desmin
C. TTR
D. Glycan

43. Spongy myocardium:
A. Noncompaction of left ventricle
B. Form of cardiomyopathy
C. Increase incidence of arrhythmias
D. All of the above

44. Poor R wave progression in chest leads is seen with:
A. AWMI
B. RBBB
C. RVH
D. RVMI

45. Which is not a secondary prevention trial?
A. Post CABG
B. WOSCOPS
C. LIPID
D. CARE

46. Sones Complex includes all *except:*
A. PDA
B. CoA
C. Subaortic stenosis
D. Parachute mitral valve

47. Goose neck deformity is seen in:
A. Complete AV canal defect
B. HOCM
C. TGA
D. Parachute mitral valve

48. A-P window: Continuous murmur is least common due to:
A. Large defect
B. PAH
C. Increase BP
D. Associated PS

49. Cortriatriatum: LAA is attached to:
A. Dorsal part
B. Ventral part
C. PV
D. Both of the above

50. Cath features of HAPE are all *except:*
A. Normal LA pressure
B. Normal LVEDP pressure
C. Increase PAP
D. Increase PCWP

51. VVI when magnet is applied converts to:
A. VOO
B. VTT
C. No effect
D. None of the above

38 D 39 C 40 C 41 B 42 A 43 D 44 A 45 B 46 A 47 A 48 A 49 B 50 D 51 A

52. VDD: Pacemaker functions by:
A. RV pacing, RA/RV sensing
B. RA/RV pacing and RA sensing
C. Both RA and RV sensing and pacing
D. None of the above

53. VDD threshold–unipolar lead with atrial threshold of:
A. < 1
B. 1-1.5
C. 1.5-2
D. > 5

54. Biventricular pacing in CCF with intraventricular conduction defects: leads are place in:
A. RA, RV, LV
B. RA, RV, CS
C. RA, RV
D. LA, RA, RV

55. Pacemaker mediated tachycardia is treated by:
A. Post ventricular atrial refractory period > VARP
B. PVARP = VARP
C. VARP > PVARP
D. None of the above

56. Serum creatinine is 8 mg% in a patient who needs digoxin. What will be dose of digoxin?
A. 0.125 mg OD
B. 0.125 mg alternate day
C. 0.25 mg OD
D. 0.182 mg OD

57. Stress echo in COPD is done by:
A. Dopamine
B. Dobutamine
C. Adenosine
D. Thallium

58. Congenital Long QT syndrome is best treated by:
A. Beta blocker
B. Amiodarone
C. Quinidine
D. Phenytoin

59. Mechanism of action of type III antiarrhythmic agents is:
A. Decrease Na
B. Decrease K
C. Decrease Ca
D. Decrease Mg

60. Long QT syndromes are not caused by:
A. Decrease K
B. Increase K
C. Decrease Ca
D. Quinidine

61. Gynecomastia is caused by:
A. Spironolactone
B. Digoxin long term
C. Both of the above
D. None of the above

62. Treatment of choice of hypertension in pregnancy is:
A. Methyl Dopa
B. Calcium channel blockers
C. ACE inhibitors
D. Losartan

63. Bisferians pulse is best felt in:
A. Carotids
B. Brachial
C. Femoral
D. Radial

64. ERP is least in:
A. Myocardium
B. SA node
C. AV node
D. Bundle of His

65. Chronic atrial fibrillation is best treated by:
A. Corridor operation
B. VDD pacemaker
C. Atrial septostomy
D. SA node ablation

52 A 53 B 54 B 55 A 56 A 57 B 58 A 59 B 60 B 61 C 62 A 63 A 64 B
65 A

66. Most specific sign of cardiac tamponade is:
A. RA diastolic collapse
B. RV collapse early diastolic
C. IVC collapse
D. None of the above

67. True about adenosine is all *except:*
A. Bronchodilatation
B. Fast i/v administration
C. Can differentiate SVT with aberration from VT
D. Contraindicated in SSS

68. SVT is differentiated from VT by:
A. Fusion beats
B. rsr in V6
C. rsr in V1
D. Monophasic R in V1

69. Adenosine is useful in all *except:*
A. SVT
B. VT
C. PPH
D. None of the above

70. Dose of reteplase is:
A. 2 bolus of 10 units 30 minutes apart
B. Single bolus of 20 units
C. Single bolus of 10 units
D. 2 bolus of 20 units 30 minutes apart

71. Spontaneous dissection of which of the following artery is commonly seen in pregnancy?
A. Coronary artery
B. Aorta
C. LIMA
D. PA

72. All are true about pheochromocytoma *except:*
A. Sweating
B. Pigmentation
C. Hypertension
D. None of the above

73. S2-OS is fixed despite cycle variation in:
A. Increase mobility
B. Decrease mobility
C. Vegetation on AML
D. Vegetation on PML

74. Ashman phenomenon: all are true *except:*
A. AF
B. Digoxin is not contraindicated
C. Long cycle followed by short cycle terminated by ectopic
D. None of the above

75. Tall 'a' and slow 'y' descent is seen in:
A. TS
B. MS
C. TR
D. Ebstein's anomaly

76. Intra-cavitary ECG showing ECG pattern of RV and pressure tracing of RA is seen in:
A. Ebstein's anomaly
B. Uhl's anomaly
C. ARVD
D. Cortriatriatum

77. Which of the following is not a contraindication to PTMR:
A. LV aneurysm
B. LVH
C. Sustained VT
D. LVEF < 25%

78. Beta blocker without ISA and membrane stabilizing action is:
A. Acebutolol
B. Bucindolol
C. Carvedilol
D. Pindolol

66 B 67 A 68 C 69 D 70 A 71 A 72 B 73 B 74 C 75 A 76 A 77 D 78 B

79. **LMWH with lowest Xa: IIa ratio is:**
A. Nadroparin
B. Dalteparin
C. Ardeparin
D. Parnaparin

80. **Compensatory mechanism in CHF includes all *except:***
A. Increased ANP
B. Increased Renin
C. Increased aldosterone
D. Increased Na

81. **Following is true about congenital complete heart block:**
A. Always familial
B. Pacemaker always required
C. Occasional bradycardia with SA nodal dysfunction and death
D. Always associated with congenital heart disease

82. **All are true about adriamycin *except:***
A. Increase QT interval
B. Cardiomyopathy
C. Pericardial effusion
D. Congestive heart failure

83. **Which is better seen, felt and heard?**
A. Opening snap
B. Atrial gallop
C. Pericardial knock
D. LVS3

84. **RHD prevalence in school children between 1984-1996 was:**
A. 3.8/1000
B. 4.8/1000
C. 5.4/1000
D. 6.8/1000

85. **Biatrial myxoma: prevalence is:**
A. 5%
B. 10%
C. 15%
D. > 15%

86. **SA nodal artery arises from RCA in what percentage of patients?**
A. 59%
B. 45%
C. 65%
D. 85%

87. **Pulmonary artery hypertension is caused by which of the following?**
A. P. vivax
B. Schistosomiasis
C. Filaria
D. Trypanosomiasis

88. **A shunt draining from SVC to RPA is:**
A. BT shunt
B. Waterston's shunt
C. Potts shunt
D. Glenn's shunt

89. **WPW–Type B causes:**
A. Reverse S2
B. Wide fixed S2
C. Wide S1
D. Single S2

90. **Normal myocardium utilizes:**
A. Free fatty acids
B. Ketones
C. Glucose
D. Amino acids

91. **Least common arrhythmia by digoxin is:**
A. First degree heart block
B. Wenckebach type I
C. Ventricular tachycardia
D. Complete heart block

79 B 80 D 81 B 82 A 83 D 84 A 85 B 86 A 87 B 88 D 89 A 90 A 91 D

92. Squatting from standing position causes:
A. Decrease in HOCM murmur
B. Murmur of AR increases
C. Murmur of MR increases
D. None of the above

93. S_4 sound in AS is heard when:
A. Pressure gradient > 70 mm Hg
B. LVEDP < 10 mm Hg
C. Vegetation on aortic valve
D. Decrease mean arterial pressure of LA

94. Phase II action potential shows:
A. Slow calcium influx
B. Fast calcium influx
C. Increase sodium influx
D. Decrease sodium influx

95. AF with bypass tract treatment of choice is:
A. Verapamil
B. Adenosine
C. Flecainide
D. Digitalis

96. Drug not used in variant angina is:
A. Calcium channel blocker
B. Beta blocker
C. Nitroglycerine
D. Alpha-blocker

97. Milrinone: true are all *except:*
A. Phosphodiesterase inhibitor
B. Was used in PROMISE trial
C. Ventricular ectopy is seen in 9% cases
D. Amrinone can be used concurrently

98. Action potential velocity is maximum of:
A. SA node
B. AV node
C. Atrial muscle
D. Purkinji fiber

99. PR interval shortening is seen with:
A. Exercise
B. Short cycle atrial pacing
C. Both of the above
D. None of the above

100. Speed of blood flow in aorta:
A. 0.6-1.2 m/s
B. 1.2-2 m/s
C. 2-2.5 m/s
D. 0.3-0.6 m/s

92 A 93 A 94 A 95 C 96 B 97 D 98 D 99 C 100 D

BHU 2003

1. **Mortality in non cardiac syncope:**
   A. 6%
   B. 6-12%
   C. 20%
   D. 30%

2. **MADIT trial; true is:**
   A. Ejection fraction <35%, status post MI
   B. 704 patients enrolled
   C. No improvement in survival
   D. Quinidine used along with AICD

3. **Pericardial knock–time after A2:**
   A. 0.08–0.09
   B. 0.06-0.09
   C. 0.09-0.12
   D. 0.14-0.18

4. **Framingham's minor criteria for CHF:**
   A. PND
   B. Neck vein distension
   C. Vital capacity decreased by 1/3 of normal
   D. Venous pressure > 16 cm of water

5. **Spironolactone was used in which trial?**
   A. RALES
   B. MERIT-HF
   C. CONSENSUS
   D. CIBIS II

6. **SOLVD trial; true is:**
   A. Lisinopril was used
   B. Enalapril ↓ mortality by 21%
   C. Lisinopril ↑ mortality by 11%
   D. Lisinopril + nitrates are better

7. **Percentage of death due to increase in CHF:**
   A. 10
   B. 20
   C. 30
   D. 40

8. **Cirrhosis shows PPH in:**
   A. 0.1%
   B. 0.3%
   C. 0.9%
   D. 0.6%

9. **Percentage of death within 1 hr in acute cor pulmonale:**
   A. 24%
   B. 40%
   C. 50%
   D. 70%

10. **Aspirin saves lives:**
    A. 24/1000
    B. 48/1000
    C. 12/1000
    D. 36/1000

1 B 2 A 3 C 4 C 5 A 6 B 7 D 8 D 9 C 10 A

11. β blocker reduced cardiovascular events post MI in:
A. 33%
B. 27%
C. 18%
D. 09%

12. WOSCOPS reduces the non fatal CHD by:
A. 11%
B. 21%
C. 31%
D. 44%

13. Which is primary prevention trial?
A. 4S
B. CARE
C. LIPID
D. AFCAPS

14. 5 mm reduction on BP decreases stroke by:
A. 42%
B. 58%
C. 60%
D. 74%

15. Normal upper limit of LVEDP:
A. –4
B. –8
C. 12
D. 18

16. HACEK infective endocarditis; treatment is:
A. Ceftriaxone 2 gm I.V OD × 4 weeks
B. Ceftriaxone 1 gm I.V OD × 4 weeks
C. Ampi 2 gm I.V OD × 4 weeks
D. Ampi 1 gm I.V OD × 4 weeks

17. Systolic murmur grading given by:
A. William Wathering
B. Paul Wood
C. Levine
D. Gruentzig

18. IE Criteria known by the name of:
A. Jones
B. Jonas
C. Dukes
D. Sones

19. Jones criteria last revised on:
A. 1944
B. 1954
C. 1992
D. 2002

20. Cyanosis becomes evident at (capillary concentration of reduced Hb):
A. 20 gm/L
B. 30 gm/L
C. 40 gm/L
D. 25 gm/L

21. RAD diagnosed after:
A. +70
B. +90
C. +100
D. +80

22. RV activation is last at:
A. Pulmonary conus
B. RV Apex
C. TV
D. Anterior papillary muscle and base of RV

23. MBC vs. MIC true is:
A. MBC decreases bacterial conc by 99.9% in 24 hours
B. Tolerance is MBC <4 times MIC
C. Tolerance = synergistic bactericidal activity
D. All of the above

24. Heparin loading dose is:
A. 40 u/kg
B. 50 u/kg
C. 60 u/kg
D. 70 u/kg

11 C 12 C 13 D 14 A 15 C 16 A 17 C 18 C 19 C 20 C 21 B 22 A 23 A 24 C

25. Enoxaparin normal loading dose in MI:
A. 0.5 mg/kg OD
B. 1 mg/kg BD
C. 1.5 mg/kg BD
D. 1 mg/kg BD

26. True about heparin:
A. Loading dose 60 U/kg
B. Maintenance dose 12 U/kg/hr
C. Anti Xa activity is measured
D. All of the above

27. Ibuprofen is used in MI pericarditis because it:
A. ↑es coronary blood flow
B. ↓es fever
C. Antioxidant effect
D. ↓es systemic vase resistance

28. True about Post MI pericarditis:
A. EF decreases upto 10 days
B. Ibuprofen is drug of choice
C. Failure of T wave inversion is suggestive of the same
D. All of above

29. A post menopausal lady suffering from MI she asks for HRT to ↓es further events. You suggest:
A. Give HRT if no contraindication
B. HRT ↑es first year mortality, therefore not to be given de novo
C. Adequate trials not available
D. All of the above

30. Balloon aortic valvuloplasty; true is:
A. Treatment of choice in children with non calcific AS
B. Treatment of choice in elderly with calcific AS
C. Low risk of recurrence
D. High risk procedure

31. Rate of restenosis in SVG graft:
A. 1% per year
B. 2% per year
C. 3% per year
D. 4% per year

32. Critical AS considered as:
A. 0.5 cm^2
B. 0.5 $cm2/m^2$
C. $0.7cm^2$
D. $0.7cm^2/m^2$

33. Criteria for operation in AR:
A. EF > 55%
B. ESV <55 ml/m^2
C. EF b/w 55-75%
D. ESV > 55 ml/m^2

34. In RHD, true about TS:
A. Hemodynamically significant in 15%
B. TR is not associated
C. Mean diastolic gradient >4 mm produces systemic venous congestion
D. Tall V wave is found

35. Abdominal jugular reflex; true is:
A. Sudden increase by 2 cm during compression
B. Sudden decrease by 2 cm during compression
C. Sudden decrease by 2 cm after release
D. Sudden decrease by 4 cm after release

36. Time frame for SCD:
A. <1 minute
B. ≤1 hour
C. ≤1 day
D. 2 days

37. Definition of cardiac arrest; incorrect is:
A. Irreversible cessation of all biological functions
B. Reversible by early intervention
C. If not corrected promptly will lead to death early
D. None of the above

25 D 26 D 27 A 28 D 29 B 30 A 31 B 32 B 33 D 34 C 35 D 36 B 37 A

38. All are given for syncope *except:*
A. β blocker
B. α blocker (prazosin)
C. Disopyramide
D. Paroxetine

39. Reversed S2 splitting due to early P2:
A. PDA
B. LBBB
C. WPW (type B)
D. Angina

40. True about Opening snap is:
A. Occurs when LV pressure falls below left atrial pressure
B. PML is responsible for OS
C. S1-OS interval 0.16 to 0.18 sec
D. A2-OS 0.03 sec

41. Anticoagulation given for ... after 1st attack of Pulmonary embolism:
A. 6 weeks
B. 6 months
C. 4 weeks
D. 12 months

42. Mortality after MVR:
A. 1%
B. 4.3%
C. 6.4%
D. 8.6%

43. HOCM: 1st degree relative echo is abnormal in:
A. 11%
B. 22%
C. 33%
D. 44%

44. β myosin HC gene (chromosome 14) in HOCM is present in:
A. 30%
B. 20%
C. 40%
D. 60%

45. True about QT:
A. Bazetts formula has very high accuracy for all rates
B. QT varies in different leads
C. Measured from beginning of QRS to beginning of T
D. None of the above

46. QT_c done by:
A. QT/RR
B. QT/RR $^{1/2}$
C. RR/QT $^{1/2}$
D. RR/QT^2

47. Criteria of LVH:
A. S in V1 + r in V5 > 35 mm
B. r in V1 + s in V5 < 35 mm
C. r in V1 + S in V5 < 35 mm
D. None of the above

48. Some penetration of contrast medium with trickling flow is:
A. TIMI 0
B. TIMI 1
C. TIMI 2
D. TIMI 3

49. Lyme carditis true is:
A. Syncope due to AV block
B. Endocarditis is common
C. Myocarditis in >50% cases
D. VT is common

50. ST/T ratio to differentiate between early repolarization and pericarditis, in favour of pericarditis:
A. <0.35
B. <0.25
C. 2.5
D. >0.25

38 B 39 C 40 A 41 B 42 C 43 C 44 A 45 B 46 B 47 A 48 B 49 A 50 D

51. Doxorubicin induced cardiomyopathy; true is:
A. Monitored by echo
B. Dose is not related to toxicity
C. Less with bolus or rapid infusion
D. $\uparrow$ed LV mass in children

52. Apical impulse in secondary MR, true is:
A. Hyperdynamic
B. Sustained
C. Apical retraction
D. Late systolic

53. Malignant carcinoid: true is:
A. Lt sided involvement only
B. Liver metastasis is necessary for cardiac involvement
C. Low output state may occur
D. PR + TS is common

54. True about PPH:
A. Incidence 2/million
B. Chest pain is commonest symptom
C. Detected in 1st or 2nd decade
D. Usually diagnosed early in course

55. True about GpIIb/IIIa receptors:
A. IIb is specific on platelets
B. 20-40,000 receptors in platelet
C. IIIa present in integrin
D. Normally exposed only in active form

56. NAME syndrome is seen in:
A. ASD
B. VSD
C. Myxoma
D. PDA

57. Diagnostic test for neurocardiogenic syncope is:
A. Holter
B. EPS
C. HUTT
D. Echo

58. Optimal diastolic BP according to JNC 6:
A. <80 mm Hg
B. <85 mm Hg
C. <90 mm Hg
D. <95 mm Hg

59. ACE inhibitors are contraindicated in pregnancy because:
A. Causes fetal abnormality
B. Cannot control BP
C. Abruptio is caused
D. Skin rashes is common

60. Stress testing false negative in which territory:
A. LMC
B. LAD
C. LCx
D. RCA

61. ASD closure true is:
A. Ideal time 3-6 yrs
B. PVRI 10
C. Shunt 1.2:1
D. Systemic saturation <85%

62. True about split S1:
A. Tricuspid component is the first sound
B. MS can cause reverse S1
C. Normal split = 40 msec
D. Found in LBBB

63. ECG characteristics of DMD; True is:
A. LVH in 100%
B. Tall R wave in right sides leads
C. Ventricular arrhythmia rare
D. Atrial (Rt) hypertrophy is common

64. Drug of choice for prevention of AF recurrence in normal heart:
A. Amiodarone
B. Propanolol
C. Sotalol
D. Class Ic

51 A 52 B 53 B 54 A 55 B 56 C 57 C 58 A 59 A 60 C 61 A 62 B 63 B 64 D

65. Valsalva manoeuvre true is:
A. Left sided murmur reverts first
B. HOCM murmur increased
C. Left sided murmur increased
D. All of the above

66. Sydenham's chorea true is:
A. Occurs in 15%
B. Secondary prophylaxis required even if no RHD
C. Carditis present
D. Short incubation period between infection and occurrence of chorea

67. PET:
A. Mismatch shows ischemia
B. Increase glucose uptake shows scar
C. Not gold standard for assessing viability
D. Matching shows ischemia

68. True in acute cor pulmonale:
A. 1st hour mortality 25%
B. Acute RV failure will occur with sudden doubling of pulmonary arterial pressure (> 50 mm Hg)
C. Caused by IPF
D. All of the above

69. For cardiac transplantation, true about VO2 max is:
A. < 10 ml/kg/min
B. 10-14 ml/kg/min
C. 14-1 8ml/kg/min
D. > 18 ml/kg/min

70. Material used on Burr of Rotational athe-rectomy:
A. Diamond
B. Nickel
C. Titanium
D. Gold

71. False about cervical venous hum is:
A. Seen in left internal jugular vein
B. Common in children
C. Continuous murmur
D. Elicited by turning head to left side

72. Pulmonary artery pressure is measured by which catheter:
A. Swan ganz
B. NIH
C. Lehman
D. Cournard

73. ASO titre increases in acute rheumatic fever in what percentage of patients?
A. 80%
B. 75%
C. 90%
D. 95%

74. Threshold for starting antihypertensive in 2nd trimester of pregnancy (DBP):
A. 90 mm Hg
B. 95 mm Hg
C. 100 mm Hg
D. 85 mm Hg

75. Classification of hypertension is from:
A. JNC-7
B. NYHA
C. CCS-2
D. IHJ-8

76. True about CPK-MB is:
A. Useful for diagnosis in less than 2 hours
B. Peak occurs at 20 hours
C. Skeletal CPK-MB shows non-plateau form
D. Single value is enough

77. Number of phases in His Purkinje fibres is:
A. 1 B. 2
C. 3 D. 5

65 B 66 B 67 A 68 B 69 B 70 A 71 A 72 A 73 A 74 C 75 A 76 B 77 D

78. True about HIV myocarditis is:
A. Clinically overt involvement in > 10%
B. Direct invasion of HIV may be responsible
C. DCMP may be seen
D. All of the above

79. Keith Wagner's Class I retinopathy, A-V ratio is:
A. 3:4 B. 1:2
C. 1:3 D. 1:4

80. True about Lenegre's disease is:
A. Primary sclerodegenerative disease of myocardial conduction system
B. Involves mitral and aortic valve
C. Septum is involved
D. None of the above

81. A 65 year old male with lone AF and without any risk factor. Treatment is:
A. Aspirin
B. Warfarin
C. Aspirin + warfarin
D. No treatment

82. True about D-dimer assessment in pulmonary embolism is:
A. > 500 ng/ml in more than 90% patients
B. Low negative predictive value
C. Levels are not raised in pulmonary infarction
D. Quantitative assessment need not be done first

83. True about bioprosthetic valve is:
A. Mechanical degeneration is low
B. Valve of choice in < 35 years of age
C. Replacement required in 30% by 10 years
D. Anticoagulation is required

84. ATPase in actin-myosin complex is located in:
A. Neck
B. Head
C. Rod
D. None of the above

85. In constrictive pericarditis, pericardial thickness is best estimated by:
A. TTE
B. TEE
C. CT scan
D. USG

86. Cut off point for surgery in thoracic aorta aneurysm is:
A. 4.5 cm
B. 5.0 cm
C. 5.5 cm
D. 6.0 cm

87. Pressure difference between pulmonary artery and left atrium is:
A. 2 cm H_2O
B. 5 cm H_2O
C. 10 cm H_2O
D. 20 cm H_2O

88. Pacemaker in bifascicular block is indicated in:
A. First degree AV block without symptoms
B. Pacing induced infrahisian block
C. H-V between 40-60 msec
D. Fascicular block with increase PR without symptoms

89. For preventing anaphylaxis before coronary angiogram, following is given:
A. i/v hydrocortisone 6 hrly + i/v avil 6 hr before the procedure
B. Oral prednisolone 6 hrly + oral avil 6 hrly + oral H_2 blocker 6 hour before the procedure
C. i/v hydrocortisone 100 mg 1 hour before + avil P.O one hour before the procedure
D. i/v hydrocortisone 500 mg 1 hour before + avil P.O one hour before the procedure

90. True about Sestamibi is:
A. Langer protocol
B. Longer imaging
C. Better image quality
D. Thallium has replaced it

78 D 79 B 80 A 81 A 82 A 83 C 84 B 85 C 86 D 87 B 88 B 89 B 90 C

91. True about 2-D echocardiography is:
A. Blue colour indicate away from probe
B. Red colour indicates towards the probe
C. Blood and pericardial fluid is seen as black
D. 8-12 MHz probes

92. Restenosis rate after intracoronary stent is:
A. 0%
B. 20%
C. 44%
D. 33%

93. All are causes of clubbing *except:*
A. Mesothelioma
B. Biliary cirrhosis
C. Cystic fibrosis
D. Non-Hodgkin's lymphoma

94. Salmonella infection is frequent in all *except:*
A. Aortic aneurysm infection in elderly
B. Infectious osteomyelitis
C. Asplenia
D. Dairy workers diarrhoea

95. Treatment of Long QT syndrome include all *except:*
A. Oral potassium supplementation
B. Nadolol
C. Sotalol
D. Nicorandil

96. All are true about polycytemia vera *except:*
A. Thrombocytosis
B. Increase erythropoietin
C. Budd Chiari syndrome
D. Pruritis

97. Most common site of brain hemorrhage is:
A. Thalamus
B. Putamen
C. Cerebellum
D. Pons

98. All are causes of vasovagal syncope *except:*
A. Beta blocker
B. Visceral pain
C. Prolonged standing
D. Fasting

99. Asymptomatic large pericardial effusion is seen in:
A. Rheumatic fever
B. Myxedema
C. Sarcoidosis
D. Hypoalbumenemia

100. All are adhesion molecules *except:*
A. Integrins
B. Matrix metalloprotein
C. VCAM
D. Selectin

91 C 92 B 93 D 94 C 95 C 96 B 97 B 98 A 99 B 100 B

BHU 2002 (February)

1. Which of the following is not seen in infants with CHF?
- **A.** Peripheral edema
- **B.** Cardiomegaly
- **C.** S3 gallop
- **D.** Tachypnea

2. LVOT gradient is measured by:
- **A.** CW Doppler
- **B.** PW Doppler
- **C.** TEE
- **D.** TTE

3. Thrombolytic therapy is contraindicated in all *except:*
- **A.** Hemorrhagic stroke > 6 month
- **B.** 3rd term pregnancy
- **C.** Aortic dissection
- **D.** Intracranial neoplasm

4. AV block in PSVT rules out:
- **A.** AVNRT
- **B.** WPW
- **C.** AF
- **D.** Atrial tachycardia

5. Spuriously increased BP is seen in all *except:*
- **A.** Small cuff size
- **B.** Obesity
- **C.** Calcified arteries
- **D.** Ausculatory gap

6. SVR in isotonic exercise:
- **A.** Decrease
- **B.** Increase
- **C.** No effect l
- **D.** Variable

7. Commonest CVS diseases in India
- **A.** HT
- **B.** TB pericarditis
- **C.** CVA
- **D.** Rh fever

8. MDM at apex is seen in all *except:*
- **A.** VSD
- **B.** ASD
- **C.** AR
- **D.** 1st episode of Rheumatic Fever

9. ASLO tittres ↑ in all *except:*
- **A.** Late onset carditis
- **B.** Pericarditis
- **C.** Subcutaneous nodules
- **D.** Arthritis

10. All are true about adenosine *except:*
- **A.** Bradycardia can be contraindication
- **B.** Not cause VF in WPW with VT
- **C.** Can be used in neonates/infants
- **D.** Used in D/D of wide QRS tachy

1 A 2 A 3 B 4 B 5 D 6 A 7 A 8 B 9 A 10 B

11. CHF is best characterised by all *except:*
A. ↓A-V O_2 difference
B. ↓CO
C. Oliguria
D. ↑EDP

12. In CHF, decrease mortality is seen with all *except:*
A. ACE I
B. Diuretics
C. β blockers
D. CCB

13. Absolute C/I for pregnancy:
A. Eisenmenger's syndrome
B. Coarctation of aorta
C. MVP
D. MR

14. Used to decrease dp/dt in dissection:
A. Propanolol
B. NTG
C. Diuretics
D. Digoxin

15. Nitroprusside is used in all *except:*
A. Ecclampsia
B. Acute hypertensive emergencies
C. Acute ICH
D. Dissection of aorta

16. CABG is definitely better in:
A. TVD with Left ventricular dysfunction
B. DVD with ischaemia on exercise
C. DVD with VPCS
D. TVD with (n) LV function

17. VPC'S in normal heart is treated by:
A. β blocker
B. CCB
C. ACE (I)
D. No treatment

18. Grade III antiarrhythmic acts on which channel:
A. K B. Na
C. Ca D. Cl

19. Familial homozygous hypercholesterolemia best responds with:
A. Statins
B. Fibrates
C. Liver Transplantation
D. Bile acid sequestration

20. RFA is used in all *except:*
A. AF
B. A flutter
C. WPW
D. RBBB

21. Hypertensive retinopathy despite long standing hypertension is seen in all *except:*
A. Pheochromocytoma
B. Coarctation of aorta
C. Bilateral renal artery stenosis
D. Essential hypertension

22. Pulmonary edema with (n) PCWP in:
A. MS
B. LVF
C. Cor triatratum
D. HAPE

23. Left axis deviation occurs in all *except:*
A. P. Atresia with intact IVS
B. Normal people
C. Rubella with peripheral pulmonary stenosis
D. Ostium primum ASD

24. ECGs in myocarditis may show all *except:*
A. LBBB
B. ↑QRS complexes voltage
C. VT
D. VF

11 A 12 D 13 A 14 A 15 A 16 A 17 D 18 A 19 C 20 D 21 B 22 D 23 A
24 B

25. Cardiotoxic effect of hyperkalemia increase by:
A. Hypernatremia
B. Hypercalcemia
C. Hypocalcemia
D. Alkalosis

26. Commonest benign tumor in children:
A. Myxoma
B. Rhabdomyoma
C. Teratoma
D. Pericardial tumor

27. Commonest cause of syncope:
A. Postural
B. Neurocardiogenic
C. Arrhythmia
D. Situational syncope

28. Confidence interval is:
A. True range of estimate in population
B. Ability to correctly identify the persons having disease
C. Standardization of estimates
D. None of the above

29. Murmur in HOCM increases by all *except:*
A. Valsalva 2nd stage
B. Leg raising
C. Inotropes
D. Digoxin

30. Surest indicator of triple vessel disease/left main on TMT:
A. ≥ 3 mm ↓ST
B. Hyoertensive response
C. VPCS
D. Fatigue

31. Definite indicator of LV Dysfunction on thallium scanning is:
A. ↑ Lung uptake
B. 2 or > region of hypo perfusion
C. Fixed defects
D. None of the above

32. Which is not true about CAD?
A. TG>500 is not associated with CAD
B. Familial apo A-1 deficiency is associated with CAD
C. Hypobetalipoproteinemia is not associated with CAD
D. Smoking cessation reduces risks of CAD

33. Continuous murmur is not seen in:
A. Peripheral P.A stenosis
B. AV Fistula
C. Unruptured sinus of Valsalva aneurysm
D. Lutembacher

34. Wide fixed S_2:
A. TAPVC
B. PAPVC
C. PDA
D. TOF

35. Bisferians best felt in:
A. Carotid
B. Brachial
C. Radial
D. Popliteal

36. ACE inhibitors in pregnancy can cause all *except:*
A. Fetal malformation
B. Polyhydramnios
C. Oliguria
D. Still birth

37. CAD occurs in all *except:*
A. Progeria
B. Hypobetalipoproteinemia
C. Hypothyroidism
D. Hyperhomocystenemia

38. CAG is not indicated in:
A. Post MI VSD
B. Post MI LV dysfunction with thrombus
C. Hotter ST depression
D. IWMI with post MI unstable angina

25 C 26 B 27 B 28 A 29 B 30 B 31 A 32 A 33 C 34 A 35 A 36 B 37 B
38 B

39. LV function overestimated by:
A. MR
B. MS
C. AR
D. TR

40. ↓ in LVEF post surgery is seen in:
A. Post MV repair
B. Post MV replacement
C. Post AV replacement for AS with MR
D. Post AV replacement for severe AS with LV dysfunction

41. Surgery not indicated in IE in:
A. Persistent fever
B. Late PVE
C. Ao root abscess
D. Recurrent embolism

42. Cong CHB in:
A. CTGA
B. TGA
C. VSD with Eisenmenger
D. Single ventricle

43. Fontan done in all *except:*
A. Tricuspid atresia
B. TOF
C. Pulmonary atresia with intact ventricular septum
D. Ebstein's anomaly

44. Eisenmenger's VSD; treatment of choice is:
A. Heart transplantation
B. Heart lung transplantation
C. Diuretics
D. PA banding

45. Eisenmenger's VSD; correct is:
A. Single second heart sound
B. Widely split S2 with increase P2
C. Narrow split S2 with increase P2
D. Paradoxically split S2 with increase P2

46. In Cyanotic spell, following is not seen *except:*
A. Absent murmur
B. Normal SO_2
C. Hypotension
D. Wide split S_2

47. SO_2 in pulmonary artery wedge position is:
A. 98%
B. 75%
C. 40%
D. 90%

48. Peak incidence of MI time:
A. 12-6 AM
B. 6-12 noon
C. 12-6 PM
D. 6-12 midnight

49. PO_2 92 mm Hg, pH 7.55; Diagnosis is:
A. Anxiety neurosis
B. DKA
C. Phenobarbiturate poisoning
D. Pulmonary oedema

50. Amiodarone therapy monitored by all *except:*
A. ECG
B. Serum level
C. TFT (thyroid)
D. LFT

51. L → R shunt is ASD is increased by:
A. PAH
B. RV dysfunction
C. Anemia
D. MR

52. SVT vs. VT differentiation include all *except:*
A. Hypotension
B. AV dissociation
C. Fusion and capture beat
D. Absent R in V5

39 A 40 C 41 B 42 A 43 B 44 B 45 A 46 A 47 A 48 B 49 A 50 B 51 D 52 A

53. Which of the following is not an antioxidant?
A. Probucol
B. Carvedilol
C. Pravastatin
D. Ethinyl estradiol

54. HV interval is increased by:
A. Digoxin
B. Amiodarone
C. Xylocaine
D. Mexiletine

55. Post MI VSD is most commonly seen on:
A. 6 hrs-48 hrs
B. 2-4 days
C. 4-7 days
D. 7-28 days

56. Post MI MR; mechanism are all *except:*
A. Papillary muscle dysfunction
B. Choral rupture
C. MV perforation
D. LV dilatation

57. Multiple (Swisscheese) VSD; treatment of choice in infants is:
A. PA banding
B. Patch closure
C. Surgical
D. Heart transplantation

58. Reversed pulses paradoxus is seen in:
A. Discrete subaortic stenosis
B. HCM
C. Supravalvular aortic stenosis
D. Valvular AS

59. Best drug for differentiating wide QRS tachycardia is:
A. Flecainide
B. Amiodarone
C. Adenosine
D. Sotalol

60. Unsynchronised DC shock is given in:
A. VT
B. AF
C. Atrial fibrillation
D. VF

61. True about unstable angina is:
A. ↑6 months mortality if trop T +ve
B. Thrombolysis in Trop T +ve
C. Myocardial revascularization indicated in all cases
D. ↓CRP

62. Systemic vascular resistance is increased by:
A. Propranolol
B. α blocker
C. Indapamide
D. Amlodipine

63. Hypertension with BPH; Drug of choice is:
A. Prazosin
B. β blocker
C. Amlodipine
D. Diuretic

64. Infant with MI at 8 weeks can be due to:
A. ALCAPA
B. ARCAPA
C. Coronary dissection
D. HLHS

65. True about atherosclerosis is all *except:*
A. Exercise increases HDL
B. 1% decrease in LDL decreases mortality by 2-3%
C. Pulses and cereals contain very little cholesterol
D. Fish liver oil decreases atherosclerosis

53 C 54 B 55 C 56 C 57 A 58 B 59 C 60 D 61 A 62 A 63 A 64 A
65 B

66. Decreased left femoral pulse is seen in all *except:*
A. Aortic dissection
B. Femoral Thromboembolism
C. Atherosclerotic peripheral vascular disease
D. Burger's disease

67. Stress testing in asthmatics is done with:
A. Adenosine
B. Dipyridamole
C. Dobutamine
D. Digoxin

68. All are true about HUTT *except:*
A. Isoprenaline is also used
B. Indicates diastolic dysfunction
C. Used for evaluation of syncope
D. Beta blocker is drug of choice

69. Loud S1 is seen in:
A. LBBB
B. WPW
C. Digoxin
D. CHF

70. Heart rate 60/min, regular atrial fibrillation means:
A. Digoxin toxicity
B. Normal sinus rhythm
C. 1st degree heart block
D. WPW syndrome

71. Treatment of heterozygous familial hyper-cholesterolemia is:
A. Atorvastatin
B. Fibric acids
C. Niacin
D. Probucol

72. LV/RV apex obliteration is seen in:
A. EMF
B. HCM
C. DM
D. Sarcoidosis

73. Hyperhomocysteinemia is seen with:
A. Vitamin B-6 deficiency
B. FA and B-12 excess
C. Deficiency of tetrahydrofolate reductase
D. Vitamin A deficiency

74. Clubbing may be seen with all *except:*
A. Within weeks of IE
B. 2 yrs with methemoglobenemia
C. Within years of central cyanosis
D. None of the above

75. All of the following are seen in pheochromo-cytoma *except:*
A. Pallor
B. Perspiration
C. Pigmentation
D. Palpitation

76. QT interval is increased in all *except:*
A. Ramano ward
B. Amiodarone
C. Hyperkalemia
D. Sotalol

77. All are true about obesity *except:*
A. ↑QT
B. ↓HDL
C. ↑LDL
D. ↑Fasting insulin

78. Predominant substrate of normal myocardium is:
A. FFA
B. Glucose
C. Amino acids
D. Acetones

79. Cardiac tamponade is most common with which of the following?
A. Bronchial carcinoma
B. Hypothyroidism
C. Rheumatic fever
D. Tuberculosis

66 D 67 C 68 B 69 B 70 A 71 A 72 A 73 C 74 B 75 C 76 C 77 C 78 A
79 A

80. All are true about diabetes mellitus *except:*
A. Increased platelet aggregability
B. Increased PAI-1
C. Decreases vwf despite vascular disease
D. None of the above

81. Drug of choice for aspirin allergy is:
A. Dipyridamole
B. Ticlopidine
C. Sulfinpyrazone
D. Clopidogrel

82. Hypertriglyceridemia is seen with all *except:*
A. Alcohol
B. Beta blockers
C. Diuretics
D. Cyclosporine

83. Morbidity and mortality in acute rheumatic carditis is due to:
A. Valvulitis
B. Myocarditis
C. Aschoff nodules
D. Arrhythmia

84. Commonest cyanotic congenital heart disease at birth is:
A. TOF
B. TAPVC
C. d-TGA
D. TA

85. Which of with following requires correction even if asymptomatic:
A. Pink TOF
B. Coarctation gradient > 10 mm Hg
C. Moderate PS
D. Moderate AS

86. Suprasystemic RV systolic pressure is seen in:
A. PS with Intact ventricular septum
B. VSD
C. PDA
D. Infundibular stenosis

87. Erectile dysfunction is caused by all *except:*
A. Lehriche's syndrome
B. Nitroglycerin
C. Beta blocker
D. Spironolactone

88. Desirable BP in diabetics is likely to be:
A. 140/90 mm Hg
B. 135/85 mm Hg
C. 150/90 mm Hg
D. 160/90 mm Hg

89. Carotid endarterectomy is required in all *except:*
A. Symptomatic hemispherical ischemia
B. High grade stenosis
C. Concurrent CABG
D. Risk of stroke > 10 % (operated)

90 Jones criteria are not required in all *except:*
A. Recurrent rheumatic fever
B. Carditis
C. Chorea
D. First attack of rheumatic fever

91. Moderate MS (MVA=1.3 cm^2), mild symptoms, pregnancy 7 months; treatment of choice is:
A. BMV
B. MVR
C. Medical follow up
D. MTP

92. Chronic fatigue syndrome; least commonly seen is:
A. Sleep disturbance
B. Headache
C. Chest pain
D. Fatigue

93. Commonest rheumatic valve lesion, alone or combined is/are:
A. MS with AR
B. AS with MS
C. MS
D. MS with MR

---

80 C 81 D 82 D 83 A 84 C 85 A 86 A 87 B 88 B 89 D 90 D 91 C 92 A
93 D

94. Correction required even if PBF is not greater than SBF in which of the following:

A. PDA
B. VSD
C. ASD with MR
D. ASD

95. Restenosis is decreased by which of the following:

A. Azithromycin
B. Clarithromycin
C. Rapamycin
D. Clopidogrel

96. Which of the following has maximum anti-staphylococcal activity:

A. Teicoplanin
B. Imipenem
C. Ceftazidime
D. Piperacillin

97. CPK is increased in all of the following *except:*

A. Cerebral infarcts
B. Limb amputation
C. Hypothyroidism
D. Duchennne's muscular dystrophy

98. Pulmonary artery hypertension is caused by:

A. Schistosomiasis
B. Paragonimiasis
C. Filariasis
D. Taenia

99. Peripheral pulmonary artery stenosis is seen in all *except:*

A. Noonan
B. Rubella
C. Alagille
D. Williams

100. Pulsus paradoxus is seen in all *except:*

A. IPPV
B. RVMI
C. Pulmonary embolism
D. COPD

94 A 95 C 96 A 97 B 98 A 99 A 100 A

BHU 2001

1. **Treatment of choice in recurrent neurocardiogenic syncope is:**
   A. Atrial pacing
   B. AV sequential pacing
   C. β blockers
   D. VVI

2. **Asplenia–polysplenia is commonly associated with:**
   A. Situs ambiguus
   B. Pulmonary AV fistula
   C. Mirror image dextrocardia
   D. Situs inversus

3. **Bounding pulse in one day old infant is:**
   A. PDA
   B. Hypoxia
   C. Systemic AV fistula
   D. Pulm AV fistula

4. **In 1st week of life which cannot be detected:**
   A. Large VSD
   B. PS
   C. AS
   D. TOF

5. **Commonest congenital anomaly presenting with cyanosis in first month:**
   A. d-TGA
   B. TOF
   C. HLH
   D. Aortic arch interruption

6. **CHF in one month old infant is due to all *except:***
   A. TAPVC (infradiaphragmatic)
   B. Truncus arteriosus
   C. Severe PS
   D. AV septal defect

7. **ACE inhibitor were used in all *except:***
   A. BHAT
   B. AIRE
   C. CONSENSUS
   D. SOLVD

8. **Congenital CHB is associated with:**
   A. c-TGA
   B. d-TGA
   C. TOF
   D. Tricuspid atresia

9. **In CONSENSUS trial, Enalapril was useful in patients with:**
   A. Severe CHF
   B. Mild CHF
   C. Asymptomatic LV enlargement
   D. CHF with high rennin levels

10. **Hypertension with prostatic enlargement: drug of choice is:**
    A. Prazosin
    B. β blocker
    C. ACE inhibitor
    D. Calcium channel blocker

1 C 2 A 3 C 4 A 5 A 6 C 7 A 8 A 9 A 10 A

11. Which of the drugs have renoprotective effect?
A. β blocker
B. Ca channel blockers
C. Diuretics
D. ACE inhibitor

12. Hypertension with IDDM; drug of choice is:
A. Captopril
B. Amlodipine
C. Atenolol
D. Chlorthiazole

13. Hypertension treatment does not reduce incidence of:
A. CAD
B. Stroke
C. CRF
D. CHF

14. Hallmark of essential hypertension is:
A. ↑ SVR
B. ↑ Cardiac output
C. ↑ Renin
D. ↑ Pulmonary vascular resistance

15. Saline infusion is helpful in:
A. Primary hyperaldosteronism
B. Pheochromocytoma
C. Cushing
D. Renovascular HT

16. Secondary hypertension is not seen in:
A. Hyponatraemia
B. Hypercalcemia
C. Cushing syndrome
D. Lead poisoning

17. Which does not cause high output failure:
A. Pregnancy
B. Paget's disease
C. Beriberi
D. Thyrotoxicosis

18. MI in 8 weeks old infant cause is:
A. ALCAPA
B. Coronary AV fistula
C. Single coronary artery
D. LCx from right coronary sinus

19. Lipid research trial drug used:
A. Cholestyramine
B. Probucol
C. Atorvastatin
D. Colestipol

20. Which does not cause Torsades de pointes?
A. Digoxin
B. Quinidine
C. Procainamide
D. Disopyramide

21. Least proarrhythmic drug amongst following is:
A. Amiodarone
B. Quinidine
C. Mexiletine
D. Procainamide

22. Wide QRS tachycardia: treatment of choice is:
A. Mexiletine
B. Propranolol
C. Procainamide
D. Adenosine

23. Amiodarone has following effect *except:*
A. ↑PR interval
B. Sinus tachycardia
C. ↑QRS
D. ↑QT interval

24. Mechanism of atrial flutter is:
A. Automaticity
B. Re-entry
C. Triggered activity
D. Parasystole

25. PSVT: drug of choice:
A. Adenosine
B. β blocker
C. Digoxin
D. Amiodarone

11 D 12 A 13 A 14 A 15 A 16 A 17 A 18 A 19 A 20 A 21 C 22 C 23 B
24 B 25 A

26. PDA can be closed by all *except:*
A. Stent
B. Coil
C. Umbrella device
D. Buttoned device

27. Mixed venous blood sampling in Fick's principle is taken from:
A. Pulmonary artery
B. SVC
C. RV
D. RA

28. Which has the least O_2 saturation?
A. Coronary sinus
B. PA
C. IVC
D. SVC

29. Which of the following is the site of insertion of the transvenous ventricular pacemaker electrodes?
A. Apical trabeculated Zone
B. Inlet of RV just below the tricuspid annulus
C. In smooth walled muscular subpulmonary canal
D. In the septal band

30. Primary PTCA is done:
A. After failed thrombolysis
B. Within 6 hours without thrombolysis
C. After successful thrombolysis
D. Combined with thrombolysis

31. Highest reperfusion rates in acute MI:
A. Primary PTCA
B. Primary rtPA
C. Streptokinase
D. Urokinase

32. In 1st 12 hours, prognosis of MI is best assessed by:
A. Serial ECG
B. Thallium
C. CPK
D. Angina

33. Reversible ischaemia in thallium is indicated by:
A. Myocardial redistribution
B. Fixed defect
C. Reverse redistribution
D. Radiotracer lung uptake

34. Pharmacological stress testing in asthmatics: which drug is used:
A. Adenosine
B. Dipyridamole
C. Dobutamine
D. None of the above

35. Which territory in thallium is least specific?
A. LCx
B. RCA
C. LAD
D. None of the above

36. Digoxin was discovered by:
A. William Withering
B. William Harvey
C. W S Thayer
D. Duke

37. BP measurement: newer concept was given by:
A. William Harvey
B. Stephen Hales
C. William Withering
D. Riva Rocci

38. ECG machine was invented by:
A. Waller
B. Einthoven
C. Levine
D. Harvey

39. Blood vessels are controlled by all *except:*
A. Sympathetic vasoconstrictive fibers
B. Sympathetic vasodilator fibers
C. Parasympathetic vasodilator fibers
D. Parasympathetic vasoconstrictive fibers

26 A **27** A **28** A **29** A **30** B **31** A **32** B **33** A **34** C **35** A **36** A **37** D **38** B **39** D

40. Wide split S2 is not seen in:
A. Truncus arteriosus
B. TAPVC
C. ASD
D. Ebstein anomaly

41. Systolic thrill in ASD in 2nd intercostal space is suggestive of:
A. PAH
B. TR
C. MS
D. AS

42. EDM is found in:
A. Fixed subaortic stenosis
B. PS
C. Acquired infundibular pulmonary stenosis
D. Valvular AS

43. Continuous murmur is found in:
A. Peripheral pulmonary artery stenosis
B. Pulmonary stenosis
C. PDA with severe PAH
D. Unruptured aneurysmal sinus of valsalva

44. Which is not teratogenic?
A. Hydralazine
B. Enalapril
C. Warfarin
D. Phenytoin

45. A patient of AF with CHB, pacemaker of choice is:
A. VVI-R
B. DDD
C. AAI
D. AAIR

46. A case of coarctation of aorta with difference in BP of upper and lower limb is seen in all *except:*
A. VSD
B. AS
C. AR
D. PDA

47. 6 weeks pregnancy with severe AS treatment of choice:
A. Balloon valvotomy
B. Medical termination of pregnancy
C. AVR
D. Medical MX

48. Unmarried female with severe MR and EF 50%: best treatment is:
A. Repair of mitral valve
B. MV replacement
C. Medical MX
D. None of the above

49. A patient with anticoagulant contraindication: valve of choice is:
A. Bioprosthesis
B. Mechanical prosthesis
C. Both of the above
D. None of the above

50. MIAMI trial used:
A. Metoprolol
B. Atenolol
C. Morphine
D. Mexiletine

51. NTG worsens pain in:
A. HOCM
B. DCMP
C. Unstable angina
D. MI

52. Following BMV, acute MR: with haemodynamic compromise treatment of choice:
A. Valve replacement
B. Diuretics
C. Digoxin
D. Vasodilator

40 A 41 C 42 A 43 A 44 A 45 A 46 D 47 B 48 A 49 A 50 A 51 A 52 A

53. On echocardiography, paradoxical septal motion is seen in:
A. RV volume overload
B. LV volume overload
C. RV pressure overload
D. VSD

54. Advantage of TEE over TTE in detecting:
A. LAA thrombus
B. LV apical thrombus
C. ASD
D. Post MI VSD

55. Which cardiac tumor is common in infancy and childhood?
A. Rhabdomyoma
B. Myxoma
C. Fibroma
D. Fibrosarcoma

56. Obtuse marginal is a branch of:
A. LCx
B. RCA
C. LAD
D. PDA

57. Eisenmenger's VSD: treatment is:
A. Heart lung transplant
B. Heart transplant
C. Lung transplant
D. Medical management

58. Pulsus paradoxus is not seen in:
A. IPPV
B. Pulmonary embolism
C. Bronchial asthma
D. Cardiac tamponade

59. Raised JVP is seen in all *except:*
A. Pyopericardium
B. Low pressure tamponade
C. CHF
D. CCP

60. Blalock Taussig shunt is:
A. MPA with subclavian
B. RPA to subclavian
C. LPA to subclavian artery
D. RPA to aorta

61. Rib notching is not seen in:
A. Pulmonary collaterals
B. Aortoarteritis
C. Coarctation of aorta
D. Blalock Taussig shunt

62. Treatment of choice for TOF at 1 year of age:
A. Total correction
B. BT shunt
C. Medical management
D. Pott's shunt

63. IABP is contraindicated in:
A. Acute AR
B. Cardiogenic shock
C. Severe ischemia
D. Severe MR

64. Amount of cyanosis in TOF correlates with:
A. Infundibular PS
B. Size of VSD
C. Aortic override
D. ASD

65. Continuous murmur is seen in all *except:*
A. Coronary AV fistula
B. ASD with left to right shunt
C. ASD with MS
D. VSD with pulmonary atresia

66. Ostium secundum ASD with MR commonest cause:
A. MVP
B. Rheumatic
C. Cleft mitral valve
D. Infective endocarditis

53 A 54 A 55 A 56 A 57 A 58 A 59 B 60 B 61 B 62 A 63 A 64 A 65 B 66 A

67. Ostium primum ASD shows:
A. Left axis deviation
B. Right axis deviation
C. North west axis
D. None of the above

68. Transcatheter closure of ASD is suitable in:
A. Small secundum ASD
B. Ostium primum
C. Sinus venous ASD
D. Large ASD

69. Mortality in Post MI patients is not decreased by:
A. Nifedipine
B. Aspirin
C. β blockers
D. ACE inhibitor

70. Antioxidant are all *except:*
A. α tocopherol
B. Carotenoid
C. Flavonoids
D. Homocysteine

71. Acute MI: following are true *except:*
A. Young smoker have recanalised vessels commonly
B. Distal IVS is more commonly ruptured following MI than proximal IVS
C. Less than 5% have normal coronaries
D. PTCA is useful only in cardiogenic shock

72. Contraindication to PTCA are all *except:*
A. Left main stenosis
B. TVD with LV dysfunction
C. SVD
D. DVD including proximal LAD

73. Which in stress test is indicative of severe disease?
A. Hypotension
B. Hypertension
C. Frequent VPCs
D. ST elevation in leads having q wave after MI

74. WPW syndrome: commonest pathway is:
A. Right posteroseptal
B. Left posteroseptal
C. Right anteroseptal pathway
D. LV free wall

75. Primordial prevention is:
A. No risk factors, no disease
B. Prevention in first degree relatives
C. Treatment of existing disorder
D. None of the above

76. Commonest cardiovascular disease in India:
A. Hypertension
B. CAD
C. DCMP
D. RHD

77. Rheumatic fever: most uncommon manifestation is:
A. Subcutaneous nodules
B. Erythema marginatum
C. Arthritis
D. Carditis

78. In cyanotic spell: which is not given:
A. Morphine
B. Diuretics
C. Phenylephrine
D. GA

79. CABG success depends most on which of the following?
A. Age
B. No. of grafted arteries
C. Angina
D. LV function

67 A 68 A 69 A 70 D 71 D 72 C 73 A 74 D 75 A 76 A 77 A 78 B 79 D

80. **CHF in infant: which is not present?**
A. Sweating
B. Failure to thrive
C. Pedal edema
D. Cardiomegaly

81. **RVSP is equal to LVSP:**
A. PS with intact LV septum
B. TOF
C. ASD
D. Restrictive VSD

82. **Least energy in DC cardioversion is used in:**
A. Atrial flutter
B. AF
C. PSVT
D. VT

83. **Which is both $\alpha + \beta$ blocker:**
A. Labetalol
B. Metoprolol
C. Bucindolol
D. Sotalol

84. **Severity of AR is assessed by all *except:***
A. Fluttering of AML
B. Width of Doppler jet
C. Pressure half time
D. Hill's sign

85. **Dobutamine vs dopamine: true is:**
A. Less vasoconstriction
B. More vasoconstrictive
C. Increase in heart rate
D. Decrease in heart rate

86. **Flecainide was found to be proarrhythmic in:**
A. CAST trial
B. GUSTO III
C. LIFE
D. None of the above

87. **Diastolic gradient between LA and PCWP is seen in:**
A. Cortriatriatum
B. AR
C. MR
D. AS with AR

88. **Technetium imaging in acute myocardial infarction shows:**
A. Red spot
B. Cold spots
C. Hot spots
D. Green spots

89. **Rate of restenosis following PTCA alone at 6 months is:**
A. 10%
B. 30%
C. 50%
D. 70%

90. **Maximum teratogenicity during pregnancy occurs at what period of gestation?**
A. 7 days
B. 7 to 18 days
C. 18 to 50 days
D. 50 days

91. **Ischemic heart disease with HT: drug of choice is:**
A. CCB
B. β blocker
C. ACE inhibitors
D. Direct vasodilator

92. **Drug to be avoided in pheochromocytoma:**
A. Prazosin
B. Phenoxybenzamine
C. Propanolol
D. Labetalol

93. **Pompe's disease all true *except:***
A. Markedly increase QRS voltage
B. Large tongue
C. Autosomal dominant
D. Hypertrophic subaortic stenosis

80 C **81** B **82** D **83** A **84** A **85** A **86** A **87** A **88** C **89** B **90** C **91** B **92** C
93 C

94. All the following are seen commonly with congestive cardiomyopathy *except:*
A. Abnormal Q waves in over 10%
B. Diastolic gallop
C. Poor X descent
D. Loud systolic murmurs

95. External carotid artery arises from which aortic arch?
A. Second arch
B. Third arch
C. Fourth arch
D. Sixth arch

96. Roth spots are seen in:
A. Bacterial endocarditis
B. Anemia
C. Scurvy
D. All of the above

97. AR can be caused by all *except:*
A. Ankylosing spondylitis
B. Richter's syndrome
C. Seropositive rheumatoid arthritis
D. Kawasaki's disease

98. Diagnosis of MS is hemodynamically best assessed by:
A. Mean gradient across mitral valve
B. Reduce LV filling pressure
C. Gradient across mitral valve in end diastole
D. Severity of pulmonary artery hypertension

99. Holt-Oram syndrome is associated with:
A. ASD
B. VSD
C. PDA
D. PS

100. Clonidine: all are true *except:*
A. Decreased sympathetic activity
B. Dryness of the mouth
C. Withdrawal syndrome
D. No sedative effect

94 D 95 B 96 D 97 D 98 C 99 A 100 D

PGI 2004

1. Breast cancer oncogene related to all *except:*
A. Myc
B. BRCA1
C. BRCA 2
D. COT

2. Warfarin levels are decreased by:
A. Sulfonamide
B. Erythromycin
C. Tetracycline
D. Rifampicin

3. In Cardiac tamponade:
A. Prominent x, absence of y descent
B. Absent x, promiment y descent
C. Square root sign present
D. a = v

4. Contraindicated in pregnancy:
A. Methyl dopa
B. Hydrallazine
C. Nifidepine
D. Ramipril

5. True about digoxin are all *except:*
A. Oral administration–rapid absorption
B. Lipid soluble
C. Metabolised by liver
D. Excreted by kidney

6. 27 year old female, BP 160/100 (lt) hemiperosis; (lt) renal bruit (rt) radial absent. Most probable diagnosis is:
A. FMD
B. Takayasu arteritis
C. Atherosclerosis
D. Atheroembolism

7. 60 year female with jaw claudication and prominent temporal arteries; Most probable diagnosis is:
A. PAN
B. Giant cell arteritis
C. Takayasu arteritis
D. Trigeminal neuralgia

8. 70 year old male, BP 90/60, chest pain for 1 hour, right femoral and left radial are absent. Most probable diagnosis is:
A. Acute MI
B. Aortic dissection
C. Acute pericarditis
D. RSOV – RV

9. All are true about transfusion associated graft versus host disease *except:*
A. Fever
B. Rosh
C. Pancytopenia
D. Extremely good response to steroids

1 A 2 D 3 A 4 D 5 C 6 B 7 B 8 B 9 C

11. AR can be caused by all *except:*
A. Ankylosing spondylitis
B. Reiter's syndrome
C. Seropositive rheumatoid arthritis
D. Kawasaki's disease

12. Muscular weakness with hypertension occurs in:
A. Congenital adrenal hyperplasia
B. Primary hyper aldosteronism
C. Pheochromocytoma
D. Renal parenchymal disease

13. Not an arteriolar vasodilator:
A. Captopril
B. Isosorbide dinitrate
C. Hydralazine
D. Phenoxybenzamine

14. Commonest side effect of ACE I:
A. Cough
B. Agranulocytosis
C. Hyperkalemia
D. Renal failure

15. Antihypertensive in pregnancy:
A. α methyl dopa
B. ACE-I
C. CCB
D. β blocker

16. HDL is decreased by:
A. Lovastatin
B. Gemfibrozil
C. Probucol
D. Niacin

17. HDL is increased by:
A. CCB
B. Prazosin
C. β blocker
D. ACEI

18. EDRF is provided by:
A. CGMP
B. CAMP
C. ATP
D. NOS

19. Absolute contraindication of BMV:
A. AF
B. Calcification
C. Restenotic valve
D. LAA clot

20. IABP is contraindicated in:
A. Acute AR
B. Ac MR
C. VSD
D. PDA

21. Rate of reperfusion is highest with:
A. Primary angioplasty
B. STK
C. STK + Aspirin
D. TPA

22. Trombolysis is contraindicated in:
A. USA
B. Ac MI
C. Pul embolism
D. PV thrombosis

23. RVSP > LVSP is seen in:
A. Eisenmenger VSD
B. Eisenmenger PDA
C. TOF with infundibular stenosis
D. Valvular PS with intact septum

24. The difference of 10 mmHg between systolic pressure of LV and RV after post ectopic beat occurs in patients with pulmonary stenosis in:
A. RV dysfunction
B. Large VSD
C. No VSD
D. Small VSD

---

11 D 12 B 13 B 14 A 15 A 16 C 17 B 18 D 19 D 20 A 21 A 22 A 23 D 24 D

25. Isotonic exercise causes:
A. Increases in heart rate
B. ↑SBP
C. ↑CO
D. ↓SVR

26. Delayed tricuspid closure occurs in:
A. TR
B. TS
C. PAH
D. RA myxoma

27. Signs and symptoms not commonly seen in LA myxoma:
A. Clubbing
B. Fever
C. Anemia
D. Thromboembolism

28. IE is least commonly seen in:
A. ASD
B. VSD
C. TOF
D. MVP with MR

29. Wide mid diastolic murmur at mitral area are seen in all *except:*
A. ASD B. VSD
C. AR D. MR

30. All of the following can be heard in unstable angina *except:*
A. Loud S1
B. Decrease splitting of S2
C. S4
D. Pansystolic murmur of MR

31. Least common manifestation of acute rheumatic fever:
A. Chorea
B. Erythema marginatum
C. Arthritis
D. Sub cutaneous nodules

32. All are symptoms of CHF in infants *except:*
A. Pedal edema
B. Hepatomegaly
C. Tachycardia
D. Sweating

33. RA tracing in TS shows:
A. Slow y decent
B. Prominent x wave
C. Rapid y decent
D. Decrease a wave

34. LA tracing in MS with AF shows:
A. Absent a waves
B. Rapid Y decent
C. Rapid X decent
D. Prominent a waves

35. TEE is better than TTE in all *except:*
A. MVP
B. LA Myxoma
C. Prosthetic valve evaluation
D. PS

36. Rate of restenosis after PTCA is significantly reduced by:
A. Coronary stent
B. Warfarin
C. Dipyridamole + aspirin
D. Direct rotational atherectomy

37. Romano Ward syndrome has:
A. Long QT interval
B. Short QT interval
C. Long PR interval
D. Short PR interval

38. Which of the following is not manifestation of digitaly toxicity:
A. AF with FVR
B. Ventricular bigeminy/trigeminy
C. PAT
D. Increase PR interval

25 D 26 B 27 A 28 A 29 A 30 A 31 D 32 A 33 A 34 A 35 D 36 A 37 A 38 A

39. LAD is seen in:
A. Ostium primum ASD
B. ASD with MVP
C. Ostium secundum ASD
D. Sinus venosus ASD

40. Paradoxical IVS motion is seen in all *except:*
A. RV overload with ASD
B. LV overload
C. CCP
D. RV overload

41. Treatment of choice in ventricular fibrillation:
A. DC cardioversion
B. IV bretylium
C. IV xylocard
D. IV amiodarone

42. Corneal opacity is the manifestation of:
A. Amiodarone
B. Carvedilol
C. Digoxin
D. Sotalol

43. CABG prolongs survival in:
A. TVD with normal LV function
B. TVD with depressed LV function
C. DVD with angina
D. SVD with normal LV function

44. Outcome of CABG depends on:
A. Angina
B. LV function
C. Age of the patient
D. Number of vessel grafted

45. Which of the following drugs doesn't reduce the mortality in AMI:
A. β blocker B. CCB
C. ASA D. STK

46. Which of the following reduces mortality in CHF?
A. ACEI
B. Calcium channel blockers
C. Digitalis
D. Anticoagulants

47. Treatment of choice in first six hours of AMI:
A. STK
B. ASA + STK
C. ASA + Heparin
D. IV heparin

48. Which of the following congenital heart disease is most incompatible with life in the first week:
A. Tricuspid atresia
B. TGA
C. TAPVC
D. PDA

49. Which of the following condition is not associated with Hypertension?
A. Renal artery stenosis
B. Carcinoid syndrome
C. Conn's syndrome
D. Hypercalcemia

50. Congenital heart disease least likely to be diagnosed clinically during first week of life:
A. Large VSD
B. TOF
C. Tricuspid atresia
D. Ebstein anomaly

51. Drug contraindicated in AF with WPW is:
A. Digoxin
B. Procainamide
C. Atenolol
D. Dilzem

52. Drug of choice for patients with exercise induced VT:
A. Propanolol
B. Amiodarone
C. Procainamide
D. Flecainide

39 A 40 B 41 A 42 A 43 B 44 B 45 B 46 A 47 B 48 B 49 B 50 A 51 A 52 A

53. **Severity of the MR can be assessed by all *except:***
A. Loudness of the murmur
B. MDM in the mitral area
C. Presence of S3
D. Wide splitting of S2

54. **Most common cardiac tumor in infant is:**
A. Rabdomyoma
B. Teratoma
C. Myxoma
D. None of the above

55. **Cyanosis in first week of life can be due to all *except:***
A. Methemoglobinemia
B. Ebstein anomaly
C. Persistant fetal circulation
D. Pulmonary AV fistula

56. **Nitrate can aggravate which of the following condition:**
A. HOCM
B. Prinzmetal angina
C. Unstable angina
D. None of the above

57. **All of the following are features of IE *except:***
A. Oslers nodes
B. Clubbing
C. Splinter hemorrhage
D. Subcutaneous nodule

58. **Which of the following is not contraindicated in TOF?**
A. Phenylephrine
B. Digoxin
C. Diuretic
D. Inotropes

59. **CHF can be associated with all *except:***
A. Oliguria
B. Increased LV filling pressure
C. Reduction in cardiac output
D. Decreased AV O_2 differences

60. **Reverse splitting in S2 can occur in all *except:***
A. DCMP B. PDA
C. HTN D. AS

61. **Multifocal atria tachycardia can be associated with:**
A. COPD
B. Hyperthyroidism
C. HTN
D. Hyperparathyroidism

62. **Drug of choice to terminate SVT:**
A. Adenosine
B. Flecainide
C. Procainamide
D. Amiodarone

63. **Ventricularization of LA tracing occurs in:**
A. Acute MR
B. VSD
C. Gerbode defect
D. Cortriatriatum

64. **High altitude pulmonary edema is associated with:**
A. ↓ PaO_2
B. ↑ PaO_2
C. Normal PaO_2
D. ↑ pH

65. **Murmur of HOCM is exaggerated with all of the following *except:***
A. Post ectopic beat
B. Standing
C. Passive leg flexing
D. Phase II of Valsalva manoeuvre

66. **Best physiological response with repair of MR is seen in:**
A. MV repair
B. MV homograft
C. Star Edward prosthesis
D. St. Jude prosthesis

53 A 54 A 55 C 56 A 57 D 58 A 59 D 60 A 61 A 62 A 63 A 64 A 65 C
66 A

67. Treatment of choice in a patient of myocardial infarction having cardiac index of 2.2 lt/min/m^2 and PCWP of 10 mmHg:
A. IV fluids
B. IABP
C. Dobutamine
D. Dopamine

68. Inverted U wave in exercise test is:
A. Non specific finding
B. Specific for LAD disease
C. Specific for RCA disease
D. Sensitive to ischemia

69. Antihypertensive of choice in a patient with old MI is:
A. Beta blocker
B. Calcium channel blocker
C. Alpha blocker
D. Diuretics

70. Antihypertensive of choice in elderly patient with benign prosthetic hypertrophy is:
A. Prazosin
B. Ramipril
C. Carvedilol
D. Diuretics

71. Protective HDL is:
A. HDL-1
B. HDL-2
C. HDL-3
D. HDL-4

72. Systemic thromboembolism can be seen with all *except:*
A. SwanGanz catheterization
B. CAG
C. BMV
D. Infective endocarditis

73. Antianginal which alters myocardial metabolism is:
A. Trimetazidine
B. Nifedipine
C. Beta blockers
D. NTG

74. Treatment of choice in unstable angina are all *except:*
A. NTG
B. Beta blockers
C. Calcium channel blockers
D. Aspirin

75. Which of the following is responsible for increase incidence of CAD in Indians?
A. Lipoprotein-a
B. HDL-3
C. Apo-β
D. IDL

76. In Fick's method, blood sample for oxygen saturation is collected from:
A. Pulmonary artery
B. RA
C. RV
D. SVC

77. Tricuspid flow murmur in ASD is seen with Qp: Qs of:
A. > 1.5:1
B. > 2:1
C. < 1.2:1
D. Qp = Qs

78. Cannon 'a' waves are seen in:
A. Junctional tachycardia
B. TS
C. CHB with pacemaker (VVI)
D. PAH

79. Sodabicarb is not used in routine CPR due to:
A. Respiratory alkalosis
B. Hyperkalemia
C. Hypercalcemia
D. Respiratory acidosis

67 A 68 B 69 A 70 A 71 B 72 A 73 A 74 C 75 A 76 A 77 B 78 C 79 D

80. Parasternal heave due to RV is less commonly seen with:
A. Eisenmenger VSD
B. Eisenmenger ASD
C. Severe MS
D. Primary pulmonary hypertension

81. Regression of atherosclerosis can occur with all *except:*
A. Life style modifications
B. Lovastatin
C. Calcium channel blocker
D. Ilial Bypass

82. A2-pericardial knock interval is:
A. 90-120 msec
B. 70-90 msec
C. 120-150 msec
D. 150-180 msec

83. A case of MS with TS in AF will have all of the following findings *except:*
A. Absent a wave
B. Blunted y descent
C. Increase a wave
D. None of the above

84. Treatment of choice for multiple VSD's with CHF is:
A. PA banding
B. VSD repair
C. Diuretics
D. Vasodilators

85. Treatment of choice in Eisenmengers complex is:
A. Heart lung transplantation
B. Heart transplantation
C. Vasodilators
D. Inotropes

86. Unilateral rib notching occurs in TOF with:
A. Aortopulmonary collaterals
B. Potts shunt
C. Blalock Tausig's shunt
D. Waterston's shunt

87. One year old infant with coarctation of aorta will have all of the following *except:*
A. Radio femoral delay
B. Rib notching
C. Figure of 3 sign on X-ray
D. Audible murmur

88. Continuous murmur is heard in all *except:*
A. PDA
B. TOF with pulmonary atresia
C. VSD with AR
D. AP window

89. All of the following features are associated with precapillary pulmonary hypertension *except:*
A. Increased PAP
B. Increased PVR
C. Increased PCWP
D. "a" wave in JVP increased

90. Neurocardiogenic syncope should be evaluated by:
A. Head up tilt test
B. EPS
C. ECG
D. SAECG

91. Prophylactic anticoagulation is not required in:
A. LA myxoma
B. Atrial fibrillation
C. Recurrent pulmonary Thromboembolism
D. None of the above

92. CHB is most commonly associated with:
A. c-TGA
B. Left isomerism
C. Tausig Bing anomaly
D. Ebstein's anomaly

80 A 81 C 82 A 83 B 84 A 85 A 86 C 87 B 88 C 89 C 90 A 91 A 92 A

93. Most common cardiac anomaly due to maternal rubella is:
A. ASD
B. VSD
C. TOF
D. PDA

94. Holt-Oram syndrome is associated with:
A. ASD
B. VSD
C. PDA
D. PS

95. Diagnosis of MS is best established by:
A. TTE
B. TEE
C. Catheterization
D. Chest X-ray

96. Drug of choice in a patient with aortic dissection and hypertension is:
A. Propranolol
B. Prazosin
C. Calcium channel blocker
D. ACE-inhibitors

97. Absolute contraindication to PTCA is:
A. Unprotected LMCA disease
B. Severe TVD
C. DVD with LV dysfunction
D. Proximal LAD disease with LV dysfunction

98. All of the following are antoxidants *except:*
A. Beta carotene
B. Vitamin C
C. α-tocopheral
D. Vitamin B_{12}

99. Diagnosis of MS is hemodynamically best assessed by:
A. Mean gradient across mitral valve
B. Reduce LV filling pressure
C. Gradient across mitral valve in end diastole
D. Severity of pulmonary artery hypertension

100. BP in lower limb is significantly more than in upper limb in:
A. Takayasu arteritis
B. CoA with AR
C. Femoral A-V fistula
D. Bilateral RAS

93 D 94 A 95 A 96 A 97 A 98 D 99 A 100 A

PGI 2004

1. Breast cancer oncogene related to all *except:*
- **A.** Myc
- **B.** BRCA1
- **C.** BRCA 2
- **D.** COT

2. Warfarin levels are decreased by:
- **A.** Sulfonamide
- **B.** Erythromycin
- **C.** Tetracycline
- **D.** Rifampicin

3. In Cardiac tamponade:
- **A.** Prominent x, absence of y descent
- **B.** Absent x, prominent y descent
- **C.** Square root sign present
- **D.** a = v

4. Contraindicated in pregnancy:
- **A.** Methyl dopa
- **B.** Hydrallazine
- **C.** Nifidepine
- **D.** Ramipril

5. True about digoxin are all *except:*
- **A.** Oral administration–rapid absorption
- **B.** Lipid soluble
- **C.** Metabolised by liver
- **D.** Excreted by kidney

6. 27 year old female, BP 160/100 (lt) hemiperosis; (lt) renal bruit (rt) radial absent. Most probable diagnosis is:
- **A.** FMD
- **B.** Takayasu arteritis
- **C.** Atherosclerosis
- **D.** Atheroembolism

7. 60 year female with jaw claudication and prominent temporal arteries; Most probable diagnosis is:
- **A.** PAN
- **B.** Giant cell arteritis
- **C.** Takayasu arteritis
- **D.** Trigeminal neuralgia

8. 70 year old male, BP 90/60, chest pain for 1 hour, right femoral and left radial are absent. Most probable diagnosis is:
- **A.** Acute MI
- **B.** Aortic dissection
- **C.** Acute pericarditis
- **D.** RSOV – RV

9. All are true about transfusion associated graft versus host disease *except:*
- **A.** Fever
- **B.** Rosh
- **C.** Pancytopenia
- **D.** Extremely good response to steroids

1 A   2 D   3 A   4 D   5 C   6 B   7 B   8 B   9 C

10. Most specific antibody for SLE:
A. Anti Sm
B. Anti dsDNA
C. Anti RO
D. Anti La

11. King's college criteria for liver transplantation in acute liver failure is:
A. ↑ed PT, ↑bilirubin, duration b/w jaundice and encephalopathy
B. CT volume of liver, S. albumin and PT, encephalitis
C. Encephalopathy grade
D. None of the above

12. Hepatitis C virus causes malignancy by all *except:*
A. Integration of viral RNA into cell RNA/DNA
B. Chronic parenchymal liver disease with abnormal regeneration
C. Extrachromosomal effects of HCV
D. Loss of microsatellite genome stability

13. Visceral leishmaniasis: treatment of choice is:
A. Amodiaquine
B. Albendazole
C. Amantadine
D. Allopurinol

14. Tick bite transmitted by:
A. Rickettsial rickettsiae
B. Spirilium minus
C. Leptospira icterohemorrhegica
D. Leishmania donovani

15. Foscarnet used in:
A. CMV retinitis
B. Lymphoma
C. AIDS pt with kaposi's sarcoma
D. SLE

16. Myocobacterium avium intracellularae: treatment is:
A. Clarithromycin
B. Cotrimoxazole
C. Ciplox
D. Chloramphenicol

17. Pregnancy: Antitubercular drug that can be given safely in 1st trimester:
A. Streptomycin
B. INH
C. Thiacetazone
D. Ethambutol

18. Warfarin induced skin necrosis is caused in patient with:
A. Protein C deficiency
B. Protein S deficiency
C. F 5 Leiden
D. Antithrombin

19. 7 year old girl with cerebral malaria on quinine on 2nd day become restless, sweating and altered sensorium most likely cause:
A. Hypoglycemia
B. Hypotension
C. Hypokalemia
D. Hypomagnesemia

20. High anion gap is seen with all *except:*
A. Ethylene glycol
B. Renal tubular acidosis
C. Carbon monoxide poisoning
D. ARF

21. Methanol poisoning: clinical symptoms produced by methanol itself and not by metabolite:
A. Vertigo
B. Convulsions
C. Coma
D. Retinal injury

22. Villonodular synovitis fluid is:
A. Hemorrhagic
B. Turbid
C. Clear
D. Amber

10 A 11 A 12 A 13 A 14 A 15 A 16 A 17 B 18 A 19 A 20 B 21 A 22 A

23. Acute gout can be treated by all *except:*
A. Aspirin
B. Colchicine
C. NSAID–Indomethacin
D. Brufen

24. 20 year old foot ball player has back pain worst in morning improves after exercise; probable diagnosis is:
A. Stress #
B. Ankylospondyloarthropathy
C. Disck prolapse
D. Caries spine

25. Treatment of septic shock proven to ↓ mortality are all *except:*
A. Anti TNFa
B. Activated protein C
C. Steroid in physiological replacement
D. Antibiotic

26. Hypermobile joint, hyperleastic skin is seen with:
A. ED syndrome
B. Pseudoxanthoma elasticin
C. Amyloidosis
D. Marfan's syndrome

27. Patient present to emergency 1 week back with unconsciousness and oral burns now–dyspnea, pulmonary rales, mild cyanosis: diagnosis is:
A. Paraquat poisoning
B. Corrosive alkali poisoning
C. OP poisoning
D. Endo sulfan poisoning

28. Sub acute sensory motor symmetric neuropathy:
A. Lead
B. Arsenic
C. Cisplantin
D. HSMN

29. All are seen in iron deficiency anemia *except:*
A. S. Ferritin <15 mg
B. TIBC > 380
C. Saturation >20%
D. Sideroblast >10%

30. Vit D resistant rickets: true is:
A. Deficiency in l-hydroxyl of 25-OH Vit D
B. Autosomal dominant
C. Late dentition
D. ↓ alkaline phosphates

31. Not found in bacterial overgrowth malabsorption syndrome:
A. Shilling Phase II
B. 24 hour fecal fat
C. D-xylose test
D. Lactose breath test

32. Neuron specific enolase increase in:
A. Neuroblastoma
B. Retinoblastoma
C. Glucagonoma
D. Pheochromocytoma

33. Cocaine causes all *except:*
A. Hypothermia
B. Seizures
C. Cardiac arrhythmia
D. Tachypnea

34. Poor prognosis in community acquired pneumonia is shown by all *except:*
A. Fever >102°F
B. Tachypnea >20/min
C. DBP <60
D. BUN >20

35. Worst prognosis in AS:
A. Angina
B. Syncope
C. CHF
D. Asymptomatic

23 A 24 B 25 C 26 A 27 A 28 D 29 C 30 C 31 C 32 A 33 A 34 B 35 C

36. Hepatic blood flow constitute what percentage of cardiac output ?
A. 50%
B. 30%
C. 20%
D. 10%

37. Hanta virus reservoir:
A. Mouse
B. Cat
C. Dog
D. Pig

38. Hyper prolactinemia causes:
A. Gynecomastia
B. Impotence
C. Hypertrichosis
D. Pigmentation

39. Sumatriptan useful in:
A. Migraine
B. Variant angina
C. Peripheral vascular disease
D. SAH

40. Beat to beat variation in BP is seen in all *except:*
A. Polymorphic VT
B. Atrial fibrillation
C. AIVR
D. CHB

41. Juvenile MS is seen:
A. Less than 12 years
B. Calcification common
C. Severe PAH often seen
D. Cause usually congenital
E. Atrial fibrillation is common

42. Five year child with Atrial fibrillation, ventricular rate of 300/min treatment of choice is:
A. I/V propanolol
B. DC shock
C. Amiodarone
D. Adenosine
E. Verapamil

43. Systemic A-V fistula; true are:
A. Bradycardia on compression
B. May cause cyanosis clubbing
C. May cause endarteritis (infective)
D. May cause CHF
E. May cause wide pulse pressure

44. dp/dt is ↑ed by:
A. Calcium infusion
B. Dopamine
C. CMP
D. Thalassemia major
E. Viral myocarditis

45. Over estimation of AS on echo:
A. Anemia
B. Pregnancy
C. PDA
D. ASD
E. Hypothyroidism

46. Brainbridge reflex:
A. Tachycardia with volume infusion
B. Bradycardia with CSM
C. Tachycardia with fright
D. Vasodilation with fright
E. Bradycardia with exercise in AS

47. Preload ↓ by
A. NTG
B. Bleeding
C. Morphine
D. Dopamine
E. RCMP

48. Evidence of heart disease in pregnancy:
A. S3
B. Pedal edema
C. MDM
D. Systolic (m) gr 2
E. PND

36 B	37 A	38 B	39 A	40 C	41 A,B,C	42 A,B,C
43 A,C,D,E	44 A,B	45 A,B,C	46 A	47 A,B,C	48 C	

49. **Pregnancy with MS; drug contraindicated is:**
A. Heparin
B. Digoxin
C. Diuretic
D. Prostaglandin
E. Ergot alkaloid

50. **1 met is equal to what oxygen consumption:**
A. 2.5 ml O_2/kg/min
B. 3.5 ml O_2/kg/min
C. 4.5 ml O_2/kg/min
D. 5.5 ml O_2/kg/min
E. 6.5 ml O_2/kg/min

51. **Therapeutic termination of pregnancy is done in:**
A. TOF
B. PPH
C. Eisenmenger
D. Peripartum CMP
E. CHF

52. **Activity involving >3 mets:**
A. Walking 5 km/hour on level ground
B. Cycling 8 km/hour on level ground
C. Sawing wood
D. Pneumatic tool
E. Climbing mountain

53. **Kearns Sayre syndrome:**
A. Tall stature
B. Epilepsy
C. Hypogonadism
D. AV block
E. Prog. Ext. opthalmoplegia

54. **Central cyanosis is seen with all *except:***
A. Pulmonary edema
B. Severe PS with (n) IAS
C. Peripheral embolism
D. Pulmonary AV Fistula
E. Eisenmenger syndrome

55. **Continuous murmur over chest:**
A. AS with AR
B. PDA with eisenmenger
C. Large PDA
D. RSOV → RV
E. BT shunt

56. **RCM seen in:**
A. Amyloid
B. Fabry's
C. MPS II
D. Hemochromatosis
E. Viral myocarditis

57. **Paradoxical splitting of S_2 may be seen in:**
A. Severe MS
B. RBBB
C. LBBB
D. Ac MR
E. HOCM

58. **HOCM:**
A. Myocardial stiffness increased
B. Chamber stiffness decreased
C. LV mass decreased
D. LV stress decreased
E. LVESV decreased

59. **Diagnosis is confirmed on endomyocardial biopsy in which of the following:**
A. Allograft rejection
B. Doxorubicin
C. Amyloidosis
D. AIDS
E. Carnitine deficienc

60. **Right heart border on chest X-ray is formed by:**
A. Asc. aorta
B. IVC
C. SVC
D. RV
E. RA

49 D,E 50 B 51 B,C 52 A,C 53 B,C,D,E 54 B,C 55 C,D,E 56 A,B,C,D
57 C,E 58 A,D,E 59 A,B,C,D 60 B,C,E

61. Patient presented in emergency with BP 60/40, PCWP 25, RA mean (15), PA: 40/20 (25), LVEDP 25 and Cardiac output of 1.2 Lt/min/m^2. Patient is likely to have:
- **A.** Pulmonary embolism
- **B.** Cardiogenic shock
- **C.** Cardiac tamponade
- **D.** Extensive MI
- **E.** ARDS

62. Torsades de pointes; true is:
- **A.** Rate 200-250
- **B.** May have (n) QT
- **C.** Pacing is helpful
- **D.** Mg may be helpful
- **E.** Isoprenaline is useful

63. In Nitroprusside toxicity earliest feature:
- **A.** $\downarrow SpO_2$
- **B.** $\downarrow$PA saturation
- **C.** Mild cyanosis
- **D.** $\uparrow$ed methemoglobin
- **E.** Metablic acidosis

64. Finding that must be present to differentiate non cardiogenic from cardiogenic pulmonary edema:
- **A.** MI on ECG (old or new)
- **B.** Cardiac enzymes
- **C.** JVP raised
- **D.** Large intrapulmonary shunt
- **E.** PCWP <18

65. GpIIb/IIIa inhibitors are:
- **A.** Abciximab
- **B.** Tirofiban
- **C.** Lamifiban
- **D.** Carvedilol
- **E.** Torcetrapib

66. Increased atherosclerosis is seen in:
- **A.** Cushing
- **B.** Diabetes mellitus
- **C.** Acromegaly
- **D.** Myxoedema
- **E.** Tangier's disease

67. Cyanosis:
- **A.** Sulfonamide
- **B.** Aniline dye
- **C.** α tocopherol
- **D.** Cytochrome reductase deficiency
- **E.** Lidocaine toxicity

68. Dissection of aorta may present with all *except:*
- **A.** MI
- **B.** Absent pulses
- **C.** AR
- **D.** MR
- **E.** Pericardial effusion

69. Peripheral PS is seen with all *except:*
- **A.** CoA
- **B.** Sub aortic membrane
- **C.** Williams
- **D.** Rubella
- **E.** Takayasu

70. Prominent 'a' waves in JVP is seen with all *except:*
- **A.** MS
- **B.** TS
- **C.** RA myxoma
- **D.** PAH
- **E.** ASD

71. Large Q waves in ECG are seen with all *except:*
- **A.** DMD
- **B.** Chronic severe AR
- **C.** Posterior wall MI
- **D.** COPD
- **E.** Infiltrative disease

61 B,D 62 A,C,D,E, 63 E 64 E 65 A,B,C 66 A,B,C,D 67 A,B,C
68 D 69 A,B 70 A,E 71 A,C

72. Favouring constrictive physiology over restrictive physiology is:
- **A.** Equalization of diastolic ventricular pressures
- **B.** Right sided failure
- **C.** Atrial fibrillation
- **D.** Mild pericardial effusion
- **E.** Pulmonary artery pressure > 50 mm Hg

73. TOF like physiology include all *except:*
- **A.** TGA with LVOT obstruction
- **B.** SV with PS
- **C.** DORV with PS
- **D.** DORV with subpulmonary VSD
- **E.** Tricuspid atresia

74. Normal pressure TR is seen with all *except:*
- **A.** IE
- **B.** CCP
- **C.** DCM
- **D.** Recurrent pulmonary embolism
- **E.** HOCM

75. Severe MS is:
- **A.** 1 cm^2
- **B.** 0.7 cm^2
- **C.** 1.25 cm^2
- **D.** 0.8 cm^2
- **E.** 0.6 cm

76. ASD is seen in all *except:*
- **A.** Turner
- **B.** TAR
- **C.** Downs syndrome
- **D.** Ellis van creveld syndrome
- **E.** Holt oram syndrome

77. Pericarditis is seen with all *except:*
- **A.** Bretylium
- **B.** Amiodarone
- **C.** Procainamide
- **D.** Methysergide
- **E.** Hydralazine

78. In NYHA class all can be seen *except:*
- **A.** Undue fatigue
- **B.** Dyspnea
- **C.** Palpitation
- **D.** Diaphoresis
- **E.** Angina

79. Prominent "y" descent seen in:
- **A.** CCP
- **B.** RCM
- **C.** Cor pulmonale
- **D.** Tamponade
- **E.** DCM

80. Normal bilateral blood pressure difference may be upto:
- **A.** 5
- **B.** 10
- **C.** 20
- **D.** 30

---

72 A,C,D 73 D,E 74 B,C,D,E 75 A,B,D,E 76 A 77 A,B 78 D
79 A,B 80 B

PGI 2003 (December)

1. Acute gouty arthritis: true are all *except:*

A. Aspirin
B. Colchicine
C. Allopurinol
D. Probenicid

2. A 25 year old diabetic female, dry hacking cough with high fever 10 days RBS-300 mg%, Hct 27mg%, BUN 9 mg% PC (n) 3.25 lac, Se iron 25, TIBC 240, Cold agglutination 1.284, RC 10%: diagnosis is:

A. SLE with hemolytic anemia
B. Drug induced hemolytic anemia
C. Infectious mononucleosis
D. Mycoplasma pneumonia

3. Thrombocytopenia with thrombosis is seen in:

A. Antiphospholipid antibody syndrome
B. ITP
C. Hypoplastic anemia
D. MDS

4. Pathological features common to all spondyloarthropathies include:

A. Enthesopathy
B. Oral ulcer
C. Bowel ulcer
D. Skin involvement

5. HLA B27 is associated with all *except:*

A. Psoriatic arthropathy
B. Reiter's
C. Ankylosing spondylitis
D. IDDM

6. Which of the following causes Pinta:

A. Treponema careteum
B. Treponema pertenue
C. Treponema pallidum
D. Fusobacterium

7. Hypokalemia may present as:

A. Twitching
B. Seizure
C. Bladder involvement
D. Quadriparesis

8. P wave is absent in:

A. Atrial fibrillation
B. A flutter
C. CHB
D. Atrial ectopics

9. True about β blockers is:

A. ↓ Cardiac output
B. ↓ Intravascular volume
C. ↑ Renin release from kidney (↓renin – 60%)
D. Blocks conversion of angiotensin I-II

10. Mitochondrial disease present as:

A. Myoclonus/Cerebellar involvement, blindness/deafness
B. Myoclonus, blindness, neuropathy
C. Autonomic neuropathy
D. Myopathy, dystonia

1 A 2 D 3 A 4 A 5 D 6 A 7 D 8 A 9 A 10 A

11. **Most common complication measles:**
A. Aseptic meningitis
B. Optic neuritis
C. Pneumonia
D. Post measles demyelination

12. **Atherosclerosis: causative organisms include all *except:***
A. CMV
B. Herpes
C. H pylori
D. Chlamydia

13. **Patient of shock; Cardiac index decreased, PCWP (N) and SVR↓: Probable diagnosis is:**
A. Cardiac tamponade
B. Septic shock
C. Cardiogenic shock
D. Hypovolemic shock

14. **Which of the following is not commonly seen in COPD?**
A. ↓DLCO
B. ↓MMEFR
C. ↓FEV_1
D. ↑Residual volume

15. **Bronchoalveolar lavage is diagnostic in:**
A. Alveolar proteinosis
B. Interstitial pulmonary fibrosis
C. Br. asthma
D. Pulmonary eosinophilia
E. PPH

16. **Recently diagnosed hyperthyroidism in a 7th month pregnant female is best treated by:**
A. Propylthiouracil
B. Stabilize with b blocker
C. Start and continue propylthiouracil until delivery
D. Induction of labour at 37 weeks

17. **Most common site of ischemic colitis is:**
A. Splenic flexure
B. Hepatic flexure
C. Caecum
D. Rectum

18. **Diabetic autonomic neuropathy is suggested by all *except:***
A. Resting bradycardia
B. Orthostatic hypotension
C. Constipation
D. Loss of sweating over one limb

19. **Cork screw oesophagus is seen in:**
A. Diffuse esophageal spasm
B. Achalasia cardia
C. Carcinoma esophagus
D. Esophagitis

20. **Malignancy is classically associated with:**
A. SLE
B. Scleroderma
C. Dermatomyositis
D. Polyarteritis

21. **Transfusion associated infections include all *except:***
A. Toxoplasmosis
B. CMV
C. Syphilis
D. Hepatitis B and C

22. **Unconjugated hyperbilirubinaemia is seen in all *except:***
A. Rotors syndrome
B. Megaloblastic anemia
C. Thalassaemia
D. Large hematoma

23. **Morphine withdrawal symptoms are seen in:**
A. 2-4 hrs
B. 8-12 hrs
C. 24-36 hrs
D. 48-72 hrs

11 C 12 B 13 B 14 A 15 A 16 A 17 A 18 A 19 A 20 C 21 A 22 A 23 B

24. β2 microglobulin is associated with:
A. Multiple myeloma
B. Chronic hemodialysis
C. Amyloidosis
D. Familial Mediterranean fever

25. Which of the following is not seen in polycythemia rubra vera?
A. Spontaneous infection
B. Hemorrhage/thrombosis
C. Progression to leukemia
D. Hyperuricaemia

26. CoA: common causes of death include all *except:*
A. Cerebral hemorrhage
B. MI
C. IE
D. Rupture of aorta

27. Acquired PS in VSD: true are all *except:*
A. Seen in 7-15%
B. 1st described by Gasul
C. Infundibular hypertrophy
D. PS is most commonly valvular

28. CDC definition of group I HIV patients is:
A. Acute HIV syndrome
B. Persistent lymphadenopathy
C. Asymptomatic infection
D. Full blown AIDS

29. Wernicke's encephalopathy: all may be seen *except:*
A. Intention tremor
B. Ataxia
C. Ophthalmoplegia
D. Mental confusion

30. Strict control of hypertension is least likely to be affected by which of the following on long term follow up?
A. Stroke
B. CHF
C. Renal failure
D. CAD

31. Octreotide:
A. Somatostatin analogue
B. Antihistamine
C. ACE I
D. MMP

32. Loss of sensation over leg, sole, side of foot, absent ankle jerk is suggestive of:
A. S1
B. L4
C. L5
D. Common peroneal involvement

33. Recent hepatitis B infection marker:
A. HBsAg
B. IgM antiHBc
C. IgM antiHBe
D. IgG AntiHBc

34. Differentiating features between CCP and RCMP:
A. Hepatic venous flow
B. Mitral inflow variation
C. RVEDP
D. Pericardial calcification
E. IVC diameter

35. Following can be used to ↑HDL:
A. Nicotinic acid
B. Clofibrate
C. Bezafibrate
D. Statins
E. Estrogen

36. ACE-inhibitors: true are all *except:*
A. Less effective in black
B. Prevents progression of DM retinopathy
C. DOC in B/L RAS
D. Improves insulin sensitivity
E. Intravenous treatment is effective in acute MI

24 B	25 A	26 B	27 D	28 A	29 A	30 D
31 A	32 A	33 B	34 A,B,C,D	35 A,B,C,E	36 B,C,E	

37. Non Q vs. Q wave MI: true are:
A. Reinfarction is more common with Non QMI
B. Infarcts smaller
C. May present with ST elevation
D. Low incidence of post MI angina
E. Thrombolytic therapy of significant benefit

38. Prinzmetal angina: drug of value:
A. Aspirin
B. α blocker (Prazosin)
C. β blocker
D. Diltiazem
E. Ramipril

39. WPW with atrial fibrillation: drug to be avoided:
A. Digoxin
B. Verapamil
C. Procainamide
D. Amiodarone
E. Cardioversion

40. α Blocking activity:
A. Bisoprolol
B. Doxazosin
C. Carvedilol
D. Labetalol
E. Metoprolol

41. Risk factor for SCD in HOCM includes:
A. Multiple VPCs
B. LBBB
C. Younger age at presentation
D. Recurrent syncope
E. Apical HOCM

42. Right aortic arch commonly seen in:
A. TGA
B. TOF
C. Truncus
D. VSD with pulmonary atresia
E. DORV

43. Marfan's syndrome: all are used for diagnosis:
A. Nitroprusside test
B. X-chromosome analysis
C. MVP
D. Dilated cistern magna
E. Inguinal hernia

44. Radiation induced cardiac injury may cause which of the following?
A. CCP
B. Coronary artery stenosis
C. DCMP
D. CHB
E. MVP

45. BAV acts as a bridge in:
A. Cardiogenic shock
B. Severe CHF
C. Peak systolic gradient >100 mm Hg
D. Associated CAD
E. Recurrent syncope

46. Balloon valvotomy has significantly good long term prognosis in all of the following *except:*
A. Rheumatic MS
B. Degenerative MS
C. Degenerative AS
D. Noonan's with PS
E. Dysplastic PS
F. Congenital PS

47. CHF within 1 week in a full term infant is seen in all *except:*
A. VSD
B. Hypocalcemia
C. PDA
D. Critical AS
E. Interrupted Aortic Arch

48. Wide split S2 is seen in all *except:*
A. Severe MR with normal LV function
B. Severe MR with LV dysfunction
C. Severe AR with normal LV function
D. Eisenmenger VSD
E. Moderate/severe PS

37 A,B,C	38 B,D	39 A,B	40 B,C,D	41 C,D	42 B,C,D	43 A,B,C
44 A,B,C,D	45 A,B	46 B,C,D,E	47 A,C	48 B,C,D		

49. TAPVC: true are all *except:*
A. Supracardiac type most common
B. Infracardiac rarely obstructive
C. Cardiac type ASD determines prognosis
D. Infracardiac type commonly opens into hepatic vein
E. Right atrial isomerism

50. MR hemodynamics: true are:
A. LV-EDV ↑ed
B. LV End syst volume ↓
C. LV End diastolic stress ↓
D. End systolic stress normal
E. LV mass increased

51. Following autosomal dominant disease may be associated with VSD:
A. Noonans
B. Treacher collins
C. Holtoram
D. Leopard
E. Myotonic dystrophy

52. Constrictive pericarditis: true are all *except:*
A. Kussmaul's sign is seen
B. Incidence of pulsus paradoxus same as tamponade
C. Intrathoracic pressure is transmitted to cardiac chambers
D. Prominent x and y descent
E. Dip and plateau in pressure tracing

53. Infective endocarditis: true are:
A. Coagulase –ve staph aureus cause early PVE
B. Streptococcus vididans causes late PVE
C. <5% culture –ve in IV drug abusers
D. >10% fungal endocarditis in IV drug abusers
E. Streptococcus fecalis is most common cause of IE in drug abusers

54. Lignocaine:
A. With verapamil causes hypotension
B. With nitrates (long acting) causes nitrate tolerance
C. Cimetidine decreases lignocaine
D. β blockers increases lignocaine
E. Halothane increases lignocaine

55. Atrial fibrillation: which of the following are true?
A. Reentry is most common mechanism
B. Ventricular response is dependent on AV conduction and not on autonomic tone
C. Pathologically, myocardial loss with fibrosis is seen
D. Hypertension is most commonly he cause
E. Digoxin is better than β blocker in controlling HR

56. Myocardial infarction following PTCA: true is:
A. 20% increase in CPKMB is cut off for screening
B. Elevation does not affect long term prognosis
C. 45% patients have more than 3 times ↑ CKMB normally with PTCA
D. 5% of patients may have q waves on ECG
E. Saphenous vein graft PTCA is rarely associated with ↑ CKMB

57. Peripartum CMP:
A. <30 yrs female
B. Multiparty is a risk factor
C. Maximum incidence in 2 months postpartum
D. 50% die or have severe CHF
E. Biopsy shows less myocarditis than patients of DCMP

58. Angiographic feature of dysplastic pulmonary valve on catheterization include:
A. Normal pulmonary annulus
B. Thickened fleshy leaflets
C. Little change in position between systole and diastole
D. Severe systolic doming
E. Post stenotic dilatation of MPA is less common

49 B,D	50 A,D,E	51 A,B,C	52 B	53 A,B,C	54 D,E	55 A , B , C
56 A,B,D	57 B,C,D,E	58 B,C,E				

59. Neurocardiogenic syncope: drugs used:

A. β blockers
B. SSRI
C. Dopamine agonists
D. Anticholinergic agents
E. Calcium channel blockers

60. Low cardiac output state hemodynamics: False statements are:

A. ↑RA pressure in RV failure
B. ↑PA pressure in hypovolemia
C. Decreased mixed venous oxygen saturation in acute pulmonary edema
D. ↑PCWP always in severe A2 pulmonary thromboembolism
E. Increase AV oxygen difference

61. Acute pulmonary embolism: true are:

A. S1Q3T3
B. Incomplete RBBB
C. 1°AV block
D. Dilated RA
E. RV ischemia

62. Coarctation syndrome in infant and neonates:

A. Hypoplastic arch and isthmus
B. LVH
C. Rib notching 4th-7th ribs
D. Left to right shunt through PDA
E. ↑RV pressures

63. CoA in a severely symptomatic infant: true are:

A. 2/3rd cases associated with PDA
B. 1/3rd cases associated with VSD
C. 25% mitral involvement (26 to 58%)
D. 15-20% has failure without associated anomaly
E. Taussig-Bing variety is not associated with CoA

64. Asplenia:

A. IVC absent
B. Right isomerism
C. ASD
D. Howel jolly bodies
E. AS

65. Arteries commonly arising from LCx include:

A. Atrial circumflex
B. Obtuse marginal
C. Septal
D. Diagonal
E. PDA

66. Procainamide: true are:

A. Prolongs APD more than ERP
B. Prolongs QT interval
C. Causes vasodilatation with hypotension
D. Used in quinidine resistant arrhythmias
E. Increases levels of digoxin

67. Congenital AS:

A. Male: Female 4:1
B. May be unicuspid/bicuspid/tricuspid
C. Peak systolic gradient >75 mmHg is suggestive of critical AS
D. Critical AS is 0.8 cm^2 with maintained cardiac output
E. Surgery is treatment of choice in infants

68. HUTT:

A. 90% specificity and gold standard
B. 10-20 min
C. 60-80° angle passive elevation 1st strep
D. Edrophonium and NTG are useful
E. Isoproterenol dose 10-20 mcg/min

69. Hypertension:

A. Newborn >80 mmHg systolic
B. 3rd - 4th week >100 mmHg systolic
C. 4th week-2 years 124/78
D. 3-12 yrs–130/80
E. 12-18 yrs–144/90 mm Hg

---

59 A,B,D   60 B,D   61 A,B,D,E   62 A,B,E   63 C   64 B,C,D   65 A,B
66 B,C,D   67 A,B,C   68 A,C,D   69 A,C,D

70. **Takayasu's arteritis: all are true *except:***
   A. Non inflammatory autoimmune disease
   B. Right subclavian (mid) is most commonly involved
   C. Syncope may occur due to common carotid involvement
   D. Aorto-iliac involvement >50% cases
   E. Histologically resembles ankylosing spondylitis aortitis

71. **Low osmolar contrast used in CAG:**
   A. Hypotension
   B. CHF
   C. Severe bradycardia and AV block
   D. Thrombus containing artery with planned stenting
   E. Acute MI

72. **A 29 year old male having renal failure and angina like chest pain, rash on hand, genitalia, buttock, mouth throughout life. Urinalysis shows casts absent and RBC present, refractile bodies. Test to clinch the diagnose is:**
   A. Direct coombs test
   B. Se electrophoresis
   C. HDL assay
   D. Alpha galacatosidase assay

73. **Tall 'R' wave in V1 is seen in:**
   A. WPW type A
   B. LAHB
   C. Posteroinferior myocardial infarction
   D. Hyperkalemia

74. **Patient presents with chest pain and ST elevation in V1-V6, ECG shows atrial fibrillation, BP-90/60 mm Hg, Pulse -110/min irregularly irregular, bilateral crepts develop 1 day later, Treatment is:**
   A. Digoxin
   B. Flecainide
   C. Amiodarone
   D. Quinidine

75. **Balloon pulmonary valvotomy: true are all *except:***
   A. It has replaced surgery
   B. Contraindicated if annulus is < 7 mm
   C. Indicated in gradient > 60 mm Hg (peak systolic)
   D. Asymptomatic infants with critical PS
   E. Highly effective in dysplastic valve

76. **Tricuspid atresia: true are:**
   A. Most commonly with normally related great arteries
   B. D-TGA in 45%
   C. L-TGA in < 10%
   D. Always associated with non restrictive VSD
   E. Is seen with PS/atresia with normally related great arteries

77. **All of the following are skin commensals *except:***
   A. Streptococcus
   B. Staphylococcus
   C. Micrococcus
   D. Corynebacterium

78. **Following drug is safe in renal failure:**
   A. INH
   B. Vancomycin
   C. Flucytosine
   D. Cotrimoxazole

79. **Casoni skin test is which type of hypersensitivity:**
   A. Type I
   B. Type II
   C. Type III
   D. Type IV

80. **Most important step in CPR is:**
   A. Defibrillation
   B. Mouth to mouth respiration
   C. Cardiac massage
   D. Intubation

70 B,D	71 A,B,C,E	72 D	73 A	74 A	75 B,E	76 A,E
77 C	78 A	79 A	80 A			

PGI 2003 (June)

1. Thrombotic thrombocytopenic purpura is caused by all *except:*
A. Ticlopidine
B. Cisplatin
C. Chlorambucil
D. Mitomycin C

2. Immune enhancing enteral diet:
A. Isoleucine
B. Valine
C. Glutamine
D. Methionine

3. Significant myocardial toxicity because of free radical formation occurs with:
A. Bleomycin
B. Cisplatin
C. Deoxycofromycin
D. Mitoxantrone

4. Chromium deficiency leads to:
A. Impaired glucose tolerance
B. Renal failure
C. Anemia
D. Cardiomyopathy

5. Decreased anion gap occurs with:
A. Bromide
B. Toluene
C. Ethyleneglycol
D. Salicylate

6. Patient with cyanosis, breathlessness due to aniline dye ingestion most important treatment is:
A. High flow O_2
B. IV methylene blue
C. Hemodialysis
D. Forced alkaline diuresis

7. 31 year old female with Ao 110/90 (mean 96), LV 110/25, RV 40/25(mean 26), RA a- 25; v-26, pulmonary artery mean pressure-30 mm Hg, PA wedge pressure- a-27, v-28, mean-25: all of the following conditions can be present *except:*
A. Tight MS
B. CCP
C. Endomyocardial fibrosis
D. Pulmonary embolism

8. Itraconazole is useful in all *except:*
A. Dermatophytosis
B. Mucormycosis
C. Aspergillosis
D. Candida

9. HTLVI causes:
A. Tropical spastic paraparesis
B. SSPE
C. Burkitts lymphoma
D. AIDS

1 C 2 C 3 D 4 A 5 A 6 B 7 A 8 B 9 A

10. Which of the following is a Prion disease?
A. SSPE
B. PM leucoencephalopathy
C. Familial fatal insomnia
D. HSP/TSP

11. Amyloid precursor protein in heart disease:
A. β2 microglobulin
B. Amyloid light chain
C. Amyloid associated protein
D. Myeloma protein

12. Pregnancy can affect ulcerative colitis in which of the following way?
A. Increase (Flare up) of disease
B. Increase extracolonic manifestation
C. Abortion
D. Fetal malformation

13. Gastric emptying increased by:
A. Propanolol
B. Imipramine
C. L-Dopa
D. Bethanechol

14. High fibre diet associated with:
A. $\uparrow$ed colonic carcinoma
B. $\uparrow$ed motility
C. Increased insulin requirement in DM
D. $\downarrow$ed residue in colon

15. Enteric organisms causing peripheral arthritis all *except:*
A. E coli
B. Y psuedotuberculosis
C. Campylobacter jejuni
D. T. Whippeli

16. Cerebellar ataxia, pigmentary retinopathy, loss of tendon jerks in presence of long standing steatorrhoea, diagnosis is:
A. Vitamin E deficiency
B. Cyanocobalamin deficiency
C. Riboflavin deficiency
D. Niacin

17. Photosensitivity occurs with all *except:*
A. Hypervitaminosis A
B. PKU
C. Niacin deficiency
D. Carcinoid

18. Endogenous inhibitor of angiogenesis:
A. Endostatin
B. Leptin
C. IL8
D. TNFα

19. JVP in pericardial tamponade; which is true:
A. Prominent 'y', absent 'x'
B. Absent 'x', absent 'y'
C. Prominent 'x' prominent 'y'
D. 'x' promintent 'y' absent

20. Growth hormone deficiency best diagnosed by:
A. Integrated GH estimation
B. Random GH assay
C. Insulin like growth factor 1 assay
D. Multiple assays of GH after L-Dopa

21. Restrictive lung disease: all are true *except:*
A. $\downarrow$TLC
B. $\downarrow$FEV1
C. $\downarrow$FVC
D. FEV1/FVC <80%

22. Most important step in CPR is:
A. Defibrillation
B. Mouth to mouth respiration
C. Cardiac massage
D. Intubation

23. Fasting hypoglycaemia occurs with:
A. Severe hepatitis
B. Post gastrectomy
C. Post gastrojejunostomy
D. Porphyria

10 C 11 B 12 A 13 D 14 B 15 A 16 A 17 A 18 A 19 D 20 D 21 D 22 A
23 A

24. **Malignant hyperthermia is:**
A. ↑temp after halothane/anesthetic agent
B. ↑ed temp after haloperidol in normal dose
C. In malignancy
D. Heat stroke (severe form)

25. **Pyruvate kinase deficiency causes:**
A. Intravascular hemolysis precipitated by oxidative stress
B. Chronic hemolysis
C. Pseudo cyanosis
D. Myelodysplasia in pregnancy

26. **Pneumonia risk increased with all *except:***
A. IgG deficiency
B. IgE deficiency
C. Cranial trauma
D. Alcohol intake

27. **Renal osteodystrophy, all are true *except:***
A. Decrease response to 25-OH cholecalciferol
B. Spontaneous fracture
C. Sub periosteal bone resoption
D. Osteosclerosis

28. **Polyarteritis nodosa: all are true *except:***
A. More in male
B. Lung involvement common
C. Renal artery aneurysm
D. PUO

29. **Sodium valproate causes:**
A. Ac pancreatitis
B. Granulocytopenia
C. Hepatotoxicity
D. Thrombocytopenia

30. **Biliary sludge occurs with:**
A. Ceftriaxone
B. Cefotaxime
C. Cefoperazone
D. Cefipime

31. **Investigation of choice in DIC in chronic liver disease is:**
A. ↑aPTT
B. ↑PT
C. ↓Factor 8
D. ↓Factor 9

32. **Phenytoin toxicity is increased with:**
A. Warfarin
B. Allopurinol
C. Isoniazid
D. Amoxycillin

33. **Significant antiadrogenic effect is found with:**
A. Nizatidine
B. Famotidine
C. Cimetidine
D. Ranitidine

34. **Activity in SLE:**
A. Leucopenia
B. ↑C3 activity
C. Stroke
D. RA factor

35. **Cryptosporidium: treatment of choice is:**
A. Cotrimoxazole
B. Parmomycin
C. Albendazole
D. Praziquantel

36. **B cell differentiated from T cells by presence of:**
A. CD3
B. CD4
C. Surface immunoglobulins
D. HLA class I

37. **Prednisone therapy beneficial in:**
A. Ducchene's muscular dystrophy
B. Limb girdle dystrophy
C. Ocular dystrophy
D. Myotonic dystrophy

24 A 25 B 26 B 27 A 28 B 29 C 30 A 31 C 32 C 33 C 34 C 35 B
36 C 37 A

38. Large vegetation with culture negative infective endocarditis: etiology is:
A. Streptococcus viridans
B. Streptococcus pneumoniae
C. E. coli
D. Haemophilus parainfluenza

39. Uncomplicated HOCM: treatment of choice is:
A. Digoxin
B. Dual chamber pacing
C. Nitrates
D. Epicardial pacing

40. Cold antibody is:
A. Mycoplasma
B. CLL
C. NHL
D. SLE

41. Wide split S2 occurs with:
A. CCP
B. Epicardial LV pacing
C. Left SVC → LA with intact septum
D. Severe pulmonary HT
E. PDA

42. Reverse split S2:
A. VSD
B. MR
C. Dual chamber pacing
D. CHF
E. Atrial tachycardia

43. Amyl nitrite accentuates murmur:
A. TOF
B. PS
C. PDA
D. MR
E. HOCM

44. BP increases by:
A. Pregnancy
B. Exercise
C. Smoking
D. Exposure to heat
E. Alcohol

45. Regarding echocardiography, true statements are:
A. LV systolic function assessed by M mode
B. LV systolic function is measured by modified Simpson's rule
C. Initial measurement of MVA by M mode
D. LV diastolic dysfunction is primarily diagnosed by PW doppler
E. MVP is diagnosed by colour doppler

46. Regarding echocardiography, true statements are:
A. Normal fractional shortening 50-60%
B. RV systolic function assessed by VTI of tricuspid valve annulus
C. SAM diagnosed by M mode
D. PLAX demonstrates coronaries

47. Severity of MS assessed by:
A. PHT
B. 2D
C. PISA
D. M Mode
E. Gorlin's formula

48. Myocardial viability is assessed by:
A. Reversed redistribution $Thal^{201}$
B. Dobutamine stress echo
C. PET
D. SAECG
E. Exercise TMT

49. High risk TMT–indicating adverse prognosis:
A. BP>180/110 mm Hg
B. ST-T/HR slope >1.6 mV/beats/min
C. Unsloping ST >1.5 mV depression at < 6 mets in greater than 5 leads and recovery in 1 min
D. Crescendo angina
E. Sustained or symptomatic VT

38 D	39 B	40 A	41 B	42 C	43 B,E	44 B,C,E
45 A,B,D	46 B,C	47 A,B,C,E	48 A,B,C	49 D,E		

50. Difficulty in interpretation of TMT with:
A. LVH on ECG
B. On Digoxin
C. On Diuretics
D. NTG given before 12 hrs
E. CCB

51. Atrial fibrillation: True are:
A. Intermediate AF predictor of stroke
B. Stroke more common in non-valvular than valvular
C. Aspirin and oral anticoagulants equal efficacy in preventing stroke
D. Biatrial pacing ↓ intermittent AF
E. Rhythm control is definitely better than rate control in non-valvular AF

52. Regarding PPI:
A. Pace maker induced tachycardia common with single chamber
B. Biatrial pacing decreases intermittent AF
C. Biventricular pacing of benefit in HOCM
D. Atrial arrhythmias less in DDD than VVI
E. VVI better than Bi ventricular pacing in CHF

53. Commonly seen in severe AS (valvular):
A. LV S4
B. 'a' waves in JVP
C. Ejection systolic murmur in mitral area
D. Soft A2
E. Family history positive

54. Severity of AR:
A. Cardiomegaly
B. S4 present
C. Pulmonary hypertension
D. Long EDM
E. Soft audible A2

55. Causes of AR:
A. Paget's disease
B. Hypertension
C. Mucopolysaccharidoses
D. PAN
E. Rheumatic MS

56. Organisms causing atherosclerosis:
A. H. pylori
B. Chlamydia pneumonia
C. Coxsackie virus
D. Pneumocystis carinii
E. CMV

57. Hyperventilation:
A. ↑PaO_2
B. ↑pH
C. ↑PCO_2
D. ↑HCO_3
E. Decrease chemoreceptor discharge

58. Young female complain of irregular palpitations, acute pain in left lower limb with MS is likely to have:
A. Variable S1
B. Normal character of pulse
C. Pulmonary edema
D. Ventricular tachycardia
E. SABE

59. Nicorandil is used in:
A. HT
B. Angina
C. CHF
D. PSVT
E. PVD (intermittent claudication)

60. 40 year male sitting in OPD with chest pain features suggesting ACS:
A. Characteristic of chest pain
B. Bedside ECG
C. Trop T
D. CPKMB
E. Bedside echo

50 A,B,C 51 A,D 52 B,D 53 A,B,C,D 54 A,D 55 B,C,D,E 56 A,B,E
57 B,E 58 A 59 A,B,C 60 A,B,E

61. Pulsus paradoxus is prominent feature in:
A. Br Asthma
B. Pulmonary embolism
C. Pregnancy
D. LA myxoma
E. Cardiac tamponade

62. Primary hyperaldosteronism:
A. Hyponatremia
B. ↓Renin
C. Hypertension
D. Hypernatremia
E. Acidosis

63. β agonist:
A. ↑Na transport
B. ↑Intracellular calcium
C. ↑cAMP
D. Decrease adenylate cyclase
E. K^+ transport

64. Wide QRS regular tachycardia with HR 200/min; drugs preferred include:
A. Verapamil
B. Digoxin
C. Adenosine
D. Cordarone
E. Metoprolol

65. PSVT with CHF most appropriate drugs are:
A. Diltiazem
B. Esmolol
C. CSM
D. Cordarone
E. Treatment of heart failure alone

66. Pre excitation: ECG finding are:
A. Delta wave
B. Short PR
C. Prolonged QRS
D. T inversion
E. Absent q waves

67. Acute pulmonary embolism: In diagnosis, most significant contribution is by:
A. FDP
B. ECG
C. CXR
D. V/Q scan
E. Peripheral venous USG

68. Negative predictive value of >50% in IE is of:
A. Echo
B. Blood c/s
C. Petichae/splinter hemorrhages
D. Clubbing
E. Palpable splenomegaly

69. Janeway lesion characteristic:
A. Tender
B. Dorsum on hand
C. Flitting
D. Macular
E. Blanch on pressure

70. Mucocutaneous lymph node syndrome: true are:
A. Erythema hand and legs
B. Cervical lymphadenopathy
C. Eosinophilia
D. Purulent conjunctivitis
E. Vesicular eruptions on trunk

71. COPD cause of HF can be:
A. Hypoxia
B. Increased work of breathing
C. TR
D. PAH
E. Hypercarbia

72. Frusemide is to be given cautiously in:
A. Sulphonamide allergy
B. Hyperuricaemia
C. Hypernephroma
D. Warfarin
E. SLE

61 A,E	62 B,C,D	63 B,C	64 C,D	65 B,D	66 A,B,C,D	67 A,D,E
68 A,B	69 D,E	70 A,B,D	71 A,C,D	72 A,B		

73. Myocardial contractility depends on:
- **A.** Pre-load
- **B.** After load
- **C.** Tachycardia
- **D.** MVO_2
- **E.** Increased calcium

74. Morphine: mechanism of benefit in acute LVF:
- **A.** Arteriolar dilatation
- **B.** Venodilatation
- **C.** Sedation
- **D.** Hypoventilation
- **E.** Analgesia

75. Nitrates post MI is given in:
- **A.** All patients for 6 months
- **B.** All pts for 3 months
- **C.** Before surgery and PTCA
- **D.** Only in presence of angina
- **E.** CHF

76. Cells seen in atheroma are:
- **A.** Platelets
- **B.** Smooth muscle
- **C.** Monocytes
- **D.** Histiocytes
- **E.** Eosinophils

77. Syncope commonly seen in:
- **A.** MS
- **B.** PPH
- **C.** Shydragger
- **D.** Adult TOF
- **E.** Cerebral thrombosis

78. SCD markedly ↑ed:
- **A.** MR
- **B.** AR
- **C.** Congestive CMP
- **D.** Cardiac amyloid
- **E.** CCP

79. TMT indications:
- **A.** Asymptomatic young male
- **B.** LBBB
- **C.** Chronotropic competence in congenital heart block
- **D.** CHF exercise capacity
- **E.** Post PTCA evaluation

80. Remodelling after MI:
- **A.** Cavity dilatation
- **B.** Hypertrophy
- **C.** Fibrosis
- **D.** Residual ischemia
- **E.** Necrosis

---

73 A,B,C,E 74 B,C 75 D,E 76 B,C 77 B,C 78 C,D 79 C,D,E
80 A,B,C

PGI 2002 (December)

1. Which of the following sounds increase in inspiration?
A. LVS_1
B. RVS 3
C. RVS 1
D. Aortic click
E. Pulmonary ejection click

2. Loud S_1 is heard in which of the following:
A. Tachycardia
B. Aortic regurgitation
C. Short PR interval
D. Acute mitral regurgitation
E. Thyrotoxicosis

3. Trans-esophageal echo is not useful in visualizing:
A. Ascending aorta
B. Arch of aorta
C. Proximal descending aorta
D. Distal descending thoracic aorta
E. Ascending aortic dissection with aortic regurgitation

4. Indications for stopping cardiac stress testing includes:
A. Grade 1 and 2 chest pain
B. ST depression of 2 mm
C. ST elevation of 1mm in leads without Q waves
D. Abnormal elevation of systolic BP
E. Ataxia

5. Increased risk in stress thallium test is seen with:
A. Increased lung uptake
B. Decreased lung uptake
C. Decreased perfusion in territory of single coronary
D. Lack of redistribution
E. Left ventricular dilatation on exercise

6. Cardiac catheterization data as follows were obtained in a case of tetralogy of fallot: systemic blood pressure 110/0 mm Hg, transpulmonary blood velocity 5 m/s. The pulmonary arterial systolic blood pressure will be:
A. 10
B. 20
C. 25
D. 30
E. 35

7. If the heart rate is 70/minute, end diastolic volume 120ml and ejection fraction of 50% what will be the cardiac output:
A. 3.0 L
B. 4.2 L
C. 4.8 L
D. 5.0 L
E. 5.8 L

1 B,C 2 A,C,E 3 B,C 4 C,D,E 5 A,E 6 A 7 B

8. During catheterization, step up in oxygen in the right atrium is seen in:

A. Total anomalous pulmonary venous connection
B. Atrial septal defect
C. Ventricular septal defect
D. Patent ductus arteriosus
E. Gerbode defect

9. During catheterization, pulmonary arterial oxygen saturation more than systemic oxygen saturation is found in which of the following conditions:

A. Transposition of great arteries
B. Taussig Bing anomaly
C. Eisenmengers syndrome
D. Ventricular septal defect
E. Inferior vena cava draining into left atrium

10. Which of the following can be seen during catheterization in a patient with AV septal defect:

A. Ostium primum atrial septal defect
B. Multiple ventricular septal defects
C. Cleft mitral valve
D. Gooseneck deformity
E. Right axis deviation

11. Which of the following are branches of the left circumflex artery:

A. PDA
B. First septal
C. AV nodal
D. Diagnonal
E. Obtuse marginal

12. Mortality rate in cardiac catheterization is doubled in:

A. Infants less than one month
B. After thrombolysis
C. Immediately after myocardial infarction
D. Left main disease
E. Atrial fibrillation

13. Renin is increased by:

A. Digoxin
B. Diuretic
C. Natriuretic peptide
D. Decreased renal perfusion
E. Sodium repletion

14. Increase in cardiac output in the supine position is caused by:

A. Digoxin
B. Dopamine
C. Volume overload
D. Atrial pacing at 120 beats per minute
E. Atropine

15. The prognosis of congestive heart failure is inversely related to:

A. Renin
B. Norepinephrine
C. Atrial natriuretic peptide
D. Ejection fraction
E. Cardiac index

16. A patient with Wolff-Parkinson white syndrome had on ECG negative delta wave and QRS in lead V_1 and negative delta wave in lead II, III and AvF. The aberrant pathway is likely to be:

A. Left rateral
B. Right posteroseptal
C. Right free wall
D. Right anteroseptal
E. Left posteroseptal

17. A patient with tachycardia bradycardia syndrome presents with complaints of palpitations, which of the following pacemarkers is best for him:

A. AAI
B. VVI
C. VVIR
D. DDD
E. DDDR

8 A,B,E 9 A,B 10 A,B,C,D 11 A,E 12 A,D 13 B,D 14 B,C,D,E
15 D,E 16 B 17 A,E

18. A patient with permanent pacemaker present with palpitations and on investigation was found to have endless loop tachycardia, which of the following maneuvers is likely to decrease his symptoms:

A. Increased ventricular refractory period
B. Increased AV nodal delay
C. Increased atrial refractory period
D. AV nodal ablation
E. Place magnet over pacemaker

19. Complication of hypertension are:

A. Coronary atherosclerosis
B. Peripheral vascular disease
C. Aortic dissection
D. Heart failure
E. Sudden death

20. Which of the following is a beta blocker with intrinsic sympathomimetic effect:

A. Sotalol
B. Oxprenolol
C. Timolol
D. Pindolol
E. Nadolol

21. Which of the following diuretics increase plasma potassium?

A. Hydrochlorothiazide
B. Amiloride
C. Bumetanide
D. Indapamide
E. Triamterene

22. Which of the following Mendelian disorders is associated with a decrease in blood pressure:

A. Fabry's disease
B. Pseudoxanthoma elasticum
C. Shy Drager syndrome
D. Dopamine β hydroxylase deficiency
E. Acute intermittent porphyria

23. Which of the following is true regarding late potentials in signal averaged ECG after MI:

A. Increase in occurrence in the 1st week after MI
B. Occurs after 3-6 months after MI
C. Decrease in amplitude with antiarrhythmics
D. 10% of patients with ventricular tachycardia have late potentials
E. Independent predictor of mortality after MI

24. Surgery in ischemic heart disease is indicated in which of the following:

A. Single vessel disease
B. Left anterior descending artery with 50% obstruction
C. Pseudo aneurysm of left ventricle
D. Acquired VSD
E. Triple vessel disease with ejection from of 17%

25. Balloon septostomy is done in:

A. Double outlet right ventricle
B. Complete transposition of great arteries
C. Pulmonary atresia
D. Tricuspid atresia
E. Tetralogy of fallot with severe pulmonary stenosis

26. Definitive treatment for transposition of great arteries in a neonate of 6 days is:

A. Balloon septostomy
B. Arterial switch
C. Glenn shunt
D. Waterston shunt
E. Blalock Taussig shunt

27. Small PDA can cause which of the following:

A. Congestive heart failure
B. Infective endoarteritis
C. Eisenmenger complex
D. Hoarseness of voice
E. Calcification

18 C,D,E | 19 A,B,C,D | 20 B,D | 21 B,E | 22 A,C,D | 23 A,C,E | 24 C,D,E
25 B,C,D | 26 B | 27 B

28. Presence of pulmonary plethora and prominent aortic knuckle with prominence of left atrium in a 7 year old child can occur in:
A. Atrial septal defect
B. Ventricular septal defect
C. Patent ductus arteriosus
D. Peripheral arteriovenous fistula
E. Rupture of Sinus of Valsalva into right atrium

29. Congestive heart failure in the first week of life is caused by:
A. Left ventricular hypoplasia
B. Transposition of great arteries
C. Hypoxia
D. Hypoglycemia
E. Large ventricular septal defect

30. Dose of propanolol for cyanotic spells in a child with Tetralogy of Fallot is:
A. 0.01 mg/kg
B. 0.04 mg/kg
C. 0.1 mg/kg
D. 0.4 mg/kg
E. 1 mg/kg

31. Left to right shunting across an ASD is increased by:
A. High altitude
B. Hypertension
C. Pulmonary hypertension
D. Isoproterenol
E. Mitral stenosis

32. Which of the following is an indication for surgery in ventricular septal defect?
A. Qp/Qs >1.8
B. Pulmonary artery resistance 12 wood units
C. Small aortic regurgitation with subpulmonic ventricular septal defect
D. Failure to thrive
E. Intractable congestive heart failure after 3 months of age

33. A 31 year old lady with asymptomatic aortic stenosis was found on echo to have a gradient of 130 mmHg across the aortic valve Which of the following would be the treatment approach:
A. Aortic valve replacement
B. Surgical valvotomy
C. Balloon valvotomy
D. Follow up
E. Digoxin, lasix and K supplementation

34. Poor prognosis in critical aortic stenosis is indicated by:
A. Angina
B. Syncope
C. Heart failure
D. Palpitation
E. Gradient >120 mmHg

35. All the following are seen in acute aortic regurgitation *except:*
A. Soft S1
B. Soft S2
C. S4 is auscultable
D. Presystolic accentuation of Austin Flint murmur
E. Peripheral ausculatory signs of aortic regurgitation

36. Infective endocarditis prophylaxis of native valve is indicated in which of the following condition:
A. Caesarean section
B. Bronchoscopy
C. Endoscopic sclerotherapy
D. Shedding of primary teeth
E. Gall bladder surgery

37. Surgery is definitely indicated in infective endocarditis in which of the following:
A. Intractable congestive heart failure
B. Unstable prosthesis
C. Perivascular abscess
D. Multiple emboli
E. Vegetation > 5 mm

28 C,E | 29 A,C,D | 30 C | 31 B,D,E | 32 A,C,D,E | 33 A | 34 A,B,C
35 D,E | 36 B,C,E | 37 A,B,C

38. In which of the following is surgery indicated for aortic dissection:

A. Proximal aortic dissection
B. 2 week stable AR syndrome
C. Saccular aneurysm
D. AR

39. Domiciliary oxygen therapy for 19 hours a day in a patient with cor pulmonale will lead to:

A. Improved survival
B. Decrease in right ventricular failure
C. Decreased pulmonary artery pressure
D. Regression of right ventricular hypertrophy
E. Oxygen toxicity

40. Which of the following is seen in cardiac tamponade?

A. Decreased cardiac pulsations on fluoroscopy
B. Presence of Kussmaul's sign
C. Increased intrapericardial pressure on inspiration
D. Wide pulse pressure
E. Diastolic collapse of right atrium

38 A,C,D 39 A,B,C,D 40 A,E

PGI 2002 (June)

Cardiology

1. Syncope is commonly seen with:
A. MS
B. PPH
C. Shy Dragger syndrome
D. Adult TOF
E. Cerebral thrombosis

2. Severity of MS indicated by:
A. Loud S1
B. A2-OS interval
C. A2-P2 interval
D. Loud P2
E. Presystolic murmur

3. Remodeling after MI: true are:
A. Fibrosis
B. Cavity dilatation
C. Myocardial necrosis
D. Hypertrophy
E. Residual ischemia

4. Digitalis toxicity is manifested by:
A. Downsloping ST in dominant ventricle
B. Short QT
C. Gynaecomastia
D. Worsening of failure
E. PAT with block

5. ECG in preexcitation: true are:
A. Short PR
B. Normal QT
C. Absent P wave
D. SVT with normal QRS
E. ST depression

6. Common finding in AS (Valvular):
A. LVS4
B. Ejection systolic murmur in mitral area
C. Soft A2
D. 'a' wave in JVP
E. Family history positive

7. Left parasternal lift is present in:
A. TR
B. PR
C. MR
D. AS
E. AR

8. Acute AR findings are:
A. Long early diastolic murmur
B. Cardiomegaly
C. Normal pulse volume
D. Pulmonary edema
E. Loud LVS4

1 B,C 2 B,C,D 3 A,B,D 4 D,E 5 A,B,D,E 6 A,B,C,D 7 C
8 C,D,E

9. Severity of AR is assessed by:
A. Long EDM
B. Soft A2
C. Cardiomegaly
D. Pulmonary HT

10. Paradoxical split S2: causes are:
A. VSD
B. MR
C. Double chamber pacing
D. Atrial tachycardia
E. CHF

11. Intensity of systolic murmur of MVP is increased by:
A. Standing
B. Squatting
C. Handgrip
D. Post VPC
E. Expiration

12. LVS3 is increased by:
A. Leg raising
B. Squatting
C. Inspiration
D. Tachycardia
E. Handgrip

13. Irregular cannon waves in JVP are present in:
A. CHB
B. AF
C. VT
D. Junctional Tachycardia
E. PSVT

14. 22 year female having irregular palpitations and having severe pain in left lower limb, CVS examination suggestive of mitral stenosis: True is:
A. Variable S1
B. Is having SABE
C. Patient is having pulmonary edema
D. Most likely having VT
E. Pulse is normal in character

15. Echo finding of MS:
A. A>E
B. PML moves posteriorly
C. IVS paradoxical
D. ↓EF slope
E. Ejection fraction normal

16. Fibrinous pericarditis: etiologies are:
A. Post MI
B. Sub acute bacterial endocarditis
C. Lithium
D. Systemic sclerosis
E. Sarcoidosis

17. SCD occurs most commonly in:
A. AR
B. MR
C. Congestive cardiomyopathy
D. Amyloidosis
E. Constrictive pericarditis

18. Pheochromocytoma diagnosis is suspected by:
A. Edema
B. Weight loss
C. Orthostatic hypotension
D. Hyperglycemia
E. Tachycardia

19. Primary hyper aldosteronism: true are:
A. Metabolic acidosis
B. Low renin
C. Accelerated hypertension
D. Increased blood volume
E. Hyponatremia

20. Hyperventilation will produce:
A. ↑ PaO_2
B. ↑ $PaCO_2$
C. ↑ pH
D. ↓ Discharge of chemoreceptors
E. ↑ HCO_3

9 A,C | 10 C | 11 A | 12 A,B,D,E | 13 A,C,D | 14 A | 15 A,D,E
16 A,D,E | 17 C,D | 18 B,C,E | 19 B,C | 20 C,D

21. Frusemide cautiously given in:
A. Sulfa allergy
B. Hyperuricaemia
C. LUPUS
D. With anticoagulants
E. Hypernephroma

22. Drug of choice in 1st time accelerated HT:
A. Oral enalpril
B. IV Beta blocker
C. S/L nifedipine
D. IV Dilzem
E. IV Lasix

23. Pulmonary edema is caused by:
A. Post lung transplant
B. Deep sea diving
C. Zero gravity
D. DIC
E. Scorpion envenomation

24. Long QT is caused by:
A. Disopyramide
B. Clonidine
C. Cetrizine
D. Trimetazidine
E. Digoxin

25. Long QT seen with:
A. Myocarditis
B. Diuretic
C. Sub arachnoid haemorrhage
D. Alkalosis
E. Hypercalcemia

26. Pulsus paradoxus occurs in:
A. Pericardial effusion
B. Bronchial asthma
C. Pulmonary embolism
D. Lt atrial myxoma
E. Pregnancy

27. Stress test: difficult to comment in patients having:
A. Receiving CCB
B. LVH
C. On diuretics
D. On digoxin
E. NTG given before 12 hours

28. Myocardial contractility depends on:
A. MVO_2
B. Preload
C. Afterload
D. Tachycardia
E. Intracellular Ca

29. Wide Complex tachycardia with rate 200/min, treatment of choice is:
A. Verapamil
B. Metoprolol
C. Adenosine
D. Digoxin
E. Amiodarone

30. CHF in DCMP is associated with:
A. Tachycardia
B. Hypotension
C. Peripheral edema
D. ↓ EF
E. Cardiomegaly

31. Not an independent risk factor for CAD:
A. Hyperthyroidism
B. Menopause
C. Pipe smoking
D. ↓ S. ferritin
E. Excessive alcohol intake

32. Less common site of angina are:
A. Jaw
B. Epigastrium
C. Substernal
D. Back
E. Right arm

21 A,B 22 B,E 23 A,B,C,D,E 24 A 25 A,B,C,D 26 B,C,E 27 B,C,D
28 B,C,D,E 29 E 30 A,B,C,D,E 31 A,B,D 32 A,B,D,E

33. Renal artery stenosis is cause of hypertension if it shows:
- A. Ipsilateral small kidney
- B. IVP–early and dense contrast in contralateral kidney
- C. Renal vein renin ratio between affected and normal kidney is > 1.4:1
- D. Significant gradient demonstrable across stenosis
- E. Cortical thinning

34. Dobutamine acts by:
- A. β1 receptor
- B. β2 receptor
- C. ANP release
- D. Renin release
- E. Stimulates dopamine receptor

35. Relief by morphine in LVF–mechanisms are:
- A. Analgesia
- B. Sedation
- C. ↓ Preload
- D. ↓ Afterload
- E. Hypoventilation

36. Cardiac involvement is commonly seen in:
- A. CA bronchus
- B. Guillian-Barre Syndrome
- C. Myasthenia gravis
- D. Gout
- E. Filariasis

37. CAD occurs following infection with:
- A. C.jejuni
- B. H. pylori
- C. CMV
- D. Chlamydia pneumoniae
- E. Coxsackie B virus

38. Right sided IE is associated with:
- A. High mortality
- B. Pulmonary valve involvement always occurs
- C. JVP always raised
- D. Pulmonary embolism
- E. Large vegetation

39. Mucocutaneous Lymph node syndrome characterized by:
- A. Cervical lymphadenopathy
- B. Purulent conjunctivitis
- C. Maculo-vesicular rashes on back
- D. Eosinophilia
- E. Erythema of hands and sole

40. Warfarin is decreased by:
- A. Sulfonamides
- B. Erythromycin
- C. Tetracycline
- D. Rifampicin

33 A,B,D 34 A,B 35 B,C,D 36 A,B 37 B,C,D 38 D,E 39 A,B,E
40 B

Medicine

1. T cell is identified by:
- **A.** Proliferative response to phytohaemagglutinin
- **B.** NBT positive
- **C.** Lymphocytic culture
- **D.** Proliferative response to concavanin A

2. IgA deficiencies is seen with all *except:*
- **A.** Asthma
- **B.** Respiratory tract infection
- **C.** NHL
- **D.** Anaphylaxis

3. Hyperglycemia occurs with:
- **A.** AZT
- **B.** Lamivudine
- **C.** Nelfinavir
- **D.** Nevirapine

4. ↑ Erythropoietin with anemia in HIV is caused by:
- **A.** AZT
- **B.** Dapsone
- **C.** Parvovirus B19
- **D.** Lamivudine

5. Pneumocystis. carinii prophylaxis is given at CDC count of:
- **A.** 200
- **B.** 250
- **C.** 300
- **D.** 350

6. Herpes simplex virus 8 in HIV causes:
- **A.** Primary CNS lymphoma
- **B.** Non cleaved small cell lymphoma
- **C.** Body cavity lymphoma
- **D.** Immunoblastic lymphoma

7. In a patient of renal insufficiency, hyperkalemia can occur with:
- **A.** Gentamicin
- **B.** Ceftriaxone
- **C.** Trimethoprim
- **D.** Dapsone

8. Acute interstitial nephritis is caused by:
- **A.** Rifampicin
- **B.** Cisplatin
- **C.** Amphotericin B
- **D.** Ciprofloxacin

9. Autosomal polycystic kidney disease is associated with:
- **A.** Pulmonary cyst
- **B.** Splenic cyst
- **C.** Retinal detachment
- **D.** MVP

10. Dysmorphic RBC's with hematuria occurs in:
- **A.** Prostatitis
- **B.** Cystitis
- **C.** Hereditary nephritis
- **D.** Renal cell Carcinoma

11. Painless voluminous diarrhea persisting on fasting; least likely diagnosis is:
- **A.** Gastrinoma
- **B.** Lactase deficiency
- **C.** Senna abuse (habitual)
- **D.** Carcinoid

12. Hb 4.5, MCV 63, ferritin 3 ugm , not responding to oral iron jejunal biopsy s/o lymphocytic infiltration, diagnosis is done by:
- **A.** Antiendomycial and antiglandin antibodies
- **B.** Duodenal fluid IgA deficiency
- **C.** Fecal fat estimation
- **D.** Schilling test

1 B 2 C 3 C 4 A 5 A 6 C 7 D 8 A 9 D 10 C 11 B 12 A

13. Mid diastolic murmur in tricuspid area occurs in:

A. VSD
B. ASD
C. PDA
D. Acute Rh Fever

14. Drug used in prevention of adriamycin toxicity:

A. Dexarozoxane
B. Probucol l
C. Dilzem
D. Verapamil

5. Minor duke's criteria are all *except:*

A. Echocardiographic evidence of vegetation
B. Roth spots
C. Janeway lesions
D. Fever

16. Patient receiving clarithromycin which drug produces major arrhythmia:

A. Astemizole
B. Aminophylline
C. Digoxin
D. Frusemide

17. Eosinophilia myalgia syndrome is caused by:

A. L-tryptophan
B. Valine
C. Lecine
D. Aspartate

18. Color of urine can be altered by intake of which drug (unrelated to O2 exposure):

A. INH
B. Riboflavin
C. PCM
D. Norflox

19. Female having pH 7.2, PCO_2 25, HCO_3-18, Na 136 Cl 100, crystalluria; diagnosis is:

A. Ethylene glycol poisoning
B. Methanol poisoning
C. Salicylate poisoning
D. Lactic acidosis

20. Rabies immunoglobulin true statement is:

A. Given IV
B. Given i/m and around wound
C. Dose–40 IV
D. Repeated on day 3

21. Antibody in Paraneoplastic encephalomyelitis is:

A. Anti Hu
B. Anti Yo
C. Anti Ri
D. Anti Ach receptor

22. Experimental animal for herpes simplex encephalitis was:

A. Mice
B. Dog
C. Cats
D. Dragon fly

23. Regarding iron toxicity: all are true *except:*

A. Hypotension
B. Hepatic dysfunction
C. Coagulopathy
D. Hyperglycemia

24. Regarding Vit A intoxication, all are true *except:*

A. Cheilosis
B. Peripheral neuropathy
C. Pseudotumour cerebri
D. Hepatic fibrosis

25. Elderly with RA factor +ve will have:

A. Less systemic involvement
B. Persistent Rh activity
C. Distal interphalangeal joint involvement
D. Self limiting

13 B 14 A 15 A 16 A 17 A 18 B 19 A 20 B 21 B 22 A 23 C 24 B 25 B

26. Migraine is precipitated by all *except:*
A. Pregnancy
B. Red wine
C. Lack of sleep
D. Menstruation

27. Indication for aspiration of amoebic liver abscess include all *except:*
A. Multiple abscesses
B. Imminent rupture of abscess
C. Severe toxemia at presentation
D. Left lobe involvement

28. Patient having flushing, diarrhea, shortness of breath and abdominal pain investigation of choice is:
A. CT abdomen
B. 5HT measurement
C. Chromogranin A measurement
D. TEE

29. Specific for SLE is:
A. Anti dsDNA
B. Anti Ss DNA
C. URNP
D. Anti Sm antibodies

30. Mixed connective tissue disorder antibodies found is:
A. Anti U1 RNP
B. Anti Ro
C. Anti Sm
D. Anti

31. Tamm Horsfall protein secreted in:
A. Thin descending loop of Henley
B. Thick ascending loop of Henley
C. Proximal convoluted tubule
D. Collecting tubule

32. Guillian Barre syndrome is associated with following infections *except:*
A. Influenza
B. C. jejuni
C. H. pylori
D. CMV

33. Malignant neurolept syndrome due to haloperidol is treated by all *except:*
A. Bromocryptine
B. Amantadine
C. Dantrolene
D. Sodium valproate

34. B/L fascial nerve palsy occurs with all *except:*
A. Sarcoidosis
B. Lyme disease
C. Melkersson syndrome
D. Diphtheria

35. Total parenteral nutrition: all are true *except:*
A. Hyperphosphataemia
B. Hypercalcemia
C. Hypokalemia
D. Hyperglycemia

36. Severe Falciparum malaria is treated by all *except:*
A. Quinine
B. Artesunate
C. Sulfadoxime-pyrimethamine combination
D. Mefloquine

37. Skin necrosis in young female receiving oral anticoagulants for DVT: likely cause is:
A. Homozygous C deficiency
B. Homozygous S deficiency
C. Factor V Leiden mutation
D. Antithrombin III deficiency

38. Folate level is decreased by:
A. Phenytoin
B. INH
C. Aspirin
D. Lamotrigine

26 A 27 A 28 B 29 D 30 A 31 B 32 A 33 D 34 C 35 A 36 C 37 A 38 A

39. Prophylaxis for pneumonic plague is given to all *except:*

A. Contacts of healthy contact
B. Close household contacts
C. Lab personnel handling samples
D. Medical personal

40. Pure red cell aplasia in multiple transfusion patients is caused by:

A. Parvovirus B19
B. HZV
C. HIV
D. HSV

39 A 40 A

PGI 2001

1. **PTCA is indicated in all *except:***
   A. Unprotected LMCA stenosis
   B. Protected LMCA
   C. Bifurcating lesion of distal LAD
   D. Proximal stenosis of SVG graft
   E. Instent restenosis

2. **On IVUS, mechanism of restenosis is:**
   A. Accelerated atherosclerosis
   B. Arterial remodelling
   C. Neo intimal hyperplasia
   D. Organization of clot
   E. Arterial remodelling & hyperplasia

3. **DCA v/s balloon PTCA: all are true *except:***
   A. Large lumen
   B. ↑ CKMB
   C. High rate of abrupt closure
   D. ↓ restenosis
   E. Better 1 year survival

4. **GpIIb/IIIa inhibitors are:**
   A. Abciximab
   B. Integrillin
   C. Tirofiban
   D. Pimobendan
   E. Ticlopidine

5. **Torsades de pointes is seen with:**
   A. Amiodarone
   B. Cisapride
   C. Terfenadine
   D. Xamiterol
   E. Adenosine

6. **ACE-inhibitor improves survival in:**
   A. Severe CHF
   B. Mild to moderate CHF
   C. MI with CHF
   D. Diastolic failure
   E. Asymptomatic LV dysfunction

7. **Benefits of thrombolytic therapy in DVT are:**
   A. Decreased incidence of PE
   B. Reduced incidence of post phlebitic syndrome
   C. Decreased recurrence of DVT
   D. Less chronic venous insufficiency
   E. Decreased need of long term anti coagulation

8. **True about Ebstein's anomaly:**
   A. R in V1 >7 mm on ECG
   B. Common preexcitation syndrome-type B
   C. No surgical treatment
   D. Ostium secundum ASD is rare
   E. On M mode, both AV valve seen simultaneously

9. **c-TGA is commonly associated with:**
   A. DORV
   B. VSD
   C. Left sided Ebstein's anomaly
   D. Unroofed coronary sinus
   E. High incidence of AV block

---

1 A | 2 B,C,E | 3 B,C,E | 4 A,B,C | 5 A,B,C | 6 A,B,C,E | 7 A,B,C
8 A,B,D | 9 B,C,E

10. Cyanosis at birth is common with:
A. d-TGA
B. TOF
C. Truncus arteriosus
D. Ostium primum ASD
E. Tricuspid Atresia

11. In CCP: haemodynamics are:
A. Low cardiac output
B. Equalisation of pressure in all 4 chambers
C. At least moderate pulmonary hypertension
D. Dip & Plateau pattern
E. Absence of overshoot in stage 4 valsalva

12. Maternal Rubella is associated with:
A. Peripheral pulmonary stenosis
B. VSD
C. Cataract
D. Myocarditis
E. Lt Axis deviation with counter clockwise rotation of QRS axis

13. Drugs contra indicated in pregnancy:
A. Hydralazine
B. Enalapril
C. Labetalol
D. α-Methyl dopa
E. Amiodarone

14. Drugs modifying the natural history of chronic severe AR:
A. Nifedipine
B. Enalapril
C. Hydralazine
D. Nitrates
E. Amiodarone

15. All are mechanical prosthetic valves *except:*
A. Carpentier Edward's
B. Medtronic Hall
C. St. Jude
D. Starr Edwards
E. Iunoescu Shiley

16. Spontaneous echo contrast in LA is seen in:
A. Severe MS
B. Dilated CMP
C. AF after D.C cardioversion
D. Large LA with chronic severe MR
E. Cardiogenic shock

17. TEE is useful in all *except:*
A. Intracardiac tumors
B. Prosthetic valve endocarditis
C. Sinus venosus ASD
D. Suspected VSD after MI
E. Dissection of aortic arch

18. Drugs used in stress echo are:
A. Adenosine
B. Dobutamine
C. Isoprenaline
D. Trimetazidine
E. Dipyridamole

19. Common organisms in IV drug abuser endocarditis:
A. Staph aureus
B. Strep viridans
C. Fungi
D. Klebsiella
E. Polymicrobial

20. True about viral myocarditis is:
A. Coxsackie B is common organism
B. PCR is important diagnostic test
C. Majority of cases develop DCMP
D. Large trials showed immunosuppressive therapy is beneficial
E. HLA DR3 is associated

21. EPILOG trial is associated with:
A. Integrellin
B. Abciximab
C. Enalapril
D. Pravastatin
E. Hirudin

10 A,B,E	11 A,B,C,D,E	12 A,B,C,D,E	13 B,E	14 A,C	15 A,E	16 A,B,C
17 D,E	18 A,B,E	19 A,B	20 A,D	21 B		

22. **True about intracardiac tumors are:**
   A. Malignant melanoma is commonest secondary tumor
   B. Rhabdomyoma common in old age
   C. Spider cell seen in rhabdomyoma
   D. Benign cystic tumors common in AV valve
   E. Angiomas common in pulmonary artery

23. **A2-OS gap in MS is:**
   A. 60-120 ms
   B. 120-240 ms
   C. 240-320 ms
   D. 40-60 msec

24. **Pulsus paradoxus is seen in:**
   A. COPD
   B. Pericardial effusion
   C. CCP
   D. Cardiac tamponade
   E. Restrictive CMP

25. **Wide pulse pressure is seen in:**
   A. Capillary dilatation
   B. Reduced compliance of arteries
   C. Paget's disease
   D. Severe AS
   E. Cardiac tamponade

26. **Beat to beat variation in B.P. seen in:**
   A. CHB
   B. Polymorphic VT
   C. Wenckbach's phenomenon
   D. AF
   E. Idioventricular rhythm

27. **Digitalis causes:**
   A. Blue vision
   B. Yellow vision
   C. Scotomas
   D. Trigeminal neuralgia
   E. Gynaecomastia

28. **Following is seen in PPH:**
   A. RVS_3
   B. Prominent a wave in JVP
   C. Clubbing frequently associated
   D. Increased CO_2 retention

29. **Warfarin acts on:**
   A. Protein C
   B. Protein S
   C. Factor VIII
   D. Factor XIII
   E. Factor II

30. **Polyarteritis Nodosa is associated with:**
   A. Acute MI
   B. CCF
   C. Aneurysm rupture
   D. Aortic root dilatation
   E. Mononeuritis multiplex

31. **High altitude pulmonary edema is associated with:**
   A. PAH
   B. ↑ PCWP
   C. Normal LA pressure
   D. ↑ LVEDP
   E. ↓ Capillary permeability

32. **Severe PS with CHF is associated with:**
   A. Loud P2
   B. Delayed P2
   C. Constant click
   D. Prominent a wave in JVP
   E. RV-S3

33. **Post streptococcal infection is diagnostic of rheumatic fever by:**
   A. Erythema nodosum
   B. Erythema multiforme
   C. Erythema marginatum
   D. Prolonged PR
   E. Subcutaneous nodules

---

22 A,C,D　23 A　24 A,C,D,E　25 A,B,C　26 A,B,D,E　27 A,B,C,D,E　28 A,B
29 A,B,E　30 A,B,E　31 A,C　32 B,D,E　33 C,D,E

34. Metabolic disorder associated with CAD are:
A. Amyloidosis
B. Homocysteinemia
C. Haemochromatosis
D. Hurler's syndrome
E. Rheumatoid arthritis

35. Drugs useful in uncomplicated HOCM are:
A. Digoxin
B. Nitrates
C. Verapamil
D. Lasix
E. Propranolol

36. Sarcoidosis of myocardium is associated with:
A. Pericardial effusion
B. A-V blocks
C. Cor pulmonale
D. ↑ G6PD deficiency
E. Ventricular aneurysms

37. LEOPARD syndrome is associated with:
A. Multiple lentigenes
B. Pulmonary stenosis
C. AS
D. Pericardial constriction
E. MR

38. Class III antiarrhythmics are:
A. Amiodarone
B. Sotalol
C. Mexiletine
D. Lignocaine
E. Bretylium

39. Heparin therapy is associated with:
A. Osteoporosis
B. Thrombocytopenia
C. ↑ ACT
D. ↓ PT
E. ↑ Factor V levels

40. Athlete's heart syndrome is associated with:
A. ↑ QRS voltage
B. QT interval prolongation
C. Prominent U wave
D. Sinus bradycardia
E. Junctional escape rhythm

41. Antisurfactant antibodies by macrophage is produced in:
A. Pulmonary alveolar proteinosis
B. Amyloidosis
C. Sarcoidosis
D. Hanta virus

42. Vertical diplopia is increased by tilting head to right side, then lesion is in:
A. Left trochlear
B. Right trochlear
C. Left ophthalmic
D. Right ophthalmic

43. CD-5 receptor is present in:
A. Mantel cell lymphoma
B. Nodal marginal lymphoma
C. Waldenstrom's macroglobulinemia
D. Histiocytosis X

44. Burkitt's lymphoma is associated with:
A. C-myc
B. p53
C. BCL
D. ABL BCR

45. Middle age man, stage 3 lymphoma, diffuse large cell without extra nodal invasion, Karnofky index 80: according to international prognostic scoring patient is in which group?
A. Low risk
B. Intermediate risk
C. High risk
D. High intermediate risk

34 B,D 35 C,E 36 A,B,C,E 37 A,B,C,E 38 A,B,E 39 A,B,C 40 A,B,C,D,E 41 A
42 B 43 A 44 A 45 C

46. DIC with septicaemia improves with:
A. Anti TNFa
B. Activated protein C infusion
C. High dose methyl prednisolone
D. Plasmapheresis

47. H. pylori is associated with all *except:*
A. Vit B12 deficiency
B. IHD
C. Adenocarcinoma stomach
D. MALT

48. Which vaccine causes encephalopathy?
A. Hepatitis B
B. Pneumococcal vaccine
C. Yellow fever vaccine
D. Acellular pertussis

49. Leukemia with DIC: chromosomal abnormality is:
A. 9:22
B. 15:17
C. 14:21
D. Inversion 16

50. HSV–8 associated with AIDS: patient on immunosuppressive treatment can result into:
A. Kaposi's sarcoma
B. Hairy leukoplakia
C. Burkitts lymphoma
D. B cell lymphoproliferative malignancy

51. Patient on clindamycin develops watery diarrhoea: drug of choice is:
A. I/V vancomycin
B. Oral metrogyl
C. I/v amikacin
D. None of the above

52. Phototoxic fluoroquinolone:
A. Sparfloxacin
B. Ofloxacin
C. Ciprofloxacin
D. Norfloxacin

53. Theophylline induced arrhythmia is associated with:
A. Clarithromycin
B. Amikacin
C. Metronidazole
D. Cefotaxime

54. Cardiac arrhythmia by astemizole is increased by:
A. Erythromycin
B. Ciprofloxacin
C. Amoxicillin
D. None of the above

55. Post transplant patient on chronic immunosuppressant drugs develops fever and cough, Chest X-ray shows multiple opacities, histology shows weak acid fast branching organisms, Then all of the following can be used *except:*
A. Cotrimoxazole
B. Minocycline
C. Ciprofloxacin
D. Amikacin

56. All are true about tuberculosis with HIV *except:*
A. Upper lobe cavity
B. Interstitial infiltrates
C. Mantoux test is highly positive
D. Intrathoracic lymph node enlargement

57. Patient of HIV receiving three drugs: AZT, Nevirapine, Indinavir has developed pulmonary tuberculosis: The drug which is contraindicated is:
A. Rifampicin
B. Streptomycin
C. Isoniazid
D. Pyrazinamide

46 B 47 A 48 C 49 B 50 A 51 B 52 A 53 A 54 A 55 C 56 C 57 A

58. Alcoholic presents with unconsciousness and nystagmus: most useful drug is:
A. Thiamine
B. Vit B12
C. Disulfiram
D. Metronidazole

59. 13 year old boy has growth retardation, hypogeusia, night blindness: treatment is:
A. Vit A
B. Zinc
C. Copper
D. Vit E

60. Child with Hb 9.6 gm% S. iron 40 μg/dl; S ferritin 400; TIBC 180: cause is:
A. Thalassaemia intermedia
B. IBD
C. PNH
D. Ancylostomiasis

61. All are causes of hypertension *except:*
A. Cocaine
B. Amphetamine
C. Barbiturates
D. MAO inhibitors

62. Angiosarcoma of liver is caused by:
A. Polyvinyl chloride
B. Chromium
C. Cadmium
D. Lead

63. Patient on haloperidol has fever with rigidity: treatment is:
A. Bromocriptine
B. Dantrolene
C. Cold sponging
D. Chlorpromazine

64. G6PD deficiency with typhoid: drug not to be given is:
A. Ciprofloxacin
B. Aztreonam
C. Ceftriaxone
D. Amoxycillin

65. Dengue shock syndrome: all are seen *except:*
A. Hemodilution
B. Ascites
C. Narrow pulse pressure
D. ↑ Capillary permeability

66. Severe falciparum malaria has shown to have no impact on mortality with:
A. High dose IV dexamethasone
B. Packed cell transfusion
C. Exchange transfusion
D. Treatment of hypoglycaemia

67. CML: drugs used are all *except:*
A. ST-5
B. Herbimycin-A
C. Homoharringtonini
D. Fludarabine

68. Patient presents with chest pain and ST elevation in V1-V6, ECG shows atrial fibrillation, BP-90/60 mm Hg, Pulse -110/min irregularly irregular, bilateral crepts develop 1 day later, Treatment is:
A. Digoxin
B. Flecainide
C. Amiodarone
D. Quinidine

69. ACE gene polymorphism is seen with all *except:*
A. LVH
B. IgA nephropathy
C. Diabetic nephropathy
D. Hypertensive retinopathy

70. Endogenous inhibitor of angiogenesis:
A. Leptin
B. IL-8
C. TNF α
D. Endostatin

58 D 59 B 60 B 61 C 62 A 63 A 64 A 65 A 66 A 67 D 68 A 69 D 70 D

71. Hantavirus reservoir is:

A. Mouse
B. Cat
C. Dog
D. Pig

72. Patient with chronic liver disease and DIC has:

A. Increase fibrinogen
B. Increase Prothrombin
C. Increase factor-7
D. Decrease factor-8

73. A 30 year old lady after receiving OCP has developed abdominal pain and paralysis of lower limbs followed by upper limb; then enzyme deficiency is:

A. Isodecarboxylase
B. ALA synthetase
C. Ferrochelatase
D. Porphobilinogen deaminase

74. Middle age men with knee joint pain, hepatomegaly, hyperpigmentation of skin, all can be given *except:*

A. Vit C
B. Diuretics
C. ACE inhibitors
D. Phlebotomy

75. Drug induced SLE: all are true *except:*

A. Decreased complement level
B. Anti histone antibodies
C. Anti ds DNA is present
D. Positive direct coomb's test

76. Hypomagnesaemia is seen with all *except:*

A. Thiazide
B. Hypoaldosteronism
C. Small bowel bypass surgery
D. Acute pancreatitis

77. Which of the following drug is contraindicated in pregnancy?

A. Ramipril
B. Hydralazine
C. Nifedipine
D. Methyl Dopa

78. Classical PAN does not involve:

A. Lung
B. Kidney
C. GIT
D. Liver

79. Aeromonas septicemia: drug of choice is:

A. Ciprofloxacin
B. Clarithromycin
C. Chloramphenicol
D. Clindamycin

80. I/v Foscarnet is used in treatment of:

A. CMV retinitis
B. HSV
C. RSV
D. Pneumocystis carinii pneumonia

71 A 72 D 73 D 74 A 75 C 76 B 77 A 78 A 79 A 80 A

PGI 2000 (December)

1. **Soft S1 is seen in :**
   A. Pulmonary hypertension
   B. MR Rheumatic
   C. Acute AR
   D. ↑ PR interval
   E. AS

2. **Wide S2 is seen in:**
   A. VSD
   B. RBBB
   C. Severe pulmonary hypertension
   D. Pulmonary stenosis
   E. Cardiac temponade
   F. Constrictive pericarditis

3. **↑ BP is a normal response in:**
   A. Pregnancy
   B. Exercise
   C. Alcohol
   D. Exposure to heat
   E. Smoking

4. **Acute chest pain in patient while sitting in OPD. Investigation which will help in diagnosis of acute coronary syndrome:**
   A. Typical characteristic of chest pain
   B. Bed side ECG
   C. Bed side echocardiography
   D. Troponin T
   E. CPKMB

5. **What causes error in measurement of BP:**
   A. Width of Cuff
   B. Length of cuff
   C. Rate of inflation
   D. Rate of deflation
   E. Level of arm

6. **Peripheral oedema in patients of heart failure is mediated by:**
   A. ↑ hydrostatic pressure
   B. Venoconstriction
   C. ↑ Catecholamines
   D. ↑ ANP
   E. Oxidative stress

7. **Nitrates are most useful after acute MI:**
   A. Within 3 month
   B. Within 6 month
   C. If angina is present
   D. CHF
   E. Prior to PTCA/CABG

8. **Nitrates act by:**
   A. Venodilatation
   B. Antioxidant
   C. Arteriodilatation
   D. Cerebral vasodilatation
   E. Coronary vasodilatation

---

1 B,C,D   2 A,B,D   3 B,C,E   4 A,B,C   5 A,B,D,E   6 A,B,C   7 C,D
8 A,C,D,E

9. True about Mild hypertension:
A. Diurnal variation is blunted
B. Pulse pressure increases
C. Tachycardia
D. ↑ in risk of stroke

10. Causes of SCD:
A. MVP
B. PDA
C. Romano Ward syndrome
D. LVH
E. CAD/HOCM

11. Central chest pain with hemodynamic changes can occur with:
A. Pulmonary embolism
B. Oesophageal pain
C. Myocarditis
D. Dissecting aneurysm
E. MVP

12. Non rheumatic MR is increased by:
A. Squatting
B. Standing
C. Isometric hand grip
D. Leg raising
E. Expiration

13. Beta agonist causes:
A. ↑ intracellular calcium
B. ↑ cAMP
C. ↑ Na transport
D. ↓ K
E. Inhibits adenylate cyclase

14. Nicorandil use is recommended in:
A. Angina
B. HT
C. CHF
D. PVD
E. PSVT

15. Patient with HT as increased risk if following are present:
A. Glycosuria
B. Labile HT
C. Grade II retinopathy
D. LVH
E. Alcohol intake

16. Hypertension is most common causative risk factor for:
A. Cardiovascular disease
B. Renal failure
C. Saccular abdominal aneurysm
D. Stroke
E. CHF

17. Drug of choice in CHF with normal sinus rhythm:
A. ACE inhibitor
B. Diuretics
C. Amiodarone
D. LMWH
E. Digitalis

18. PSVT with heart failure is managed by:
A. Esmolol IV
B. Dilzem IV
C. Amiodarone IV
D. Carotid massage
E. Management of CHF

19. ACE inhibitors are contraindicated in:
A. Left renal artery stenosis
B. Dehydration
C. AS
D. Dissecting aneurysm
E. COPD

20. Hypotension with acute MI which is true:
A. Morphine
B. NTG
C. Pain
D. Sweating
E. Tachycardia

9 A,D	10 A,C,D,E	11 A,C,D	12 A,C,D	13 A,B	14 A,B,C	15 A,C,D,E
16 A,B,D,E	17 A,B	18 A,C,D,E	19 B,C	20 C,D,E		

21. Thrombolysis is done in:
A. Non QMI
B. Re infarction in 1 week
C. Hyper acute ECG changes without symptoms
D. Atypical symptoms without ECG changes
E. ↑ing enzymes level

22. TMT after MI is done:
A. After 1 week
B. After 3 weeks
C. If Angina is present
D. Ventricular tachycardia
E. Persistent ST elevation

23. Early angiography is indicated in:
A. CHF
B. PSVT
C. Angina
D. Embolism of coronary artery

24. Pulmonary embolism-significant contribution to diagnosis is provided by:
A. ECG
B. CXR
C. FDP level
D. V/Q scan
E. Venogram

25. Negative predictive value is high in IE with:
A. Echocardiography
B. Blood culture
C. Janeway lesions
D. Splenomegaly
E. Splinter hemorrhage

26. Janeway lesion: true are:
A. Tender
B. Fleeting
C. Blanching
D. Macular
E. Dorsum of hand

27. At high altitude: adaptation are:
A. ↑ V/Q
B. Hypoventilation
C. ↓ diffusion capacity
D. ↓ tidal volume
E. Hyperventilation

28. Pulmonary oedema-causes of hypoxia are:
A. V/Q mismatch
B. ↓ diffusion of gases
C. Capillary leak
D. Constriction of capillaries
E. Wall stress

29. Fatigability in chronic heart failure is caused by:
A. ↓ O_2 in blood
B. ↓ metabolism
C. Stimulation of J receptor in muscle
D. ↓ Cardiac output
E. ↓ AVP

30. Methyldopa interacts significantly with:
A. Haloperidol
B. Levodopa
C. Amlodipine
D. Disopyramide

31. Statins interact with:
A. Warfarin
B. Digoxin
C. Gemfibrozil
D. Oral hypoglycemics

32. Causes of AR:
A. Polyarteritis nodosa
B. Paget's disease
C. Rheumatic MS
D. Mucopolysaccharidoses
E. HT

21 B,C	22 A,B	23 A,C	24 A,B,D,E	25 A,B	26 D	27 A,E
28 A,B,C	29 A,D	30 A,B	31 A,B,C	32 A,B,C,D,E		

33. Activities not advised in patients of chronic sable angina:
A. Cycling
B. Jogging
C. Push ups
D. Moving a static vehicle
E. Sexual activity

34. CHF with normal sinus rhythm caused by ischaemic heart disease drug of choice
A. Digoxin
B. Beta blocker
C. Nitrates
D. Hydralazine
E. Spironolactone

35. In COPD causes of CHF:
A. TR
B. Pulmonary hypertension
C. ↑ work of breathing
D. Hypoxia
E. Intrapulmonary Shunts

36. In patients of congestive cardio myopathy CHF increases with:
A. Myxedema
B. Chest infection
C. AV asynchrony
D. ↑ apoptosis

37. Diagnosis of WPW on ECG is done by:
A. ↑ QRS duration
B. Absent Q waves
C. ↓ PR interval
D. Inverted T waves
E. Delta waves

38. To differentiate PSVT and VT what favours PSVT:
A. RBBB
B. Left axis deviation
C. Presence of p wave
D. Capture beat
E. Reduction by carotid massage

39. Cells seen in atherosclerotic plaque:
A. Platelet
B. Monocytes
C. Histiocytes
D. Smooth muscle cells
E. Eosinophils

40. Theophylline levels are decreased by:
A. Isoniazid
B. Phenytoin
C. Cimetidine
D. Erythromycin

41. Common site of involvement in Takayasu arteritis:
A. Subclavian
B. Internal carotid
C. Renal
D. Aorta
E. Iliac arteries

33 C,D | 34 B,C,E | 35 A,B,C,D | 36 A,B,C,D | 37 C,D,E | 38 A,E | 39 B,D
40 B | 41 A,C,D

PGI 2000 (June)

1. Infant with coarctation of aorta:
- **A.** Hypoplasia of aortic arch and isthmus
- **B.** PDA is present in 2/3rd of cases
- **C.** VSD is seen in 50% of cases
- **D.** Rib notching is seen from 4th to 7th rib
- **E.** LV hypertrophy on ECG is seen

2. Right aortic arch is present in
- **A.** DORV
- **B.** TOF
- **C.** VSD with pulmonary atresia
- **D.** Truncus arteriosus
- **E.** TGA

3. CHF in first week of life is seen in all *except:*
- **A.** VSD
- **B.** PDA
- **C.** Critical PS
- **D.** Critical AS
- **E.** Coarctation of aorta

4. CCP is characterised by all *except:*
- **A.** Kussmaul's Sign
- **B.** Pulsus paradoxus
- **C.** Dip & plateau
- **D.** Increase 'y' descent
- **E.** Respiratory variation in mitral inflow velocities

5. Noonan syndrome is associated with:
- **A.** VSD
- **B.** PS
- **C.** ASD
- **D.** CoA
- **E.** HOCM

6. Common organisms in IV drug abuser endocarditis:
- **A.** Staph aureus
- **B.** Strep viridans
- **C.** Fungi
- **D.** Klebsiella
- **E.** Polymicrobial

7. All are true about TAPVC *except:*
- **A.** Infradiaphragmatic is not associated with obstruction
- **B.** Infradiaphragmatic drains into hepatic vein
- **C.** Supradiaphragmatic type is most common
- **D.** Associated with wide splitting of S_2
- **E.** Figure of eight appearance on chest X-ray

8. Balloon pulmonary valvuloplasty is indicated in all *except:*
- **A.** Valvular PS
- **B.** Dysplastic pulmonary valve
- **C.** Subvalvular pulmonary stenosis
- **D.** Peripheral pulmonary artery stenosis
- **E.** TOF

9. True about CPK level following PTCA:
- **A.** 1% patient leads to myocardial infarction
- **B.** CPK does not increase in PTCA of venous graft
- **C.** Small amount of CPK is generally increased after PTCA
- **D.** 300% increase in CPK is used as criteria for diagnosis of MI
- **E.** Mild elevation of CPK does not affect the prognosis

1 A | 2 A,B,C,D | 3 A,B | 4 B | 5 A,B,C,E | 6 A,B | 7 A,B
8 B,C,E | 9 A,C,D,E

10. Non ionic dye is preferred over ionic dye in following conditions:
A. AMI
B. Hypotension
C. Coronary stenting
D. CHF
E. Heart blocks

11. Aortic Balloon valvuloplasty is often used as a bridge to AVR in following conditions:
A. Patients with severe CHF
B. Critical AS in infant
C. Gradient >100mmHg
D. Pregnant women with critical AS
E. Extremely high operative risk

12. Statements true about IE are:
A. Streptococcus viridans is seen in prosthetic valve endocarditis
B. More than 10% IV drug abusers have fungal infection
C. I/V drug abusers have <5% seronegative blood culture
D. In PVE, 3% have fungal infection
E. In PVE, 10% have culture negative on investigation

13. Which of the following statements are true about AS:
A. Congenital AS may be because of unicuspid/ bicuspid/tricuspid value
B. Male to female ratio is 4:1
C. Area 0.8 cm^2/m^2 represent critical AS
D. Gradient ≥ 75 mmHg indicates critical AS
E. Balloon aortic valvuloplasty can be used successfully in infants

14. Systemic hypertension is labelled as:
A. Neonates systolic BP >80 mmHg
B. 2-4 months >100 mmHg
C. 2-12 years >130/80
D. 2-4 years >120/74
E. Three consecutive reading at three different times at least 30 minutes apart is considered as significant

15. All can be seen in pulmonary embolism *except:*
A. ↑ PCWP in massive pulmonary embolism
B. ↑ RAE
C. $S_1Q_3T_3$ pattern
D. Incomplete RBBB
E. 1st degree AV block

16. Wide splitting of second sound is heard in all *except:*
A. Severe MR with CHF
B. VSD with right to left shunt
C. Moderate MR with normal LV function
D. AR with normal LV function
E. TAPVC

17. Which of the following is not used in patients with AF in WPW syndrome:
A. Digoxin
B. Verapamil
C. Xylocaine
D. Procainamide
E. Flecainide

18. Poor prognostic factors of HOCM are:
A. Frequent VPC
B. Recurrent syncope
C. Age < 30 years
D. Family history of sudden cardiac death
E. Aborted sudden cardiac death
F. Nonsustained VT

19. Seen in MR:
A. ↑ EDV
B. ↑ LV mass
C. ↑ LA pressure
D. ↑ Ejection Fraction
E. ↑ EPSS in normal LV function

20. Lp(a) can be treated by:
A. Estrogen
B. Bezafibrate
C. Statins
D. Clofibrate
E. Stanazolol

10 A,B,D,E 11 A,D,E 12 A,C,D,E 13 A,B,D,E 14 A,E 15 A,E 16 A,B,D
17 A,B,C 18 B,C,D,E,F 19 A,B,D 20 A,B,E

21. Following statements are true about HUTT in Neurocardiogenic syncope:
- **A.** Passive inclination to 60-80°
- **B.** Wait for 10-15 minutes
- **C.** Edrophonium to be given to ↑ response
- **D.** IV isoprenaline used upto 10-20 μg/minute
- **E.** Specificity of test is 90%

22. All are true about ACE inhibitors:
- **A.** Not much effective in blacks
- **B.** Use in bilateral renal artery stenosis
- **C.** Improve insulin sensitivity
- **D.** Regress ventricular hypertrophy
- **E.** Should be started as early as possible after MI

23. α blocker property is seen with:
- **A.** Bisoprolol
- **B.** Metoprolol
- **C.** Labetalol
- **D.** Bucindolol
- **E.** Carvedilol

24. Following statements are true about Marfan syndrome:
- **A.** Positive nitroprusside test
- **B.** X chromosome analysis
- **C.** Hyperflexible joints are seen
- **D.** Aortic root dilatation of more than 5.5 cm is an indication for surgery
- **E.** Cystic medial necrosis is seen pathologically

25. All are true about Takayasu arteritis *except:*
- **A.** Most common in right med subclavian artery
- **B.** Iliofemoral involvement in > 50% cases
- **C.** Auto immune, non infectious, inflammation are the possible etiologies
- **D.** More common in females
- **E.** HT is the common presentation in childrens

26. Following drugs can be used in Prinzmetal angina:
- **A.** β blocker
- **B.** α blocker
- **C.** Ca channel blocker
- **D.** ACE Inhibitors
- **E.** Aspirin

27. Following statements are true about Peri-partum cardiomyopathy:
- **A.** Seen in multiparous lady
- **B.** Generally seen in less than 30 yrs of age
- **C.** More common with twin presentation
- **D.** 50% die because of CHF
- **E.** Most commonly seen in second month of post partum

28. Following are useful in differentiating CCP from RCMP:
- **A.** Pericardial calcification
- **B.** Kussmaul's sign
- **C.** IVC collapse of < 50% on inspiration
- **D.** Pulmonary artery pressure is > 50 mmHg
- **E.** Respiratory variation of mitral inflow velocity

29. Radiation can cause:
- **A.** Restrictive cardiomyopathy
- **B.** MVP
- **C.** CHB
- **D.** Pericarditis
- **E.** CAD

30. VSD is seen in following conditions:
- **A.** Holt Oram syndrome
- **B.** Noonan syndrome
- **C.** Leopard syndrome
- **D.** Myotonic dystrophy
- **E.** Treacher Collins syndrome

31. Following statements are true about atrial fibrillation *except:*
- **A.** Reentry is the mechanism for arrhythmia
- **B.** Ventricular response depends on property of AV node conduction than of SA node
- **C.** Can be successfully ablated in more that 80% of cases
- **D.** Pulmonary veins are one of the possible source of AF origin
- **E.** Class 1B drugs can be used successfully for prevention of recurrence

---

21 A,C,E 22 A,C,D,E 23 C,D,E 24 A,B,D,E 25 A,B 26 B,C 27 A,C,D,E
28 A,B,C,E 29 A,B,C,D,E 30 A,B,E 31 C,E

32. Following statements are true about Procainamide:
- **A.** Causes more prolongation of Action Potential duration than effective refractory period
- **B.** Vasodilatation and hypotension
- **C.** Effective in quinidine resistant arrhythmia
- **D.** Increase serum digoxin level
- **E.** Prolongs QT interval

33. Following statements are true regarding cardiac catheterization:
- **A.** PCWP is always increase in massive pulmonary embolism
- **B.** RA pressure is increase in severe PS
- **C.** a = v wave in ASD
- **D.** Mortality rate is > 2%
- **E.** Upper limit of normal LVEDP is 12

34. True statement regarding dysplastic pulmonary valve:
- **A.** Fleshy and thickened leaflets
- **B.** Normal subvalvular apparatus
- **C.** Normal systolic and diastolic leaflet movement
- **D.** Soft P2
- **E.** Balloon pulmonary valvuloplasty is treatment of choice

35. Asplenia:
- **A.** IVC absent
- **B.** Right isomerism
- **C.** ASD
- **D.** Howell jolly bodies
- **E.** AS

36. Cyanosis:
- **A.** Sulfonamide
- **B.** Aniline dye
- **C.** α tocopherol
- **D.** Cytochrome reductase deficiency
- **E.** Lidocaine toxicity

37. Pericarditis is seen with all *except:*
- **A.** Bretylium
- **B.** Amiodarone
- **C.** Procainamide
- **D.** Methysergide
- **E.** Hydralazine

38. c-TGA is commonly associated with:
- **A.** DORV
- **B.** VSD
- **C.** Left sided Ebstein's anomaly
- **D.** Unroofed coronary sinus
- **E.** High incidence of AV block

39. Athlete's heart syndrome is associated with:
- **A.** ↑ QRS voltage
- **B.** QT interval prolongation
- **C.** Prominent U wave
- **D.** Sinus bradycardia
- **E.** Junctional escape rhythm

40. A2-OS gap in MS is:
- **A.** 60-120 ms
- **B.** 120-240 ms
- **C.** 240-320 ms
- **D.** 40-60 msec

41. Muscle involvement is not seen in which glycogen storage disorder:
- **A.** Type I
- **B.** Type II
- **C.** Type III
- **D.** Type IV

42. Following is characteristic of spondyloarthropathy:
- **A.** Enthesitis
- **B.** Bursitis
- **C.** Urethritis
- **D.** None of the above

43. Ischemic colitis: most commonly involved site is:
- **A.** Splenic flexure
- **B.** Hepatic flexure
- **C.** Rectum
- **D.** Ileum

---

32 B,C,E	33 B,C,E	34 A,B,D	35 B,C,D	36 A,B,C	37 A,B	38 B,C,E
39 A,B,C,D,E	40 A	41 A	42 A	43 A		

44. β blocker causes
A. ↓ Cardiac output
B. ↑ Heart rate
C. ↑ flushing
D. ↓ Lipoprotein(a)

45. Corkscrew oesophagus is seen in:
A. Diffuse esophageal spasm
B. Achalasia cardia
C. Esophagitis
D. None of the above

46. Recurrent hepatic infection in Hepatitis B will show:
A. ↑ IgM antiHBc
B. ↓ IgM antiHBc
C. Decreased bilirubin
D. None of the above

47. Following can be seen in polycythemia vera *except:*
A. Severe spontaneous infection
B. Massive splenomegaly
C. Hyperuricemia
D. Venous or arterial thrombosis

48. Following are seen in Wernicke syndrome *except:*
A. Intention tremor
B. Ophthalmoplegia
C. Global confusion
D. Ataxia

49. Tall R wave in ECG in V_1 is seen in:
A. WPW type A
B. COPD
C. Anteroseptal MI
D. None of the above

50. Atherosclerosis caused by all *except:*
A. H. pylori
B. CMV
C. C. Pneumonia
D. Influenza

51. A patient 40 years of age, BP 90/60 mmHg, PCWP normal, decreased peripheral vascular resistance, decreased cardiac index; diagnosis is:
A. Septic shock
B. C. tamponade
C. Hypovolemic shock
D. Cardiogenic shock

52. Pinta is caused by:
A. T. pallidum
B. T. pallidum pertenue
C. T.pallidum endemicum
D. T.Carateum

53. Hypokalemia causes all *except:*
A. Twitching
B. Seizure
C. Quadriparesis
D. Hemiparesis

54. Disease transmitted by blood transfusion are all *except:*
A. Syphilis
B. CMV
C. Hepatitis B & C
D. Toxoplasmosis

55. Thrombocytopenia with thrombosis occurs in:
A. Myeloproliferative disorder
B. ITP
C. Antiphospholipid antibody syndrome
D. None of the above

56. Bronchoalveolar lavage is helpful in all *except:*
A. Bronchial asthma
B. Hypersensitivity pneumonitis
C. Pulmonary alveolar proteinosis
D. Diffuse alveolar haemorrhage syndrome

44 A 45 A 46 A 47 A 48 A 49 A 50 D 51 A 52 D 53 D 54 D 55 C 56 A

57. Young female with fever cold antibody >250 IU, reticulocyte count 1.5%, diagnosis is:
A. Mycoplasma infection
B. Infectious mononucleosis
C. CMV
D. SLE

58. VSD with secondary pulmonary stenosis all true *except:*
A. Valvular PS
B. Infundibular PS
C. Pulmonary stenosis regresses after surgery
D. Katz-Watchel phenomenon can be seen

59. HELLP syndrome include all *except:*
A. Hemolysis
B. Low platelet
C. Elevated liver enzyme
D. Pancreatitis

60. 40 year old male, TLC 40000, DLC P59 L35, M5 platelet 325000 joint pain and fever, rashes on mucocutaneous region, genitalia, family history in first degree relatives positive diagnostic investigation is:
A. Anti nuclear antibody
B. a glucosidase estimation in plasma
C. Plasma homocysteine
D. None of the above

61. Unconjugated hyperbilirubinaemia:
A. Dubin Johnson syndrome
B. Crigler Najjar Syndrome
C. Rotor syndrome
D. Familial intrahepatic cholestasis

62. HIV grade I is:
A. CDC category disease
B. Persistent generalized lymphadenopathy
C. Acute HIV syndrome
D. Asymptomatic

63. Which is a mitochondrial disease?
A. Kearns sayre syndrome
B. MERRF
C. MELAS
D. Mycoclonic epilepsy
E. All of the above

64. In gout arthritis, drug not used is:
A. Piroxicam
B. Ibuprofen
C. Aspirin
D. Naproxen

65. Common complication of mumps in children:
A. Aseptic meningitis
B. Orchitis
C. Myocarditis
D. Nephritis

66. In COPD, lung function test: all are true *except:*
A. ↓ diffusion capacity
B. ↓ FEV1
C. ↓ Residual volume
D. None of the above

67. 7 month pregnancy with thyrotoxicosis, treatment of choice:
A. Surgery
B. Radioactive iodine
C. Propylthiouracil
D. Induction of labor

68. P wave absent in:
A. AF
B. Atrial tachycardia
C. Sinus nodal re-entry
D. CHB

69. Morphine withdrawal syndrome appears after– hours after last dose
A. 2-4 hrs
B. 8-12 hrs
C. 24-36 hrs
D. 48-72 hrs

57 A 58 A 59 D 60 B 61 B 62 C 63 C 64 C 65 A 66 C 67 C 68 A 69 B

70. Octreotide is:
A. Somatostatin
B. Somatostatin analogue
C. Growth hormone
D. IGF-1

71. HLA B27 all are associated *except:*
A. Ankylosing spondylosis
B. Reiter syndrome
C. IDDM
D. Psoriasis

72. Good control of hypertension, decreases incidence of:
A. Stroke
B. CAD
C. Renal failure
D. CHF

73. Patient with ST elevation in V1-V6 with S3 gallop with B/L crepts with H/R of 140/mm with irregular pulse, treatment of choice:
A. Digoxin
B. Amiodarone
C. β blocker
D. Diltiazem

74. Diabetic autonomic neuropathy all are true *except:*
A. Constipation
B. Bradycardia
C. Postural hypertension
D. Impotence

75. In coarctation of aorta, cause of death are all *except:*
A. Infective endocarditis
B. CHF
C. MI
D. Stroke

76. Which drug is safe in renal failure?
A. INH
B. Vancomycin
C. Pyrazinamide
D. Gentamicin

77. Sensory lose with pain in ulnar side of foot with plantar flexor and absent ankle jerk, diagnosis is:
A. S1 radiculopathy
B. L5 radiculopathy
C. Common peroneal nerve involvement
D. Tibial nerve involvement

78. All are salt wasting nephropathy *except:*
A. Ch. Pyelonephritis
B. Tubulointerstitial disease
C. Medullary cystic disease
D. Ch. glomerulonephritis

79. p-ANCA is present in all *except:*
A. Polyarteritis nodosa
B. Wegner's granulomatosis
C. Chrugstrauss syndrome
D. Good pasture syndrome

80. All drugs causes hepatic granuloma *except:*
A. Sulphonamide
B. Allopurinol
C. Quinidine
D. Amiodarone

70 B 71 C 72 A 73 A 74 B 75 C 76 A 77 A 78 D 79 B 80 C

PGI 1999

1. **Coronary ischemia is caused by:**
   A. Cisplatin
   B. Cocaine
   C. 5FU
   D. Verapamil
   E. Nifedipine

2. **Activity matching with ≥ 3 MET**
   A. Raking leaves
   B. Golf
   C. Exterior carpentry
   D. Strip and make bed
   E. Clean window

3. **Central cyanosis occurs with:**
   A. Reduced hemoglobin >3 gm%
   B. Reduced hemoglobin >5 gm%
   C. Saturation <90%
   D. Saturation <85%
   E. Methaemoglobin > 0.5 gm%

4. **Which increases with inspiration:**
   A. RVS3
   B. RVS4
   C. MR
   D. TR
   E. LVS3

5. **TEE is better than TTE in:**
   A. MS
   B. Left atrial Appendage clot
   C. Poor echo window
   D. Emphysema
   E. LV clot

6. **True regarding Constrictive pericarditis are:**
   A. Intrapericardial pressure is not transmitted to chambers
   B. Equalization of pressure in all cardiac chambers
   C. Most common cause in India is tuberculosis
   D. Dip and plateau pattern
   E. 'X'-descent prominent 'Y'-descent blunted

7. **ECG findings in acute pulmonary embolism:**
   A. S1Q3T3
   B. Incomplete RBBB
   C. In V1 R more than S
   D. LAHB
   E. Prominent S wave in V6

8. **ECG in RVMI in presence of IWMI:**
   A. ST elevation in V1 and ST depression in V2
   B. 1mm Q wave in V4 R
   C. RBBB
   D. 2nd degree heart block
   E. ST elevation in lead 1 and AVL

9. **Indications of termination of TMT are:**
   A. Abnormal increase of systolic blood pressure > 240 mm Hg
   B. Grade 1 chest pain
   C. > 2 mm ST elevation in non Q wave leads
   D. Ataxia
   E. Ischemic ST depression = 2 mm

1 A,B,C 2 A,B,C 3 B,D,E 4 A,B,D 5 B,C,D 6 A,B,C,D 7 A,B,C
8 A,B,C 9 A,C,D

10. Hemodynamic data in low cardiac output state, true are:
A. Mixed venous oxygen decreased
B. SVR decreased in presence of MR
C. PCWP decreased in hypovolumic shock
D. PCWP grossly elevated
E. RA and RV pressure elevated

11. Torsades de pointes true are:
A. Rate 200-250 per minute
B. QTC always prolonged
C. QTC may be normal
D. IV magnesium is treatment of choice
E. Overdrive Pacing can also be used

12. In High risk perfusion imaging after acute MI is indicated by:
A. Decreased lung uptake
B. High lung uptake
C. LV cavity dilatation
D. Visualisation of RV at rest
E. Large perfusion defect

13. Prominent left parasternal heave is present in:
A. PPH
B. Pulmonary stenosis
C. RV pressure overload
D. RV volume overload
E. Severe MR

14. Mortality in CHF is inversely related to:
A. Norepinephrine
B. ANP
C. Renin
D. Cardiac output
E. EF

15. All are true regarding Lignocaine:
A. Given I/V bolus 60 mg to terminate VT
B. Cimetidine reduces clearance
C. β blockers can decrease Lignocaine concentration
D. Can cause neuropsychiatric manifestations
E. Metabolized by liver

16. Treatment of endless loop tachycardia:
A. Magnet application
B. Increase post ventricular atrial refractory period
C. Decreased post ventricular atrial refractory period
D. Ablation
E. Shorter A-V interval

17. Clinical feature of PPH:
A. Raynaud's phenomenon
B. Cyanosis
C. Clubbing
D. LV enlargement
E. Left to right shunt

18. Pregnancy is contraindicated in:
A. Eisenmenger's syndrome
B. PPH
C. TOF
D. ASD
E. VSD

19. Regarding JNC 6 true statements are:
A. Optimal blood pressure is 120/80 mmHg
B. Total stages are three
C. Used to assess HT in >18 years of age
D. Drug treatment is required in all stages
E. Diabetes is not considered as risk factor

20. Autosomal dominant condition:
A. Holt Oram syndrome
B. Noonan syndrome
C. Myotonia dystrophica
D. Duchene's dystrophy
E. Wilson's disease

21. Treatment of hypoxic spells are all *except*:
A. Propranolol
B. NTG
C. Nifedipine
D. Methoxamine
E. Morphine

---

10 A,C 11 A,C,D,E 12 B,D,E 13 A,B,C,E 14 B,D,E 15 A,B,D,E 16 A,B,E
17 A,B,C 18 A,B,C 19 A,B,C 20 A,B,C 21 B,C

22. Goose neck deformity is found in:
- **A.** Ostium primum ASD
- **B.** Complete AV canal defect
- **C.** Ebstein anomaly
- **D.** Truncus arteriosus
- **E.** TGA

23. Indication of surgery in VSD:
- **A.** Small supracristal subaortic VSD with small AR
- **B.** Intractable CHF
- **C.** PVR less than 12 woods
- **D.** Shunt 1.5:1
- **E.** Failure to thrive

24. Coarctation of aorta true are:
- **A.** PDA in 2/3 of cases
- **B.** VSD in 1/3 of cases
- **C.** Tausig Bing anomaly can be associated
- **D.** 40% of patients without associated anomalies develop CHF
- **E.** Most commonly CHF occurs during infancy

25. Regarding aortic stenosis true statements are:
- **A.** Male: female 4:1
- **B.** Critical AS is 0.8 cm^2/m^2 body surface area
- **C.** Valve morphology Unicuspid > bicuspid > tricuspid
- **D.** Mortality after onset of angina is within 5 years
- **E.** BAV is preferred treatment modality for adult severe aortic stenosis

26. Beat to beat variation in the blood pressure is seen in:
- **A.** AF
- **B.** MAT
- **C.** CHB
- **D.** Idioventricular rhythm
- **E.** Second degree AV block Wencheback

27. Pulmonary artery saturation more than systemic artery saturation is found in:
- **A.** d-TGA
- **B.** Taussig Bing Anomaly
- **C.** Truncus arteriosus
- **D.** LTGA
- **E.** DORV

28. Kearns Sayre syndrome true are:
- **A.** Conduction blocks
- **B.** Seizures
- **C.** Pigmentary retinopathy
- **D.** Ophthalmoplegia
- **E.** Cardiomyopathy

29. Indication of BMV all *except:*
- **A.** Loud S1
- **B.** Presence of LVS3
- **C.** Short A2-OS interval
- **D.** Pliable valve
- **E.** LA thrombus

30. S1 is loud in:
- **A.** Sinus tachycardia
- **B.** Short PR interval
- **C.** Mitral stenosis
- **D.** MR
- **E.** Aortic stenosis

31. BAV can be done in:
- **A.** Patient with critical AS with cardiogenic shock
- **B.** As bridge to aortic valve replacement
- **C.** In patients having associated CAD
- **D.** Patient with severe CHF
- **E.** Critical AS with pregnancy

32. Prosthetic valve endocarditis: true statements are:
- **A.** After 1 year most common cause is streptococcus viridans
- **B.** In early post-operative period; common cause is coagulase negative staphylococci.
- **C.** Fungal endocarditis occurs in more than 10% of patients
- **D.** Antibiotic treatment required is for 4-6 weeks
- **E.** Unstable prosthesis is a relative indication for surgery

---

22 A,B　23 A,B,E　24 C,E　25 A,D　26 A,C,D　27 A,B,C　28 A,C,D,E
29 A,B,E　30 A,B,C　31 A,B,D,E　32 A,B,D

33. Risk factor for CAD are:
A. HDL <35 mg%
B. HDL >35 mg%
C. Serum triglyceride >200 mg%
D. LDL cholesterol without CAD > 160 mg%
E. Estrogen

34. In patients having PCWP 18 mm Hg, LVEDP 25 mm Hg, Blood pressure of 90/60 mm Hg and cardiac index <1.6; diagnosis is:
A. ARDS
B. Eisenmengers syndrome
C. Cardiogenic shock
D. Pulmonary embolism
E. Hypovolemia

35. Following drug is safe in renal failure:
A. INH
B. Vancomycin
C. Flucytosine
D. Cotrimoxazole

36. HOCM true statements are:
A. Increased End diastolic volume
B. Increased myocardial stiffness
C. Increased wall stress
D. Increased LV mass
E. Increased end systolic volume

37. Pre-capillary hypertension is present in:
A. PTE
B. MS
C. Cortriatriatum
D. Pulmonary venous obstructive disease
E. COPD

38. Prominent LVS4 is present in all *except:*
A. PPH
B. MS with PAH
C. ASD Eisenmenger's
D. VSD Eisenmenger's
E. LV apical aneurysm

39. True about Loop diuretics:
A. Causes Hypokalemia
B. Acts on Na^+-K^+ 2Cl transport
C. Acts mainly on ascending thick limb of loop of Henle
D. Frusemide contraindicated in patients having sulpha allergy
E. Acts on thin descending limb of loop of Henle

40. Pheochromocytoma causes:
A. Pigmentation
B. Pallor
C. Palpitation
D. Orthostatic hypertension
E. Weight loss

33 A,C,D 34 C 35 A 36 B,D 37 A,E 38 E 39 A,B,C,D
40 B,C,D,E

PGI 1998

1. Shone syndrome: which of the following are seen:
- **A.** Coarctation
- **B.** Parachute mitral valve
- **C.** PS
- **D.** ASD
- **E.** Tricuspid atresia
- **F.** Supravalvular mitral ring

2. Echo features of CCP are:
- **A.** Pericardial thickening
- **B.** Septal bounce
- **C.** Abrupt increase in RV volume with decrease in LV volume on inspiration
- **D.** IVC collapse of > 50%

3. Cardiac tamponade true are:
- **A.** Stroke volume is reduced
- **B.** Atrial and venous pressures are reduced
- **C.** Bradycardia in setting of pulsus paradoxus
- **D.** Despite ↓ S.V., BP may be maintained

4. Beat to beat variation in blood pressure is seen in:
- **A.** VT
- **B.** VF
- **C.** Pulsus alternans
- **D.** Heart block

5. JVP:
- **A.** 'a' wave due to LA Contraction
- **B.** 'a' wave due to RA Contraction
- **C.** 'v' wave in RV diastole
- **D.** 'y' descent when TV opens
- **E.** 'c' wave d/t abrupt opens up of AV valve

6. Reverse splitting of S_2 is not seen in:
- **A.** Complete LBBB
- **B.** Hypertension
- **C.** WPW type A
- **D.** LV paced beat

7. HOCM murmur increases with:
- **A.** Sudden standing
- **B.** Valsalva strain phase
- **C.** β agonist
- **D.** Isometric hand grip
- **E.** Leg raising
- **F.** Squatting

8. Double apical impulse is seen in:
- **A.** HOCM
- **B.** LV aneurysm
- **C.** MR
- **D.** AR
- **E.** VSD

9. Pericarditis is common in:
- **A.** Tumor
- **B.** TB
- **C.** Viral
- **D.** Injury

1 A,B,F 2 A,B,C 3 A,D 4 A,B,C,D 5 B,D 6 C,D 7 A,B,C
8 A,B 9 A,B,C,D

10. Chest X-ray in MS not seen:
- **A.** Cephalisation of venous circulation
- **B.** Cardiomegaly with straightening of left heart border
- **C.** Acute carinal angle
- **D.** Left atrial enlargement
- **E.** LVH

11. Cardiogenic shock occurs when:
- **A.** > 40% of loss of myocardium
- **B.** 100% LAD obstruction
- **C.** Unstable angina present
- **D.** MR due to papillary muscle necrosis

12. IABP is not used in:
- **A.** AR with arrhythmias
- **B.** Post op LV dysfunction
- **C.** To increase diastolic coronary flow
- **D.** Aortic dissection

13. True about IABP:
- **A.** Femoral artery route and placed distal to subclavian artery
- **B.** Augments systolic BP
- **C.** Decreases SVR
- **D.** Increases CO
- **E.** Helpful in AR

14. Increased risk of death in HOCM is associated with:
- **A.** Age <30 year
- **B.** Severe LVOT gradient
- **C.** Family h/o SCD
- **D.** Massive hypertrophy

15. SCD risk is increase in:
- **A.** AR
- **B.** MR
- **C.** DCMP
- **D.** Amyloidosis
- **E.** CCP

16. Single S_2 heard in:
- **A.** TOF
- **B.** Pulmonary atresia
- **C.** VSD
- **D.** AR
- **E.** Eisenmenger's syndrome

17. CXR in coarctation of aorta shows:
- **A.** LV enlargement
- **B.** Narrowing of aortic arch
- **C.** Enlarged pulmonary artery
- **D.** 'E' sign on barium filled esophagus
- **E.** Rib notching

18. Rib notching is seen in:
- **A.** Aortoarteritis
- **B.** B-P collaterals
- **C.** Pulmonary AV fistula
- **D.** SVC & IVC obstruction
- **E.** Neurofibromatosis

19. Ostium primum ASD: all are true *except:*
- **A.** Right → Left shunt at atrial level
- **B.** RVH & RAD on EKG
- **C.** Cleft in AML
- **D.** AV conduction defect
- **E.** Gooseneck deformity on cath (AP view)

20. LVS_3 increases in:
- **A.** Inspiration
- **B.** Leg raising
- **C.** Isometric handgrip
- **D.** Tachycardia

21. Opening snap is heard in:
- **A.** Rheumatic MS
- **B.** Rheumatic MR
- **C.** DORV
- **D.** HOCM
- **E.** VSD
- **F.** Ebstein's anomaly
- **G.** TS

10 C,E	11 A,B,D	12 A,D	13 A,C,D	14 A,C	15 C,D	16 A,B,E
17 A,D,E	18 A,B,E	19 A,B	20 B,C	21 A,B,E,F,G		

22. Counter-clockwise rotation occurs in:
A. Single atrium
B. Pulmonary atresia
C. AV canal defects
D. DORV with PS

23. True about AR in VSD is:
A. 25-30% of outlet VSD
B. 8-10% are trabecular VSD
C. Herniation of right coronary & non coronary cusp
D. Loses of support of right coronary cusp
E. Defective development of non coronary cusp

24. Ductus dependant circulation is:
A. Interrupted aortic arch
B. TGA with intact IVS and IAS
C. PA with intact IVS
D. DORV

25. Juxtaposed atrial appendages are seen in:
A. TOF
B. Tricuspid atresia
C. C-TGA (anatomically corrected TGA)
D. Pulmonary atresia

26. Presystolic pulsation of liver is seen in:
A. TR
B. PS
C. CCP
D. Right sided restrictive cardiomyopathy
E. TS

27. DC shock (defibrillation) which is true:
A. Current is DC
B. Duration is 50 msec
C. Paddle size in 10-13cm
D. Pressure on paddle is 2.5lb
E. Always should be done at end expiration (to minimize transthoracic impendence)

28. Cystic medial necrosis causing CAD in:
A. Marfan's syndrome
B. TOF
C. Behcet's syndrome
D. DORV

29. Complication of small PDA:
A. CHF
B. IE
C. Recurrent chest infection
D. PAH

30. Difference in BP between right and left arm in:
A. AR
B. Valvular AS
C. Coarctation of aorta
D. Aberrant subclavian artery
E. Aortoarteritis

31. Digitalis toxicity causes:
A. Vertigo
B. Yellow vision
C. ST ↓ in all leads
D. QT prolongation

32. Digitalis does not cause:
A. 1°HB common
B. Mobitz type II block
C. Bundle branch block
D. Junctional premature complexes
E. Paroxysmal junctional tachycardia

33. Equation of diastolic pressure of all chambers of heart is seen in:
A. CCP
B. Restrictive CMP
C. EMF
D. DCMP

34. Pulsus paradoxus seen in:
A. CCP
B. COPD
C. Rest CMP
D. DCMP
E. Absence of pericardium

22 A,C,D	23 C,D,E	24 A,B,C	25 B,C	26 E	27 A,B,C,D,E	28 A
29 B	30 C,D,E	31 A,B,C	32 B,C	33 A	34 A,B,C	

35. CPR is not useful in:
- **A.** Pulmonary embolism
- **B.** VF
- **C.** Chest wall deformity
- **D.** Cardiac tamponade
- **E.** Pacing failure

36. HDL is not decreased by:
- **A.** Smoking
- **B.** Exercise
- **C.** Fibric acid derivatives
- **D.** Stanozolol
- **E.** Probucol

37. WPW syndrome: which is not true?
- **A.** 0.7-3.5/1000 in healthy population
- **B.** Male > female
- **C.** Increased frequency of arrhythmia with age
- **D.** Right sided necessary pathway commonest
- **E.** Majority have normal CVS

38. Myxomas of heart; which is not true:
- **A.** 86% in LA
- **B.** 50% sporadic
- **C.** Familial myxoma is autosomal recessive 70% in male
- **D.** 70% occurs in female
- **E.** 30-50% of all cardiac tumors

39. Which of the following are useful for cardioplegia?
- **A.** Hypothermia
- **B.** Hyperthermia
- **C.** Potassium permanganate
- **D.** Infusion of cardioplegia solution from aortic side

40. CT ratio on CXR: which is true:
- **A.** Assessed in PA view
- **B.** RV enlargement easily seen
- **C.** Most sensitive for LV enlargement
- **D.** Sequential films are not useful
- **E.** CTR > 50% is abnormal

41. Syncope associated with:
- **A.** Hypoglycemia
- **B.** CA myxoma
- **C.** Autonomic insufficiency
- **D.** Hypercarbia
- **E.** Alcohol

42. In mucocutaneous lymph node syndrome seen:
- **A.** Polymorphous vesicular rash on trunk
- **B.** Cervical lymph node enlargement
- **C.** Erythema of hand and feet
- **D.** Purulent conjunctivitis

43. Wrong about contrast medial nephrotoxicity:
- **A.** Increase in DM
- **B.** Increase in MM
- **C.** Non ionic dye more nephrotoxic than ionic
- **D.** Pre-catheterization hydration has no role to play
- **E.** Nifedipine given pre procedure decreases incidence

44. Dermatomyositis which is true:
- **A.** Heliotrope rash
- **B.** Photosensitivity
- **C.** Asymmetrical proximal muscle weakness
- **D.** Elevated muscle enzymes

45. High dose immunoglobulins given in:
- **A.** Kawasaki's disease
- **B.** Guillian Barre syndrome
- **C.** ITP
- **D.** Myocarditis

46. Opsoclonus is seen in:
- **A.** Neuroblastoma
- **B.** Nephroblastoma
- **C.** Ovarian Ca
- **D.** Breast Ca
- **E.** Bronchogenic Ca

35 A,D	36 B,C	37 D	38 BC	39 A,C,D	40 A,C	41 A,B,C
42 B	43 C,D,E	44 ABD	45 ABC	46 ADE		

47. Behcet's syndrome which are true:
A. Iritis
B. HLA B27
C. Arthritis
D. Pulmonary embolism

48. Direct Coombs test is positive in:
A. Hodgkin's lymphoma
B. Leukemia
C. Hemolytic anemia
D. Idiopathic thrombocytopenia

49. HTLV-I causes:
A. TSP
B. AIDS
C. SSPE
D. Burkitts lymphoma
E. Cutaneous T cell lymphomas

50. Microscopic polyangiitis: which of the following is true?
A. p-ANCA is positive
B. Glomerulonephritis is very rare
C. Medium sized artery involvement
D. Lung is spared

51. Transplant rejection; which is true:
A. Humoral immunity involved in hyperacute rejection
B. Cellular component
C. Cyclosporine causes decrease endothelin
D. Mycophenolate increases atherosclerosis

52. Botulism which are true:
A. Diarrhoea
B. Third nerve palsy
C. Pupillary abnormality
D. Honey is protective

53. Food poisoning due to preformed toxins:
A. Bacillus cereus
B. Cholera
C. Clostridium perfringens
D. Salmonella

54. Lyme disease: which of the following are true?
A. Heart block is uncommon
B. Arthritis is the common manifestation
C. Caused by Borrelia burgdorferi
D. Drug of choice is doxycycline

55. Plasmapheresis can be used as treatment in:
A. GBS
B. Hemochromatosis
C. Waldenstrom's macroglobulinemia
D. Multiple myeloma

56. True about Cheyne-stokes breathing is:
A. Cerebellar hemorrhage
B. Brainstem hemorrhage
C. Severe CHF
D. Sleep apnea syndrome
E. Cortical lesion

57. Morphine useful in acute LVF by:
A. Venodilatation
B. Arteriolar dilation
C. Decreased respiratory rate
D. Sedation

58. Acromegaly which are true:
A. Spinal canal stenosis
B. Decreased incidence of colonic cancer
C. Heart size normal
D. Macroadenoma

59. Cryoglobulinaemia is seen in:
A. Malaria
B. Syphilis
C. Hepatitis A
D. Hepatitis C

47 A	48 ABC	49 A	50 A	51 A	52 C	53 A
54 C	55 ACD	56 BCDE	57 A	58 D	59 D	

60. Seen with ageing:
A. Increased total body fat
B. Decrease BP
C. Decrease ADH
D. Increase total body water

61. Absent ankle jerk with up going planters is seen in:
A. SACD
B. Friedrichs ataxia
C. Brown Sequard syndrome
D. Cauda-equina syndrome

62. True about adult polycystic kidney disease:
A. Chromosome 15
B. Berry aneurysms presence is criteria for diagnosis
C. Colonic diverticulosis
D. Mitral stenosis

63. True about crescentric glomerulonephritis is:
A. Type II commonest in India
B. SLE
C. Cyclophosphamide causes thrombosis
D. Wire loop lesions have best prognosis

64. Classification basis of porphyrias:
A. Erythropoiesis
B. Photosensitivity
C. Neurological
D. Hematological

65. Hemolytic anemia:
A. Tauri disease
B. Glucose-6 P deficiency
C. Hexaminidase deficiency
D. Numan Pick's disease

66. Protein losing enteropathy seen in:
A. Whipples disease
B. Abetalipoproteinaemia
C. Lymphoma
D. Severe anemia

67. Indications for closed tube thoracostomy:
A. Pleural fluid pH >7.2
B. Pleural fluid leucocyte count < 500
C. Pus cells + in pleural fluid
D. Bacteria + in pleural fluid

68. All are dystonias *except:*
A. Writers cramp
B. Hemifacial spasm
C. Gilles de la tourette syndrome
D. Tandine dyskinesia

60 A 61 B 62 C 63 B 64 B 65 A 66 A 67 C 68 C

Jaipur 2004

1. **Narrow PR interval is seen in all *except:***
   - **A.** WPW syndrome
   - **B.** Carditis
   - **C.** Low atrial pacemaker
   - **D.** Infant < 1 year

2. **Normal PR interval is:**
   - **A.** < 1
   - **B.** 1-1.6
   - **C.** 1.6-2.0
   - **D.** > 2.0

3. **Dome and dart p in V1 is seen in:**
   - **A.** Ectopic LA rhythm
   - **B.** Ectopic RA rhythm
   - **C.** Tricuspid valve dysplasia
   - **D.** Uhl's anomaly

4. **Collapsing pulse is seen in all *except:***
   - **A.** Pregnancy
   - **B.** Anemia
   - **C.** AR
   - **D.** AS with AR

5. **True about P is all *except:***
   - **A.** P terminal force in V1 > 0.04 msec
   - **B.** P mitrale is classically seen in lead II
   - **C.** Tall bifid p with 2nd hump larger is suggestive of RAE
   - **D.** Normal duration of P is 0.06s

6. **All of the following can bee seen in hyperkalemia *except:***
   - **A.** Wide QRS
   - **B.** Increase QT interval
   - **C.** Tenting of T with ST elevation
   - **D.** Decrease height of P wave

7. **Best noninvasive screening for CAD is done by:**
   - **A.** EBCT
   - **B.** Multislice CT
   - **C.** MRI
   - **D.** Angioscopy

8. **Bisferians pulse is best palpated in:**
   - **A.** Carotid
   - **B.** Femoral
   - **C.** Brachial
   - **D.** Radial

9. **HOCM gradient in increased by all *except:***
   - **A.** Increase preload
   - **B.** Decrease afterload
   - **C.** Valsalva maneuver
   - **D.** Increase contractility

10. **Brockenbrough phenomenon is:**
    - **A.** Decrease systolic pressure in post-ectopic beat
    - **B.** Decrease pulse pressure in post ectopic beat
    - **C.** Decrease diastolic pressure in post ectopic beat
    - **D.** Decrease aortic systolic pressure in post ectopic beat

1 B 2 B 3 A 4 D 5 C 6 B 7 A 8 A 9 A 10 B

11. Septal ablation with alcohol in HOCM: true is:
- **A.** For symptomatic benefit in resting gradient > 30 mm Hg in symptomatic patients
- **B.** For symptomatic benefit in resting gradient > 50 mm Hg in symptomatic patients
- **C.** Decrease arrhythmias
- **D.** For all provocable gradients

12. Gradient depends on all *except:*
- **A.** Site of hypertrophy
- **B.** Severity of hypertrophy
- **C.** Increase adrenergic activity
- **D.** Increase peripheral resistance

13. Loud P2 in Eisenmenger's syndrome is seen in all *except:*
- **A.** Single ventricle
- **B.** DORV
- **C.** Truncus arteriosus
- **D.** c-TGA

14. Wide S2 is heard in all *except:*
- **A.** AS
- **B.** PS
- **C.** Eisenmenger's syndrome
- **D.** MR

15. Fixed S2 is heard in all *except:*
- **A.** RV failure
- **B.** Pulmonary embolism
- **C.** PS
- **D.** TAPVC

16. For split S2 to be audible, A2-P2 interval should be:
- **A.** 0.01 sec
- **B.** 0.02 sec
- **C.** 0.2 sec
- **D.** 0.04 sec

17. Vasodilator imaging is done with all *except:*
- **A.** Adenosine
- **B.** Dipyridamole
- **C.** Dobutamine
- **D.** Dopamine

18. Adenosine is used for treatment for:
- **A.** Pulmonary hypertension
- **B.** DCMP
- **C.** Angina
- **D.** Myocarditis

19. Drug used in pulmonary hypertension are all *except:*
- **A.** Sildenafil
- **B.** NO
- **C.** PGI_2
- **D.** All of the above

20. Moderate AS (valvular), with peak instant gradient on doppler is in:
- **A.** Early systole
- **B.** Mid systole
- **C.** Late systole
- **D.** Equal in all

21. Gallaverdin's phenomenon is:
- **A.** Valvular AS, any etiology
- **B.** Atherosclerotic AS
- **C.** Subvalvular AS
- **D.** Supravalvular AS

22. Most common cause of CHF at birth is:
- **A.** Hypoplastic left heart syndrome
- **B.** Preductal coarctation
- **C.** TGA
- **D.** TAPVC

23. First episode of acute RF, echo shows all *except:*
- **A.** MS
- **B.** MR
- **C.** Pleural effusion
- **D.** Nodular swelling of mitral valve

11 A 12 B 13 C 14 A 15 B 16 B 17 D 18 A 19 D 20 B 21 B 22 A 23 A

24. Marfan's syndrome: Most specific criteria is:
A. Increase homocysteine
B. Musculoskeletal defects
C. Aorto-annular dilatation
D. Lens subluxation on slit lamp examination

25. Which of the following is best tolerated on pregnancy:
A. MR/AR
B. MS
C. AS
D. PAH

26. Mitral stenosis with pulmonary edema is most likely at:
A. 16-20 weeks
B. 28 weeks
C. Full term
D. Immediately post delivery

27. Beta blockers causes all *except:*
A. Decrease heart rate
B. Decrease contractility
C. Decrease size
D. Decrease arrhythmia

28. Increase survival in post MI LV dysfunction is seen with:
A. Beta blockers
B. Sotalol
C. Aspirin
D. Amiodarone

29. Treatment for NSTEMI includes all *except:*
A. Thrombolysis
B. Antiplatelets
C. Beta blockers
D. Anticoagulants

30. TIMI-3 flow within 90 minutes is achieved maximum with:
A. Prehospital thrombolysis
B. Half thrombolysis + half GpIIb/IIIa inhibitor
C. Half thrombolysis + full GpIIb/IIIa inhibitor
D. Full thrombolysis + full GpIIb/IIIa inhibitor

31. Protocol used for Abciximab include all *except:*
A. Without PCI (bolus + 2 hour infusion)
B. Bolus + 12 hour infusion followed by PCI
C. Bolus + 12 hour infusion starting 1 hour before PCI
D. Waiting for PCI

32. Oral GpIIb/IIIa inhibitors are all *except:*
A. Orafiban
B. Sibrafiban
C. Lamofiban
D. Xemolifiban

33. Mechanism of action of clopidogrel is:
A. Inhibiting ADP receptor
B. Inhibiting thrombin receptor
C. Inhibit thromboxane A2 synthesis
D. Inhibit GpIIb/IIIa receptors

34. Effective platelet inhibition for GpIIb/IIIa inhibitors requires what percentage of receptor blockage?
A. < 50%
B. 50-80%
C. > 80%
D. 100%

35. Pleotropic effects of statins include all *except:*
A. Increase endothelin
B. Increase EDRF
C. Decrease PAI -1
D. Decrease fibrinogen

36. Maximum cholesterol reduction with statin is:
A. 35-45%
B. 25-35%
C. 45-55%
D. 55-65%

24 C 25 A 26 B 27 C 28 A 29 A 30 C 31 C 32 C 33 A 34 C 35 A 36 A

37. Which is not a secondary trial?
A. Post CABG
B. WOSCOPS
C. LIPID
D. CARE

38. Normal LDL cholesterol were used in which trial?
A. CARE
B. WOSCOPS
C. AFCAPS
D. 4S

39. RVH in TGA at birth is defined by:
A. Monomorphic R in V1
B. T upright in V1 after 1 week
C. R/S < 1 in V6
D. Incomplete RBBB

40. Decrease of which of the following indicates increase CAD mortality?
A. HDL
B. LDL
C. IDL
D. VLDL

41. Increase of which of the following increases mortality?
A. Small dense LDL
B. Large buoyant LDL
C. Apo A
D. HDL

42. All of the following are true about syndrome X *except:*
A. Hypertension
B. Increase triglycerides
C. Overt diabetes mellitus
D. Abdominal obesity

43. NIDDM: true are all *except:*
A. Aspirin reverses platelet aggregation
B. Risk of CAD doubled
C. Increase waist-hip ratio
D. Increase blood glucose

44. Equivalent of CAD is:
A. > 2 risk factors without CAD; 10 year risk = 10-20%
B. PVD
C. Abdominal aortic aneurysm
D. DM

45. Cholesterol content of egg is:
A. 100 mg%
B. 200 mg%
C. 70 mg%
D. 400 mg%

46. Monounsaturated and saturated fatty acids are best found in:
A. Coconut
B. Nuts
C. Fish oil
D. Fruits

47. PEP/LVET in failing heart is:
A. Increased
B. Decreased
C. Same
D. Initially increased and then decreases

48. EECP: true are all *except:*
A. Increase NO
B. Increase VEGF
C. Increase ANP
D. Increase endothelin

49. Tricuspid valve is histopathologically involved in what percentage of cases of RHD?
A. < 70%
B. 50%
C. 30%
D. > 70%

37 B 38 A 39 B 40 A 41 A 42 C 43 A 44 A 45 C 46 A 47 A 48 D 49 C

50. Which of the following vitamin is not useful for CAD?
A. Carotene
B. Vitamin B1
C. Vitamin C
D. Vitamin E

51. Shone syndrome: all are true *except:*
A. PDA
B. CoA
C. Parachute mitral valve
D. Subaortic stenosis

52. Scimitar syndrome has all of the following *except:*
A. Right lower lobe atelectasis
B. Ostium primum ASD
C. Mediastinal shift to right
D. PAPVC

53. PA dilatation in chest X ray is seen in all *except:*
A. Pulmonary valve stenosis
B. Absent pulmonary valve stenosis
C. Infundibular pulmonary stenosis
D. Large left to right shunt

54. All of the following are true about rib notching *except:*
A. Uncommon in aortoarteritis
B. Present in preductal coarctation
C. Classical BT shunt is unilaterally on opposite side can cause it
D. Present unilaterally in aberrant right subclavian artery

55. Infective endocarditis is least common in:
A. Large VSD
B. Small PDA
C. Severe MR
D. Bicuspid aortic valve with mild AS

56. All of the following are high risk markers in acute coronary syndrome *except:*
A. CD-40
B. Myoglobin
C. CRP
D. Troponin T

57. Right aortic arch is most commonly seen in:
A. Truncus arteriosus
B. TOF
C. Tricuspid atresia
D. Pulmonary atresia with VSD

58. Truncal valve most commonly:
A. Hexacuspid
B. Bicuspid
C. Tricuspid
D. Quadricuspid

59. JNC VII includes which of the following stages?
A. Optimal, Normal, Prehypertension, stage1 and 2
B. Normal, Prehypertension, stage1 and 2
C. Normal, Prehypertension, stage1, 2 and 3
D. Optimal, prehypertension, stage 1 and 2

60. JNC VII: best statement is:
A. Stepped therapy is with beta blocker ± diuretic
B. Among many, combination with one being diuretic
C. First time patients calcium channel blocker/ ACE inhibitors
D. Start with one drug: increase upto tolerance and then add another

61. ACE-inhibitor is contraindicated in:
A. U/L renal artery stenosis
B. Bilateral renal artery stenosis
C. Renal failure with 2-3 mg%
D. Diabetic nephropathy

50 B 51 A 52 B 53 C 54 B 55 D 56 B 57 A 58 D 59 B 60 B 61 B

62. WPW with PSVT: which of the following is not to be used?
A. Adenosine
B. Amiodarone
C. Digoxin
D. Procainamide

63. Single S2 is seen in all *except:*
A. Truncus arteriosus
B. Small VSD with severe PS
C. Large VSD with severe PAH
D. c-TGA

64. Beta blocker with intrinsic sympathomimetic activity is:
A. Pindolol
B. Propanolol
C. Metoprolol
D. Atenelol

65. Selective beta blocker are all *except:*
A. Bisoprolol
B. Carvedilol
C. Acebutalol
D. Pindolol

66. Most common single ventricle relation with great arteries is:
A. Transposition
B. Malposed with side to side
C. Double outlet
D. Normal

67. PDA dependent circulation are all *except:*
A. Truncus arteriosus
B. TGA with intact IVS
C. Tricuspid atresia with pulmonic atresia
D. Pulmonary atresia with intact IVS

68. Age for Fontan's surgery is:
A. < 1 year
B. 1-2 year
C. 2-4 year
D. > 4 year

69. Arterial switch surgery is best dome at:
A. < 3 weeks
B. 3-6 weeks
C. 6-12 weeks
D. > 12 weeks

70. TPI in AWMI is done in all *except:*
A. RBBB with LAHB
B. Transient 2 : 1 block
C. Transient CHB
D. AMI with LBBB

71. NHANES: Hypertension is well controlled with drugs in what percentage of population:
A. 33%
B. 50%
C. 25%
D. 75%

72. RVH in corpulmonale is:
A. Type A
B. Type B
C. Type C
D. None of the above

73. Hypertension: which of the following is false in elderly?
A. Elderly > 70 years: 60-70% are hypertension
B. Systolic pressure increases and more risk factor for CAD
C. Diastolic pressure increases till 50 years then decreases
D. Pulse pressure is not a risk factor

74. 4S trial: true is:
A. Decrease total cholesterol
B. Decrease nonfatal MI but not total mortality
C. Decrease total mortality that commensurate with LDL decrease
D. Increase non-cardiac mortality

62 C 63 C 64 A 65 B 66 A 67 A 68 C 69 A 70 B 71 A 72 C 73 D 74 C

75. Graham Steels murmur is:
A. Normal TR
B. Hypertensive TR
C. Normal PR
D. Hypertensive PR

76. c-TGA: all can be seen *except:*
A. VSD
B. Ebstein's anomaly (right sided)
C. Congenital CHB
D. PS

77. Most common paroxysmal narrow complex tachycardia is:
A. AVNRT
B. AVRT
C. SNRT
D. Ectopic atrial tachycardia

78. ASH: true are all *except:*
A. Valvular PS
B. Valvular AS
C. Amyloidosis
D. Post wall MI

79. CoA: all of the following can be seen *except:*
A. Papilloedema
B. Feeble right subclavian
C. Aortic bruit
D. Collateral murmur

80. All of the following are oral modalities to treat PPH *except:*
A. Tadanafil
B. Sildenafil
C. Beraprost
D. Iloprost

75 D 76 B 77 A 78 D 79 A 80 D

Jaipur 2003

1. **Features of typical angina:**
   A. Relieved by antacids
   B. Left precordial pain
   C. Caused by emotional exertion
   D. Prolonged, repeated

2. **In NYHA classification following is not a symptom:**
   A. Angina
   B. Cyanosis
   C. Dyspnea
   D. Palpitation

3. **Phasic ejection click of aortic valve is seen in:**
   A. PS
   B. TOF
   C. Systemic hypertension
   D. AS

4. **Wide split second heart sound is seen in:**
   A. LV pacing
   B. PDA
   C. LVOT obstruction (severe)
   D. LSVC to LA with intact septum

5. **Wide pulse pressure is seen in:**
   A. PDA with PR
   B. Severe hypertensive TR
   C. Adult TOF
   D. AS with MR

6. **Early systolic murmur is seen in all *except:***
   A. MVP with MR
   B. Small VSD
   C. Acute severe MR
   D. Normotensive TR

7. **Normotensive TR is seen in all *except:***
   A. Carcinoid
   B. MS with functional TR
   C. IE
   D. Tricuspid valve prolapse

8. **BP in lower limbs is significantly more than in upper limb:**
   A. Takayasu arteritis
   B. Coarctation of aorta with AR
   C. Femoral AV fistula
   D. Bilateral RAS

9. **Cannon "a" wave is seen in:**
   A. VVI
   B. DDD
   C. Severe TS
   D. PSVT

10. **Effort syncope is seen in:**
    A. Severe LMCA stenosis
    B. Straight back syndrome
    C. Pulmonary AV fistula
    D. Persistent LSVC to LA

1 C   2 B   3 B   4 A   5 A   6 A   7 B   8 A   9 A   10 A

11. Syncope is not a characteristic manifestation of:
A. HOCM
B. Severe PS
C. CoA
D. MS

12. Nocturia is seen in all *except:*
A. Diabetes Mellitus
B. CHF
C. Hypertension
D. VSD

13. R in V1 is seen in all *except:*
A. VSD
B. Duchenne's muscular dystrophy
C. Posterior wall MI
D. Situs inversus with dextrocardia

14. ACE-inhibitors cause abrupt increase in Serum Creatinine in:
A. Hypotension
B. CHF
C. B/L RAS
D. All of the above

15. True about ACE-Inhibitors is all *except:*
A. Increase renin
B. Increase angiotensin-1
C. Decrease renal blood flow
D. Increase bradykinin

16. Digoxin toxicity is seen in all *except:*
A. Hypokalemia
B. Acidosis
C. Hypomagnesemia
D. Decrease intravascular volume

17. Digoxin level is increased in all *except:*
A. Phenytoin
B. Amiodarone
C. Erythromycin
D. Verapamil

18. Cardioselective beta blocker is:
A. Sotalol
B. Bisoprolol
C. Nadolol
D. Pindolol

19. RV impulse is prominent in:
A. MS with severe PAH
B. Ebstein's anomaly
C. Tricuspid atresia
D. TOF with pulmonary atresia

20. K^+ channel activator is:
A. Adenosine
B. Amiodarone
C. Labetalol
D. Sotalol

21. Drug to be given in first 24 hours of MI:
A. ACE-inhibitor
B. CCB
C. Statin
D. Digoxin

22. Drug beneficial in mortality in CHF:
A. Digoxin
B. Spironolactone
C. Oral anticoagulants
D. All of the above

23. Antioxidant effect is seen with all *except:*
A. Carvedilol
B. Vitamin D
C. Allopurinol
D. Probucol

24. Statin may cause all *except:*
A. Decreased stent thrombosis
B. Stablizes plaque
C. Decrease senile osteoporoisis
D. Improves endothelial function

11 C 12 D 13 A 14 D 15 C 16 D 17 A 18 B 19 A 20 A 21 A 22 B 23 B 24 A

25. Smoking causes atherogenesis by all *except:*
A. Antioxidant effect
B. Decreased HDL
C. Increased platelet aggregation
D. Endothelial dysfunction

26. Anterolateral papillary muscle is supplied by:
A. LAD and LCx
B. LAD
C. LCx
D. RCA

27. Not a branch of RCA:
A. OM
B. Acute marginal
C. Conus
D. PDA

28. Vein draining into RA through coronary sinus are all *except:*
A. Thebesian vein
B. Small cardiac vein
C. Anterior cardiac vein
D. Vein of Marshall

29. Vein used for LV pacing:
A. Posterolateral vein
B. Anterior cardiac vein
C. Small cardiac vein
D. Thebesian vein

30. Most common stenotic valve (Aortic) at birth is:
A. Unicuspid
B. Bicuspid
C. Tricuspid
D. Quadricuspid

31. Spontaneous contrast in LA is seen in:
A. RCM
B. Acute MI
C. Severe TS
D. RA myxoma

32. Superior axis deviation is seen in all *except:*
A. RSOV to RV
B. TOF with large inlet VSD
C. ECD
D. Tricuspid atresia

33. Coronary AV fistula most commonly drain in:
A. RV
B. RA
C. LV
D. Pulmonary artery

34. Penetrating injury most commonly affects:
A. RV
B. LV
C. RA
D. IVS

35. Bisferins pulse best felt in:
A. Carotid
B. Brachial
C. Abdominal aorta
D. Radial

36. Cyanosis with decreased blood flow is seen in:
A. Ebsteins anomaly
B. Tricuspid atresia with nonrestrictive VSD without PS
C. Tausig Bing anomaly
D. TGA

37. Pulsus paradoxus is seen in:
A. COPD
B. HOCM
C. Cardiac tamponade with AR
D. Severe TR

38. Enlarged LA is seen in:
A. Lutembacher's syndrome
B. ASD-OS
C. Corpulmonale
D. Ebstein's anomaly

25 A 26 A 27 A 28 A 29 A 30 A 31 A 32 A 33 A 34 A 35 A 36 A 37 A 38 A

39. Oxygen step up in RV is seen in:
A. PDA with PR
B. RSOV into LA
C. Sinus venosus ASD
D. Cortriatriatum

40. Adult survival is expected in:
A. PS
B. TGA
C. Ostium primum ASD
D. TOF with pulmonary atresia

41. Down's syndrome: most commonly associated with:
A. ECD
B. TOF
C. PS
D. Pulmonary artery stenosis

42. Which of the following is an incorrect match:
A. AS-Ross
B. TGA-Banding PA
C. TOF-BT
D. Pulmonary atresia- Unifocalisation

43. CHF in first week of life is seen in all *except:*
A. Severe MR
B. Coarctation of aorta
C. VSD
D. Congenital MS

44. WPW in congenital heart disease is associated with:
A. RSOV
B. TGA
C. Ebstein's
D. Uhl's anomaly

45. Markers of myocardial infarction are all *except:*
A. Troponin C
B. Myosin light chain
C. LDH
D. CK-MB

46. RVMI: true is all *except:*
A. Increased RA pressure
B. Normal PA pressure
C. Increased PCWP
D. Increased RV diastolic pressure

47. CHF: true is all *except:*
A. Reduced norepinephrine
B. Reduced cardiac output
C. Increased arteriovenous difference (oxygen)
D. Increased filling pressure

48. Pericarditis is seen with:
A. Methysergide
B. Lithium
C. Protamine
D. Indomethacin

49. In diabetes mellitus: Goal of Anti-lipid therapy is (without CAD):
A. LDL <100 and TG< 150 mg%
B. LDL <100 and TG < 200 mg%
C. LDL < 130 and TG < 200 mg%
D. LDL < 160 and TG < 150 mg%

50. MVA in echo is assessed by all *except:*
A. Gorlin's formula
B. PISA
C. Planimetry
D. PHT

51. True in echo for aortic valve disease:
A. Velocity of 2.5 m/s s/o mild AS
B. Peak instantaneous pressure in echo has good correlation with peak to peak pressure in cath
C. Mean aortic pressure in echo is invariably lower than that in cath
D. Gradual deceleration in gradient indicates severe AR

39 A 40 A 41 A 42 B 43 C 44 C 45 A 46 C 47 A 48 A 49 A 50 A 51 A

52. True in echo is all *except:*
A. Fractional shortening is 50-60%
B. PLAX for coronary artery
C. RV systolic function assessed by tricuspid annular velocity
D. LA contrast in mitral stenosis

53. Acute severe AR: true are all *except:*
A. Absent S4
B. Austin flint murmur
C. Absent peripheral signs
D. Soft S1.

54. Which of the following is true:
A. Diastolic murmur graded from 1 to 6
B. Gallavardin phenomenon is seen in noncalcific AS
C. Carvallo's sign in TR with RVF
D. Austin flint murmur is absent in mild AR

55. Pregnancy: Following are suggestive of heart disease:
A. Diastolic murmur at apex
B. LVS3
C. Systolic murmur-grade2/6 in pulmonary area
D. Edema

56. Poor prognosis in pregnancy is seen in:
A. PPH
B. CoA
C. OS-ASD
D. MR

57. Most dangerous coronary anomaly:
A. ALCAPA
B. Left coronary from right aortic sinus with interarterial course
C. LAD from right aortic sinus with retroaortic route
D. RCA from Lt aortic sinus

58. Amyl nitrate inhalation increases murmur of:
A. HOCM
B. TOF
C. PDA
D. MR

59. Cyanotic spell is maximum in TOF:
A. Less than 2 month
B. 2-6 months
C. > 6 months
D. 1-2 years

60. Treatment of cyanotic spell is all *except:*
A. Morphine
B. Esmolol
C. Phenylephrine
D. Frusemide

61. SCD in athlete: most common cause is:
A. HOCM
B. CAD
C. Coronary abnormality
D. Idiopathic ventricular tachycardia

62. Pacing: true is:
A. Pacemaker mediated tachycardia is seen in VVI pacing
B. DDD pacing causes less of atrial arrhythmia than VVI
C. Biventricular pacing in HOCM is beneficial
D. VVI is useful in CHF

63. Atrial fibrillation: true is:
A. Risk of thromboembolism is more in nonvalvular than valvular
B. Biatrial pacing is useful in prevention of intermittent AF
C. Rhythm control is definitely better than rate control
D. Aspirin and warfarin are equally efficacious in preventing stroke

52 B 53 A 54 D 55 A 56 A 57 B 58 A 59 B 60 D 61 A 62 B 63 B

64. Infective endocarditis: Highest risk is associated with:
- **A.** Bicuspid aortic valve
- **B.** Ebstein's anomaly
- **C.** PPH
- **D.** OS-ASD

65. IE: indication for surgery are all *except:*
- **A.** Unstable prosthesis
- **B.** Intractable CHF
- **C.** NVE relapse after optimal antimicrobial treatment
- **D.** Vegetation > 10 mm with embolic phenomenon

66. Myocardial viability is assessed with all *except:*
- **A.** SAECG
- **B.** PET
- **C.** Dobutamine stress
- **D.** Stress Thallium

67. Findings in stress thallium s/o multivessel CAD are all *except:*
- **A.** Transient LV dilatation
- **B.** Increase RV uptake
- **C.** Uptake lung/heart <0.45
- **D.** Defect in more than 2 coronary artery territory

68. Which of the following findings are suggestive of strongly positive TMT:
- **A.** Exercise duration less than 8 min
- **B.** Exercise induced LBBB
- **C.** Recurrent sustained symptomatic VT
- **D.** Peak exercise BP more than 180 mm Hg

69. Not an indication of TMT:
- **A.** Advanced CHB
- **B.** Congenital asymptomatic CHB
- **C.** To diagnose IHD in chest pain patient
- **D.** Final assessment in valvular heart disease

70. BMV balloon size:
- **A.** Height of person in cm/10 + 10 mm
- **B.** Height of person in cm/10 + 5 mm
- **C.** Height of person in mts + 10 mm
- **D.** Height of person in cm/8 + 10 mm

71. IABP: Absolute contraindication:
- **A.** Severe AR
- **B.** Cardiogenic shock with aortic aneurysm
- **C.** Acute MI with VSD
- **D.** Severe MR

72. Characteristic pathology in Marfan's in aorta:
- **A.** Cystic medial necrosis
- **B.** Annuloaortic ectasia
- **C.** Fibrinoid degenration
- **D.** Plexiform arteriopathy

73. Primary hyperaldosteronism: true are all *except:*
- **A.** Urine K < 30 meq
- **B.** Hypertension
- **C.** Hypokalemia
- **D.** Decreased rennin

74. Primary prevention trial is:
- **A.** AFCAPS
- **B.** 4S
- **C.** CARE
- **D.** LIPID

75. Indication of thrombolysis in pulmonary embolism:
- **A.** Paradoxical emboli
- **B.** LV dysfunction
- **C.** RV dysfunction/hypokinesia/hypotension
- **D.** All of the above

76. Familial myxoma: true are all *except:*
- **A.** Endocrine disorder
- **B.** Present in elderly
- **C.** Multiple
- **D.** Biatrial

64 A 65 C 66 A 67 C 68 C 69 A 70 A 71 A 72 A 73 A 74 A 75 C 76 B

77. Mechanism of hemoptysis in MS are all *except:*

A. Acute pulmonary edema
B. Chest infection
C. Recurrent laryngeal nerve paralysis
D. Pulmonary thromboembolism

78. Most common complication of catheterization:

A. Local vascular complications
B. Azotemia
C. Ventricular tachycardia
D. Acute MI

79. Cyanosis is seen in:

A. Common atrium
B. RSOV to RV
C. VSD with AR
D. Coronary AV fistula

80. Lp(a): true are all *except:*

A. Important risk factor in Asian Indians
B. Inhibit endogenous fibrinolysis
C. Homologous to fibrinogen
D. Decreased by niacin

77 C 78 A 79 A 80 C

Jaipur 2002

1. **All are true about CHF *except:***
   A. Decreased AV O_2 difference
   B. Decreased Cardiac output
   C. Increased filling pressure
   D. Oliguria

2. **Gynaecomastia is produced by:**
   A. Triamterene
   B. Spironolactone
   C. Amiloride
   D. Frusemide

3. **Calcific pericarditis; Investigation of choice is:**
   A. CT
   B. TEE
   C. TTE
   D. MRI

4. **Echo finding in severe AR are all *except:***
   A. AML flutter
   B. ↑ EPSS
   C. Decreased LVESD
   D. Diastolic reversal in descending thoracic aorta

5. **All are true about severity of AR *except:***
   A. Loudness of murmur
   B. Length EDM
   C. Cardiomegaly
   D. S/o wide pulse pressure

6. **Aging is associated with:**
   A. ↓Basal life
   B. ↑Lung closing volume
   C. ↓GFR
   D. ↑SBP

7. **Trop T is preferred over CPK in all *except:***
   A. 4 days after MI
   B. 2 hrs after MI
   C. Post CABG
   D. Bedside diagnostic marker

8. **Familial hypercholesterolemia is differentiated from combined hypercholesterolemia by:**
   A. Tuberous xanthoma
   B. Tendon xanthoma
   C. Xanthelesma
   D. Arcus senilis

9. **All are true about PAH *except:***
   A. Schistosamiasis
   B. Toxic oil
   C. Progress primary systemic sclerosis
   D. Argemone Mexicana poisoning

10. **All are true about reversed split S2 *except:***
    A. LBBB
    B. LV apical pacing
    C. Angina
    D. LVOT obstruction

11. **RA > PA saturation is seen in:**

1 A 2 B 3 A 4 C 5 A 6 B 7 B 8 B 9 D 10 B

A. RVMI
B. LVF
C. ASD
D. Normal hemodynamics

12. Child SBP 90 mmHg, 4 m/sec velocity across perimembranous VSD, Pulmonary artery pressure is:
A. Normal PAP
B. Moderate PAP
C. Severe PAH
D. Increased PVR

13. Square root response is seen in all *except:*
A. Post transplant
B. ASD
C. CHF
D. HOCM

14. MVP is seen in all *except:*
A. Rheumatic fever
B. HOCM
C. Marfan's syndrome
D. Straight back syndrome

15. MDM at apex is heard in all *except:*
A. Ac Rheumatic fever
B. ASD
C. VSD
D. AR

16. Cardiac tamponade is excluded if following is absent:
A. Hypertension
B. Heart sounds are decreased
C. Pulsus paradoxus
D. Increased intrapericardial pressure

17. All are true about cyanide poisoning *except:*
A. Cherry red blood
B. Increased mixed venous O_2 sat
C. Response to Na thiosulphate
D. Lactic acidosis

18. All are true about secondary hyperaldosteronism *except:*
A. Pregnancy
B. Conn's syndrome
C. RAS
D. Hypertension

19. All are true about hyponatremia *except:*
A. Diuretic
B. Diabetis inspidus
C. Polyuric phase of tubular necrosis
D. CHF

20. Exudative retinopathy:
A. Pheochromocytoma
B. Takayasu type I
C. Conn's syndrome
D. Coarctation of aorta

21. All are used in unstable angina *except:*
A. rtPA (front loaded)
B. IV heparin
C. GpIIb/IIIa inhibitors
D. NTG

22. Cardiogenic shock is best managed by:
A. PTCA
B. IABP
C. GpIIb/IIIA inhibitors
D. Thrombolysis

23. Kussmaul's sign is not seen in:
A. Cardiac tamponade
B. RVMI
C. Pulmonary embolism
D. CCF

24. Not to be given in cardiac tamponade is:
A. Isoprenaline
B. Diuretics
C. Fluids
D. Dobutamine

11 C 12 A 13 D 14 A 15 B 16 D 17 A 18 B 19 B 20 A 21 A 22 A 23 A
24 B

25. **All are true about fetal CHF *except:***
A. Supraventricular tachycardia
B. CHB
C. Anemia
D. Severe CoA, GA

26. **Drugs contraindicated in pregnancy are all *except:***
A. Enalapril
B. Adenosine
C. Na nitroprusside
D. ARB

27. **In CHF all prolong survival *except:***
A. ACE I
B. Digoxin
C. Spiranolactone
D. β blockers

28. **Cyanosis with clubbing with normal splitting is seen in:**
A. Pulmonary A-V fistula
B. TOF
C. c-TGA with VSD with PS
D. TAPVC

29. **Wide fixed split S2 is heard in:**
A. TAPVC
B. PAPVC
C. Straight back syndrome
D. Peripheral pulmonary artery stenosis

30. **Normal splitting of S2 is heard in all *except:***
A. TAPVC
B. LSVC to LA
C. Methemoglobinaemia
D. Pulmonary A-V fistula

31. **Continuous murmur is heard in all *except:***
A. RSOV → LV
B. TAPVC
C. Coronary arterial fistula
D. PDA

32. **Continuous murmur is not heard in:**
A. A-P window
B. Intercostal AV fistula
C. Peripheral pulmonary artery stenosis
D. Coronary AV fistula

33. **Continuous murmur is more prominent in diastole in all *except:***
A. Small PDA
B. A-V fistula
C. Coronary A-V fistula
D. RSOV

34. **Rib notching is seen in all *except:***
A. Modified ST shunt
B. Neurofibromatosis
C. CoA
D. Intercostal AV fistula

35. **MI in presence of LBBB is diagnosed by all *except:***
A. >3 mm ST ↑ in V_1V_2
B. q in I avL, V_5V_6
C. Slurring upstroke in V_3 V_4
D. Primary SI-T changes in V_5 V_6

36. **R wave in V1 > 10 mm is seen in all *except:***
A. TOF
B. WPW-type B
C. Duchhene's dystrophy
D. d-TGA

37. **Pregnancy is well tolerated in all *except:***
A. CoA
B. Mod PS
C. MVP
D. Moderate MR

38. **DC shock is not effective in all *except:***
A. Atrial tachycardia
B. Junctional tachycardia
C. Atrial flutter with varying block
D. Chronic AF

25 D 26 B 27 B 28 A 29 A 30 A 31 A 32 A 33 A 34 A 35 A 36 B 37 A
38 C

39. HV interval is increased with all *except:*
A. Propafenone
B. Amiodarone
C. Xylocaine
D. Disopyramide

40. Most common cause of AS in India in a 10 year old child is:
A. Biscuspid AS
B. Unicuspid AS
C. Rheumatic AS
D. None of the above

41. According to current data, drug not to be used to treat hypertension in CAD is:
A. Doxazocin
B. Slow release diltiazem
C. Diuretic
D. Amlodipine

42. Pulmonary oedema with normal PCWP is seen in all *except:*
A. HAPE
B. Narcotic overdose
C. B/L renal artery stenosis
D. Post CABG

43. Clinical pulmonary edema can be seen with all *except:*
A. Narcotic overdose
B. Hypoalbuminemia
C. Hemorrhagic peritonitis
D. Severe MS

44. Increase PCWP is seen in all *except:*
A. Anaphylactic shock
B. Septic shock
C. Hypotension
D. Cardiac tamponade

45. Primary TR is seen with all *except:*
A. Pulmonary embolism
B. Ebsteins anomaly
C. IE of TV
D. Traumatic TR

46. LBBB can be seen with all *except:*
A. Digoxin
B. Hyperkalemia
C. Lev's disease
D. WPW syndrome

47. Poor prognostic factors for SCD in HOCM are:
A. Age <30 yrs
B. VT on Holter
C. Family history positive
D. Severity of gradient across LVOT

48. Least likely finding in pulmonary embolism is:
A. Normal CXR
B. Normal Perfusion scan
C. Normal ABG
D. None of the above

49. BP Control of 220/130 with developing stroke should be:
A. 110/80 (if feasible)
B. 180/105
C. 140/95
D. No measures

50. Commonest cause of syncope:
A. Vasovagal
B. Orthostatic
C. CHB
D. β blockers

51. Orthostatic hypotension is seen with all *except:*
A. Essential HT
B. Pheochromocytoma
C. Diuretic
D. Shy dragger syndrome

52. Child within one week of d-TGA: treatment of choice is:
A. Arterial switch
B. Atrial switch
C. Pulmonary artery banding
D. BT shunt

39 C 40 B 41 A 42 C 43 B 44 C 45 A 46 A 47 D 48 B 49 B 50 A 51 A
52 A

53. Which of the following does not increase in CHF:
- **A.** Arginine
- **B.** Na^+
- **C.** Aldosterone
- **D.** Endothelin

54. All of the following about ACE inhibitors are true *except:*
- **A.** ↑Renin
- **B.** ↑Bradykinin
- **C.** ↓GFR
- **D.** Ventricular hypertrophy

55. Bioprosthetic valve preferred over mechanical valve in:
- **A.** Young female
- **B.** Elderly
- **C.** Children
- **D.** Recurrent PVTE

56. Following are consequences of aging *except:*
- **A.** Bacteriuria
- **B.** DM
- **C.** CHF
- **D.** HTN

57. Following are pre requisites for cardiac transplantation *except:*
- **A.** Lymphocyte matching
- **B.** CMV
- **C.** HLA matching
- **D.** ABO matching

58. Normal healthy myocardium uses which substrate for energy:
- **A.** Fatty acid
- **B.** Glucose
- **C.** Amino acid
- **D.** Ketones

59. Exercise induced VT may be seen in all of the following *except:*
- **A.** Brugada syndrome
- **B.** Romano Ward syndrome
- **C.** RVOT tachycardia
- **D.** Ischemic VT

60. Least likely in structurally normal heart is:
- **A.** Atrial flutter
- **B.** VT with LBBB
- **C.** PSVT
- **D.** VPC's

61. Best measure of prevention of SCD in a community is:
- **A.** AICD
- **B.** β blocker
- **C.** Advanced life support
- **D.** Decrease coronary risk factors

62. Hemoptysis is seen with:
- **A.** Hereditary hemorrhagic telangiectasia
- **B.** Peripheral pulmonary artery stenosis
- **C.** Pulmonary A-V fistula
- **D.** All of the above

63. Normal anion gap acidosis is seen with:
- **A.** DKA
- **B.** CRF
- **C.** RTA
- **D.** Ethylene glycol

64. Best marker of myocardial oxygen requirement is:
- **A.** LVESD
- **B.** LVEDD
- **C.** HR
- **D.** Contractility

65. Best mortality predictor after MI:
- **A.** TVD
- **B.** LM disease
- **C.** EF
- **D.** VPC

53 B 54 D 55 B 56 A 57 C 58 A 59 A 60 A 61 D 62 D 63 C 64 C 65 C

66. Prinzmetal angina treatment include all *except:*
A. β blocker
B. CCB
C. Nitrates
D. ∝ blockers

67. All are HMG CoA reductase inhibitors *except:*
A. Rosuvastatin
B. Atorvastatin
C. Ezitimibe
D. Fluvastatin

68. LDL-C value following CABG should be what?
A. < 15 mg%
B. < 120 m%
C. < 100 mg%
D. < 70 mg%

69. G protein is the mediator in action of mechanism of all of the following *except:*
A. Insulin
B. ACTH
C. Adenosine
D. NO

70. Following is not included in NYHA classification:
A. Angina
B. Cyanosis
C. Dyspnea
D. Palpitation

71. Wide pulse pressure is seen in:
A. PDA with PR
B. Severe hypertensive TR
C. Adult TOF
D. AS with MR

72. Normal anion gap acidosis is seen with all *except:*
A. DKA
B. RTA
C. Diarrhoea
D. Potassium sparing diuretics

73. Which of the following is a feature of typical angina:
A. Relieved by antacids
B. Left precordial pain
C. Caused by emotional exertion
D. Prolonged, repeated

74. Prominent Y descent is seen in:
A. Cardiac tamponade
B. CCP
C. RVMI
D. None of the above

75. NTG worsens chest pain in:
A. HOCM
B. Unstable angina
C. MI
D. None of the above

76. CPK is not raised in:
A. Hypothyroidism
B. Muscular dystrophy
C. Cerebral infarcts
D. Carnitine deficiency

77. GpIIb/IIIa deficiency occurs in:
A. Bernard Soulier syndrome
B. Glanzmann's thrombesthenia
C. Scott's syndrome
D. Giant platelets

78. Maximum mortality after MI is seen with:
A. Primary VF
B. Secondary VF
C. Aneurysm
D. Mitral regurgitation

66 A 67 C 68 D 69 A 70 B 71 A 72 A 73 C 74 B 75 A 76 D 77 B 78 B

79. **Tall R wave in V1 is seen in all *except:***
   A. Friedrich's ataxia
   B. TOF
   C. Muscular dystrophy
   D. WPW Type B syndrome

80. **ST elevation in V1 is seen in all *except:***
   A. Pulmonary embolism
   B. Brugada syndrome
   C. Septal infarct
   D. Pericarditis

79 D 80 A

Jaipur 2001

1. **Bisferian pulse is best felt in:**
   A. Carotid
   B. Brachial
   C. Radial
   D. Femoral

2. **Murmur of HOCM is increased by all *except:***
   A. Valsalva
   B. Amyl nitrate
   C. Post VPC
   D. Leg raising

3. **Omega 3 fatty acid present in all *except:***
   A. Mustard oil
   B. Canola oil
   C. Soya oil
   D. Walnut oil

4. **Serum cholesterol is increased by all *except:***
   A. Trans saturated Fatty acid
   B. MUFA
   C. PUFA
   D. Diet cholesterol

5. **Which of the following statement is wrong:**
   A. Mortality ↑ by 2% with 1% ↑ in serum cholesterol
   B. Walking ↑ses HDL-C
   C. Type II DM associated with ↑TG
   D. Insulin resistance syndrome associated with ↑ LDL

6. **ACE inhibitor is contraindicated in:**
   A. B/L renal artery stenosis
   B. CHF with S. creatinine 1.5
   C. DM nephropathy
   D. None of the above

7. **In CHF all prolongs life *except:***
   A. ACEI
   B. Digoxin
   C. Spironolactone
   D. β blockers

8. **Increased chance of brain abscess is in**
   A. R-L shunt
   B. L-R shunt
   C. Anemia
   D. AS

9. **Treatment of Eisemenger syndrome is:**
   A. Heart lung transplant
   B. Heart transplant
   C. Lung transplant
   D. None of the above

10. **CI <1.8, PCWP 10mmHg; treatment of choice is:**
    A. IV fluids
    B. Dopamine
    C. β blocker
    D. Diuretics

1 A 2 D 3 A 4 C 5 A 6 A 7 B 8 A 9 A 10 A

11. **CHB seen in:**
 A. cTGA
 B. dTGA
 C. AV canal defect
 D. Ebsteins anomaly

12. **In patients of AMI, TPI is indicated in all *except:***
 A. RBBB
 B. LBBB
 C. RBBB with ↑ PR with Left axis deviation
 D. Mobitz type II

13. **Na nitroprusside is indicated in all *except:***
 A. Eclampsia
 B. Aortic dissection
 C. HT emergency
 D. Co-arctation aorta

14. **In myocardial ischemia all can be seen *except:***
 A. Tachycardia
 B. Hypertension
 C. ST-T changes
 D. Loud S1

15. **False statement regarding RHD in India is:**
 A. ↑MV calcification
 B. Tricuspid involvement is seen
 C. Mitral valve involvement is most commonly seen
 D. None of the above

16. **In athelets heart all can be seen *except:***
 A. Bradycardia
 B. Mobitz type II block
 C. Systolic murmur
 D. Diastolic murmur

17. **ASH seen in all *except:***
 A. HOCM
 B. AS
 C. Post MI
 D. PPH

18. **In PPH, true statement is:**
 A. Exertional dyspnea
 B. Clubbing occurs very early
 C. Cyanosis is severe
 D. More common in males

19. **Wide splitting of S2 is heard in all *except:***
 A. TAPVC
 B. PAPVC
 C. Pulmonary stenosis
 D. RBBB

20. **Angiotensin-II receptor blocker is:**
 A. Losartan
 B. Pimobendan
 C. Vesnarinone
 D. Fosnopril

21. **Commonest cause of sudden pericardial tamponade is:**
 A. Ca Lung
 B. Uremia
 C. Hypothyroidism
 D. Ankylosing spondylitis

22. **Least common cause of constrictive pericarditis is:**
 A. RHD
 B. TB
 C. Viral
 D. Drugs

23. **Poor outcome of pregnancy is seen with:**
 A. PPH
 B. Bicuspid aortic valve
 C. Coarctation
 D. ASD

24. **Asynchronized DC shock is given in:**
 A. VF
 B. VT
 C. SVT with aberrancy
 D. Atrial flutter

11 A 12 A 13 A 14 D 15 A 16 D 17 C 18 A 19 B 20 A 21 A 22 A 23 A
24 A

25. Mechanism involved in SCD:
A. VF
B. Asystole
C. Electromechanical association
D. None of the above

26. Obliteration of cardiac apex is seen with:
A. Endomyocardial fibrosis
B. Sarcoidosis
C. SLE
D. Amyloidosis

27. In myocarditis all are seen *except:*
A. STT changes
B. Increased QRS voltage
C. Sinus tachycardia
D. Q waves

28. In young patient with calcific AS velocity of 5m/sec, treatment of choice is:
A. Aortic valve replacement
B. Observation
C. Valve repair
D. Balloon aortic valvuloplasty

29. IABP is contraindicated in:
A. Acute AR
B. AMI with CHF
C. AMI with MR
D. Refractory ischemia

30. Which of the following gives best outcome of PTCA in MI?
A. Stent
B. DCA
C. Rotational atherectomy
D. Laser

31. Parasternal heave is seen in all *except:*
A. ASD with eisenmenger
B. VSD with eisenmenger
C. Severe MR
D. MS with PAH

32. Single S2 is seen with:
A. Ebstein
B. VSD Eisenmenger complex
C. CTGA
D. TAPVC

33. Wide splitting of S2 is seen in all *except:*
A. MVP
B. TAPVC
C. ASD
D. PS

34. In LV diastolic dysfunction, all are seen *except:*
A. S4
B. A>E
C. Cardiomegaly
D. ↑ LVEDP

35. Which of following mechanism is not see in production of MR following myocardial infarction?
A. Perforation of valve leaflet
B. Rupture of chordae
C. Dilatation of annulus
D. Papillary muscle dysfunction

36. Continuous murmur is seen in all *except:*
A. RSOV → RV
B. Peripheral PS
C. VSD with AR
D. Lutembacher's syndrome

37. R wave in V_1 seen in all *except:*
A. RBBB
B. Tricuspid atresia
C. Pulmonary atresia
D. DMD

38. LAA thrombus is best seen with:
A. TEE
B. TTE
C. CT scan
D. CW doppler

25 A 26 A 27 B 28 A 29 A 30 A 31 B 32 B 33 A 34 C 35 A 36 C 37 B
38 A

39. In HT which of the following mechanism is not seen:
A. ↑ Venous capacitance
B. ↑ Smooth muscle tone
C. ↑ PVR
D. ↑ Aldosterone

40. Calcium channel blocker is not indicated in which of the following:
A. Unstable angina with VPC's
B. AMI
C. CHF
D. Diabetic nephropathy

41. All are antioxidant *except:*
A. Probucol
B. Pantothenic acid
C. Vitamin E
D. None of the above

42. Drugs that decreases homocysteine is:
A. Folic acid
B. Thiamine
C. Vitamin E
D. Vitamin C

43. Atrial infarction is indicated by:
A. ↑ PR segment
B. ↑ PR interval
C. ↓ PR segment
D. ↓ PR interval

44. In TOF all drugs are given *except:*
A. Propranolol
B. Digoxin
C. Morphine
D. O_2

45. Pulmonary edema with normal PCWP:
A. High altitude pulmonary oedema
B. Pul edema with renal artery stenosis
C. Pul edema with aortic dissection
D. Pul edema with DCMP

46. NYHA class III is:
A. Dyspnea with less than ordinary activity
B. Dyspnea with ordinary activity
C. Dyspnea on undue efforts
D. None of the above

47. Primordial prevention:
A. No risk factors
B. Prevents initiation of disease
C. Is to be done to prevent complication
D. Not the Best way for health promotion

48. In patients with normal ECG with VPC, treatment of choice:
A. β blockers
B. Observation
C. Aspirin
D. Life style changes

49. Commonest side effect of ACE inhibitor:
A. Cough
B. Agranulocytosis
C. Teratogenicity
D. Angioedema

50. In patient with cardiogenic shock; best treatment is:
A. IABP
B. PTCA
C. Conservative
D. Thrombolysis

51. Commonest cardiovascular disease in India is:
A. HTN
B. RHD
C. CAD
D. Dyslipidemia

52. Drug contraindicated in DM nephropathy + CCF:
A. Captoril
B. Metformin
C. Fosinopril
D. β blocker

39 A 40 B 41 B 42 A 43 A 44 B 45 A 46 A 47 A 48 B 49 A 50 B 51 A 52 B

53. Left axis deviation is seen with which ASD:
A. Septum primum
B. Septum secondum
C. Coronary sinus
D. Sinus venosus

54. Normal pressure TR is not seen with:
A. Pulmonary embolism
B. Ebstein
C. Infective endocarditis
D. Carcinoid heart disease

55. In which condition, MDM is not heard at apex:
A. ASD
B. VSD
C. MS
D. AR

56. In acute AR; true is:
A. ↑LVEDP
B. ↓Pulse pressure
C. ↑Systolic pressure
D. None of the above

57. In treatment of unstable angina all are given *except:*
A. Thrombolysis
B. CABG
C. Heparin
D. Gp IIb/IIIa inhibitors

58. Post stenotic dilatation is seen in:
A. Valvular PS
B. TOF
C. Peripheral pulmonary stenosis
D. Carcinoid

59. All of the following shows ↑ severity of MR *except:*
A. Duration of murmur
B. Loudness of murmur
C. Wide split S2
D. LVS3

60. Pain due to NTG is ↑ in:
A. HOCM
B. Angina
C. AMI
D. Prinz metal

61. MI in infant at 8 weeks is seen in:
A. ALCAPA
B. Retro aortic course of coronary arteries
C. HOCM
D. Anomalous origin of LCx from RCA

62. In AF, regular heart rate of 60/min is seen with:
A. Digitalis toxicity
B. Occurrence of CHB
C. Myocarditis
D. None of the above

63. Gynecomastia is seen with:
A. Spironolactone
B. Warfarin
C. Aspirin
D. Ranitidine

64. Commonest cause of syncope:
A. Vasovagal
B. AS
C. VT
D. Carotid stenosis

65. In HT all are beneficial *except:*
A. Salt <2 g/day
B. Isometric exercise
C. Walk
D. Diet control

66. Regression of LVH is seen with all *except:*
A. ACE inhibitors
B. Beta blockers
C. ARB's
D. Hydralazine

53 A 54 A 55 A 56 A 57 A 58 A 59 B 60 A 61 A 62 A 63 A 64 A 65 B
66 D

67. All are true about classical angina *except:*
- **A.** Last for 40-50 mins duration
- **B.** Gets relieved by sublingual sorbotrate within 2-5 mins
- **C.** More common in early morning hours
- **D.** Increases on exertion

68. Nonsynchronized DC shock is given in:
- **A.** VF
- **B.** AF
- **C.** VT
- **D.** VPC's

69. All can be given in pregnancy *except:*
- **A.** Methyldopa
- **B.** Hydralazine
- **C.** ACE inhibitors
- **D.** None of the above

70. Which of the following drug decreases preload:
- **A.** NTG
- **B.** Dobutmine
- **C.** Hydralazine
- **D.** Calcium channel blockers

71. Which of the following is not seen in a structurally normal heart:
- **A.** Atrial flutter
- **B.** VPC's
- **C.** APC's
- **D.** AF

72. Dyspnoea in CHF can occur due to all of the following *except:*
- **A.** Decrease lung compliance
- **B.** Hypoxia
- **C.** Increase airway resistance
- **D.** Anxiety

73. Drug having beneficial effect on serum cholesterol is:
- **A.** Prazosin
- **B.** Beta blockers
- **C.** Diuretics
- **D.** None of the above

74. All of the following decreases mortality in MI *except:*
- **A.** Calcium channel blockers
- **B.** ACE-Inhibitors
- **C.** Beta blockers
- **D.** Aspirin

75. Conduction abnormality is seen with which of the following valvular lesion ?
- **A.** AS
- **B.** AR
- **C.** MS
- **D.** MR

76. Infective endocarditis is least likely seen with:
- **A.** ASD
- **B.** PS
- **C.** HOCM
- **D.** VSD

77. Reverse pulsus paradoxus is seen with:
- **A.** IPPV
- **B.** Cardiac Tamponade
- **C.** COPD
- **D.** CCP

78. ACE inhibitors were not used in which trial:
- **A.** BHAT
- **B.** AIRE
- **C.** CONSENSUS
- **D.** SOLVD

79. Systolic thrill in ASD in second left intercostals space indicate presence of:
- **A.** PAH
- **B.** TR
- **C.** MS
- **D.** AS

80. Treatment of choice for TOF at one year of age is:
- **A.** Total surgical correction
- **B.** BT shunt
- **C.** Conservative
- **D.** Pott's shunt

67 A 68 A 69 C 70 A 71 A 72 D 73 A 74 A 75 A 76 A 77 A 78 A 79 C 80 A

Jaipur 2000

1. **Radio frequency ablation is highly successful in:**
   A. AF
   B. WPW
   C. VT
   D. Atrial flutter

2. **A patient present with wide QRS tachycardia with QS in lead VI: which of the following is not a possible mechanisms:**
   A. SVT with LBB morphology
   B. Mahaim conduction
   C. Left free accessory pathway with antidromic conduction
   D. Idiopathic VT from Right ventricle

3. **Patient with known AF with regular heart rate of 60 min; diagnosis is:**
   A. Digitalis toxicity
   B. Sleep
   C. Sinus node dysfunction
   D. Hypothyroidism

4. **On echo attenuati›n of LV ɿnd RV apex is characteristic of:**
   A. EMF
   B. Amyloidois
   C. Carcinoid
   D. Sarcoidosis

5. **Commonest side effect of ACE inhibitor:**
   A. Cough
   B. Hypotension
   C. Angio edema
   D. Rash

6. **Most common lesion alone or in combination in RHD:**
   A. MS
   B. MS-MR
   C. MR-AR
   D. MS-AR

7. **Most common lesion in carcinoid heart disease:**
   A. PS
   B. PS-TR
   C. TR-MR
   D. MS with AR

8. **What can aggravate L-R shunt in ASD:**
   A. Anemia
   B. MR
   C. PAH
   D. RV dysfunction

9. **Cause of mortality in adults with PDA:**
   A. IE
   B Aneurysmal rupture
   C. CCF
   D. Reversal of shunt

1 B 2 C 3 A 4 A 5 A 6 B 7 B 8 B 9 C

10. Cyanosis in hands with pink toes:
A. TGA with PDA with coarctation with reversal
B. Methemoglobinaemia
C. Peripheral circulatory failure
D. CoA

11. All of the following drugs are contraindicated in cyanotic spell *except:*
A. NTG
B. Captopril
C. Digitalis
D. Propanolol

12. Unusual in a cyanotic spell are all *except:*
A. Absent murmur
B. Hypotension
C. Normal PaO_2
D. Split S_2

13. Commonest primary malignant tumor of the heart:
A. Angiosarcoma
B. Rhabdomyosarcoma
C. Teratocarcinoma
D. None of the above

14. Most likely to cause tamponade:
A. Bronchial carcinoma
B. Melanoma
C. Hypothyroidism
D. Acute rheumatic fever

15. NTG aggravate the chest pain in:
A. HOCM
B. Subendocardial ischemia
C. Coronary artery spasm
D. HTN

16. True about cholesterol are all *except:*
A. Cholesterol ↓ mortality by 2% if there is 1% reduction in cholesterol
B. Lovastatin is HMG CO-A reductase inhibitor
C. Exercise increase HDL-C
D. Most cereals and pulses contain low cholesterol

17. Confidence interval gives:
A. Probability range of true estimate
B. Correction factor applied to obtain true prevalence
C. Validity of survey method
D. Age/sex standardization of study

18. Commonest cause of syncope:
A. Vasovagal
B. Postural hypotension
C. Drug induced
D. CHB

19. Diagnosis of vasovagal syncope is made by:
A. Tilt test
B. EEG
C. ECG
D. EChocardiography

20. Diagnosis of reversible ischemia is best established by:
A. Stress thallium
B. MUGA
C. TMT
D. Echocardiography

21. Investigation of choice for ischemia in LBBB:
A. Stress echo
B. Lactate levels
C. TMT
D. Holter

22. Most potent simulus for PAH in COPD:
A. Hypoxia
B. LV dysfunction
C. Alveolar membrane destruction
D. Obliteration of pulmonary vasculature

10 A 11 D 12 A 13 A 14 A 15 A 16 A 17 A 18 A 19 A 20 A 21 A 22 A

23. Commonest lesion associated with conduction defects:
A. MS B. AS
C. MR D. AR

24. Most useful to reduce mortality in AMI within 6 hrs:
A. Aspirin
B. Aspirin + thrombolysis
C. Beta blocker + thrombolysis
D. Thrombolysis alone

25. Pulses paradoxus is seen in all *except:*
A. DCMP
B. COPD
C. CCP
D. Cardiac tamponade

26. Pulses paradoxus is seen in all *except:* (repeat)
A. COPD
B. CCP
C. Cardiac tamponade
D. Positive pressure ventilation

27. Treatment of wide QRS tachycardia of unknown origin:
A. Procainamide
B. Adenosine
C. Lignocaine
D. Flecainide

28. Indicated for HT in pregnancy:
A. Hydralazine
B. Sodium nitroprusside
C. Diuretics
D. Captopril

29. Which of the following heart disease is not hazardous in pregnancy?
A. Marfan
B. MVP
C. CoA
D. Eisenmenger

30. Not seen in HIV:
A. TB effusion
B. Kaposi
C. Myocarditis
D. Staphylococcal IE

31. CPK is increased in all *except:*
A. Hypothyroidism
B. Stroke
C. Limb amputation
D. Duchenne's dystrophy

32. All of the following are teratogenic *except:*
A. Warfarin
B. Retinoic acid
C. Lithium
D. Alcohol

33. Parasite causing pulmonary hypertension is:
A. Schistosomiasis
B. Filariasis
C. Paragonimiasis
D. None of the above

34. Asymmetrical septal hypertrophy is seen with all *except:*
A. HOCM
B. PAH
C. Post MI
D. AS

35. HV interval is not increased by all *except:*
A. Amiodarone
B. Digitalis
C. Lidocaine
D. Propranolol

36. Indication of thrombolysis (STK) are all of the following *except:*
A. Recent administration of STK about 3 weeks back
B. Pulmonary embolism
C. Pulmonary venous thrombosis
D. Deep vein thrombosis

23 B 24 B 25 A 26 D 27 A 28 A 29 B 30 D 31 C 32 C 33 A 34 C 35 A
36 A

37. All of the following will record high systolic BP *except:*
A. Obesity
B. Small cuff
C. Calcific arteries
D. Auscultatory gap

38. MI with CI of 1.8 l/min/m^2 and PCWP of 10 mm Hg; treatment is:
A. IV fluids
B. IABP
C. Inotropic support
D. Digoxin

39. If pH 7.2, PO2 85, PCO2 20; diagnosis is:
A. DKA
B. Phenobarbiturate poisoning
C. Pulmonary oedema
D. Anemia

40. Cause of wide fixed split:
A. TAPVC
B. PAPVC
C. Peripheral pulmonary artery stenosis
D. Straight back syndrome

41. True about β blocker is:
A. Decrease renin
B. Decrease conversion of Angiotensin I to II
C. Decrease cardiac output
D. Decrease vascular volume

42. Granulomatous hepatitis is caused by:
A. Oestrogen
B. Amiodarone
C. Allopurinol
D. Methyldopa

43. True about mycoplasma pneumonia are all *except:*
A. Bilateral infiltrate on X-ray
B. Organism is usually not isolated
C. Responds to cefuroxime
D. Serology is important in diagnosis

44. True about polycythemia vera are all *except:*
A. Increase incidence of thrombosis/haemorrhage
B. Hyperuricemia
C. Increase spontaneous infections
D. Increased incidence of leukaemia

45. Following are used in carcinoma prostate *except:*
A. Estrogen
B. Luperotide
C. Adrenalectomy
D. Somatostatin anlogue

46. Glycogen storage disorder without muscle involvement:
A. Type I
B. Type II
C. Type III
D. Type IV

47. Common to all spondyloarthropathies:
A. Enthesopathy
B. Pigmentation
C. Oral ulcer
D. None of the above

48. Cause of osteomyelitis in drug abusers:
A. Pseudomonas
B. Staphylococcus
C. Candida
D. Tuberculosis

49. HIV positive patient with diffuse lymhadenopathy:
A. TB
B. Kaposi's sarcoma
C. Lymphoma
D. All of the above

37 D 38 A 39 C 40 A 41 A 42 C 43 C 44 C 45 D 46 A 47 A 48 B 49 D

50. Not to be used in renal failure:
A. Trimethadone
B. Procainamide
C. Phenytoin
D. Propranolol

51. Seen in Wernicke's encephalopathy are all *except:*
A. Confusion
B. Ataxia
C. Ophthalmoplegia
D. Intention tremor

52. Hypercalcemia in Ca bronchus is seen with:
A. Small cell carcinoma
B. Squamous cell
C. Large cell carcinoma
D. Adenocarcinoma

53. Commonest site for Osler nodes is:
A. Digital pad of finger and toes
B. Palm and sole
C. Upper chest
D. Sacral region

54. Seen in lead poisoning are all *except:*
A. Increase protoporphyrin
B. Megaloblastic anemia
C. Microcytic hypochromic anemia
D. Fanconi like haemolytic anemia

55. Corkscrew esophagus is seen in:
A. Diffuse esophageal spasm
B. Oesophagitis
C. Achalsia cardia
D. Diffuse malignancy

56. Decrease in IgG is seen in all *except:*
A. Wiskot Aldrich syndrome
B. Common immunodeficiency syndrome
C. Di George syndrome
D. Selective IgA deficiency

57. Mousy odour of skin is seen in:
A. Phenylketonuria
B. Homocystenemia
C. Malonic aciduria
D. Ketoacidosis

58. Treatment of asymptomatic isolated VPC in healthy individual is:
A. No treatment
B. Anxiolytics
C. Digitalis
D. Phenytoin

59. Increased amylase in pleural effusion is seen in:
A. TB
B. Malignancy
C. Pulmonary infarction
D. RA

60. Swelling of costochondral junction is seen in all *except:*
A. Scurvy
B. Rickets
C. Marfans
D. Costochondral dystrophy

61. Following rhythm is least likely in normal heart:
A. PVC
B. Atrial flutter
C. PSVT
D. VT with LBBB morphology

62. Drug contraindicated in 60 year old male with NIDDM with bilateral renal artery stenosis is:
A. Enalapril
B. Beta blocker
C. Nifedipine
D. OHA

63. Mechanism of action of digoxin is:
A. Release of Ca^{++} from sarcoplasmic reticulum
B. Opening of Ca^{++} channels
C. No effect on Ca^{++} channels
D. None of the above

50 B 51 D 52 B 53 A 54 B 55 A 56 D 57 A 58 A 59 C 60 C 61 B 62 A 63 A

64. **Virus with retroviral activity are all *except:***
A. HIV
B. Retrovirus
C. HSV
D. None of the above

65. **Highest IE among all of the following is caused by:**
A. VSD
B. Pulmonary stenosis
C. Subvalvular aortic stenosis
D. MS

66. **Most common change on histology in nephrotic syndrome caused by bronchogenic carcinoma is:**
A. Minimal change disease
B. Membranous
C. Membranoproliferative
D. None of the above

67. **IE is least likely in:**
A. ASD
B. MVP
C. Small VSD
D. TOF

68. **Hyperpigmentation is seen in all *except:***
A. Addison's disease
B. Whipple's disease
C. Celiac sprue
D. Tropical sprue

69. **Most common cause of diarrhoea in AIDS is:**
A. CMV
B. MAC
C. Cryptosporidium
D. None of the above

70. **Pancreatitis is caused by all *except:***
A. Sodium valproate
B. Ciprofloxacin
C. Azathioprine
D. Thiazides

71. **Pseudolymphoma like picture is seen with:**
A. Sjogren's syndrome
B. PSS
C. SLE
D. Behcet's disease

72. **All are true about cholinergic system *except:***
A. Bradycardia
B. Reverse by catecholamine
C. Increase perspiration
D. None of the above

73. **Drug contraindicated in CRF is:**
A. Furosemide
B. Bumetanide
C. Ethcrynic acid
D. Triamterene

74. **All are causes of palpable purpura *except:***
A. ITP
B. Serum sickness syndrome
C. Henoch Schonlein purpura
D. Wegner granulomatosis

75. **Ketanseran is:**
A. 5 HT blocker
B. Beta blocker
C. 5 HT blocker + alpha blocker
D. Alpha blocker

76. **All are seen in Conn's syndrome *except:***
A. Hypokalemia
B. Increase perspiration
C. Weakness and paralysis
D. Polyuria and nocturia

77. **True about Conn's syndrome is:**
A. Low renin
B. Hyponatremia
C. Hypotenison
D. Acidosis

64 C 65 A 66 B 67 A 68 D 69 C 70 B 71 A 72 D 73 D 74 A 75 C 76 B 77 A

78. Normotensive TR is seen with all *except:*
A. Pulmonary embolism
B. Ebstein's anomaly
C. Trauma
D. Right sided EMF

79. Most specific of recent HBV infection is:
A. HBsAg
B. IgM AntiHBs
C. IgM Anti HBc
D. Anti HBc

80. All of the following can be seen in CHF *except:*
A. Decrease A-V O_2 difference
B. Increase A-V O_2 difference
C. Increase serum norepinephrine
D. None of the above

78 A **79** C **80** A

Jaipur 1999

1. Right isomerism is characterized by all *except:*

A. Bilateral morphologic Right Bronchi
B. Wandering spleen
C. Howel jolly bodies
D. Asplenia

2. Most important EKG feature of c-TGA is:

A. q-wave absent in 1, av1, v5, v6
B. q-wave absent in II, III, av F
C. Equiphasic complexes in midprecordial leads
D. 2:1 heart block

3. Most accepted indication of balloon angioplasty in coarctation of aorta is:

A. Restenosis after surgical repair
B. Restenosis after angioplasty
C. Co-arctation in infants
D. Co-arctation

4. Brugada's syndrome is characterized by:

A. ST elevation in VI with rsR pattern
B. ST elevation in VI with qR pattern
C. ST depression on VI with rsR pattern
D. ST elevation in V2 with rsR pattern

5. Indication of AICD implantation:

A. Atrial fibrillation with fast ventricular rate
B. Ventricular tachycardia with hemodynamic compromise
C. Incessant ventricular tachycardia
D. Primary ventricular tachycardia

6. Drugs shown to reverse endothelial dysfunction are all *except:*

A. Estrogen
B. Progestrone
C. ACE-inhibitors
D. Lovastatin

7. ACEI should be started after Ac MI after:

A. As soon as patient stabilizes
B. 10 hrs
C. 24 hrs
D. 48 hrs or more

8. Right atrial enlargement with LAD in a cyanotic heart disease is characterized by:

A. Ebstein anomally
B. Pulmonic stenosis with R-L shunt
C. Pulmonary atresia with VSD
D. Tricuspid atresia

9. Probable cure for Eisenmenger syndrome is:

A. Heart lung transplant
B. Cardiac transplantation
C. Lung transplantation
D. Not possible

10. Newer risk factors for CAD include all of the following *except:*

A. Fibrinogen
B. Homocysteinemia
C. Lipoprotein (a)
D. Calcium

1 B 2 A 3 A 4 A 5 B 6 B 7 A 8 D 9 A 10 D

11. Use of Simvastatin in 4S study increased HDL levels by:
A. 2%
B. 20%
C. 8%
D. 30%

12. Differential diagnosis of linear echo in LA includes all *except:*
A. Dilated Coronary sinus
B. TAPVC
C. Cortriatriatum
D. Left pulmonary artery

13. ELITE trial compared..................in CCF patients:
A. Losartan with Felodipin
B. Enalapril with Quinapril
C. Losartan with captopril
D. Digoxin with Diuretics

14. VAQWISH Trial concluded that in patients with Non Q-MI:
A. Angioplasty is superior to medical therapy
B. Medical (conservative) treatment is better than radical
C. CABG is superior to angioplasty
D. Stress thallium is must before coronary angiography

15. I year survival in patient with cardiac transplant:
A. > 85%
B. > 70%
C. > 50%
D. > 40%

16. ATLAS trail concluded:
A. Low dose lisinopril is more effective than high dose in reducing mortality in patients with CCF
B. High does lisinopril is more effective than low dose in reducing mortality in patients with CCF
C. No difference in mortality rates with use of different doses of lisinopril in patients with CCF
D. High dose lisinopril is effective in reducing mortality in elderly with CCF but not in the young

17. Spontaneous dissection of the following artery is typically described in pregnancy:
A. Aorta
B. Coronary
C. Carotid
D. Pulmonary

18. Small Aorta with small PA is a cardiological feature of:
A. Criss Cross heart
B. Home's heart
C. Ebstein's heart
D. Cretinism

19. Arterial switch procedure in d-TGA is done within:
A. 2 wks of life
B. 4 wks of life
C. 6 wks of life
D. 8 wks of life

20. Drug contra indicated in pregnancy–3rd trimester:
A. ACE Inhibitors
B. Lignocaine
C. Phenytoin
D. Warfarin

21. Indicators of surgery in a patient with aortic regurgitation with no symptoms:
A. NYHA II
B. LVESD > 45 mm
C. LVEF < 70%
D. LVEDD > 52 mm

11 C 12 D 13 C 14 B 15 A 16 B 17 B 18 C 19 A 20 A 21 B

22. Drug which has been shown to retard progression of aortic regurgitation conclusively is:
A. Digoxin
B. Enalapril
C. Nifedipine
D. Prazosin

23. Best management of atrial flutter in a patient with 32 wks pregnancy:
A. Digoxin
B. Verapamil
C. DC shock
D. β blockers

24. Cause of paradoxical splitting of S2:
A. LV dysfunction
B. Severe MR
C. Large VSD
D. Severe TR

25. Incidence of involvement of plumonary value in RHD is less than ....in autopsy series:
A. 1%
B. 2%
C. 3%
D. 7%

26. 52 years old male diabetic, hypertensive, suffered Ac, inferior wall MI complicated by 2:1 AV block on day 2, recovery was uneventful. Best modality for risk stratification would be:
A. Pre discharge TMT
B. TMT at 6 weeks
C. Coronary angiogram before discharge
D. Coronary angiography and EPS before discharge

27. 45 years old male diabetic, hypertensive for 10 years, developed severe acute retrosternal chest pain with EKG showing ST depression from VI-V4; Best management is:
A. Coronary angiography and angioplasty
B. Medical management only
C. Medical management followed by revascularization if symptoms not controlled
D. Immediate thrombolysis

28. BARI trial showed that CABG is superior to PTCA in:
A. All patients
B. Diabetics
C. Patients with two vessel disease and LV dysfunction
D. Patient with high lipids

29. Incidence of toxemia in patients with Coarctation of aorta (as compared to general population):
A. Highest
B. Same
C. Lower
D. Invariably present

30. Which statement is false regarding VSD with acquired PS?
A. Occurs in 7-15% cases of VSD
B. Was first described by Gasul
C. Usually due to infundibular hypertrophy
D. PS is valvular in location

31. Severity of TOF is decided by:
A. Infundibular PS
B. VSD
C. Overriding of aorta
D. RVH

32. SA node is supplied by:
A. RCA in 60%
B. LCx in 60%
C. Diagonals
D. Septal artery

33. RFA is highly successful in:
A. AVNRT slow pathway
B. AVNRT fast pathway
C. Concealed accessory pathway
D. Atrial fibrillation

22 C 23 C 24 A 25 C 26 A 27 A 28 B 29 B 30 D 31 A 32 A 33 A

34. Complication is least in ablation of which of the following?
A. Left lateral pathway
B. Left anteroseptal pathway
C. Right posteroseptal pathway
D. Left posteroseptal pathway

35. Which of the following manifestations of rheumatic fever hasn't been described in Indians?
A. Arthritis
B. Subcutaneous nodules
C. Chorea
D. Erythema marginatum

36. Device closure is done in all *except:*
A. ASD (20 mm)
B. PFO (R → L)
C. Supracristal VSD 4 mm
D. PDA 5 mm

37. CoA collateral involve all *except:*
A. 1st intercostals artery
B. 3rd intercostals artery
C. Hypogastric artery
D. Inferior epigastric artery

38. Commonest valvular lesions associated with conduction defect is:
A. MS
B. MR
C. AS
D. AR

39. NTG increases the pain in:
A. HOCM
B. Variant angina
C. Intramyocardial bridging
D. MI

40. Pulses paradoxus is seen in all *except:*
A. COPD
B. IPPV
C. CCP
D. Cardiac tamponade

41. Most potent LDL reducer is:
A. Fluvastatin
B. Lovastatin
C. Simvastatin
D. Atorvastatin

42. LBBB is seen with all *except:*
A. Digitalis
B. Hyperkalemia
C. Lev's disease
D. WPW syndrome

43. CHF in utero can occur in all *except:*
A. Ebstein's anomaly
B. D-TGA
C. Anaemia
D. PSVT

44. High output failure occurs in all *except:*
A. Multiple myeloma
B. Ruptured aneurysm of Galen
C. Hemangioma of liver
D. RSOV

45. Freidrich's sign is seen in which of the following?
A. Severe Right heart failure
B. Left ventricular failure
C. CCP
D. Cardiac tamponade

46. Primordial prevention means:
A. Prevention in persons with no risk factor
B. Prevention in communities with risk factor
C. Prevention in persons with only risk factors for disease
D. Antenatal prevention measures

47. All prolong QT *except:*
A. Digoxin
B. Amiodarone
C. Class Ia drugs
D. Hypocalcemia

34 A 35 D 36 C 37 A 38 C 39 A 40 B 41 D 42 A 43 B 44 B 45 A 46 A
47 A

48. Recurrent pulmonary embolism is least likely with:
- **A.** Normal ECG
- **B.** Normal TEE
- **C.** Normal pulmonary scan
- **D.** Normal Chest X-ray

49. ↑ RA pressure with (n) PCWP:
- **A.** RVMI
- **B.** MS
- **C.** IE
- **D.** CHF

50. Side effect of adenosine are all *except:*
- **A.** Bronchospasm
- **B.** SVT
- **C.** Bradycardia
- **D.** Anginal chest pain

51. Contrast echo visualizes best:
- **A.** Right to left shunt
- **B.** Left to right shunt
- **C.** Regurgitant lesion
- **D.** Stenotic lesion

52. Drug of choice for wide QRS tachycardia is:
- **A.** Adenosine
- **B.** Lignocaine
- **C.** Procainamide
- **D.** Flecainide

53. HEYDE syndrome is:
- **A.** Angiodysplasia of colon with AS
- **B.** Angiosarcoma of rectum with AS
- **C.** Angiodysplasia of colon with AR
- **D.** None of the above

54. S2 in large PDA is frequently:
- **A.** Narrow split
- **B.** Wide split
- **C.** Paradoxical split
- **D.** None of the above

55. CCP is differentiated from RCMP by:
- **A.** Variation in mitral inflow velocities
- **B.** TR
- **C.** AR
- **D.** LVEF < 45%

56. Most common type of aortoarteritis in India is:
- **A.** Type I
- **B.** Type II
- **C.** Type III
- **D.** Type IV

57. The most unsaturated venous blood is:
- **A.** IVC
- **B.** Coronary Sinus
- **C.** SVC
- **D.** Hepatic vein

58. Most specific echocardiographic feature of cardiac tamponade is:
- **A.** RVOT diastolic collapse
- **B.** RA diastolic collapse
- **C.** Distension of IVC
- **D.** Paradoxical septal motion

59. Echo findings of MS are all *except:*
- **A.** Decrease EF slope
- **B.** PHT < 50 sec
- **C.** Elevated LA gradient
- **D.** Anterior movement of PML

60. Most common lesion in rheumatic heart disease is:
- **A.** AS + MR
- **B.** MS + MR
- **C.** MS + AR
- **D.** TS + TR

48 C 49 A 50 B 51 A 52 C 53 A 54 C 55 A 56 C 57 B 58 A 59 B 60 B

UP DM 2003

1. **Epigastric pulsations are felt in all *except:***
   A. LVH
   B. Pregnancy
   C. Aortic aneurysm
   D. All of the above

2. **Migratory polyarthritis in child: Diagnosis can be established by:**
   A. ASLO
   B. ESR
   C. Pharyngeal throat swab culture
   D. ECG

3. **Culture negative endocarditis: investigation of choice is:**
   A. Repeat blood culture
   B. Urine culture
   C. Echocardiography
   D. CXR

4. **Embolism: most common cause is:**
   A. Tight MS with AF
   B. AS
   C. TR
   D. AR

5. **Low voltage complex on ECG is seen in:**
   A. Hypothyroidism
   B. Schizophrenia
   C. Barbiturate poisoning
   D. Creutzfeld Jacob disease

6. **CCP is not found in:**
   A. Rh fever
   B. TB
   C. Malignant involvement of pericardium
   D. Legionaieres disease

7. **Elevated apex with round contour of left heart border on Chest X-ray is seen in:**
   A. RVE
   B. LVH
   C. LAE
   D. MS

8. **AMI with RBBB with LAHB: treatment is:**
   A. IV atropine
   B. Prophylactic pacing
   C. Isoprenaline infusion
   D. No treatment

9. **Changing murmur with embolism diagnosis is:**
   A. SABE
   B. Rh fever
   C. MS
   D. AR

10. **Most common manifestation of Rh fever:**
    A. Polyarthritis
    B. Pancarditis
    C. Erythema marginatum
    D. Chorea

1 A 2 A 3 C 4 A 5 A 6 A 7 A 8 B 9 A 10 A

11. **Migratory polyarthritis in a small child; probable diagnosis is:**
A. Rh fever
B. RA
C. Reiter's syndrome
D. Kawasaki's disease

12. **Ten days high grade fever in a 5 year old child with splenomegaly and swelling of joints of four months duration; Diagnosis is:**
A. Syphilis
B. Malaria
C. RA
D. Rh Fever

13. **Causes of joint pains in younger child < 5 years are all *except:***
A. Growing pains
B. Rheumatoid arthritis
C. Neuroblastoma
D. Leukemia

14. **Reversed split of S_2 is heard in all *except:***
A. PS
B. PDA
C. HOCM
D. LBBB

15. **Step up of oxygen in right atrium is seen in:**
A. Gerbode defect
B. ALCAPA
C. LSVC persistent
D. A-P window

16. **PA saturation > aorta is seen in:**
A. d-TGA
B. VSD
C. Triology of Fallot
D. TOF

17. **Infective endocarditis is least common in:**
A. ASD
B. PDA
C. TOF with BT shunt
D. MR

18. **Thrombosis of prosthetic valve is more common in which position ?**
A. Mitral
B. Aortic
C. Pulmonary
D. Tricuspid

19. **Sudden dyspnea, hypotension, PCWP=10, RV 56/18, PA 54/12, RA=18. The diagnosis is:**
A. Cardiac tamponade
B. Pulm embolism
C. Acute MI with LVF
D. Biventricular failure

20. **Acute MI with Cardiac index of 1.8, PCWP 06, SBP 80 mm Hg. Treatment of choice is:**
A. I/v Fluids
B. Dopamine
C. Dobutamine
D. Isoprenaline

21. **Atrial fibrillation with CHB: pacemaker of choice is:**
A. VVIR
B. VVI
C. DDD
D. AAI

22. **Causes of mid diastolic murmur are all *except:***
A. MR
B. PR (hypertensive)
C. VSD
D. CHB

23. **Early systolic murmur is heard in all *except:***
A. Acute severe MR
B. TR (IE in drug abuser)
C. TR with PAH
D. Large VSD with PAH

11 A 12 C 13 C 14 A 15 A 16 A 17 A 18 D 19 B 20 A 21 A 22 B 23 C

24. Increased heart rate causing increased contraction is:
A. Treppe effect
B. Anrep effect
C. Woodworth phenomenon
D. Laplace Law

25. A patient of heart failure with specific activity scale class III symptoms will complete following activities:
A. ≤ 2 mets
B. ≥ 4 mets
C. ≥ 5 mets
D. ≥ 7 mets

26. Maximum systolic tension develops at sarcomere length of:
A. 2.4 mm
B. 2.2 mm
C. 2.5 mm
D. 0.3 mm

27. All are seen in CHF *except:*
A. Decreased pulse pressure
B. Decreased cardiac output
C. Decreased A-V oxygen difference
D. Oliguria

28. Dp/Dt decrease in aortic dissection is achieved by:
A. Hydralazine
B. Sodium nitreprusside
C. β blocker
D. Nifedipine

29. HV interval is increased by:
A. Digoxin
B. Verapamil
C. Dofetilide
D. Bisoprolol

30. Contraindication of IABP are all *except:*
A. Severe PVD
B. Severe Ao iliac disease
C. Severe AS
D. Severe AR

31. IABP is indicated in all *except:*
A. Refractory acute coronary syndrome
B. Acute severe MR
C. Post MI VSD
D. Proximal Ao dissection

32. Drug used in Heart protection study was:
A. Simvastatin
B. Pravastatin
C. Atorvastatin
D. Fenofibrate

33. Obligatory coronary vasodilator are all *except:*
A. Acetylcholine
B. Hypoxia
C. NO
D. NTG

34. All are seen in apical HOCM *except:*
A. Spade like appearance on LV angiogram
B. Giant T inversion in precordial leads
C. No intraventricular gradient
D. Marked symptoms/malignant course

35. All are true about myxoma *except:*
A. 90% solitary
B. 86% LA
C. Valve myxoma not reported
D. Arises most commonly from fossa ovalis

36. LMWH monitoring requires:
A. aPPT
B. ACT
C. Anti Factor Xa activity
D. Russel viper venom time

24 A 25 A 26 B 27 C 28 C 29 C 30 C 31 D 32 A 33 D 34 D 35 C 36 C

37. All are given in Non-Q myocardial infarction *except:*
A. Urokinase
B. LMWH
C. NTG
D. Aspirin

38. GbIIb/IIIa inhibitor act by inhibiting platelet:
A. Aggregation
B. Adhesion
C. Activation
D. Secretion

39. Most successful advancement in management of Restenosis is:
A. Drug eluting stents
B. Brachytherapy
C. Antiproliferative drugs
D. Statins

40. Cyanotic spells are managed with all *except:*
A. Digoxin
B. Morphine
C. Phenylephrine
D. Bicarbonate

41. Congenital long QT syndrome: Treatment of choice is:
A. β blocker
B. Permanent pacing
C. Amiodarone
D. Mg

42. Most common Valvular lesion with conduction block:
A. AS
B. Tight calcific MS
C. AR
D. MR

43. Normal PCWP:
A. 0-2
B. 2-6
C. 6-12
D. 12-18

44. Normal portal venous pressure:
A. 0-20 cm of H_2O
B. 25-35 cm of H_2O
C. 100-120 cm of H_2O
D. 140-180 cm of H_2O

45. Vitamin B-12 level in chronic myeloid leukaemia is:
A. Normal
B. Increased
C. Decreased mildly
D. Severely decreased

46. All are true about PNH *except:*
A. Hypocellular marrow
B. Hemosiderinuria
C. Decreased alkaline phosphatase
D. Pancytopenia

47. Elderly patient with refractory anemia with peripheral smear showing ring sideroblast, 15% blast cells and pancytopenia; Diagnosis is:
A. MDS
B. AML
C. CML
D. Malignant infiltration of bone marrow

48. Late response in Br asthma:
A. Mast cell
B. Eosinophil
C. Macrophages
D. Neutrophils

49. Fiberoptic bronchoscopy is useful in:
A. BAL
B. Endobroncial biopsy
C. Massive hemoptysis
D. All of the above

37 A 38 A 39 A 40 A 41 A 42 A 43 C 44 A 45 B 46 A 47 A 48 A 49 A

50. Crushman's spirals:
A. Br Asthma
B. Bronchitis
C. Bronchiectasis
D. Emphysema

51. True for pancoast tumor is:
A. Radicular pain in UL
B. Left lower lobe
C. Recurrent LN palsy
D. Cerebral pseudo tumor

52. Not seen in pancreatic insuffiency in a patient of chronic pancreatitis:
A. Decreased absorption of iron
B. B12 deficiency
C. Steatorrhoea
D. Calcification

53. Saint's triad include all *except:*
A. Gall stones
B. Cirrhosis
C. Diverticulosis
D. Hiatus hernia

54. Best prognosis in pancreatitis:
A. Gall stone
B. Traumatic
C. Idiopathic
D. Alcoholic

55. Azoospermia (obstructive) is seen in:
A. Munierkhan syndrome
B. William Campbell syndrome
C. Young syndrome
D. Yellow nail syndrome

56. All are true about Addison's disease *except:*
A. HT
B. Low NL
C. Pigmentation
D. Autoimmune is most common etiology

57. Ectopic ACTH in small cell lung carcinoma usually presents with:
A. Hypopigmentation
B. DMS oral +ve (8mg)
C. Hypokalemia alkalosis
D. Cushing features common

58. Post lumbar puncture headache is due to all *except:*
A. Early mobilisation
B. Dehydration
C. CSF pressure changes
D. Rapid change of blood volume

59. 25 year old young, pulling car has BP 150/100 mm Hg headache, positive Kernig, subhyaloid hemorrhage on fundus; Diagnosis is:
A. SAH
B. Cerebral hemorrhage–CVA
C. Meningitis
D. Vascular headache

60. First 2 days after methyl isocyanate poisoning, all are seen *except:*
A. Hemoptysis
B. Lacrimation
C. Chest pain
D. None of the above

61. CNS lymphoma; False statement is:
A. Seen in HIV
B. Multicentric–diffuse histiocytic appearance
C. CSF spread
D. Poorly responsive to RT/CT

62. All are true about Spastic paraplegia *except:*
A. MND
B. Cervical spondylosis
C. Chronic lead poisoning
D. Lathyrism

50 A 51 A 52 A 53 B 54 A 55 C 56 A 57 C 58 D 59 A 60 C 61 D 62 C

63. Prophylactic in intermittent febrile seizures:
A. Diazepam
B. Carbamazepine
C. Phenobarbitone
D. Valproate

64. Bromocriptine is a:
A. D1 Agonist
B. D1 Antagonist
C. D2 Agonist
D. D2 Antagonist

65. Least common site of meningioma is:
A. Falx
B. Sphenoid wing
C. Tentorium
D. Choroid plexus

66. Neurofibroma is not seen with:
A. Pigmentation
B. Meningocoele
C. Cerebral aneurysm
D. Meningioma

67. True for brainstem glioma are all *except:*
A. Brain biopsy required for diagnosis
B. Surgery is difficult
C. MRI delineates well
D. Treatment of choice is radiotherapy

68. Histology in Neumen pick:
A. Foam cells
B. Granules in cytoplasm
C. Multinucleate cells
D. Eosinophils

69. All of the following conditions are autosomal dominant *except:*
A. Tuberous sclerosis
B. Cystic fibrosis
C. Polyposis coli
D. Myotonia dystrophica

70. Melphalan is used in:
A. Myeloma
B. AML
C. Neuroblastoma
D. CML/ALL

71. Nickel is responsible for which carcinoma?
A. Nasopharyngeal
B. Larynx
C. Lung
D. Ethmoid

72. All can be seen in Hodgkin's lymphoma *except:*
A. Lymphocytes
B. Eosinophilia
C. Thrombocytopenia
D. Neutropenia

73. Transplacental transmission is not seen with:
A. CMV
B. Herpes zoster
C. Hepatitis
D. Toxoplasmosis

74. Phenylketonuria is diagnosed by:
A. Gerhardt's test
B. Ferric chloride test
C. Guthre test
D. VMA in urine

75. % of burns calculated from neck, head and face constitutes what percentage in infants?
A. 10
B. 14
C. 15
D. 13

63 C 64 C 65 D 66 C 67 D 68 A 69 B 70 A 71 A 72 C 73 B 74 C 75 B

76. 5 year old with history of fever 10 days with negative physical examination; Differential diagnosis will include all *except:*
A. Polio
B. UTI
C. RA
D. TB complex

77. All are seen in trisomy 18 *except:*
A. Normal intelligence
B. Flexion fingers
C. Rocker bottom foot
D. Prominent occiput

78. Streptococcal vaginitis in child:
A. Local gentian violet
B. Systemic penicillin
C. Estrogen
D. Estrogen + penicillin

79. Malignancy in childhood are all *except:*
A. AML
B. ALL
C. Retinoblastoma
D. Wilm's tumor

80. In children, anabolic steroid are not given because of:
A. Premature closure of epiphysis
B. Hirsutism
C. Precocious puberty
D. None of the above

81. Most common chromosomal abnormality:
A. Trisomy 13
B. Trisomy 18
C. Trisomy 21
D. Fragile X syndrome

82. All are true about Downs syndrome *except:*
A. Commonest cause of mental retardation in children
B. Incidence 1:1300
C. Epicanthal fold
D. Acetabulum rudimentary

83. Reduced calcium:
A. Respiratory acidosis
B. Respiratory alkaiosis
C. Metabolic acidosis
D. Metabolic alkalosis

84. True about chromosomes:
A. Short chromosome denoted as p
B. Triploidy means 3 chromosomes
C. 1st stage meiosis produces haploid cells
D. Chromosomal size increased with group

85. 6 weeks infant will have all *except:*
A. Head holding
B. Fixed gaze
C. Pincer grasp
D. Turning head on sound

86. Infant sits with support at:
A. 4 months
B. 5 months
C. 6 months
D. 7 months

87. Infant sits without support at:
A. 3-5 month
B. 6-8 month
C. 10-12 month
D. 13 months

88. Walking on tip toes begin at:
A. 2.5 yrs
B. 3.5 yrs
C. 2 yrs
D. 1.5 yrs

89. 8 months old child:
A. Sits without support
B. Speaks mama/papa
C. Stands without support
D. None of the above

76 A 77 A 78 B 79 A 80 A 81 C 82 B 83 B 84 A 85 C 86 A 87 B 88 A 89 A

90. Deciduous teeth appear:
A. 9-12 months
B. Stopping bottle feed
C. 5-9 month
D. < 5 months

91. Adolescence behaviour is best described as:
A. Paradoxical
B. Belligerent
C. Aggressive
D. Dominating

92. Nocturnal emission:
A. Psychiatric counselling after puberty
B. Counselling not required
C. Test for hyperthyroidism
D. None of the above

93. Liver abscess is best diagnosed by:
A. USG
B. Exploratory laprotomy
C. Stool ova test
D. Liver enzymes

94. Essentially common to all nephritic syndromes is:
A. Oedema
B. Hypertension
C. Severe proteinuria
D. Hypoproteinemia

95. Tamm Horsfell protein is:
A. Tubular protein
B. Not detected by dipstick
C. Component of serum albumin
D. None of the above

96. Number of parathyroid glands are:
A. 1
B. 2
C. 4
D. 6

97. Most common cause of impotence is:
A. Psychogenic
B. Syphilis
C. Diabetes Mellitus
D. Leriche's syndrome

98. Most common organism causing osteomyelitis is:
A. Staphylococcus
B. Streptococcus
C. Tubercle bacilli
D. Spirochetal organisms

99. Most common valve involved in rheumatic fever is:
A. Mitral
B. Tricuspid
C. Aortic
D. Pulmonic

100. Which s not a phase of Diastole?
A. Isovolumic relaxation
B. Diastasis
C. Atrial contraction
D. Isovolumic contraction

90 C 91 A 92 A 93 A 94 C 95 A 96 C 97 A 98 A 99 A 100 D

UP DM 2001

1. **In patient with post MI VSD, most useful in diagnosis is:**
   A. Large V wave
   B. Palpable thrill
   C. Murmur (systolic)
   D. O2 step up in RV

2. **All are true about acute MR *except:***
   A. Loudness does not indicate severity
   B. IE should be rule out
   C. ECG s/o acute MI
   D. LV systolic pressure is ↑

3. **All are true about acute MR *except:***
   A. Large LA
   B. Normal heart size
   C. ↑ LA pressure
   D. ↑ PAP

4. **Bisferians pulse can be seen in all *except:***
   A. AR
   B. AS with AR
   C. HOCM
   D. CHF

5. **Weak low volume pulse is seen in all *except:***
   A. VSD
   B. Card tamponade
   C. CCF
   D. AS

6. **Which is most characteristic of chronic severe AR?**
   A. Traube's sign
   B. Quincke's sign
   C. Pistol shot
   D. Duroziez sign

7. **Contrast echo is useful in diagnosis of:**
   A. Regurgitant lesion
   B. Stenotic lesion
   C. R → L shunt
   D. L → R shunt

8. **Essence trial used:**
   A. Dalteparin
   B. Enoxaparine
   C. Nadroparine
   D. Fraxiparine

9. **Diagnosis of pericardial effusion is best established by:**
   A. Angiography
   B. Echocardiography
   C. Serial X-ray
   D. Cine angiocardiography

10. **All of the following drugs are used for stress echo *except:***
   A. NTG
   B. Adenosine
   C. Dipyridamole
   D. Dobutamine

1 D 2 D 3 A 4 D 5 A 6 D 7 C 8 B 9 B 10 A

11. Incidence of ARF after streptococcal pharyngitis:
A. 0.3-3%
B. 10-20%
C. 50-60%
D. 80-90%

12. Aschoff nodule is seen in all *except:*
A. RV free wall
B. Atrial appendage
C. IVS
D. LV lat wall

13. ↑ ASO is least likely to be seen in all *except:*
A. Carditis
B. Chorea
C. Arthritis
D. SC nodule

14. IE is most common in:
A. PS
B. Floppy valve with MR
C. MS
D. CAD

15. Pregnancy is least tolerated in all *except:*
A. Marfan
B. CoA
C. MVP
D. PPH

16. All of the following is used as adjunctive with PTCA + stent *except:*
A. Acitrom
B. Clopidogrel
C. Ticlopidine
D. Aspirin

17. All are true about Clopidogrel *except:*
A. Glycoprotein IIb/IIIa inhibition through ADP
B. Severe BM depression
C. Single dose
D. As effective as ticlopidine

18. Restenosis will be least with:
A. Concentric lesion< 10 mm
B. >10 mm
C. Prox graft stent (SVG)
D. Total occlusion

19. ↑ recurrence following PTCA/stent is seen with all *except:*
A. ↑ plaque burden
B. Small vessel size
C. Ostial lesion
D. Increase MLD

20. Stent is useful for:
A. Dissection
B. ↓ Heart attack
C. ↓ Restenosis
D. Decreasing mortality

21. AH jump is characteristic of:
A. AVNRT
B. AVRT
C. WPW
D. Atrial tachycardia

22. Carotid sinus massage decrease rate in all *except:*
A. AVRT
B. AVNRT
C. Atypical AVNRT
D. Atrial tachycardia

23. Decrease QT is seen with all *except:*
A. Hypercalcemia
B. Hyperkalemia
C. Digitalis
D. Astemizole/terfenadine

24. In HOCM, all are effective *except:*
A. VVI
B. DDD
C. Amiodarone
D. β blocker

11 A 12 A 13 B 14 B 15 C 16 A 17 B 18 A 19 D 20 A 21 A 22 D 23 D 24 A

25. All are true about torsades de pointes *except:*
A. Axis and amplitude alternating around baseline
B. Class 1A & 1 c is use for treatment
C. Prolong QT predisposes to torsades
D. Bradycardia with CHB can lead to torsades

26. All are true about VT of arrhythmogenic right ventricular dysplasia *except:*
A. LBBB
B. RAD
C. Increase T wave amplitude in precordial leads
D. RFA may be effective

27. Magnet application over demand pacemaker leads to:
A. Reversion to fixed mode
B. Slows underlying rhythm
C. Ventricular fibrillation
D. Loss of cardiac capture

28. AAI pacing is indicated in:
A. SSS
B. CHB (Acq)
C. CHB (congenital)
D. Trifascicular block

29. All are true about sexual side effects of beta blockers *except:*
A. Vasodilator can be useful
B. Dose related
C. Can improve by decreasing dose
D. 1-2% incidence

30. All are true about RVMI *except:*
A. ↑RV systolic pressure
B. ↑RV filling pressure
C. Normal LV filling pressure
D. ↓ CO

31. All are true about mitral stenosis *except:*
A. Presystolic murmur indicate severe MS
B. MS with MR with long MDM indicate severe MS
C. Severity is assessed by duration of murmur
D. MDM is a low pitch murmur

32. All are true about orthostatic hypotension *except:*
A. ↑parasympathetic outflow
B. Occurs with upright posture
C. Dizziness and syncope with upright posture
D. ↓venous return

33. Constrictive pericarditis: etiology is:
A. Tubercular
B. Fungal
C. Postpyocardium
D. All of the above

34. Paradoxical split is seen with all *except:*
A. WPW type B
B. PPH
C. LBBB
D. HOCM

35. Post stenotic aortic root dilatation is seen with all of the following *except:*
A. Rheumatic AS
B. Cong AS
C. Subaortic membrane stenosis
D. HOCM

36. AR because of valve and aorta involvement is seen in:
A. Marfan
B. Ankylosing spondylitis
C. Syphilis
D. IE

37. Negative delta wave in I, aVl indicate:
A. Left lateral pathway
B. Right lateral pathway
C. Right posteroseptal pathway
D. Left posteroseptal pathway

25 B 26 C 27 A 28 A 29 D 30 A 31 A 32 A 33 D 34 B 35 D 36 B 37 A

38. All are true about ACE-I *except:*
- **A.** Low dose as effective as high dose
- **B.** 1st drug of choice in systolic dysfunction
- **C.** High and low dose well tolerated
- **D.** None of the above

39. Hemodynamic burden is associated with all compensatory mechanism *except:*
- **A.** ↓ venous return
- **B.** Vent hypertrophy
- **C.** ↑ NE/E release from adrenergic nerve ending and adrenal medulla
- **D.** On the maximum of Frank Starlings curve

40. AF is least likely to convert in following conditions *except:*
- **A.** Large LA
- **B.** AF of recent onset
- **C.** AF of more than one year duration
- **D.** Long standing MS

41. Electrical defibrillation is treatment of choice in:
- **A.** VF
- **B.** VT
- **C.** AF
- **D.** Atrial tachycardia

42. Isolated primary TR is seen in following condition *except:*
- **A.** Rheumatic
- **B.** IE
- **C.** Ebstein's anomaly
- **D.** Carcinoid syndrome

43. All are true about thromboembolism of mechanical prosthesis *except:*
- **A.** Aortic more common than mitral
- **B.** 1-3% per year
- **C.** 1-2 % incidence of CNS complications
- **D.** Higher incidence with tricuspid valve prosthesis

44. Bioprosthetic valve is:
- **A.** Bjork Shiley valve
- **B.** Starr Edward
- **C.** Carpentier Edward
- **D.** Omniscience

45. Pulmonary wedge pressure injection is done in:
- **A.** Pulmonary atresia
- **B.** TAPVC
- **C.** Pulmonary venoocclusive disease
- **D.** ASD

46. ↑PCWP is seen in all *except:*
- **A.** MS
- **B.** LVF secondary to MI
- **C.** COPD
- **D.** VSD large

47. Pseudoaneurysm is diagnosed by:
- **A.** Size of neck
- **B.** Site
- **C.** Thrombus
- **D.** Wall thickness

48. All are reperfusion arrhythmias *except:*
- **A.** AIVR
- **B.** Atrial flutter
- **C.** Sinus Bradycardia
- **D.** NSVT

49. All are mechanism of action of statins *except:*
- **A.** Improve endothelial function
- **B.** ↑macrophage, T cell apoptosis
- **C.** ↓Platelet aggregation
- **D.** Decrease smooth muscle proliferation

50. Most common cause of sudden cardiac death is:
- **A.** Kawasaki disease
- **B.** CAD
- **C.** AS
- **D.** HOCM

38 A 39 A 40 B 41 A 42 A 43 A 44 C 45 A 46 C 47 A 48 B 49 B 50 B

UP DM 2000

1. Normal A_2-OS interval is:
- **A.** 60-120 msec
- **B.** 120-140 msec
- **C.** 200-320 msec
- **D.** 300-400 msec

2. Normal S1–S3 interval is:
- **A.** 60-120 msec
- **B.** 120-240 msec
- **C.** 300-400 msec
- **D.** 240-300 msec

3. Worst prognosis in increasing frequency in AS is:
- **A.** Angina < syncope < failure
- **B.** Syncope > angina > failure
- **C.** Failure < syncope < angina
- **D.** Syncope > angina < failure

4. Which of the following is useful in treatment of uncomplicated HOCM?
- **A.** Dual chamber pacing–Epicardial leads over LA and LV
- **B.** NTG
- **C.** Digoxin
- **D.** Dual chamber pacing - Endocardial leads in RA and RV

5. All are seen in acute MR *except:*
- **A.** Normal LV size
- **B.** Normal LV pressure
- **C.** Acute MI
- **D.** IE is the cause

6. BMV is indicated in all *except:*
- **A.** Wide A_2-OS
- **B.** Loud OS
- **C.** Loud S1
- **D.** LVS_3

7. HAPE is associated with:
- **A.** ↑ LVEDP
- **B.** ↑ PCWP
- **C.** Decrease pulmonary capillary permeability
- **D.** Normal LA pressure

8. Best to beat variation in BP is seen in all *except:*
- **A.** Polymorphic VT
- **B.** CHB
- **C.** Idioventricular rhythm
- **D.** AF

9. All can be seen in PS with CHF *except:*
- **A.** Loud P_2
- **B.** Delayed P_2
- **C.** Large a wave
- **D.** RVS_3

10. Abnormal in >45 year age:
- **A.** Grade 1/3 LPH
- **B.** LVS3
- **C.** $A_2 > P_2$
- **D.** Absent P2 in mitral area

1 A 2 C 3 A 4 D 5 B 6 D 7 D 8 C 9 A 10 B

11. All are true about PPH *except:*
- **A.** Hoarseness of voice
- **B.** Syncope
- **C.** Squatting
- **D.** Hemoptysis

12. All are true about PPH *except:*
- **A.** ↑ PCO_2 in arteries
- **B.** Large a wave
- **C.** Constant ejection clicks
- **D.** Palpable P_2

13. All are true about sarcoidosis *except:*
- **A.** Pericardial effusion
- **B.** Ventricular aneurysms
- **C.** Conduction abnormality
- **D.** G6PD deficiency

14. CAD is associated with all of the following *except:*
- **A.** Amyloidosis
- **B.** Rheumatoid arthritis
- **C.** Hurler's syndrome
- **D.** Homocystinuria

15. All can be seen in digitalis toxicity *except:*
- **A.** Yellow vision
- **B.** Scotoma
- **C.** Gynecomastia
- **D.** Erythema marginatum

16. Digitalis toxicity can cause all *except:*
- **A.** 1° heart block
- **B.** CHB
- **C.** Wenckbach
- **D.** VT

17. Pulsus paradoxus is seen in all *except:*
- **A.** Pericardial effusion
- **B.** Constrictive pericarditis
- **C.** Cardiac tamponade
- **D.** COPD

18. Wide split S2 is heard in:
- **A.** Moderate MR
- **B.** LBBB
- **C.** AS
- **D.** HOCM

19. A patient is admitted to emergency with digitalis toxicity showing trifascicular block with a heart rate of 45/min. His serum potassium is 3.5 meq/L. His BP is 90/60 mm Hg and ejection fraction is 22%. The treatment would include all *except:*
- **A.** Potassium correction i/v
- **B.** Injection xylocaine
- **C.** Temporary cardiac pacing
- **D.** Stop digoxin

20. P2 is not heard in all *except:*
- **A.** Severe PS
- **B.** Pulmonary atresia
- **C.** Peripheral pulmonary artery stenosis
- **D.** Absent pulmonary valve syndrome

21. Wide pulse pressure is seen in all *except:*
- **A.** PDA
- **B.** A-V fistula
- **C.** RSOV
- **D.** MS with AR

22. LEOPARD syndrome has:
- **A.** Pulmonary stenosis
- **B.** Eye abnormalities
- **C.** Oral ulcers
- **D.** None of the above

23. TEE is superior to TTE in all *except:*
- **A.** LA thrombus
- **B.** Assessing severity of MS
- **C.** LAA clot
- **D.** Poor echo window

11 C 12 A 13 D 14 A 15 D 16 A 17 A 18 A 19 A 20 C 21 D 22 A 23 B

24. Patient with recurrent V ' with increased QT interval. Treatment is:
A. i/v Magnesium
B. Pacing
C. Lignocaine
D. Beta blocker

25. Acute AF in pregnancy; treatment of choice is:
A. DC cardioversion
B. Amiodarone
C. Xylocaine
D. Digitalis

26. Class III antiarrhythmic is:
A. Amiodarone
B. Bretylium
C. Mexiletine
D. Xylocaine

27. Oxygen step up in RA is due to:
A. VSD with TR
B. AP window
C. PDA
D. Eisenmenger syndrome

28. Warfarin does not affect which of the following factors:
A. II
B. VII
C. IX
D. XII

29. P2 component of second heart sound in TOF may be audible with all of the following *except:*
A. Pink TOF
B. Excessive bronchopulmonary collaterals
C. Bilateral pulmonary artery stenosis
D. Malposition of great arteries

30. Chordae tendinae rupture is not found in:
A. ASD
B. HOCM
C. AR
D. RHD

31. In a case of PDA with Qp:Qs of 1.5 and RV 30/15, the operation is done to prevent:
A. CHF
B. AF
C. Eisenmengers syndrome
D. IE

32. Which of the following is not seen in situs solitus?
A. Hyparterial right bronchus with trilobed lung
B. Hyparterial left bronchus with bilobed lung
C. Right atrium on right and left atrium on left
D. IVC on right and aorta on left

33. Which of the following are true with respect to right aortic arch?
A. Associated congenital cardiac malformation in 95% cases
B. Occurs in 25% cases of tricuspid atresia
C. Occurs in 5% cases of TOF
D. Occurs in 5% cases of truncus arteriosus

34. Warfarin causes carboxylation of all the following factors *except:*
A. Protein C
B. Protein S
C. Factors VIII
D. Factor II

35. Opening snap is not heard in:
A. Ebsteins anomaly
B. ASD
C. Pure MR
D. Severe MS

36. Smoking is not associated with:
A. Increased free fatty acid mobilisation
B. Angina
C. Shift of oxygen dissociation curve to right
D. Catecholamine excess

24 B 25 A 26 C 27 A 28 D 29 B 30 C 31 D 32 B 33 A 34 C 35 B 36 C

37. Oxygen dissociation curve is shifted to right by all *except:*

A. Increase CO_2
B. Increase Temperature
C. Acidosis
D. Increase pH

38. Teratogenic drugs are all *except:*

A. Alcohol
B. Labetalol
C. Lithium
D. Retinoic acid

39. Balloon atrial septostomy is done in all *except:*

A. TOF
B. TGA
C. TA
D. MA

40. Following can be seen in hypothermia *except:*

A. Osborn wave
B. Elevation of J point
C. Sinus bradycardia
D. VT

41. True about athlete heart is:

A. Sinus bradycardia
B. High incidence of CHD
C. Predisposes for SCD
D. VT is generally seen

42. Which of the following is true?

A. Malignant melanoma has highest propensity for metastasis to pericarditis
B. RA myxoma is more common than LA myxoma
C. Angiosarcoma is most common in children
D. None of the above

43. Plain X-ray chest in a 2 year old child with coarctation of aorta not in CHF, which of the following radiological signs would be seen?

A. Rib notching
B. Cardiomegaly
C. E Sign
D. Normal Heart size

44. Cyanosis with increase pulmonary blood flow is seen in:

A. Truncus Arteriosus
B. Tricuspid atresia
C. TOF
D. RSOV

45. BP difference of > 5 mm Hg in upper limbs is seen with:

A. Supravalvular AS
B. Subaortic stenosis
C. Valvular AS
D. None of the above

46. Which of the following would you use in Phase IV of Korotkoff sounds as an index of diastolic blood pressure?

A. Aortic stenosis
B. Riley Day Syndrome
C. Severe Aortic regurgitation
D. Mitral stenosis

47. The survival of a population in years is given below. What is the median survival of this population? (2,3,3,4,4,4,5,5,6,7,7,8,9)

A. 4 years
B. 4.7 years
C. 5 years
D. 5.7 years

48. Following are the side effects of heparin *except:*

A. Osteoporosis
B. Thrombocytopenia
C. Increase level of factor V
D. Prolonged activated clotting time

37 D 38 B 39 A 40 D 41 A 42 A 43 D 44 A 45 A 46 C 47 C 48 C

49. All are true about PAN *except:*

A. MI
B. CHF
C. Aortic root dilatation
D. Mononeuritis multiplex

50. During cardiac catheterization of a 3 years old child with VSD, the following data are obtained: Saturation PA-88%, Ao-91%, RA-60%, Pulmonary vein 90%. His arterial blood gases show PaO_2=67, $PaCO_2$=56 and pH=7.3. Most likely cause of low aortic saturation is:

A. Right to left shunt a atrial level
B. Eisenmengers complex
C. Presence of chest infection
D. Sedative overdose

49 C 50 D

CMC Vellore 2004

1. Differentiating feature of acute MR from chronic AR is:
- **A.** Normal heart size
- **B.** No holosystolic murmur
- **C.** Murmur radiating to neck
- **D.** Normal JVP

2. Which of the following is not useful in unstable angina:
- **A.** Aspirin
- **B.** Heparin
- **C.** Hirudin
- **D.** Thrombolytic therapy

3. GpII/IIIa receptors are encoded on which chromosome:
- **A.** 13
- **B.** 14
- **C.** 15
- **D.** 17

4. HOCM is encoded on which chromosome?
- **A.** 1
- **B.** 14
- **C.** 15
- **D.** All of the above

5. Normal intraventricular pressure (no gradient) with spade shaped ventricular cavity on echocardiography with deep T wave inversion on ECG is suggestive of:
- **A.** Apical HOCM
- **B.** ARVD
- **C.** DCMP
- **D.** RCMP

6. True is:
- **A.** Increase in serum potassium increases AV junctional delay
- **B.** Potassium is used for treatment of mild CHF in elderly
- **C.** HF causes increase serum potassium
- **D.** ACE-inhibitors cause low potassium

7. Post MI primary prevention of VF-ICD trials is:
- **A.** MADIT
- **B.** CASH
- **C.** AVID
- **D.** CIDS

8. GUSTO I-β angio subset showed TIMI III flow at 90 minutes with streptokinase in:
- **A.** 22%
- **B.** 33%
- **C.** 54%
- **D.** 70%

1 A 2 D 3 D 4 D 5 A 6 A 7 A 8 B

9. Thirty four year old female, PA 100/48 mm Hg (68 mm Hg), RV-100/18 mm Hg, RA mean–18 mm Hg, PCWP-18 mm Hg, CI–2.0 Lt/min/m^2: diagnosis is:
- A. Pulmonary venocclusive disease
- B. PPH
- C. RVF
- D. Pulmonary AV fistula

10. Transpulmonary gradient is:
- A. 2 mm Hg
- B. 10 mm Hg
- C. 45 mm Hg
- D. 63 mm Hg

11. Pulmonary vascular resistance index is:
- A. 20
- B. 40
- C. 60
- D. 80

12. A 13 year old patient with pressure half time of 150 msec at heart rate of 65/min, transmitral gradient of 5 mm Hg at heart rate of 72/min, PCWP 11 mm Hg: calculated MVA of 0.9 cm^2: Diagnosis is:
- A. Mild MS
- B. Moderate MS
- C. Severe MS
- D. Indeterminate

13. Treatment of the above mentioned patient is:
- A. Medical
- B. BMV
- C. Surgery
- D. Either of them

14. Follow up should be done after how much time?
- A. 1 year
- B. 2 year
- C. 6 weeks
- D. 6 months

15. Renal transplant was done in a patient 1 year back with prior IWMI. He received kidney from sister. Lipids- total cholesterol-280 mg%, HDL-50 mg%, Tg-100 mg%, creatinine-0.8 mg%: Patient is on prednisolone and cyclosporine. treatment for this patient is:
- A. Atorvastatin
- B. Simvastatin
- C. Lovastatin
- D. Pravastatin

16. LDL goal in this patient is:
- A. <100 mg%
- B. <130 mg%
- C. <160 mg%
- D. <200 mg%

17. Repeat lipid profile should be done at:
- A. 6-8 weeks
- B. 6-12 weeks
- C. 4 months
- D. 6 months

18. 54 year old female with uncomplicated IWMI 3 weeks back is on aspirin, ACE-inhibitors and beta blockers. Treatment is:
- A. Exercise training thrice weekly
- B. Cardiac rehabilitation
- C. Vitamin E 400 mg/day
- D. TMT after 3 weeks

19. PA saturation of 75%, FA saturation of 99%, BP-120/80 mm Hg- After giving a drug PA saturation is 85% and FA saturation is 99% with BP-110/60 mm Hg. Which of the following drug is given:
- A. Bisoprolol
- B. Norepinephrine
- C. Verapamil
- D. Dobutamine

9 A 10 A 11 B 12 B 13 A 14 A 15 D 16 A 17 A 18 D 19 C

20. Diagnosis is:
A. Left to right shunt
B. PPH
C. Pulmonary AV fistula
D. Right to left shunt

21. Troponin in post MI patient: true is:
A. Peak after 24 hours
B. Elevated for 10-20 days
C. Troponin I is typically elevated upto 10 times
D. Elevated < 2 hours

22. Inverted p in II, III and aVF is seen in:
A. Low atrial rhythm
B. Coronary sinus rhythm
C. Atrial flutter
D. All of the above

23. A 6 year old child with history of multiple episodes of tinnitus, deafness. Younger sister had sudden cardiac death. Probable diagnosis is:
A. Jervell Lange Nielsen syndrome
B. Romano ward syndrome
C. Barlow syndrome
D. None of the above

24. Following emboli are of cardiac origin:
A. Cholesterol
B. Holenhurst plaque
C. Fibrin and platelets
D. Calcium

25. A patient had cardiac arrest and monitor showed ventricular tachycardia. Treatment is:
A. Lidocaine
B. Monitor for 2-5 minutes
C. DC shock 200 J
D. Any of the above

26. After the above treatment, patient developed ventricular fibrillation: treatment is:
A. Shock 3 times
B. Shock once of 360 J
C. i/v epinephrine
D. None of the above

27. Discharge rate from hospital for such patients is:
A. 90%
B. 67%
C. 10%
D. 20%

28. Which of the following is true about contrast nephropathy:
A. Routine monitoring is important to prevent
B. Best treatment is saline infusion
C. Incidence is high with contrast volume < 100 ml
D. Non ionic has less thrombogenicity

29. MR is treated surgically when LVESD is greater than:
A. 45 mm
B. 55 mm
C. 47-52 mm
D. 40 mm

30. Graham Steel murmur of PAH:
A. Increases in expiration
B. Increases in inspiration
C. No change with respiration
D. Decrease with inspiration

31. Nonhypertensive severe TR: true is:
A. Holosystolic murmur with normal RV pressure
B. High frequency in IE
C. Giant v wave
D. None of the above

32. RVMI in anterior wall MI is seen in:
A. Rare
B. Impossible
C. 13%
D. 25%

20 A 21 A 22 D 23 A 24 C 25 C 26 B 27 B 28 B 29 A 30 B 31 B 32 A

33. Abdominal aortic aneurysm in patients with CAD is seen in:
- A. 1%
- B. 5%
- C. 10%
- D. 15%

34. TS murmur: true is:
- A. Best heard at left sternal border
- B. Increase in inspiration
- C. Present in AF
- D. Present in sinus rhythm
- E. All of the above

35. Reperfusion causes all *except:*
- A. Congestion necrosis
- B. Accelerated myocardial necrosis
- C. Hemorrhagic infarct
- D. Limits infarct size

36. A 75 year old male with continuous chest pain radiating to back and BP of 190/90 mm Hg. Treatment of choice is:
- A. IV metoprolol or i/v nitroprusside
- B. Direct admission in a medical emergency
- C. ECG is useful in diagnosis
- D. None of the above

37. Which of the following favors RCMP rather than CCP:
- A. LVEDP = RVEDP
- B. 80% filling occur in early diastole
- C. Apical impulse is palpable
- D. Prominent S3

38. Symptoms in HOCM are due to:
- A. Hypertrophy
- B. Ischemia
- C. Diastolic dysfunction
- D. Obstruction
- E. All of the above

39. Post pericardiotomy syndrome is seen in all *except:*
- A. PDA closure
- B. CoA repair
- C. ASD closure
- D. MVR

40. Diaphragmatic paralysis: true is:
- A: Confirmed by snuff test
- B. Following open heart surgery is not reversible
- C. Bilateral palsy is treated with pacing
- D. None of the above

41. Current hypertension classification is:
- A. JNC 6
- B. JNC 5
- C. JNC 7
- D. JNC 8

42. Regarding BMV; true is:
- A. Echo before BMV for suitability
- B. Mortality is 5%
- C. Subvalvular anatomy is not important
- D. All of the above

43. Primary APLS: true are all *except:*
- A. Recurrent arterial thrombosis
- B. NBTE
- C. LV thrombosis
- D. Conduction system disease

44. Least lipid soluble beta blocker is:
- A. Propanolol
- B. Metoprolol
- C. Carvedilol
- D. Nadolol

45. Which of the following does not cause atherosclerotic CAD?
- A. SLE
- B. PAN
- C. MVP
- D. Aortic stenosis

33 B 34 E 35 B 36 A 37 C 38 E 39 A 40 A 41 C 42 A 43 D 44 D 45 C

46. A 45 year old businessman with retrosternal chest pain immediately on lying down, relieved by nitrates after 10-20 minutes: Diagnosis is:
A. Reflux oesophagitis
B. Variant angina
C. Variable threshold angina
D. None of the above

47. Exudative pleural effusion is characterized by:
A. Fluid: serum LDH > 60%
B. Fluid: serum LDH > 80%
C. Fluid: serum LDH > 40%
D. Fluid: serum LDH is not relevant

48. Abciximab dose is:
A. 160 mg bolus followed by 50 mg/hour
B. 0.25 mg/kg i/v bolus followed by 0.125 μg/kg/min infusion
C. 0.50 mg/kg i/v bolus followed by 0.125 μg/kg/min infusion
D. Two bolus of 0.25 mg/kg i/v 10 minutes apart followed by 0.125-10 μg/kg/min infusion

49. Renovascular hypertension: true is:
A. MRI is 100% sensitive for diagnosis
B. Post captopril PRA > 12 IU is diagnostic
C. Captopril Tc99 DTPA is 90% sensitive
D. None of the above

50. Temporal arteritis; true is:
A. Small artery disease
B. Jaw and tongue claudicated
C. Stenosis is severe only if it lasts for 3 weeks
D. None of the above

51. Holiday heart syndrome: most common abnormality is:
A. Atrial fibrillation
B. Atrial ectopics
C. Ventricular tachycardia
D. Ventricular fibrillation

52. In Frederickson classification, type with increased triglyceride levels are all *except:*
A. IV
B. V
C. III
D. IIa

53. Tangier's disease: true are all *except:*
A. Enlarge yellow tonsil
B. Increased HDL
C. Is due to abnormal efflux in skin fibroblast
D. None of the above

54. In ARVD, ECG shows:
A. Epsilon wave
B. LBBB
C. LAHB
D. LPHB

55. Most common arrhythmia in preexcitation is:
A. PSVT
B. AF
C. Atrial flutter
D. VT

56. To provoke vasospasm in variant angina, which of the following is used:
A. Ergonovine
B. Methacholine
C. Hyperventilation
D. All of the above

57. In depression, which of the following is true:
A. Decrease heart rate variability
B. TCA decrease AV block
C. SSRI increases warfarin levels
D. A + C

58. Thrombolysis in elderly causes:
A. Less mortality
B. Same incidence of intracranial hemorrhage in elderly as young
C. Is an absolute contraindication
D. None of the above

46 A 47 A 48 B 49 C 50 B 51 A 52 D 53 B 54 A 55 A 56 D 57 C 58 D

59. Which of the following is true about AIDS:
A. ELISA is the best screening test
B. P24 antigen capture is confirmatory
C. Western blot is also for screening
D. All of the above

60. Needle stick injury in cath lab from a known HBsAg + patient. Best treatment modality is:
A. HBIG 0.06 ml/kg followed by HB vaccine 2 weeks later
B. HBIG 0.03 ml/kg only
C. Full hepatitis-B vaccine course
D. Any of the above

61. Roth spots are seen in:
A. Anemia
B. Leukemia
C. IE
D. All of the above

62. Intraventricular conduction defect in myocardial infarction: True is:
A. LAHB in 20%
B. LBBB in 15%
C. LPHB in 20%
D. LPHB denotes extensive damage

63. Animal with maximum coronary collaterals is:
A. Pig
B. Dog
C. Rabbit
D. Guinea pig

64. Angiogenesis is:
A. Sprouting of new collaterals from existing collaterals
B. Conversion of existing blood vessels into collaterals
C. Insertion of SVC graft by surgeon
D. None of the above

65. Increase collateral blood flow: true is:
A. Endogenous vasodilatation
B. Collaterals more in males
C. Collateral formation occurs when stenosis is more than 50%
D. All of the above

66. Large vegetation prone to embolisation is seen in:
A. Enterococci infection
B. Fungal infection
C. Staphylococcus aureus infection
D. HACEK infection

67. Enterococcal endocarditis: true are all *except:*
A. Cephalosporins are treatment of choice
B. Synergistic action between cell wall agent and aminoglycoside is required for treatment
C. Sensitive to penicillin G
D. Treatment for 6 weeks

68. IE: true is:
A. Two blood cultures should be taken from two separate venipuncture site
B. Arterial or venous sample does not influence culture positivity
C. Two separate sample 12 hours apart should be positive
D. All of the above

69. IE: major criteria are all *except:*
A. New Regurgitant murmur
B. Increase in existing Regurgitant murmur on chest examination
C. Partial valve ring dehiscence
D. Culture positive in a sample sent 12 hours apart

70. ACE inhibitors in MI: true is:
A. I/v enalapril is to be given < 24 hours
B. Should be given for minimum 6 weeks in STEMI
C. Oral to be given within 24 hours
D. All of the above

59 A 60 A 61 D 62 D 63 D 64 B 65 B 66 B 67 A 68 D 69 B 70 C

71. Trial showing decreased mortality with spironolactone is:
A. RALES
B. ELITE
C. SOLVD
D. EMERALD

72. Ibutilide is which type of antiarrhythmic:
A. I
B. II
C. III
D. IV

73. Which is a class III antiarrhythmic?
A. Amiodarone
B. Lidocaine
C. Procainamide
D. Quinidine

74. All of the following are seen in hypertensive crisis *except:*
A. Diastolic BP > 140 mm Hg
B. Proteinuria
C. Normal sensorium
D. Retinal hemorrhage

75. Best valve in tricuspid position is:
A. Porcine heterograft
B. St Judes prosthesis
C. Caged ball valve
D. None of the above

76. Regarding bioprosthetic valve degeneration, true is:
A. Is directly proportional to age of the valve
B. Maximum in aortic position
C. Porcine graft shows maximum degeneration
D. Homograft

77. Maximum thrombogenicity is seen with:
A. Ball and cage valves
B. St Jude prosthesis in mitral position
C. St Jude prosthesis in aortic position
D. Bioprosthesis in aortic position

78. Regarding bioprosthetic valve, true is:
A. 30% degeneration at 10 years
B. Requires anticoagulation after 3 months
C. Valve failure is slower in children
D. All of the above

79. Significant transvalvular gradient for TS is:
A. 1 mm Hg
B. 2 mm Hg
C. 3 mm Hg
D. 4 mm Hg

80. TR jet velocity is 4 m/sec, RA pressure is 4 mm Hg, RVSP is:
A. 64 mm Hg
B. 68 mm Hg
C. 70 mm Hg
D. 72 mm Hg

81. Constrictive pericarditis with calcification extending into the myocardium and epicardial coronaries; clinical feature is:
A. Pseudo infarct with deep 'q' waves
B. Atrial fibrillation
C. Conduction block
D. Ventricular tachycardia

82. Pericardial calcification: true is:
A. Most commonly involves diaphragmatic surface
B. Calcification can occur without hemodynamic compromise
C. Thickening and calcification can cause CCP
D. Isolated involvement of one ventricle can occur

83. In unstable angina, obstruction in angiography is present in:
A. 25%
B. 15%
C. 85%
D. 50%

71 A 72 C 73 A 74 C 75 A 76 A 77 A 78 A 79 B 80 B 81 C 82 B 83 C

84. Cardiac free wall rupture following MI, True are all *except:*

A. More common in males
B. Less common with multiple myocardial infarctions
C. Occur with > 20% of myocardial involvement
D. More common with anterior than inferior wall MI

85. Brugada syndrome: true is:

A. RBBB with ST elevation
B. Cause of VT
C. 10% of idiopathic VT
D. VT never occurs during sleep

86. Myocardial oxygen consumption is dependant on all *except:*

A. Contractility
B. Stroke volume
C. Heart rate
D. Wall stress

87. In clinical setting, most common cause of stunning is:

A. Exercise induced ischemia
B. Post cardiac surgery
C. Unstable angina
D. Post MI

Hibernation is determined by all *except:*

A. Post extrasystolic potential
B. Dobutamine echocardiography
C. PET scan
D. Nuclear imaging

89. Definitive indication for endomyocardial biopsy is in diagnosis of:

A. Myocarditis
B. Rejection of graft
C. AIDS
D. All of the above

90. Amyloidosis with cardiac disease is best detected by:

A. Endomyocardial biopsy
B. Rectal biopsy
C. Abdominal fat pad aspiration
D. None of the above

91. Endomyocardial biopsy: grading is used according to which criteria:

A. Dallas criteria
B. Duke's criteria
C. Sone's criteria
D. Seller's criteria

92. IE: diagnostic criteria used are:

A. Duke's criteria
B. Jones criteria
C. Dallas criteria
D. None of the above

93. Post surgery recurrence is more with:

A. Sporadic myxoma
B. Familial myxoma
C. Both of the above
D. None of the above

94. Bisferians pulse: true is:

A. Tidal and percussion wave
B. Seen in HOCM
C. Seen in AS with AR
D. Same as dicrotic pulse

95. Post MI: true is:

A. Beta blocker decrease ventricular ectopy and decrease mortality
B. Calcium channel blocker decrease mortality
C. Amiodarone indicated in asymptomatic VPC's
D. All of the above

96. Most common reperfusion arrhythmia is:

A. AIVR
B. Sinus bradycardia
C. Atrial fibrillation
D. Ventricular fibrillation

84 A 85 A 86 B 87 B 88 A 89 B 90 C 91 A 92 A 93 B 94 C 95 A 96 A

97. Vitamin K dependent factors are all *except:*

A. V
B. VII
C. IX
D. Protein C

98. Methods to assess severity of MS by echo include all *except:*

A. Pressure half time
B. Mean transvalvular gradient
C. Peak transvalvular gradient
D. Pulmonary venous flow

99. Isovolumic contraction index:

A. Dp/Dt max
B. VEF mean
C. Both of the above
D. None of the above

100. Pleural effusion is most common with:

A. RVF
B. LVF
C. AR
D. PR

101. Early PVE: most common organism is:

A. Staph aureus
B. Staph epidermidis
C. Strep viridians
D. Gram negative bacteria

102. Type I silent ischemia is:

A. No associated angina
B. Angina with silent ischemic episodes
C. Occur at night
D. All of the above

103. Before PTCA, which of the following is given:

A. Aspirin
B. Clopidogrel
C. Heparin
D. Hirudin
E. All of the above

104. After valve replacement, patient has low grade fever for 3 weeks with anemia. What investigation will you do to confirm your clinical impression:

A. Blood culture
B. Blood count
C. Echocardiography
D. None of the above

105. Duration of treatment will include:

A. 6-8 weeks
B. 3-6 weeks
C. 4-8 weeks
D. Only 4 weeks

97 A 98 D 99 A 100 B 101 B 102 A 103 E 104 A 105 A

CMC Vellore 2002

1. **Pulsus paradoxus occurs in:**
   A. Cardiac tamponade
   B. RCMP
   C. AR
   D. HOCM

2. **In secondary MR, apical impulse is:**
   A. Hyperdynamic
   B. Sustained
   C. Delayed
   D. Retraction of apex

3. **With mitral valve replacement mortality is:**
   A. 4.32%
   B. 6.4%
   C. 0.02%
   D. 12.7%

4. **Mortality due to non cardiac causes of syncope is:**
   A. 0.1%
   B. 1%
   C. 6%
   D. 8%

5. **Investigation of choice in syncope:**
   A. HUTT
   B.. Blood sugar
   C. Echo
   D. CT scan (head)

6. **Treatment of choice to prevent recurrence of atrial fibrillation after normal sinus rhythm:**
   A. Type Ic drugs
   B. Amiodarone
   C. Digoxin
   D. Calcium channel blockers

7. **Treatment in lone atrial fibrillation:**
   A. No treatment
   B. Warfarin
   C. Amiodarone
   D. DC Shock

8. **Critical AS:**
   A. 0.5 cm^2
   B. 0.5 cm^2/m^2
   C. 0.7 cm^2
   D. 0.7 cm/m^2

9. **Indication of surgery in AR is:**
   A. ESV >55 ml/m^2
   B. EDD <55 mm
   C. EF >50%
   D. Asymptomatic moderate AR

10. **NAME syndrome is associated with:**
   A. Atrial myxoma
   B. Amyloidosis
   C. Brugada's syndrome
   D. Atrial flutter

1 A 2 B 3 B 4 C 5 A 6 A 8 B 7 A 9 A 10 A

11. Aortic aneurysm: In symptomatic patients surgery is indicated at:
- **A.** 4.5 cm
- **B.** 5.0 cm
- **C.** 5.5 cm
- **D.** 6.0 cm

12. ECG changes in pericarditis: true is:
- **A.** PR segment depression
- **B.** PR segment elevation
- **C.** No serial changes
- **D.** AF present

13. Dressler's syndrome all are true *except:*
- **A.** Fever and Pain
- **B.** Pericardial effusion
- **C.** Auto immune
- **D.** Steroid beneficial

14. In MADIT trial true is:
- **A.** ICD indicated if EF <35%
- **B.** ICD indicated if EF >35%
- **C.** Amiodarone better if EF >35%
- **D.** Amiodarone better if EF <35%

15. Which is a primary prevention trial:
- **A.** WOSCOPS
- **B.** Helsinki heart study
- **C.** LIPID
- **D.** CARE

16. Aspirin in secondary prevention, all are true *except:*
- **A.** Reduction of mortality
- **B.** Anti inflammatory
- **C.** Anti platelet
- **D.** Not beneficial in endothelial dysfunction

17. 5 mmHg reduction of BP decreases risk of stroke by:
- **A.** 42%
- **B.** 36%
- **C.** 48%
- **D.** 32%

18. Regarding atrial gallop, true is:
- **A.** 80% incidence in MI
- **B.** Present in hyperdynamic circulation
- **C.** Present in normal elderly male
- **D.** Present in pericardial effusion

19. Regarding TR all are true *except:*
- **A.** Holosystolic in pulmonary embolism
- **B.** Holosystolic in normal pressure TR
- **C.** Early systolic in MS
- **D.** Early systolic in TV infective endocarditis

20. Hypertension associated with hypokalemia true is:
- **A.** Renal artery stenosis
- **B.** Essential HT
- **C.** CRF
- **D.** ↑ Intra-cranial pressure

21. Female on OCP's develops HT:
- **A.** Essential
- **B.** Renal
- **C.** OCP induced
- **D.** All of above

22. Pregnancy-induced hypertension: indication of treatment at diastolic BP of:
- **A.** ≥ 80 mmHg
- **B.** ≥ 90 mmHg
- **C.** ≥ 100 mmHg
- **D.** ≥ 110 mmHg

23. Criteria for hypertension is:
- **A.** JNC VII
- **B.** JNC VIII
- **C.** ACC
- **D.** AHA

24. Optimal diastolic B.P. is:
- **A.** < 80 mmHg
- **B.** < 85 mmHg
- **C.** < 90 mmHg
- **D.** < 95 mmHg

11 D 12 A,D 13 D 14 A 15 A 16 B,D 17 A 18 A,C 19 B,C 20 A 21 D 22 C
23 A 24 A

25. Keith Wagener's classification is for:
A. HT
B. DM
C. CAD
D. USA

26. Not used in treatment of neurocardiogenic syncope:
A. β blocker
B. α blocker
C. ↑ salt intake
D. Propanolol

27. CoA at 2 yrs true is:
A. Mortality at 30 yrs
B. Notching of Ribs
C. Immediate surgery
D. Intermittent claudication

28. ASD repair: true is:
A. Optimal age 3-6 yrs
B. Qp/Qs > 1.2:1
C. PVR 10 WU
D. Saturation <85%

29. Cyanosis occurs when reduced Hb concentration in blood:
A. 3 gm%
B. 4 gm%
C. 5 gm%
D. 6 gm%

30. Regarding rheumatic TS true is:
A. Not accompanied by TR
B. 4mmHg of gradient causes venous congestion
C. Incidence 28%
D. 2mmHg gradient is diagnostic

31. Regarding carcinoid: true is:
A. Heart involvement occurs only after hepatic metastasis
B. Hyperdynamic circulation
C. Lesion in left side is common
D. Poor prognosis

32. S2-pericardial knock interval is:
A. 10-20 msec
B. 40-60 msec
C. 60-70 msec
D. 70-90 msec

33. Normal A2-OS interval is:
A. 20-40 msec
B. 40-80 msec
C. 60-120 msec
D. 120-180 msec

34. Normal HV interval:
A. 30-40 msec
B. 35-55 msec
C. 40-60 msec
D. 60-80 msec

35. Indication of pacing in bifacsicular block is:
A. With prolonged PR, no symptoms
B. With no AV block, no symptoms
C. With pacing induced infrahision block
D. With syncope

36. Class III anti arrhythmic is:
A. Amiodarone
B. Lignocaine
C. Phenytoin
D. Quinidine

37. Holt Oram syndrome: associated cardiac defect is:
A. ASD
B. VSD
C. PDA
D. MR

38. Sestamibi vs. thallium: true regarding sestamibi is:
A. Long time
B. Long protocol
C. Thallium better
D. Better image quality

25 A 26 B 27 A 28 A 29 B 30 BD 31 A 32 D 33 C 34 B 35 CD 36 A 37 A 38 D

39. Wide split S2 with clubbing is seen in:
A. TAPVC
B. TOF
C. Pulmonary hypertension
D. CHF

40. Duchenne's muscular dystrophy true is:
A. Tall R wave V_1
B. Tall S wave V_1
C. Associated with AF
D. Responds to steroid

41. Stress test may have false negative results in:
A. RCA disease
B. LAD disease
C. LCx disease
D. LMCA disease

42. Regarding Echo true is:
A. In adults transducer frequency used is 8-10 MHz
B. In colour doppler, blue is blood flow away from transducer
C. In color Doppler red is blood flow away from transducer
D. In children transducer frequency is 10-20 MHz

43. Cardiac sources of emboli are all *except:*
A. Calcium
B. Fibrin & platelet
C. LV clot
D. Atherosclerotic plaque

44. Rotablator chips are made up of:
A. Diamond
B. Platinum
C. Gold
D. Silver

45. In PET scan, mismatch indicates:
A. Ischaemia
B. Necrosis
C. Poor prognosis
D. Good prognosis

46. In myosin heavy chain, site of energy formation is:
A. Neck
B. Rod like portion
C. Globular portion
D. Head

47. Incidence of HOCM due to β MHC is about:
A. 10%
B. 20%
C. 30%
D. 40%

48. In acute right heart failure due to cor pulmonale, mortality is:
A. 50%
B. 40%
C. 60%
D. 30%

49. In which trial spironolactone decreased mortality in CHF:
A. RALES
B. SPIRAL
C. CADILLA
D. GLOBUS

50. Mortality in heart failure is reduced by which drug:
A. Captopril
B. Aspirin
C. Nitrates
D. Digoxin

51. Primary cardiac arrest survivors maximum incidence of re-arrest occurs at:
A. <15 days
B. 1-6 month
C. 6-18 month
D. 2 years

39 A 40 AC 41 C 42 B 43 D 44 A 45 A 46 D 47 C 48 A 49 A 50 A 51 C

52. True about cardiac arrest is:
- **A.** Irreversible form
- **B.** Reversible
- **C.** Comatose state
- **D.** Vegetative form

53. Mortality reduction in WOSCOPS trial is:
- **A.** 27%
- **B.** 17%
- **C.** 31%
- **D.** 20%

54. Nitrate effect in MVP:
- **A.** ↑ murmur
- **B.** ↓ murmur
- **C.** No effect on murmur
- **D.** Murmur delayed and louder

55. Patient of uraemic cardiac tamponade true is:
- **A.** Increase in systemic venous pressure
- **B.** Increase in pulmonary venous pressure
- **C.** Decrease in systemic venous pressure
- **D.** Decrease in pulmonary venous pressure

56. Nitrate in heart failure: true is:
- **A.** Reduced congestion
- **B.** Increases C.O
- **C.** No change in C.O
- **D.** Decreases C.O

57. Regarding pericarditis true is:
- **A.** Serial ST changes present
- **B.** ST elevation
- **C.** ST depression
- **D.** T wave inversion

58. Aspirin in CAD patients reduces mortality by:
- **A.** 18%
- **B.** 25%
- **C.** 12%
- **D.** 15%

59. Thyrotoxicosis with AF, which drug is contra-indicated:
- **A.** Digoxin
- **B.** ACE inhibitor
- **C.** Esmolol
- **D.** Neomercazole

60. Atrial infarction true statement is:
- **A.** More common on right side
- **B.** PR segment depression
- **C.** Incidence 20%
- **D.** More with anterior infarction

61. Regarding Multifocal Atrial Tachycardia (MAT) true statement is:
- **A.** Different P wave morphology in 3 consecutive beats
- **B.** Associated with MI
- **C.** Poor prognosis
- **D.** Respond to propanalol

62. In Framingham heart criteria which is not a major criteria:
- **A.** PND
- **B.** ↑ JVP
- **C.** ↓ Vital capacity
- **D.** S3

63. Venous hum: all are true *except:*
- **A.** Heard in supraclavicular fossa
- **B.** Present in healthy children
- **C.** Increases in diastole
- **D.** Present in A-V fistulae

64. Heart principally contains which LDH:
- **A.** LDH1
- **B.** LDH2
- **C.** LDH4
- **D.** LDH5

65. Restenosis rate after coronary stenting is:
- **A.** 33%
- **B.** 12%
- **C.** 50%
- **D.** 20%

52 B 53 C 54 A 55 A 56 A 57 A 58 B 59 A 60 A 61 A 62 C 63 D 64 A 65 D

66. Effect of nitrates in Ischemic MR is:
- **A.** ↑ MR
- **B.** ↓ MR
- **C.** ↑ Mortality
- **D.** ↓ Mortaltiy

67. Primary VF during AMI is:
- **A.** 30% incidence
- **B.** Higher incidence in AWMI
- **C.** Higher incidence in IWMI
- **D.** Poor prognosis

68. LPHB true is:
- **A.** Presence of q wave in leads I/AV_L/V5/V6
- **B.** Presence of rS complex in leads II/III/avF
- **C.** Presence of qR complex in leads II/III/ avF
- **D.** Seen in LBBB

69. Indication of anticoagulation with infarct in convalescent period is:
- **A.** AMI
- **B.** Inferior wall infarction
- **C.** Clot in left atrium
- **D.** Hibernating myocardium

70. HRT after MI: true is:
- **A.** No conclusive evidence
- **B.** ↑ CV event in 1st year
- **C.** ↓ mortality
- **D.** Indicated in women with MI

71. Regarding nitrate patch: all are true *except:*
- **A.** ↑ exercise tolerance for 24 hrs
- **B.** Antiischemic effect for 12 hours
- **C.** Free interval not required
- **D.** Rebound phenomenon does not occur

72. Regarding aortic valvuloplasty, true is:
- **A.** Indicated in children with severe AS with pliable valves
- **B.** Increased incidence of restenosis
- **C.** ↑ mortality
- **D.** Indicated in elderly with calcified valves

73. Opening snap true is:
- **A.** Soft in calcified anterior mitral leaflet (both tip and body)
- **B.** Occurs when LA pressure is more than LV pressure
- **C.** Occurs before S2
- **D.** Indicate beginning of mitral valve opening

74. Normal LVEDP is:
- **A.** 9 mmHg
- **B.** 18 mmHg
- **C.** 24 mmHg
- **D.** 32 mmHg

75. Aortic aneurysm–diagnosis is made by:
- **A.** CT & MRI
- **B.** TEE
- **C.** TTE
- **D.** TEE investigation of choice in ruptured aneurysms

76. Increase in murmur with standing occurs in:
- **A.** HOCM
- **B.** MR
- **C.** MVP
- **D.** AS

77. Murmur 2nd day of birth all are true *except:*
- **A.** TAPVC
- **B.** Pulmonary A-V fistulae
- **C.** Systemic A-V fistulae
- **D.** VSD

78. Early systolic murmur occurs in:
- **A.** Very small VSD
- **B.** VSD with early Eisenmenger
- **C.** TR (low pressure)
- **D.** MR

79. Single S2 occurs in:
- **A.** TOF
- **B.** Pulmonary atresia
- **C.** Eisemenger's syndrome
- **D.** TAPVC

---

66 B **67** B **68** C **69** C **70** A **71** A **72** A,B **73** A **74** A **75** A **76** A,C **77** D
78 A,B,C **79** A,B,C

80. Drive force for moving 5 lit/m of blood from pulmonary artery to LA is:
A. 20 mmHg
B. 30 mmHg
C. 80 mmHg
D. 12 mmHg

81. Catheter used in pulmonary artery is:
A. Swan Ganz catheter
B. RCA catheter
C. Amplatz catheter
D. Judkins catheter

82. Bioprosthetic valve true is:
A. Used in children
B. Low rate of degradation
C. High rate of degradation
D. Valve of choice in tricuspid position

83. Enterococcal endocarditis: all are true *except:*
A. No response to penicillin
B. Difficult to treat
C. Not associated with septicemia
D. Large/prolonged course of antibiotic required

84. Oedema is caused by:
A. Minoxidil
B. Prazosin
C. Calcium channel blocker
D. Metolazone

85. Lyme's myocarditis true is:
A. Syncope due to conduction blocks
B. Prolonged treatment
C. Responds to penicillin
D. In A-V block pacemaker not required

86. Incidence of ASO titre elevation within 1st attack of rheumatic fever:
A. 80%
B. 85%
C. 90%
D. 95%

87. TR with inspiration true is:
A. Murmur decreases
B. No effect on murmur
C. Murmur disappears
D. Murmur increases

88. Energy required for terminating SVT:
A. 50 J
B. 100 J
C. 150 J
D. 200 J

89. S_4 sound in AS is heard when:
A. Pressure gradient > 70 mm Hg
B. LVEDP < 10 mm Hg
C. Vegetation on aortic valve
D. Decrease mean arterial pressure of LA

90. Biatrial myxoma: prevalence is:
A. 5%
B. 10%
C. 15%
D. > 15%

80 D 81 A 82 C,D 83 A 84 A,C 85 A,B,C,D 86 A 87 D 88 A 89 A 90 B

CMC Vellore 2001

1. **Not seen in Down's syndrome is:**
   A. MVP
   B. TGA
   C. Truncus arteriosus
   D. Ostium primum ASD
   E. AV canal defect

2. **Children with PDA are most commonly born in:**
   A. March
   B. December
   C. June
   D. May
   E. None of the above

3. **In Down's syndrome translocation of chromosome 21 is likely when maternal age is:**
   A. <30
   B. >35
   C. >45
   D. <20
   E. None of the above

4. **In Cri du chat syndrome there is involvement of chromosome:**
   A. 5P
   B. 21
   C. 18
   D. Xp
   E. 9q

5. **O_2 Step up in right atrium during catheterization is seen in all *except:***
   A. Outlet VSD
   B. VSD with TR
   C. TAPVC
   D. Ostium primum
   E. LV to RA defect

6. **ASD device closure is done when:**
   A. Superior margin is at least 5mm
   B. Inferior margin 22mm
   C. Ostium primum ASD
   D. Correction < 1 year
   E. AV canal defect

7. **36 weeks pregnancy on Warfarin with INR 2.9 with Bjork shelly valve treatment of choice:**
   A. Continue Warfarin
   B. Heparin after labour
   C. Natural delivery
   D. Emergency caesarean if labor not terminated
   E. Omit warfarin and add heparin

8. **All are true about anticoagulation in Bjork Shelly valve *except:***
   A. Chance of thromboembolism 2.5%
   B. Double with stoppage of anticoagulation
   C. One episode of thromboembolism carries high risk for recurrent embolization
   D. Highest risk from 6 months to 1 year after surgery

1 B 2 B 3 B 4 A 5 A 6 A 7 D 8 D

9. Which is not present in vegetation of IE?
A. Platelet
B. Fibrin
C. Vascular channel
D. Infective organisms
E. WBC

10. HACEK organisms include all *except:*
A. Haemophilus
B. Actinobacillus
C. E. Coli
D. Kingella
E. Cardiobacterium

11. Incidence of drainage of TAPVC in left innominate vein:
A. 11%
B. 15%
C. 23%
D. 27%
E. 33%

12. Ibuprofen used in Dressler's syndrome because of:
A. Antioxidant effect
B. Positive inotropic effect
C. Decreases fever rapidly
D. ↓ systemic vascular resistance

13. Streptokinase acts through:
A. Fibrin
B. Plasminogen
C. Thrombin
D. Plasmin

14. Warfarin acts on all of the following coagulation factors *except:*
A. Factor II
B. Factor VII
C. Factor IX
D. Factor X
E. Factor III

15. About LWM heparin all are true *except:*
A. Action on factor IIa
B. Causes less thrombocytopenia
C. More bioavailability
D. Less adverse effect
E. Does not bind to plasma protein

16. All are true about ticlopidine *except:*
A. Does not prevent restenosis
B. Acts through ADP
C. Inhibits GbIIb/IIIa through ADP receptors
D. Decreases fibrinogen binding to GbIIb/IIIa through ADP

17. Angiographically diagnosis of restenosis in a patient of PTCA is established by:
A. >70% ↓ in luminal diameter
B. > 40% of loss in the gain achieved
C. <0.73 mm diameter
D. All above
E. None of above

18. b blockers decreases mortality by ....% in post MI patients:
A. 18%
B. 53%
C. 23%
D. 27%
E. 35%

19. Primary prevention trial with lipid lowering with statins is:
A. 4S
B. CARE
C. LIPID
D. AFCAPS
E. WHO

20. Mortality decreased in WOSCOPS by:
A. 11%
B. 31%
C. 42%
D. 24%
E. 56%

9 C 10 C 11 E 12 C 13 D 14 E 15 E 16 D 17 D 18 A 19 D 20 B

21. For 5-6mm decrease of BP, risk of stroke is decreased by:
- **A.** 12%
- **B.** 24%
- **C.** 42%
- **D.** 50%
- **E.** 10%

22. WPW is a .... disease:
- **A.** Congenital
- **B.** Idiopathic
- **C.** Acquired
- **D.** degenerative
- **E.** None of the above

23. In a patient of hypotension, GI bleed, fever and lobar pneumonia, the drug of choice is:
- **A.** CP + Gentamicin
- **B.** Azithromycin
- **C.** Tetracycline
- **D.** Cephalosporin + Amikacin + ceftazidime
- **E.** Ciprofloxacin

24. Hypotension with PCWP 13mm Hg, -CVP in a patient of RVMI the treatment of choice is:
- **A.** IV fluids
- **B.** Frusemide
- **C.** Dobutamine
- **D.** Digoxin
- **E.** IABP

25. Pulmonary wedge angiography is done in all *except:*
- **A.** ASD
- **B.** MS
- **C.** PAH
- **D.** Pulmonary venocclusive disease

26. In Antiphospholipid antibody syndrome, all are true *except:*
- **A.** Test for SLE always positive
- **B.** False positive test for syphilis
- **C.** Anticoagulants are of benefit
- **D.** Valvular involvement occurs
- **E.** Stroke is a complication

27. Severe thiamine deficiency occurs in:
- **A.** Pellagra
- **B.** Angular stomatitis
- **C.** Korsakoff syndrome
- **D.** Motor peripheral neuropathy

28. Central apnea is characterized by:
- **A.** Decrease airflow with increased respiratory effort
- **B.** ↑ airflow with ↓ respiratory effort
- **C.** No airflow, no respiratory effort
- **D.** Normal airflow with ↓ respiratory effort
- **E.** None of the above

29. Which of the following does not occur in a patient of MS with AF?
- **A.** Diastolic murmur
- **B.** Presystolic accentuation
- **C.** OS
- **D.** Loud S1
- **E.** Loud P2

30. All can be seen with SLE *except:*
- **A.** RBC cast
- **B.** Granular cast
- **C.** Microscopic hematuria
- **D.** Massive hemoptysis
- **E.** Nephrotic syndrome

31. Following are true about sarcoid *except:*
- **A.** Endomyocardial biopsy is useless
- **B.** Cardiac lesion manifestation occurs in 5% cases
- **C.** Chest X-ray shows parenchymal infiltrates
- **D.** Commonest presentation is acute
- **E.** Facial nerve involvement is the most common CNS manifestation

21 C 22 A 23 D 24 A 25 A 26 A 27 C 28 C 29 B 30 B 31 A

32. All are true about doxorubicin induce cardiomyopathy *except:*
- **A.** Dose 300-400 mg/m^2
- **B.** Most common age <40 years
- **C.** Male > female
- **D.** Radiation adds to the toxicity
- **E.** I/V bolus dose is given to avoid toxicity

33. About adenosine, which of the following are true?
- **A.** Adenilic acid deaminase level is high in myocardium
- **B.** Inosine and hypoxanthine are ways in which it enters directly into myocardium
- **C.** A-2 receptors mediate vasodilatation
- **D.** Acts on A2 receptors for ischemic preconditioning
- **E.** Acts on A2 receptors for AV block

34. All are true about megaloblastic anemia *except:*
- **A.** Thrombocytopenia
- **B.** Increased reticulocyte count
- **C.** Splenomegaly
- **D.** Macrocytosis
- **E.** Hyperbilirubinaemia

35. All are true about subendocardial ischemia *except:*
- **A.** Increase LVEDP→↑ subendocardial flow
- **B.** ↓LVEDP→↑ subendocardial flow
- **C.** No effect of LVEDP in subendocardial flow
- **D.** None of the above

36. Increase coronary blood flow with increased LV contractility effect is known as:
- **A.** Greg effect
- **B.** Anrep effect
- **C.** Treppe effect
- **D.** Salisbury

37. ACE related cough; true is:
- **A.** Males 20% incidence
- **B.** Females 10% incidence
- **C.** Stops within 24 hours stoppage of drugs
- **D.** Caused by bradykinin

38. In cor-pulmonale, role of digoxin is in:
- **A.** RV failure
- **B.** Pulmonary artery pressure is 25 mmHg
- **C.** Cardiac index > 2.5
- **D.** Assessment of LV failure

39. COPD: arrhythmias are commonest in:
- **A.** Morning
- **B.** Night
- **C.** Noon
- **D.** Evening

40. Long QT syndrome is associated with all *except:*
- **A.** I_{Kr}
- **B.** I_{KS}
- **C.** Mink
- **D.** Herg
- **E.** Sodium

41. Patient of MS with AF develops regular rhythm; cause is:
- **A.** A-V block with junctional escape
- **B.** Idioventricular rhythm
- **C.** Flutter with 3:1 block
- **D.** Flutter with 4:1 block
- **E.** Digitalis effect

42. DC shock in ventricular tachycardia, true is:
- **A.** First shock of 200 J is given
- **B.** Second shock of 200-300 J is given
- **C.** Third shock of 360 J is given if there is no response
- **D.** If there is VF after cardiac arrest, then directly 360 J is given
- **E.** All of the above

43. Three continuous VPC on ECG is known as:
- **A.** Quadrigeminy
- **B.** Bigeminy
- **C.** VT
- **D.** VF

32 E 33 A,B,C 34 B 35 D 36 D 37 D 38 A 39 A 40 B 41 A 42 E 43 C

44. PSVT: treatment of choice are all *except:*
A. Verapamil
B. DC Shock
C. Digoxin
D. Adenosine

45. All are true about wenkebach's phenomenon *except:*
A. Progressive lengthening of PR with drop of a P wave
B. Progressive ↑ in RR interval
C. Doesn't affect survival
D. Occurs in AV nodal ischemia
E. Usually narrow complex

46. PCWP increase is seen in:
A. Pulmonary venoocclusive disease
B. Pulmonary embolism
C. Cor-pulmonale
D. Pulmonary stenosis
E. PPH

47. All are true about BNP *except:*
A. Present in ventricular myocardium
B. Acts through ventricles
C. Synergistic action with ANP
D. Increase in Heart failure
E. None of the above

48. Central venous pressure 13 mm Hg , velocity 4m/sec across tricuspid valve, pulmonary artery systolic pressure is:
A. 32
B. 40
C. 64
D. 80
E. None of the above

49. RVMI with right coronary disease: least likely ECG change is:
A. ST elevation in V_3V_4 R
B. Q in V1 and V2
C. Q in V4, V5, V6
D. Q in II, III, aVF

50. Arm lead reversal leads to inversion of P waves in:
A. Lead I
B. Lead II
C. Lead III
D. aVF

51. In situs inversus heart, is on the:
A. Left side
B. Right side
C. Normal structurally
D. In midline

52. 2 year old child died of arrhythmias, biopsy shows spider cell; diagnosis is:
A. Papillary fibroelastoma
B. Rhabdomyosarcoma
C. Myxoma
D. Lipoma

53. All are true about primary cardiac tumors *except:*
A. Pericardial effusion associated with malignancy
B. Myxoma is the commonest tumor
C. Malignant tumor more common on left side
D. Angiosarcoma and rhabdomyosarcoma commonest among malignancies

54. Smooth muscle migration in pulmonary arterial hypertension is caused by:
A. Abronectin
B. Tenasin
C. β-TGF
D. Angiotensin II

55. β myosin heavy chain mutation in HOCM is seen in:
A. 30%
B. 11%
C. 15%
D. 60%

44 C 45 B 46 A 47 E 48 D 49 C 50 A 51 A 52 B 53 C 54 C 55 A

56. All are true about hypothyroidism *except:*
A. Decreased exercise tolerance
B. Increased ejection time
C. Decrease capillary permeability
D. Low voltage ECG

57. Digoxin toxicity is not associated with:
A. Hypercalcemia
B. Hypothyroidism
C. Hydrochlorothiazide
D. Hypokalemia
E. Hepatic disease

58. QT interval is increased by all *except:*
A. Quinidine
B. Disopyramide
C. Amiodarone
D. Flecainide
E. Lidocaine

59. In hepatic encephalopathy; earliest sign is:
A. Left right dissociation
B. Constructional apraxia
C. Slurred speech
D. Asterixis
E. Extensor planter

60. Quinidine induced syncope; treatment of choice is:
A. Temporary pacing
B. IV magnesium
C. Isoproterenol
D. All of the above

61. Torsades treatment of choice:
A. IV Mg
B. Cardiac pacing
C. β blockers
D. Isoproterenol
E. All of the above

62. Which of the following has least a adrenergic activity?
A. Norepinephrine
B. Epinephrine
C. Isoprenaline
D. Dopamine
E. Dobutamine

63. Levels of noradrenaline associated with increased mortality in CHF:
A. <400 pg/ml
B. 400-800 pg/ml
C. >800 pg/ml
D. All of the above

64. QRS duration with RBBB is:
A. <0.9 sec
B. >0.11 sec
C. >0.24 sec
D. >0.03 sec
E. <0.12 sec

65. Carvedilol; true is:
A. High dose has a + b blocking activity
B. Trials have shown no survival benefit
C. COPERNICUS trial was done in severe CHF
D. Has no antioxidant activity
E. Increased survival by 52% at 1 year in CHF

66. High pitched brief sound near apex is:
A. Ejection click
B. A2
C. P2
D. OS
E. S4

67. Major criteria for rheumatic fever are all *except:*
A. Arthralgia
B. Arthritis
C. Carditis
D. Subcutaneous nodules
E. Chorea

56 C 57 C,E 58 E 59 B 60 B 61 E 62 C 63 C 64 B 65 C 66 A,D
67 A

68. Balloon aortic valvuloplasty; true is:
- **A.** Restenosis rate- 50% at 6 months
- **B.** Best approach through trans-septal puncture
- **C.** Best entered via subclavian vein
- **D.** ASD (significant) occurs in 40% patients
- **E.** AR occurs in 50% of patients

69. Correlation of CW Doppler gradient in AS is best with:
- **A.** Peak to peak gradient
- **B.** Peak instantaneous gradient
- **C.** Mean gradient
- **D.** None of the above

68 A 69 B

CMC Vellore 2000

1. **In Goldman's specific activity scale grade I, patient can complete activity**
   A. $\leq$ 7 METS
   B. $\geq$ 5
   C. $\geq$ 2
   D. $\geq$ 2

2. **Clubbing occurs in cyanosis after:**
   A. At appearance
   B. 1-2 years
   C. 2-4 years
   D. 5-6 years

3. **Still's murmur is:**
   A. Early systolic
   B. Early diastolic
   C. Mid systolic
   D. Mid diastolic

4. **Cardiorespiratory murmur is heard in:**
   A. Left angle of scapula
   B. Right clavicle
   C. Aortic area
   D. All of the above

5. **In MVP, amylnitrate inhalation will cause:**
   A. Increase prolapse
   B. Decrease prolapse
   C. Increase papillary muscle ischemia
   D. Decrease papillary muscle ischemia

6. **GpII/IIIa receptors are encoded on which chromosome:**
   A. 13
   B. 14
   C. 15
   D. 17

7. **Maximum warfarin toxicity in pregnancy may occur at which period of gestation:**
   A. 2-6 weeks
   B. 6-9 weeks
   C. 9-12 weeks
   D. More than 12 weeks

8. **Vitamin D toxicity causes:**
   A. Supravalvular AS
   B. ASD
   C. VSD
   D. All of the above

9. **Hypertension is caused by all *except:***
   A. Cocaine
   B. Cyclosporine
   C. Erythropoietin
   D. NO

10. **Leptospirosis causes:**
    A. Myocardial necrosis
    B. Increase PR interval
    C. Bradycardia
    D. All of the above

---

1 A 2 B 3 C 4 A 5 A 6 D 7 B 8 A 9 D 10 D

11. Sinus arrhythmia true is:
- **A.** P wave morphology varies
- **B.** PR interval varies
- **C.** PR interval is 100 msec
- **D.** Maximum sinus length–minimum cycle length > 120 msec

12. Radiation causes all *except:*
- **A.** Myocardium is most commonly affected
- **B.** LV dysfunction can occur 5-20 years after radiation
- **C.** Constrictive pericarditis
- **D.** Myocardial infarction

13. Most common metastasis to pericardium is from:
- **A.** Bronchogenic carcinoma
- **B.** Mesothelioma
- **C.** Seminoma
- **D.** Breast cancer

14. RV infarct causes:
- **A.** Gross elevation of ANP
- **B.** ST depression in V5R
- **C.** RV diastolic pressure is not raised
- **D.** All of the above

15. Good indicator of thrombolysis:
- **A.** Early CPKMB peak
- **B.** Increase troponin T
- **C.** VPC's
- **D.** Relief of chest pain

16. Streptokinase decreased mortality in FTT trial by:
- **A.** 33%
- **B.** 20%
- **C.** 45%
- **D.** 18%

17. Mortality is improved after MI by:
- **A.** STK
- **B.** Beta blocker
- **C.** Aspirin
- **D.** All of the above

18. Number of components in pericardial rub are:
- **A.** 4
- **B.** 3
- **C.** 2
- **D.** 1

19. On phonocardiogram S1 has how many components:
- **A.** 4
- **B.** 3
- **C.** 2
- **D.** 1

20. Streptococcal infective endocarditis with MIC <0.1 μg/ml standard treatment regimen are all *except:*
- **A.** Vancomycin–4 weeks
- **B.** Crystalline penicillin 4 weeks
- **C.** CP + Gentamicin 4 weeks
- **D.** Ceftriaxone 2 weeks

21. Normal waist hip ratio:
- **A.** 0.7
- **B.** 0.85
- **C.** 0.6
- **D.** 0.9

22. Hypokalemia with hypertension occurs in all *except:*
- **A.** Patient treated with lasix and thiazide diuretics
- **B.** Malignant hypertension
- **C.** Pheochromocytoma
- **D.** Renal artery stenosis

23. Regarding hypothyroidism, true are all *except:*
- **A.** Increase incidence of hypertension
- **B.** Treating hypothyroidism decrease BP
- **C.** Severe hypothyroidism causes low BP
- **D.** Increase in only systolic BP

11 D 12 A 13 A 14 A 15 A 16 D 17 D 18 B 19 A 20 C 21 B 22 C 23 D

24. Left parietal infarct, anticoagulation indication in 75 year old person having:
A. ASD
B. AF
C. MI
D. HT

25. Risk factor for atrial fibrillation is:
A. DM
B. HT
C. MS
D. All of the above

26. Streptokinase is a:
A. Enzyme
B. Protein
C. Glycoprotein
D. Hormone

27. HERO-2 trial:
A. Hirudin
B. Streptokinase + Hirudin
C. GP IIb/IIIa inhibitor + streptokinase
D. Hirulog

28. Gp IIb/IIIa antagonists all *except:*
A. Clopidogrel
B. Eptifibatide
C. Tirofiban
D. Abciximab

29. St Jude valve true is:
A. 3 discs
B. 4 struts
C. Made upof titanium
D. Especially useful in children

30. Mechanical valve preferred over bioprosthetic valve in:
A. Pregnancy
B. Patient taking anticoagulation regularly
C. Old age person not having risk factor for thromboembolism
D. Tricuspid position

31. A patient had cardiac arrest and monitor showed ventricular tachycardia. Treatment is:
A. Lidocaine
B. Monitor for 2-5 minutes
C. DC shock 200 J
D. Any of the above

32. Korotkoff sounds 4 & 5 have difference in B.P. of:
A. 5 mmHg
B. 10 mmHg
C. 40 mmHg
D. 30 mmHg

33. NTG can be given in AMI till:
A. Systolic BP upto 105 mmHg
B. Systolic BP decreases 15 mmHg from starting
C. Systolic BP 90 mmHg
D. No relation with systolic BP

34. NTG is used in:
A. Large anterior infarct
B. Severe bradycardia
C. CCF
D. Severe hypertension

35. Angiotension II causes hypertension by:
A. AT 1 receptor
B. AT II receptor
C. Endothelin receptor
D. All of the above

36. Endopeptidase inhibitor causes:
A. Potentiate natriuretic peptide
B. Decreases natriuretic peptide
C. No effect
D. None of the above

37. Atrial infarction: true are all *except:*
A. Occurs in 40% of AMI
B. Mostly site is right atrium
C. Causes atrial arrhythmias
D. Associated with increase secretion of natri-uretic peptide

24 B 25 D 26 B 27 D 28 A 29 D 30 B 31 C 32 B 33 C 34 A,C,D 35 A
36 A 37 A

38. Which is class III antiarrhythmic?
A. Amiodarone
B. Quinidine
C. Xylocaine
D. All of the above

39. All causes Torsades de pointes *except:*
A. Sotalol
B. Ibutilide
C. Mexiletine
D. Terfenadine

40. Emetine causes all *except:*
A. QT prolongation
B. Myocardial necrosis
C. ECG changes disappears within 2-3 days
D. Most common ECG finding is T wave inversion

41. Chagas disease true is:
A. Apical aneurysm
B. Focal myocardial necrosis
C. Right sided heart failure
D. All of the above

42. After 30 min of chest pain immediate investigation of choice:
A. CK-MB
B. Trop-T
C. Lipid profile
D. None of the above

43. Saphenous vein graft; patency rate after 10 years of CABG:
A. 40%
B. 60%
C. 90%
D. 20%

44. Rupture of heart after MI: true are all *except:*
A. Most commonly occurs after 1-4 days post MI
B. 90% mortality with medical management
C. More frequent in woman with infarction
D. 50% of patient has new murmur

45. Cocaine causes:
A. Sudden death
B. Increased atherosclerosis
C. Contraction band necrosis
D. All of the above

46. Uremic pericarditis all are true *except:*
A. Moslty hemorrhagic
B. Dialysis is treatment
C. Heparin use during dialysis may exacerbate pericarditis
D. Cardiac tamponade is very rare

47. ECG changes in pericarditis true is:
A. ST elevation in all leads except AVR and V1
B. ST segment axis between 30-60°
C. Mechanism of ST elevation is flow of current from epicardium to thorax and back to heart
D. All of the above

48. Normal pericardial fluid amount:
A. 15 ml
B. 60 ml
C. 70 ml
D. None of the above

49. Regarding familial atrial myxoma, true is:
A. Age > 50 years
B. Autosomal dominant
C. Seen only in LA
D. 80% of total myxomas

50. Osteogenesis imperfecta, all are true *except:*
A. Blue sclera
B. Osteopenia
C. Pregnancy leads to remission
D. Hearing loss

51. HOCM worst prognosis with chromosome:
A. Chromosome 1
B. Chromosome 15
C. Chromosome 11
D. Chromosome 14

38 A 39 C 40 C 41 D 42 D 43 A 44 D 45 D 46 D 47 D 48 A 49 B 50 C
51 A

52. Regarding amyloidosis: all are true *except:*
A. LV wall thinning
B. Low voltage ECG
C. Pericardial effusion common
D. Orthostatic hypotension

53. Regarding subendocardial perfusion true is:
A. Less in systole than subepicardium
B. Increased LVEDP leads to decreased perfusion in subendocardium than subepicardium
C. Subendocardial: subepicardial flow ratio can be increased by elevation in aortic pressure.
D. All of the above

54. DCMP with syncope with 40% EF with S3 gallop with intraventricular conduction defects with normal EP study, next action is:
A. Sotalol
B. Amiodarone
C. ICD
D. Holter monitoring (loop recorder)

55. In DCMP decreased mortality is seen by all *except:*
A. Isosorbide dinitrate + Hydralazine
B. Digoxin
C. Carvedilol
D. ACE inhibitor

56. DCMP: all are used for treatment *except:*
A. Batista procedure
B. Morrow procedure
C. Carvedilol
D. Multisite pacing

57. Best method to detect coronary calcification:
A. Cine CT
B. MRI
C. Fluoroscopy
D. Angiography

58. S2 paradoxical splitting occurs in all *except:*
A. Angina
B. LBBB
C. VSD
D. LVOT obstruction

59. Hypoxic spell: true are all *except:*
A. Related to degree of cyanosis
B. Initiated by feeding, crying
C. Do not occur in pulmonary atresia
D. Child becomes in limp position

60. TOF with pulmonary atresia: all are true *except:*
A. Continuous murmur
B. QRS widening
C. Single 2nd heart sound
D. Aortic ejection sound varies with respiration

61. TOF after corrective surgery; true are all *except:*
A. Sudden death after 10 years is common
B. Rate of arrhythmia is 10-15% after 20 years
C. Most common arrhythmia is AF
D. Upto 1/3rd of all death are arrhythmic in origin

62. Lutembacher's syndrome: all are true *except:*
A. Clinical features of mitral stenosis are obscured
B. Pulmonary venous hypertension occurs early
C. Predominantly in female
D. Continuous murmur may be heard

63. TAPVC: all are true *except:*
A. O_2 saturation is equal in all chambers
B. Infradiaphragmatic is usually obstructive
C. X-ray chest shows snowman appearance
D. Clinical manifestation does not depend on interatrial communication

64. Early systolic murmur is heard in:
A. Acute severe MR
B. TR (low pressure)
C. Very small VSD
D. All of above

52 A 53 D 54 D 55 B 56 B 57 A 58 C 59 C 60 B 61 A 62 B 63 D 64 D

65. In ASD cyanosis is not seen in:
- **A.** Common atrium
- **B.** ASD with PAPVC
- **C.** Complete AV septal defect
- **D.** ASD with transient R-L shunt after birth

66. Ebstein anomaly; all are true *except:*
- **A.** Type A WPW
- **B.** LV predominant
- **C.** Small aorta & PA
- **D.** Mild cyanosis

67. In pulmonary stenosis; all are true *except:*
- **A.** Most commonly unicommissural
- **B.** Post stenotic dilatation present
- **C.** BPV is treatment of choice
- **D.** Size of the balloon more than annulus

68. Pulmonary stenosis (dysplastic), all are true *except:*
- **A.** Associated with Noonan's syndrome
- **B.** Due to fusion of commissure
- **C.** All three valve cusps thickened and dysplastic
- **D.** Post stenotic dilatation not common

69. Down syndrome; all are true *except:*
- **A.** Hypotonia
- **B.** Clockwise axis rotation
- **C.** Left axis deviation
- **D.** Endocardial cushion defects

70. About cotton wool spots in hypertension; all are true *except:*
- **A.** Nerve fiber layers
- **B.** Retinal infarct
- **C.** Characteristic of hypertensive retinopathy
- **D.** Cytoid body

71. In CoA; all are true *except:*
- **A.** Fig of 'E' due to aorta above and below coarctation in X-ray chest
- **B.** Brachiofemoral delay
- **C.** B/L rib notching
- **D.** CCF common in infancy

72. Congenital aortic stenosis; all are true *except:*
- **A.** Commonly bicuspid
- **B.** Mostly males
- **C.** Severity proportional to post stenotic dilatation
- **D.** PDA and COA are frequently associated lesions

73. "Snap" terminology given by:
- **A.** W.S Thayer
- **B.** Duke
- **C.** Bernard
- **D.** Goldman

74. Arrhythmogenic RV dysplasia all are true *except:*
- **A.** MRI is a promising tool
- **B.** RV type arrhythmia
- **C.** Enodcardial fibrosis
- **D.** Male predominance

75. LVS4 occurs in:
- **A.** Acute MI
- **B.** AS
- **C.** Systolic HT
- **D.** All of the above

76. COPD: all of the following are true *except:*
- **A.** MAT may be seen
- **B.** Digoxin is the first line of therapy
- **C.** Can cause RVF
- **D.** None of the above

77. Quinidine induced polymorphic VT; all are true *except:*
- **A.** Hypokalemia is a prominent feature
- **B.** Normal QT interval
- **C.** Mg is Treatment of choice
- **D.** Quinidine causes Torsades de pointes in 1 to 3% of patients

65 B 66 A 67 A 68 B 69 B 70 C 71 A 72 C 73 A 74 C 75 D 76 B 77 B

78. Lithium causes:
A. SA node dysfunction
B. AV node dysfunction
C. VT
D. All of the above

79. Most common reperfusion arrhythmia is:
A. AIVR
B. Sinus bradycardia
C. Atrial fibrillation
D. Ventricular fibrillation

80. Anrep effect; all are true *except:*
A. Not a true inotropic effect
B. When aortic pressure is elevated abruptly, a positive inotropic effect follows
C. Independent of muscle length
D. Na^{+}/Ca^{++} exchange mediated

81. Atrial fibrillation during AMI: all are true *except:*
A. 10 to 15% incidence during acute MI
B. Commonly right atrium affected
C. Least common arrhythmia
D. Marker of poor prognosis

82. In what percentage of patients pleural effusion is seen on chest X-ray in constrictive pericarditis:
A. 40%
B. 60%
C. 90%
D. 100%

83. 6 weeks treatment for infective endocarditis is required in all *except:*
A. Enterococcus
B. Staphylococcal endocarditis
C. Prosthetic valve staph endocarditis
D. HACEK

84. For LDL calculation, following are used:
A. HDL
B. TG
C. Total cholesterol
D. All of the above

85. Myxedema causes all *except:*
A. Increased atherosclerosis
B. Treating hypothyroidism decreased angina
C. Cardiomegaly
D. T wave changes

86. Definitive indication for endomyocardial biopsy is in diagnosis of:
A. Myocarditis
B. Rejection of graft
C. AIDS
D. All of the above

87. Significant transvalvular gradient for TS is:
A. 1 mm Hg
B. 2 mm Hg
C. 3 mm Hg
D. 4 mm Hg

88. Resting membrane potential true is:
A. I Na
B. I K_1
C. I Ca-T
D. IK (Ach)

89. Homocysteinemia all true *except:*
A. Mental retardation
B. Platelet dysfunction causes thrombosis
C. Due to deficiency of cystathione B synthase
D. Patient advised to take pyridoxine rich diet

90. Restrictive vs. constrictive pattern favors restrictive if all of the following are present *except:*
A. Pulmonary artery pressure <50 mmHg
B. 5 mmHg difference in LV & RV pressure
C. RVEDP less than 1/3rd of RV end systolic pressure
D. RV shows dip and plateau pattern

78 A 79 A 80 A 81 C 82 B 83 D 84 D 85 B 86 B 87 B 88 B 89 D 90 A

91. Calcification of aortic valve may be seen in all *except:*
   A. Increased serum calcium
   B. Homocystinuria
   C. Marfan's syndrome
   D. All of the above

92. Aspirin in AMI reduces death by:
   A. 33%
   B. 20-25%
   C. 45%
   D. 60%

93. Down's syndrome: all are true *except:*
   A. Most common cardiac lesion is endocardial cushion defect
   B. TGA is common
   C. TOF is not a common lesion
   D. Hypotonia

91 D 92 B 93 B

Jayadeva 2002

1. **LVH in ECG is a good predictor of mortality in:**
   A. Men
   B. Women
   C. Men with strong family h/o CAD
   D. Women with strong family h/o CAD

2. **In elderly control of both stroke and CAD is achieved by:**
   A. Reduction in systolic BP
   B. Reduction of diastolic BP
   C. Control of Homocysteinemia
   D. Control of Hyperglycemia

3. **T wave alternans in a patient is present with:**
   A. Beat to beat variation
   B. (L) Cervical Sympathetic stimulation
   C. (R) cervical sympathetic stimulation
   D. Hypokalemia

4. **LAD is caused by (-30°–90°):**
   A. Hypernatraemia
   B. Hypomagnesaemia
   C. Hypokalemia
   D. Hyperkalemia

5. **Drug effective in smoking cessation programme:**
   A. Bupropion
   B. Buprenorphine
   C. Nicotinic acid
   D. Methadone

6. **Circle of vieussens is formed by anastomosis between:**
   A. RCA to LAD
   B. RCA to LCx
   C. LCX to LAD
   D. PA to LAD

7. **Vein of Marshall is situated between:**
   A. Left SVC to coronary sinus
   B. Left IVC to coronary sinus
   C. Right SVC to coronary sinus
   D. IVC to SVC

8. **Myocardial non compaction leads to:**
   A. ARVD
   B. WPW
   C. CHB in child
   D. LBBB in adults

9. **IABP is C/I in:**
   A. AR
   B. MR
   C. VSD
   D. Cardiogenic shock

10. **Brugada syndrome; mechanism of VT:**
    A. Re-entry
    B. Triggered activity
    C. ↑Automaticity
    D. Parasystole

1 D 2 A 3 D 4 D 5 A 6 A 7 A 8 D 9 A 10 A

11. Digitalis toxicity psychiatric manifestation appear (in elderly):
- **A.** Levels >2
- **B.** Therapeutic levels
- **C.** Sub therapeutic
- **D.** Suicidal dose

12. EADS is responsible for:
- **A.** TDP
- **B.** Dig Toxicity
- **C.** RVOT VT
- **D.** Bundle branch re-entry tachycardia

13. Holt Oram syndrome is associated with:
- **A.** ASD with conduction defects
- **B.** Ostium primum ASD
- **C.** Coronary sinus ASD
- **D.** Sinus venosus ASD

14. HLA B27 is associated with:
- **A.** AV conduction defect
- **B.** SA nodal exit block
- **C.** Bundle branch re-entrant tachycardia
- **D.** ARVD

15. Fetal gene induction:
- **A.** Heart failure
- **B.** EMF
- **C.** HOCM
- **D.** DCM

16. Spade like configuration:
- **A.** Apical HOCM
- **B.** RCM
- **C.** DCM
- **D.** Aortic stenosis

17. Elephant trunk surgery:
- **A.** Dissection & thoracic aortic aneurysm surgery
- **B.** Removal of long saphenous vein
- **C.** Coronary bypass surgery-off pump
- **D.** Multivalve replacement surgery

18. Corridor procedure is used in:
- **A.** Chronic atrial fibrillation
- **B.** RFA of accessory pathway
- **C.** Homologous heart transplant
- **D.** Heterologous heart transplant

19. Incidence has increased two fold in recent year (due to unknown reasons) of:
- **A.** ASD
- **B.** VSD
- **C.** MVP
- **D.** TOF

20. Transient LV dilatation in thallium stress test suggests:
- **A.** Proximal LAD stenosis
- **B.** Left main stenosis
- **C.** Proximal RCA stenosis
- **D.** Proximal LCX stenosis

21. Radiation can cause:
- **A.** Coronary ostial stenosis
- **B.** Dissection
- **C.** Aneurysm
- **D.** VSD

22. Patient of variant angina on treatment with calcium channel blocker and long acting nitrate, next drug is:
- **A.** β blocker
- **B.** Aspirin
- **C.** Clonidine
- **D.** Reserpine

23. Chronotbiological response is used for treatment by:
- **A.** Verapamil
- **B.** Nifedipine
- **C.** Amlodipine
- **D.** Felodipine

11 B 12 A 13 A 14 A 15 A 16 A 17 A 18 A 19 A 20 B 21 A 22 C 23 A

24. Paget schotter syndrome:
- **A.** Traumatic obstruction to subclavian vein
- **B.** Thoracic inlet syndrome
- **C.** Genetic predisposition present
- **D.** Left lower lobe hypoplasia

25. Distichiasis is associated with:
- **A.** Superficial vein thrombosis
- **B.** Venous haemangiomas
- **C.** Recurrent pulmonary embolism
- **D.** Varicose vein

26. Mondor's disease:
- **A.** Superficial vein thrombosis of anterior chest wall
- **B.** Mountain sickness
- **C.** Costochondritis
- **D.** Variant angina

27. Waxy papules on eyelid bleeds to pinch is found in:
- **A.** Hurler syndrome
- **B.** Amyloidosis
- **C.** Type II hyperlipidemia
- **D.** Hunter syndrome

28. Tangier's disease: true is:
- **A.** Orange lobulated tonsils
- **B.** Cerebellar manifestations
- **C.** Recurrent bleeding
- **D.** Pericarditis

29. Herceptin antibody causes:
- **A.** DCMP
- **B.** EMF
- **C.** HOCM
- **D.** CCP

30. Non immune hydrops fetalis is most commonly caused by:
- **A.** SVT
- **B.** CHB
- **C.** VT
- **D.** Sinus bradycardia

31. Most common arrhythmia causing morbidity and mortality is:
- **A.** AF
- **B.** VF
- **C.** VT
- **D.** PSVT

32. Nicoladani Branham sign is found in:
- **A.** AV fistula
- **B.** Paget's disease
- **C.** Beriberi
- **D.** Pregnancy

33. Most common valve damaged in blunt and penetrating trauma:
- **A.** TV
- **B.** AV
- **C.** PV
- **D.** None of the above

34. Mahaim fibres on ECG shows:
- **A.** Wide QRS with LBBB
- **B.** Wide QRS with RBBB
- **C.** Narrow QRS with RAD
- **D.** Narrow QRS with LAD

35. Interrupted IVC is not seen in:
- **A.** Polysplemia
- **B.** Asplenia
- **C.** B/L left sidedness
- **D.** None of the above

36. Termination of atrial fibrillation is most effective by:
- **A.** Ibutilide
- **B.** Amiodarone
- **C.** Flecainide
- **D.** Sotalol

24 A 25 D 26 A 27 B 28 A 29 A 30 A 31 A 32 A 33 B 34 A 35 B 36 A

37. Mulibrey nanism:
- **A.** Constrictive pericarditis
- **B.** Acute pericarditis
- **C.** Hypothyroidism
- **D.** Hyperparathyroidism

38. Postprandial hypotension and syncope: treatment are all *except:*
- **A.** Octreotide
- **B.** Fluoxetine
- **C.** Sertraline
- **D.** Disopyramide

39. Treatment of type II hyperthyroidism in amiodarone toxicity:
- **A.** β blockers
- **B.** Steroids
- **C.** Radio iodine
- **D.** Propylthiouracil

40. Catch 22 association is seen with:
- **A.** Conotruncal anomaly
- **B.** Down's syndrome
- **C.** Coarctation of aorta
- **D.** Bicuspid aortic valve

41. Cardiovascular complication of CRF: true is:
- **A.** Complete heart block
- **B.** HCM
- **C.** AF
- **D.** Atrial flutter

42. Confluence of pulmonary veins in TAPVC:
- **A.** Intrapericardial
- **B.** Extrapericardial
- **C.** Extrapleural
- **D.** Intrapleural

43. Myocyte slippage is mechanism for:
- **A.** Ventricular dilatation
- **B.** Ventricular remodelling
- **C.** Negative remodelling after PTCA
- **D.** Graft arteriopathy

44. Saphenous vein graft v/s native coronary atherosclerosis:
- **A.** Concentric
- **B.** Eccentric
- **C.** Diffuse
- **D.** Multifocal

45. Contraction band necrosis is seen in:
- **A.** Thrombolysis and reperfusion
- **B.** Border of ischaemic myocardium
- **C.** Redistribution
- **D.** Myocarditis

46. Regional and global ventricular dysfunction after ischemia and reperfusion:
- **A.** Stunning
- **B.** Hibernation
- **C.** Ischemic preconditioning
- **D.** Necrosis

47. Nitroglycerin withdrawal is caused by:
- **A.** Endothelium derived hyperpolarizing factor
- **B.** Adenosine
- **C.** NO
- **D.** Endothelin

48. Most potent vasoconstrictor:
- **A.** Angiotensin II
- **B.** Endothelin
- **C.** Norepinephrine
- **D.** Dopamine

49. In a pressure volume curve when does pressure volume relation normalised to a pressure of zero:
- **A.** Ventricular elastance
- **B.** Ventricular compliance
- **C.** Preload
- **D.** Afterload

---

37 A 38 A 39 B 40 A 41 B 42 B 43 A 44 C 45 A 46 A 47 D 48 B 49 A

50. Post Fontan procedure can cause:
A. Protein losing enteropathy
B. Complete heart block
C. RV tachycardia
D. LV tachycardia

51. Pulmonary hypertension is most common in the following blood group:
A. A
B. B
C. AB
D. O

52. Pulmonary vasodilation without effect on systemic vascular resistance:
A. Adenosine
B. O_2
C. Prostacyclin
D. NO

53. Post partum bromocriptine can cause:
A. Severe hypertension
B. LV dysfunction
C. Coronary spasm
D. Arrhythmia

54. Gestational hypertension definition:
A. Beginning after 20 weeks and ending before 6th post partum week
B. Beginning after 10 weeks and ending before 4th post partum week
C. Beginning after 30 weeks and ending before 4th post partum week
D. Beginning after 40 weeks and ending before 4th post partum week

55. Doxorubicin toxicity is prevented by:
A. Dexrazoxane
B. Mesna
C. N acetyl cysteine
D. Dexpheroxamine

56. IE within 60 days after prosthetic valve replacement: commonest cause is:
A. Staph. aureus
B. Staph. epidermidis
C. Strep. viridans
D. Fungus

57. Primary APLA cause:
A. Thrombosis in coronary artery
B. Myocarditis
C. Pericarditis
D. Pericardial effusion

58. Cytoid bodies:
A. SLE
B. Hypertension and retinal infarction
C. IE
D. Coarctation of aorta

59. Angiod streaks:
A. Pseudo xanthoma elasticum with AR
B. Infective endocarditis
C. Acute rheumatic fever
D. Amyloidosis

60. Hollen horst plaque:
A. Atheroembolic
B. Hypertension
C. Retinal embolism
D. Diabetes mellitus

61. Incidence of RF in endemic areas:
A. 3%
B. 0.3%
C. 5%
D. 0.5%

62. Difference between UFH & LMWH:
A. LMWH has greater activity against Xa
B. LMWH has equal activity
C. LMWH doesn't causes HIT
D. LMWH is only given intravenously

50 A 51 A 52 D 53 C 54 A 55 A 56 B 57 A 58 B 59 A 60 A 61 A 62 A

63. Middle aged obese, hypertensive male with TG 274, S. cholesterol 247 mg%, HDL 31 mg%, LDL 162 mg%: diagnosis is:
A. Familial combined hyperlipidemia
B. Type II hyperlipidemia
C. Type I hyperlipidemia
D. Secondary hyperlipidemia

64. Difference of chordae tendinae of MV & TV is:
A. MV chordae is shorter
B. MV chordae is longer
C. Chordae of mitral valve does not attach to the interventricular septum
D. None of the above

65. MV opens earliest in:
A. Severe MS
B. MR
C. Normal
D. Ebstein's of tricuspid valve

66. Acute AR: characteristic finding is:
A. Soft to absent S1
B. Reversed split S2
C. Wide split S2
D. S3 and S4

67. Wide HV interval is seen:
A. Myotonic dystrophy
B. Ducchene's dystrophy
C. Friedrichs ataxia
D. Familial hypercalcemic paralysis

68. Typical ventriculo-phasic arrhythmia:
A. Children
B. Complete heart block
C. Digoxin
D. Amiodarone

69. In pressure of LA and RA:
A. 'a' > 'v' in LA
B. 'a' > 'v' in RA
C. 'a' = 'v' in RA
D. 'a' = 'v' in LA

70. Normal coronary artery not responding to pharmacological agents and stress is:
A. Prinzmetal angina
B. Microvascular angina
C. Linked angina
D. Epicardial stenosis

71. Apoptosis staining is done with:
A. Tc Annexin
B. Sestamibi
C. Tetraphosmin
D. Indium

72. Cardiac sympathetic innervation, detection in diabetics in myocardium:
A. MIBG
B. Guanabenz
C. Dopamine
D. Reserpine

73. Phase 2 current show:
A. Inward Na
B. Inward CL
C. Inward PO_4^-
D. Outward K

74. Mumps gene is seen in:
A. Kawasaki
B. EMF
C. Endocardial fibroelastosis
D. HOCM

75. Biventricular pacing in heart failure is useful in:
A. LBBB with PR prolongation with MR
B. LBBB
C. LBBB with PR prolongation
D. LBBB with short PR interval

76. True about ARDS is:
A. Alveolocapillary membrane abnormality
B. PCWP > 25 mmHg
C. Inhaled NO is a modality of treatment
D. Ventilation in lateral position is most effective

63 A 64 C 65 A 66 A 67 A 68 B 69 B 70 B 71 A 72 A 73 D 74 C 75 A 76 A

77. Normal values:
A. PCO_2 : 35-45 mmHg
B. pH:7.45-7.55
C. PaO_2 : 70 mmHg
D. HCO_3^- : 16

78. ACIP-TIPI: time independent predictor of:
A. Ventricular arrhythmia
B. Long QT
C. UA/MI
D. DCM

79. Autosomal dominant with severe HTN:
A. Liddle's syndrome
B. Pheochromocytoma
C. Renovascular hypertension
D. Barter's syndrome

80. Left ventricular assist device: most common disadvantage is:
A. Immune response↑due to T cell activation
B. Not portable
C. ↑ apoptosis
D. Hypersensitivity

81. Means Lerman scratch is heard in:
A. Hyperthyroidism
B. Hyperparathyroidism
C. Growth hormone deficiency
D. Paget's disease

82. Potassium channel openers are all *except:*
A. Molsidomine
B. Nicorandil
C. Cromakalim
D. Pinacidil

83. Diuretic long term used causes increased Na absorption is known as:
A. Braking effect
B. Counter current
C. Rebound effect
D. Aliasing effect

84. Non cardiac surgery with highest risk:
A. TURP
B. GB surgery
C. Abdominal aneurysm surgery
D. Carcinoma breast

85. Factors V Leiden is associated with:
A. Activated protein C resistance
B. Protein C deficiency
C. Bleeding tendency
D. VWF defect

86. Nitroprusside side effect in hypertensive crisis:
A. ↑ICT
B. ↓sed systolic pressure
C. ↓diastolic pressure
D. Severe hypotension

87. Mill wheel sound is heard in:
A. Hydropneumopericardium
B. Hyperparathyroidism
C. Post cardiac transplant
D. Post CABG

88. Erythema migrans:
A. Lyme arthritis
B. Rheumatic fever
C. Sleeping sickness
D. Rickettsias

89. Myocardial hypertrophy after MI:
A. Eccentric
B. Concentric
C. Reactive
D. Immunogenic

90. In LA myxoma fever, malaria, arthralgia is due to:
A. IL-6
B. IL-4
C. Vasculitis
D. TNF a

77 A 78 C 79 A 80 A 81 A 82 A 83 A 84 C 85 A 86 A 87 A 88 A 89 B
90 A

Miscellaneous I

1. **Branches of the left coronary artery are all *except:***
   A. Anterior descending artery
   B. One to three diagnonal branches
   C. Circumflex artery
   D. Conus artery

2. **All the veins drain directly into the right atrium *except:***
   A. Thebesian veins
   B. The anterior cardiac vein
   C. Coronary sinus
   D. Oblique vein of Marshall

3. **True about P cell is:**
   A. Large size
   B. Well developed sarcoplasmic reticulum
   C. Abundant glycogen
   D. Empty appearing cytoplasm

4. **All of the following statements apply to Vmax *except:***
   A. Shortening of the contractile element
   B. Isometric contraction
   C. Lengthening of the series elastic element
   D. Not affected by increases in heart rate

5. **Which of the following decrease myocardial contractility:**
   A. Cardioglobulin
   B. Serotonin
   C. Paired electrical stimulation
   D. Lidocaine

6. **Blood vessels are controlled by all *except:***
   A. Sympathetic vasoconstrictive fibers
   B. Sympathetic vasodilator fibers
   C. Parasympathetic vasodilator fibers
   D. Parasympathetic vasoconstrictive fibers

7. **Which of the following would characterize the arterial pulse of the radial artery as compared to that of the subclavian artery?**
   A. Less steep initial upstroke
   B. More prominent anacrotic pulse
   C. Earlier and higher dicrotic notch
   D. Systolic maximum becomes peaked and increased in magnitude

8. **All of the following are major cardiac substrates *except:***
   A. Ketone bodes
   B. Pyruvate
   C. Lactate
   D. Amino acids

9. **Which of the following are associated with osteogenesis imperfecta?**
   A. Marked bowing of the legs, saber shine, and pseudarthrosis
   B. Calcification of arteries
   C. Kyphoscoliosis
   D. Aortic regurgitation
   E. All of the above

1 D 2 D 3 D 4 D 5 D 6 D 7 D 8 D 9 E

10. Friedreich's ataxia is associated with:
A. Hammertoes
B. Sinus node artery occlusion
C. Equinovarus
D. A + C
E. All of the above

11. Hurler's syndrome is associated with all *except:*
A. Deafness
B. Mucopolysaccharide deposits in the heart valves, coronary arteries and aorta
C. Coarse features
D. Absent eyebrows

12. Enlarged tongue:
A. Amyloid
B. Hurler's syndrome
C. Down's syndrome
D. All of the above

13. Hurler's syndrome is associated with:
A. Mucopolysaccharide deposition in the coronary arteries
B. Endocardial fibroelastosis
C. Valvular thickening
D. All of the above

14. Sickle cell disease may result in:
A. Cardiomegaly
B. Pulmonary infarction
C. Diastolic murmur
D. A + B
E. All of the above

15. Aortic regurgitation is seen in:
A. Rheumatoid spondylitis
B. Polychondritis
C. Morquio's syndrome
D. All of the above

16. Abnormalities involving which of the following chromosomes have been described with congenital heart disease:
A. 1
B. 9
C. 11
D. All of the above

17. All the following apply to a bisferiens pulse *except:*
A. Percussion and tidal wave
B. Idiopathic hypertrophic subaortic stenosis
C. Aortic stenosis and regurgitation
D. Same as dicrotic pulse

18. Which of the following might accentuate pulses alternans?
A. Nitroglycerin
B. Tourniquets applied the extremities
C. The upright position
D. All of the above

19. Which of the following may be seen in the jugular venous pulse?
A. H wave
B. A wave
C. Z point
D. A + B
E. All of the above

20. All of the following would tend to accentuate the H wave *except:*
A. Constrictive pericarditis
B. Bradycardia
C. Tricuspid regurgitation
D. Hyperthyroidism

21. True about X wave:
A. Is prominent during tricuspid regurgitation
B. Is accentuated in the presence of atrial fibrillation
C. May be more prominent than the Y wave in constrictive pericarditis
D. Is not related to atrial relaxation

10 E 11 D 12 D 13 D 14 E 15 D 16 D 17 D 18 D 19 D 20 D 21 C

22. Polydactyly is associated with:
A. Ellis-van Creveld syndrome
B. Laurence Moon Biedl Bardet syndrome
C. Trisomy 13-15 syndrome
D. All of the above

23. Regarding Holt Oram syndrome all true *except:*
A. Autosomal recessive
B. Longer than normal thumbs
C. Short forearms
D. Hypoplastic thumbs

24. Rubinstein Taybi syndrome all true *except:*
A. Patent ductus arteriosus
B. Atrial septal defect
C. Ventricular septal defect
D. Small thumbs

25. Trisomy 18 syndrome all true *except:*
A. Ventricular septal defect
B. Patent ductus arteriosus
C. Abnormal valves
D. Normal hands

26. Cornelia de Lange syndrome:
A. Phocomelia
B. Hirsutism
C. Associated with a ventricular septal defect
D. All of the above

27. Pseudoxanthoma elasticum:
A. Plucked chicken skin
B. Angina pectoris
C. Aortic and mitral valvular disease
D. All of the above

28. Generalized lentigo characterized by:
A. Brown macules
B. Left axis deviation
C. T wave changes
D. Subvalvular stenosis
E. All of the above

29. Klippel Feil syndrome:
A. Bony deformities
B. Ventricular septal defect
C. Webbing of the neck
D. All of the above

30. Non valvular Aortic regurgitation is seen in:
A. Aorto arteritis
B. Marfan's syndrome
C. Syphilis
D. All of the above

31. Which of the following would be associated with absent phase V of the Korotkoff sounds?
A. Anemia
B. Thyrotoxicosis
C. Arteriovenous fistulas
D. All of the above

32. Peripheral mechanisms causing increased pulse pressure:
A. Arteriolar shunts
B. Capillary vasodilatation
C. Decreased distensibility of arteries
D. All of the above

33. Congenital heart diseases which may cause a greater than 5 mmHg difference in blood pressure between the right and left arms are all *except:*
A. Coarctation of the aorta
B. Aberrant subclavian artery
C. Supravalvular aortic stenosis
D. Patent Ductus Arteriosus

34. All of the following may cause a paradoxical pulse *except:*
A. Constrictive pericarditis
B. Chronic obstructive lung disease
C. Restrictive cardiomyopathy
D. Pericardial effusion

22 D 23 A 24 D 25 D 26 D 27 D 28 E 29 D 30 D 31 D 32 D 33 D 34 D

35. All of the following may cause wide splitting of the first sound *except:*
A. Right bundle branch block
B. Right atrial myxoma
C. Ebstein's anomaly
D. LBBB

36. All of the following would suggest suitability for a closed mitral Valvulotomy *except:*
A. Normal first sound
B. Loud opening snap
C. Diastolic murmur
D. Loud first sound

37. Fixed splitting of the second heart sound is seen in all *except:*
A. Atrial septal defect
B. Constrictive pericarditis
C. Right ventricular failure
D. Anomalous pulmonary venous return

38. All of the following would result in fixed splitting of the second heart sound *except:* ?
A. Right bundle branch block
B. Right ventricular failure
C. Total anomalous pulmonary venous return
D. Atrial septal defect

39. Which of the following would be an unexpected finding after closure of an atrial septal defect?
A. Respiratory variation in the splitting of the second heart sound
B. Delay in pulmonary closure
C. Abnormal electrocardiogram
D. Diastolic murmur

40. Tetralogy of Fallot following are true:
A. P2 is usually absent
B. P2 may be present but delayed in acyanotic infants
C. The position and anatomy of the valve are two factors which may play a role in an audible P2
D. All of the above

41. Wide splitting of the second sound is caused by all *except:*
A. Right bundle branch block
B. Mitral insufficiency
C. Aortic stenosis
D. Ventricular septal defect

42. Reversed splitting of the second sound may be caused by all *except:*
A. Wolff Parkinson White syndrome
B. Incomplete left bundle branch block
C. Systolic hypertension
D. Pulmonary stenosis

43. All of the following would be abnormal in a 40 year old man *except:*
A. Split second sound at the mitral area
B. P2 louder than A2 in the second left interspace
C. Palpable second sound in the pulmonic area
D. Absent pulmonic second sound in the mitral area

44. Single second heart sound can be seen in:
A. Pulmonary atresia
B. Single ventricle
C. Eisenmenger's ventricular septal defect
D. All of the above

45. In tricuspid insufficiency true is:
A. Positive Carvallo's sign with advanced right ventricular failure
B. Holosystolic murmur when there is normal right ventricular systolic pressure.
C. High frequency murmur when secondary to bacterial endocarditis
D. Giant V wave

46. Early systolic murmur may occur in:
A. Mitral incompetence
B. Tricuspid incompetence
C. Large ventricular septal defect with pulmonary hypertension
D. All of the above

35 D 36 A 37 B 38 A 39 D 40 B 41 C 42 D 43 D 44 D 45 D 46 D

47. In pulmonary insufficiency without pulmonary hypertension true is:
A. High pitched murmur
B. Murmur ends well before the first heart sound
C. Early diastolic murmur
D. Decrescendo murmur

48. Which of the following murmurs will become louder after pressor amine infusion?
A. Cyanotic tetralogy of Fallot
B. Ventricular septal defect
C. Mitral regurgitation
D. All of the above

49. Left anterior hemiblock all true *except:*
A. Q waves in leads I and AVL
B. May mimic anteroseptal infarction
C. Clockwise rotation
D. Right axis deviation

50. In chronic tricuspid regurgitation all true *except:*
A. Lymphocytosis
B. Normal albumin
C. Associated gastrointestinal disease
D. Normal bilirubin

51. Which of the following contribute to the anterior heart border in the right anterior oblique position?
A. Right ventricle
B. Right atrium
C. Pulmonary artery
D. Left atrium
E. A + C

52. All of the following help form the posterior border of the heart in the left anterior oblique projection *except:*
A. Left ventricle
B. Left atrium
C. Atrioventricular groove
D. Right ventricle

53. All of the following will obliterate the postero-inferior recess of the hear in the lateral view *except:*
A. Left ventricular hypertrophy
B. Pericardial effusion
C. Left atrial enlargement
D. Right atrial enlargement

54. Pericardial calcification all are true *except:*
A. Found in about one half of patients with constrictive pericarditis
B. Usually confined to one ventricle
C. Most commonly along the diaphragmatic aspect of the ventricles
D. May be found in patients without clinical evidence of constrictive pericarditis

55. Which of the following is an absolute indication to stop an exercise test:
A. Development of bundle branch block
B. ST depression of greater than 2 millimeters
C. Persistent bigeminy
D. Blood pressure falling below usual resting level

56. Slow EF slope may occur in:
A. Left atrial tumor
B. Pulmonary hypertension
C. IHSS
D. All of the above

57. The echocardiogram in IHSS all true *except:*
A. Ratio of septal wall to posterior wall thickness greater than 1.3:1 in diastole
B. ASH
C. Rapid posterior motion of the mitral leaflet in systolic
D. SAM

47 B 48 D 49 D 50 C 51 E 52 D 53 D 54 B 55 D 56 D 57 C

58. Causes of paradoxical motion of the interventricular septum all *except:*
A. Right ventricular volume overload
B. Constrictive pericarditis
C. Coronary artery disease involving the right coronary artery
D. Various conduction abnormalities

59. A ventricular pressure curve showing an early diastolic dip followed by a sudden rise to a high end diastolic pressure plateau could indicate:
A. Myocardial failure
B. Endocardial fibroelastosis
C. Constrictive pericarditis
D. All of the above

60. Which of the following are true in a dilated heart?
A. Myocardial fiber tension less for given pressure within the ventricle
B. Myocardial fiber tension progressively decreases during ejection
C. Increase in rate of myocardial fiber shortening
D. Oxygen requirement is increased

61. Heart failure is frequently seen with a normal sized heart in all *except:*
A. Acute myocardial infarction
B. Mitral stenosis
C. Acute renal failure
D. Hypertension

62. Kerley 'B' lines may be seen in:
A. Hemochromatosis
B. Infiltration by tumor
C. Heart failure
D. All of the above

63. Kerley 'A' lines characterized by:
A. Longer than Kerly 'B' lines
B. Seen in HF
C. Extended peripherally from the hilum
D. All of the above

64. Which of the following are toxic effects of digitalis?
A. Diarrhoea
B. Abdominal pain
C. Delirium
D. All of the above

65. Which of the following have been associated with Digitalis administration?
A. Trigeminal neuralgia
B. Gynecomastia
C. Bluish vision
D. All of the above

66. Which of the following are of value in the treatment of digitalis toxicity when there is a atrial tachycardia with 3:1 AV block:
A. Lidocaine
B. Potassium
C. Quinidine
D. Discontinuing digitalis

67. All of the following drugs act in the ascending limb of the Loop of Henley *except:*
A. Hydrochlorthiazide
B. Frusemide
C. Bumetanide
D. Ethacrynic acid

68. Which of the following diuretics act on the proximal tubule?
A. Hydrochlorthiazide
B. Aldactone
C. Triamterene
D. Mannitol

69. All of the following characterize sinus node depolarization *except:*
A. Well developed phase 1
B. Well developed phase 3
C. Absent phase 2
D. Relatively slow phase 0

58 C 59 D 60 D 61 D 62 D 63 D 64 D 65 D 66 D 67 A 68 D 69 A

70. All of the following apply to vasodepressor syncope *except:*
- **A.** May occur when vagal activity is blocked by atropine
- **B.** Decreased cerebral resistance
- **C.** Decreased renal blood flow
- **D.** Increased blood flow to the skin

71. Concerning electrical cardioversion of atrial fibrillation all true *except:*
- **A.** Over digitalization predisposes to serious arrhythmias
- **B.** Anticoagulation is thought to help prevent peripheral embolization
- **C.** Peripheral embolization occurs in about 10%
- **D.** Pulmonary edema is a recognized complication

72. All of the following are seen normally with standing *except:*
- **A.** Acceleration of the heart rate
- **B.** Increase in plasma catecholamine
- **C.** Decreased intrathoracic pressure
- **D.** Drop in diastolic blood pressure

73. Disease of the blood vessels supplying the SA and AV nodes is seen in:
- **A.** Muscular dystrophy
- **B.** Marfan's syndrome
- **C.** Primary pulmonary hypertension
- **D.** All of the above

74. True about Duchenne's type of muscular dystrophy:
- **A.** Late age of onset
- **B.** Slow progression
- **C.** Atrophy
- **D.** Sex-linked recessive

75. Following are seen in Duchenne's type of muscular dystrophy:
- **A.** Heart failure
- **B.** EKG evidence of myocardial infarction
- **C.** Tall R wave in V-1
- **D.** All of the above

76. True about myotonia dystrophica:
- **A.** Autosomal recessive inheritance
- **B.** Early onset of symptoms
- **C.** Testicular hypertrophy
- **D.** Baldness and cataracts

77. All of the following are seen in type II hyperlipoproteinaemia *except:*
- **A.** Corneal arcus
- **B.** Tendinous xanthomas
- **C.** Increased beta lipoprotein
- **D.** Autosomal recessive gene

78. All of the following apply to type I hyperlipoproteinaemia *except:*
- **A.** Autosomal dominant
- **B.** Hepatosplenomegaly
- **C.** Xanthoma
- **D.** Deficiency of lipoprotein lipase

79. All of the following apply to type IV hyperlipoproteinaemia *except:*
- **A.** Increased pre-beta lipoprotein
- **B.** Carbohydrate induced
- **C.** Increased presence of arteriosclerosis
- **D.** Stringent fat restriction is indicated

80. Which of the following is true about Tangier's disease?
- **A.** Hypercholesterolemia
- **B.** Atrophic tonsils
- **C.** Beta lipoprotein deficiency
- **D.** Familial

81. All of the following apply to beta lipoprotein deficiency *except:*
- **A.** Acanthocytic red blood cells
- **B.** Neurologic degeneration
- **C.** Steatorrhoea
- **D.** Autosomal dominant

70 D 71 C 72 D 73 D 74 D 75 D 76 D 77 D 78 A 79 D 80 D 81 D

82. Atrial septal defects may be:
A. At the fossa ovalis
B. Inferior to the fossa ovalis
C. Superior to the fossa ovalis
D. Posterio-inferior to the fossa ovalis
E. All of the above

83. Which of the following are complications of a large patent ductus arteriosus?
A. Pulmonary hypertension
B. Hoarseness
C. Aneurysm of the pulmonary artery
D. All of the above

84. Which of the following are seen in anomalous origin of the left coronary artery?
A. Myocardial infarction
B. Endocardial fibroelastosis
C. Mitral insufficiency
D. All of the above

85. Which of the following are true of ruptured aortic sinus anuerysms:
A. Posterior sinus ruptures into the right atrium
B. Right aortic sinus ruptures into the right ventricle
C. Left sinus rarely involved
D. All of the above

86. All of the following are associated with a bicuspid aortic valve *except:*
A. Polycystic kidneys
B. Coarctation of the aorta
C. Bacterial endocarditis
D. Equal size of the two cusps

87. All of the following are associated with aortic atresia *except:*
A. Retrograde filling of the proximal aorta
B. Atrial septal defect
C. Pulmonary venous obstruction
D. Predominantly in females

88. Uhl's anomaly all true *except:*
A. Parchment heart
B. Right ventricular hypertrophy
C. May be confused with Ebstein's anomaly
D. Less common than Ebstein's anomaly

89. All of the following are related to persistent left superior vena cava *except:*
A. Azygos vein joins right innominate vein
B. Hemiazygos vein joins left superior vena cava
C. Left superior vena cava empties into coronary sinus
D. Atrophic coronary sinus

90. Which of the following apply to ventricular septal defects of less than 0.5cm²/m²:
A. Elevated right ventricular pressure
B. Large left to right shunt
C. Congestive heart failure
D. Bacterial endocarditis

91 All of the following apply to ventricular septal defects of greater than 1 cm²/m²:
A. Congestive heart failure
B. Equal pressure in the ventricles
C. Increased pulmonary vascular resistance
D. Left to right shunt depends on the size of the defect

92. All of the following are associated with Ebstein's malformation *except:*
A. Pulmonary valve usually abnormal
B. Malposition of posterior cusp of the tricuspid valve
C. Tricuspid regurgitation
D. Right to left shunt

93. All of the following are seen with large ventricular septal defects *except:*
A. Left lower lobe atelectasis
B. Diastolic murmur
C. Pulmonary oedema
D. Soft first heart sound

82 E 83 D 84 D 85 D 86 D 87 D 88 B 89 D 90 D 91 D 92 A 93 D

94. True about truncus arteriosus:
A. Widely split second heart sound
B. Narrow pulse pressure
C. Characteristic EKG findings and chest X-ray
D. Right aortic arch in 1/3 of cases

95. All of the following are true about right sided aortic arch *except:*
A. Occurs in 15% of cases of tricuspid atresia
B. Occurs in 25% of cases of tetralogy of fallot
C. Occurs in 33% of persistent truncus arteriosus cases
D. Associated congenital cardiac abnormalities in 95%

96. All of the following are seen on the chest X-ray in coarctation of the aorta *except:*
A. 'E' Sign
B. Poststenotic dilatation
C. Normal heart size
D. Rib notching in infants

97. All of the following are related to discrete fibrous subvalvular aortic stenosis *except:*
A. Ejection sound is usually not heard
B. Aortic insufficiency murmur frequently heard
C. Post stenotic dilatation of the ascending aorta usually absent
D. Symptoms usually occur earlier than that with valvular stenosis

98. Which of the following is true about transposition of the great vessels:
A. More common in females
B. Low birth weight
C. Posterior aorta
D. Most frequent cause of congestive heart failure in the first two months of life

99. All of the following apply to transposition of the great vessel *except:*
A. Box shaped heart
B. Egg on side contour to heart
C. Higher oxygen saturation in the pulmonary artery than in the aorta
D. Right ventricular hypertrophy

100. All of the following are seen in the electrocardiogram with total anomalous pulmonary venous connection *except:*
A. RVH
B. qR pattern in right precordial leads
C. Enlarged p waves
D. LVH

101. Single ventricle all true *except:*
A. Usually morphologically left ventricle
B. Transposition is present in eighty five percent
C. Anoxic spells do not occur
D. Cyanosis is common

102. In partial anomalous pulmonary venous connection all true *except:*
A. Most common form is that associated with sinus venosus defect
B. All veins of the right lung may return to the inferior vena cava
C. All the veins of the left lung may connect to the left brachiocephalic vein
D. When one lung drains anomalously, the left to right shunt is about 25 percent

103. Double outlet right ventricle all true *except:*
A. May mimic tetralogy of Fallot
B. May mimic ventricular septal defect
C. Is called Taussig Bing heart if the ventricular septal defect is subpulmonary
D. Cyanosis is usually severe even without pulmonic stneosis

104. Which of the following apply to aneurysms of the sinus of valsalva?
A. Those of the right sinus rupture into the right ventricle
B. Those of noncoronary sinus rupture into the right atrium
C. Continuous murmur
D. Mortality of 20% if operated

94 D 95 A 96 D 97 D 98 D 99 A 100 D 101 C 102 D 103 D 104 D

105. Aortopulmonary window all true *except:*
A. Patients usually have a continuous murmur
B. Severe pulmonary hypertension
C. Defect is usually small
D. Surgery should be done before the age of 2 years

106. All of the following apply to palliative operations for tetralogy of Fallot *except:*
A. Blalock anastomosis
B. Waterston procedure
C. Pott's operation
D. Mustard procedure

107. Truncus arteriosus: true is:
A. A main pulmonary artery is seen in type II
B. The pulmonary arteries arise from the posterior aspect in type III
C. The right and left pulmonary arteries arise separately from the respective sides in type II
D. A right aortic arch is present in about thirty percent of cases

108. All of the following have been used in the treatment of Ebstein's malformation *except:*
A. Closure of the foramen ovale
B. Anastomosis of the superior vena cava to the right pulmonary artery
C. Replacement of the tricuspid valve by a prosthesis
D. Mustard procedure

109. All of the following apply to the Taussing Bing malformation *except:*
A. Resembles transposition of the great arteries
B. Double outlet right ventricle
C. Subpulmonic ventricular septal defect
D. Subaortic ventricular septal defect

110. All of the following are true of Aschoff bodies *except:*
A. Specific for rheumatic carditis
B. Fragmentation of interstitial collagent
C. Multinucleated cells and monocytes
D. Marked destruction and loss of myocardial fibers

111. Which of the following apply to aortic regurgitation:
A. Mild tachycardia usually has a deleterious effect
B. Pressure over-load of the left ventricle
C. With heart failure, the murmur is usually louder
D. Functional mitral regurgitation may occur

112. All of the following murmurs are seen characteristically with acute rheumatic fever *except:*
A. Mitral systolic murmur
B. Mitral mid diastolic rumble
C. Aortic diastolic murmur
D. Aortic systolic murmur

113. Which of the following are true of Sydenham's chorea:
A. Usually an early manifestation of acute rheumatic fever
B. Handwriting unaffected
C. Permanent neurological residual is common
D. Incidence has decreased

114. The echocardiogram may simulate mitral stenosis (slow EF slope) in:
A. Aortic stenosis
B. Idiopathic hypertrophic subaortic stenosis
C. Severe pulmonary hypertension
D. Barlow's syndrome

115. Which of the following apply to spontaneous isolated rupture of the chordae tendineae:
A. Most common in females
B. Usually involves the anterior leaflet
C. Markedly enlarged left atrium
D. Preservation of normal sinus rhythm

105 A 106 D 107 D 108 D 109 D 110 D 111 D 112 D 113 D 114 B 115 D

116. An opening snap may be seen in:
A. Ebstein's anomaly
B. ASD
C. Mitral regurgitation
D. Tricuspid stenosis
E. All of the above

117. All the following are true about precordial honks *except:*
A. Louder with expiration
B. May originate in tricuspid valve
C. Loudest after standing
D. Louder after amyl nitrite

118. Which of the following apply to the electrocardiogram in patients with late systolic clicks and murmurs?
A. Short QT interval
B. T wave abnormalities most common anteriorly
C. Standing tends to improve the changes
D. Marked T wave inversions may develop

119. All of the following apply to calcification of the mitral annulus *except:*
A. Elderly males
B. Ejection murmur
C. Relation to diabetes and hypercalcemia
D. Patients frequently asymptomatic

120. All of the following circumstances may disguise the characteristic slow ascent of the pulse in aortic stenosis *except:*
A. Atheromatous vessels
B. Elderly patient
C. Concomitant aortic insufficiency
D. Palpation of the carotid pulse only

121. Which of the following is true about the murmur of tricuspid stenosis?
A. Lower pitched than that of mitral stenosis
B. Best heard to the right of sternum
C. The murmur is unaffected by respiration
D. Murmur presystolic in sinus rhythm

122. True about Morquio's syndrome is:
A. Mental deficiency, usually severe
B. Aortic regurgitation is rare
C. Bone changes usually minimal
D. Corneal clouding

123. All of the following apply to Ehlers-Danlos syndrome *except:*
A. Mitral regurgitation
B. Cigarette paper scars
C. Autosomal recessive
D. Aortic rupture

124. All of the following apply to familial hypercholesterolemia *except:*
A. Fredrickson's type II
B. Increased beta lipoproteins
C. Xanthoma tendinosum
D. Turbid fasting serum

125. Fredrickson's type III hyperlipoproteinaemia all *except:*
A. Broad beta lipoprotein band
B. Abnormal glucose tolerance
C. Clofibrate useful
D. Increase in plasma chylomicrons

126. Type V hyperlipoproteinaemia: true statement is:
A. PHHA is always very low
B. Accelerated atherosclerosis
C. Obesity is unusual
D. Eruptive xanthomas

127. Which of the following may mimic a myocardial infarction on an electrocardiogram?
A. Friedrichs ataxia
B. Progressive muscular dystrophy
C. Cardiomyopathies
D. All of the above

116 E 117 D 118 D 119 A 120 D 121 D 122 D 123 C 124 D 125 D 126 D 127 D

128. All are true about chronic constrictive pericarditis *except:*
- **A.** M pattern of right atrial pressure pulse
- **B.** Early diastolic dip
- **C.** Mean right atrial pressure equals wedge pressure
- **D.** Cardiac output usually diminished

129. All the following can result in severe early coronary artery disease *except:*
- **A.** Necrotizing arteritis of infancy
- **B.** Coarctation of the aorta
- **C.** Supravalvular aortic stenosis
- **D.** Aortic atresia

130. Endocrine secretions of the kidney are all *except:*
- **A.** Renin
- **B.** Erythropoietin
- **C.** Blood pressure reducing agents
- **D.** Aldosterone

131. Which of the following would be unusual in primary aldosteronism?
- **A.** Malignant hypertension
- **B.** Hyponatremia
- **C.** Tumor weighing greater than 6 grams
- **D.** Low serum magnesium levels

132. Ethacrynic acid all *except:*
- **A.** Transient hearing loss
- **B.** Fatal agranulocytosis
- **C.** Hyperuricaemia
- **D.** Frequent diabetes

133. Reserpine causes all *except:*
- **A.** Bradycardia
- **B.** Colitis
- **C.** Constipation
- **D.** Parkinsonism

134. Clonidine: all are true *except:*
- **A.** Decreased sympathetic activity
- **B.** Dryness of the mouth
- **C.** Withdrawal syndrome
- **D.** No sedative effect

135. Prostaglandins all *except:*
- **A.** Hypotensive action
- **B.** Induce natriuresis
- **C.** Those in the E and A classes have predominantly cardiovascular action
- **D.** Those in the F class have predominantly cardiovascular action

136. Bradykinin all true *except:*
- **A.** Dilates pulmonary arteries
- **B.** Constricts the umbilical arteries and veins
- **C.** Constricts the ductus arteriosus
- **D.** Formed from inactive precursor kallikrein

137. In high altitude pulmonary edema all true *except:*
- **A.** The heart is enlarged
- **B.** Normal left atrial pressure
- **C.** Normal pulmonary artery wedge pressure
- **D.** Pulmonary hypertension is a consistent finding

138. In high altitude pulmonary edema all occur *except:*
- **A.** Widespread intravascular fibrin deposits
- **B.** Normal wedge pressure
- **C.** Patchy pulmonary edema is characteristic on the X-ray
- **D.** Removal to a lower altitude is necessary after an acute attack

139. Primary pulmonary hypertension all true *except:*
- **A.** Hoarseness
- **B.** Prominent A waves
- **C.** Systolic ejection click
- **D.** Frequent clubbing of the fingers

128 D 129 D 130 D 131 D 132 D 133 C 134 D 135 D 136 D 137 A 138 D 139 D

140. Which of the following may occur with acute cor pulmonale?

A. Giant A waves
B. Giant V waves
C. Left ventricular failure
D. All of the above

141. All of the following are causes of general alveolar hypoventilation *except:*

A. Sedative drugs
B. Extreme obesity
C. Deformity of the thoracic musculoskeletal system
D. Emphysema

142. Which of the following are true about vegetations in bacterial endocarditis:

A. Middle layer composed primarily of fibrin
B. Outer layer composed primarily of bacteria
C. In atrial septal defects, vegetations are usually located on the atrial wall
D. Vegetations may be large enough to obstruct the valve orifice

143. Roth spots are seen in:

A. Bacterial endocarditis
B. Anemia
C. Scurvy
D. All of the above

144. All of the following may be helpful in treating carcinoid *except:*

A. Cyclophosphamide
B. Digoxin
C. Valve replacement
D. Bradykinin

145. Endomyocardial fibrosis all true *except:*

A. Digitalis of little value
B. May be related to carcinoid
C. Often stimulates constrictive pericarditis
D. Embolic phenomena are frequent (over 50%)

146. In Chronic Chagas's disease all true *except:*

A. Positive Machado Guerreiro complement fixation test
B. Precordial pain
C. Positive xenodiagnostic study
D. There is marked cardiac muscle destruction

147. Which of the following are seen with chronic Chagas disease:

A. Mitral insufficiency
B. Tricuspid insufficiency
C. Mural thrombosis
D. All of the above

148. Toxoplasmosis true is:

A. Myocardial involvement is rare
B. Complete recovery from Toxoplasma myocarditis is the rule
C. Clinical cardiac disease is invariable
D. Pyrimethamine and sulfonamides are useful

149. Trichinosis all true *except:*

A. Periorbital edema
B. Eosinophilia
C. Muscle tenderness
D. Chronic heart disease is the rule

150. In congestive cardiomyopathy,, all the following murmurs may be heart commonly *except:*

A. Mitral insufficiency
B. Pulmonary insufficiency
C. Tricuspid insufficiency
D. Aortic insufficiency

151. All the following are seen commonly with congestive cardiomyopathy *except:*

A. Abnormal Q waves in over 10%
B. Diastolic gallop
C. Poor X descent
D. Loud systolic murmurs

140 D **141** D **142** D **143** D **144** D **145** D **146** D **147** D **148** D **149** D **150** D **151** D

152. Idiopathic hypertrophic subaortic stenosis all true *except:*
A. Elevated left atrial mean pressure in 50% of patients
B. Left ventricular end diastolic pressure usually elevated
C. Marked variability in hemodynamic findings in the same patient
D. Pulse pressure increases in the beat following a premature ventricular contraction

153. All of the following will intensify the obstruction in IHSS *except:*
A. Isuprel
B. Nitroglycerin
C. Digitalis
D. Phenylephrine

154. All of the following will intensify the obstruction in IHSS *except:*
A. Methoxamine
B. Exercise
C. Standing
D. Valsalva maneuver

155. All of the following are seen in the angio-cardiogram in IHSS *except:*
A. Mitral insufficiency
B. Hypertrophied papillary muscles
C. Abnormal position of the anterior leaflet during systole
D. Large left ventricular cavity

156. Myocardial sarcoidosis all true *except:*
A. Corticosteroid indicated
B. Ventricular arrhythmias may occur
C. Electrocardiogram may resemble myocardial infarction
D. More common in males

157. Following statements after thiamine treatment for beriberi heart disease true *except:*
A. Hypertension
B. Pulmonary edema
C. Sudden increase in peripheral vascular resistance
D. Myocardial lesion responds more rapidly than the peripheral lesion

158. Pompe's disease all true *except:*
A. Markedly increase QRS voltage
B. Large tongue
C. Autosomal dominant
D. Hypertrophic subaortic stenosis

159. Which of the following is the largest and strongest component of Cardiac skeleton?
A. Rt Fibrous Trigone
B. Lt Fibrous trigone
C. Membranous septum
D. Intervalvular fibrosa

160. Mitral Valvular annular dilatation affects which of the following structures maximally?
A. Posterior mitral leaflet
B. Anterior Mitral leaflet
C. Both leaflets are affected equally
D. Depends on etiology of annular dilatation

161. Which of the following best differentiates congenital clefts from true commissures of a mitral valve?
A. Location of the cleft
B. Number of clefts
C. Presence of underlying papillary muscle in commissures
D. Long length of the commissures

162. All of the following are true about chordae of atrioventricular valve *except:*
A. They are inserted on the ventricular surface of the anterior leaflet
B. May calcify with age
C. Tricuspid chordae but not mitral valve chordae may insert on ventricular septum
D. Characterized by absence of cardiac muscle

152 D 153 D 154 D 155 D 156 D 157 D 158 C 159 A 160 A 161 C 162 D

163. All of the following are true about structure of Aortic valve *except:*

A. Has three half-moon cusps forming pocket like avascular tissue flaps
B. Nodule of Arantis is present at closing edges
C. It contains a well defined tensing apparatus
D. Lunular fenestrations in the Aortic valve are not associated with Aortic regurgitation

164. All of the following are true about Lambl's Excrescences *except:*

A. Most commonly found on Aortic valve
B. They are diagnosed only on postmortem examination
C. Occur due to thickening of Nodule of Arantis
D. They can cause cardio embolic stroke

165. All of the following are true about fat accumulation in heart *except:*

A. Excess fat in right ventricle may be associated with arrhythmogenic Right ventricular cardiomyopathy
B. Fat accumulation in atrial septum is associated with lipomatous hypertrophy
C. Fat accumulation prevents cardiac rupture after transmural infarction
D. Atrioventricular grooves is the most common site of fat accumulation in epicardium

166. Which of the following is the site of insertion of the transvenous ventricular pacemaker electrodes?

A. Apical trabeculated Zone
B. Inlet of RV just below the tricuspid annulus
C. In smooth walled muscular subpulmonary canal
D. In the septal band

167. All of the following are true about Crista Supraventricularis *except:*

A. Parietal band, infundibular band and septal band are the three components
B. Separates TV from PV
C. Moderator Band extends from septal band to anterior tricuspid papillary muscle
D. Parietal Band separates right and left ventricular outflow tracts

168. All of the following are true about ventricular structure *except:*

A. In a hypertrophied heart, left ventricular apex is much more trabeculated than right ventricular apex
B. Maximum thickness of the LV is at base
C. Normally, ventricular septum bulges to the right
D. Mitral Valve and AV share continuity but TV and PV are separated

169. All of the following are true about pseudotendons in heart *except:*

A. They are normal anatomical variants present in 50% of hearts.
B. They are never attached to Mitral Leaflets
C. Can cause innocent systolic musical murmurs
D. Much more common in females

170. Patent foramen ovale is found in how much percentage of cases?

A. 5%
B. 15%
C. 25%
D. 35%

171. Which of the following is the anatomical hallmark of right atrium?

A. Crista terminalis
B. Fossa ovalis
C. Right atrial appendage
D. Eustachian valve

172. Most common site of drainage of left persistent Superior venacava is:

A. Left Atrium
B. Right Atrium
C. Coronary sinus
D. Right SVC

163 C 164 D 165 C 166 A 167 D 168 A 169 D 170 D 171 B 172 C

173. The part of right atrium that is most prone to perforation is:
A. Free wall between pectinate muscles
B. Crista terminalis
C. Right atrial appendage
D. Interatrial septum

174. Which of the following statements is not true about Myocardial bridges:
A. Can be seen in 25% of children
B. Associated with intramural LAD
C. 10% of general population has Myocardial bridging
D. May cause sudden death due to systolic luminal narrowing

175. SVC receives azygous vein:
A. Anteriorly
B. Posteriorly
C. Laterally
D. Either anterior or posterior–50% each

176. Chiari net is formed:
A. By Oblique vein of Marshall
B. At the site of communication of azygous vein with SVC
C. By fenestrated Thebasian valve
D. At the site of entrance of SVC into RA

177. All of the following are true about oblique vein of Marshall *except:*
A. It is generally seen as a ligamentous remnant
B. Derived from Left common cardinal vein
C. It is present as a communication between Left persistent SVC and right atrium
D. Both veins and ligament are potentially arrhythmogenic

178. All of the following are the site of collaterals in coronary circulation *except:*
A. Ventricular apex
B. Posterior right ventricular free wall
C. Cardiac crux
D. Anterolateral LV free wall

179. Veins which drain directly into the right atrium are all *except:*
A. Thebasian veins
B. Oblique vein of Marshall
C. Anterior cardiac vein
D. Coronary sinus

180. Which of the following is not a branch of right coronary artery:
A. Intermediate artery
B. Conus artery
C. Right half of Vieussen's ring
D. Three to four right ventricular branches

181. All of the following are branches of left coronary artery *except:*
A. Ramus intermedius
B. Circumflex artery
C. Diagonal branches
D. Conus artery

182. Which of the following is not a branch of left anterior descending artery:
A. Small artery curving about the pulmonary conus
B. Septal perforating branches
C. Branches to left ventricular free wall
D. Marginal branch

183. Which of the following structure may be supplied by Left circumflex artery:
A. AV node
B. SA node
C. Left bundle branch
D. Posteromedial papillary muscle

184. All of the following conditions may be associated with small coronary artery disease (due to hereditary medial necrosis) *except:*
A. Freidrich's ataxia
B. Pompe's disease
C. Progressive muscular dystrophy
D. Primary pulmonary Hypertension

173 A 174 C 175 B 176 C 177 C 178 B 179 B 180 A 181 D 182 D 183 B 184 B

185. Wenckebach's bundle is:
A. Middle internodal tract
B. Anterior internodal tract
C. Interfascicular bundle
D. Interatrial bundle

186. All of the following are true about left main coronary artery *except:*
A. Arises from the inferior portion of the left aortic sinus
B. Judkins catheter is most frequently used to engage LCA
C. It is best viewed in AP projection with slight caudal angulation
D. LM disease is best managed by CABG

187. Right dominance is found in what percentage of cases?
A. 55%
B. 65%
C. 75%
D. 85%

188. All of the following are true about right coronary artery *except:*
A. Ideal angiographic projection for right coronary artery is LAO cranial
B. Gives rise to sinoatrial node artery in 60% cases
C. Upto 25% of cases of RCA dominance may have a double PDA
D. Conus artery arises from RCA in 70% cases

189. Codominant circulation is seen in how many of cases?
A. 3.5%
B. 7.5%
C. 15%
D. 20%

190. All of the following are true about SA node *except:*
A. Spindle shaped structure
B. Supplied by left circumflex in 40% cases
C. Is subendocardial in location
D. P cells are responsible for impulse formation

191. All of the following are true about triangle of Koch *except:*
A. Inferior boundary is formed by septal leaflet of tricuspid valve
B. AV node lies at the base of the triangle
C. Tendon of Todaro lies superiorly
D. Coronary sinus forms the base of the triangle

192. Vascular system starts developing at what gestational age in embryo:
A. Third week
B. Sixth week
C. Eighth week
D. Tenth week

193. Roots and proximal portion of Aorta and Pulmonary artery arise from:
A. Proximal portion of Bulbus Cordis
B. Conus cordis
C. Distal portion of Bulbus cordis
D. Mid portion of Bulbus cordis

194. What percentage of congenital heart disease is associated with chromosomal aberrations?
A. Less than 2 %
B. 6-10%
C. 15-20%
D. 23%

195. Earliest pacemaker of heart is which of the following structures?
A. Sinus venosus
B. AV node
C. Cranial part of left cardiac tube
D. Caudal part of left cardiac tube

185 A 186 A 187 D 188 D 189 B 190 C 191 B 192 A 193 C 194 B 195 D

196. Which of the following statements best describes the formation of Persistent Truncus Arteriosus:

A. It is due to fusion of dorsal and ventral swellings of conus cordis

B. It is present when conotruncal septum fails to follow its normal apical course and runs straight down.

C. It occurs when conotruncal region fails to fuse and descends towards ventricles.

D. It is due to unequal division of the conus because of anterior displacement of cono-truncal septum.

197. All of the following are true about aortic sac *except:*

A. It is the most distal part of Truncus arteriosus

B. Aortic arches-I, II, III, IV and VI arise from aortic sac

C. Gives rise to three horns–Right, left and central

D. Right horn gives rise to Brachiocephalic artery

198. Which of the Aortic arch is also known as pulmonary arch?

A. Second arch

B. Third arch

C. Fourth arch

D. Sixth arch

199. External carotid artery arises from which aortic arch?

A. Second arch

B. Third arch

C. Fourth arch

D. Sixth arch

200. Ductus arteriosus arises from:

A. Proximal part of right sixth aortic arch

B. Distal part of right sixth aortic arch

C. Distal part of left sixth aortic arch

D. Proximal part of left sixth aortic arch

201. Double aortic arch arises from:

A. Persistent right dorsal aorta

B. Abnormal origin of right subclavian artery

C. Persistent Fifth aortic arch

D. Right third aortic arch

202. All of the following are true about umbilical arteries *except:*

A. Form Internal iliac arteries

B. They are paired ventral branches of Aorta

C. Oxygen Saturation of blood is approximately 70%

D. Distal part is obliterated to form medial umbilical ligament

203. All of the following are true about umbilical veins *except:*

A. They originate from chorionic villi

B. Left umbilical vein is connected to right hepatic cardiac vein by Ductus venosus

C. They are responsible for oxygen supply to the embryo

D. Right umbilical vein forms ligamentum venosum

204. Azygos vein arises from:

A. Left supracardinal vein

B. Right supracardinal vein

C. Left posterior cardinal vein

D. Right common cardinal vein

205. Double IVC represents:

A. Persistent left subcardinal vein

B. Persistent right subcardinal vein

C. Persistent right sacrocardinal vein

D. Persistent left sacrocardinal vein

206. Left superior vena cava is derived from:

A. Left supracardinal vein

B. Left anterior cardinal vein

C. Proximal right anterior cardinal vein

D. Right common cardinal vein

196 C 197 C 198 D 199 B 200 C 201 A 202 C 203 D 204 B 205 D 206 B

207. Functional closure of Ductus Arteriosus occurs mostly:
A. Within 2-3 minutes in most cases
B. Within 4 days in most cases
C. Within 1 week in most cases
D. Within 2-3 months

208. Following thrombolysis between 12 hrs–24 hrs in MI, which trial showed mortality benefit?
A. ISIS-4
B. LATE
C. EMERAS
D. None of the above

209. In GUSTO angiographic substudy, 90 minute patency rate in the infarct related artery was highest in which of the four treatment arms?
A. Accelerated tpA
B. tPA+Streptokinase
C. Streptokinase+ IV heparin
D. Streptokinase + SC heparin

210. In GUSTO angiographic substudy, the 180 minute patency rate was highest in which of the treatment arms?
A. Accelerated tpA
B. Streptokinase + IV Heparin
C. Streptokinase + SC Heparin
D. There was no significant difference in different treatment arms

211. In GUSTO study, the incidence of intracranial haemorrhage was higher in which of the following treatment arms?
A. Accelerated tpA
B. Streptokinase + IV heparin
C. Streptokinase + SC heparin
D. There was no difference

212. Regarding 30 day mortality in angiographic substudy of GUSTO trial, following statements are true *except:*
A. 6.3% in accelerated tpA group
B. 6.1% in tpA + Streptokinase group
C. 7.4% in Streptokinase and IV heparin group
D. 7.2% in streptokinase and SC heparin group

213. Absolute contraindication of thrombolysis in MI are following:
A. History of haemorragic cerebrovascular accident
B. Active peptic ulcer disease
C. Pregnancy
D. None of the above

214. In acute MI, following statements are true *except:*
A. Troponin T increases within 3 hours of chest pain and returns to normal within 3 days
B. Trophonin T increases within 3 hours of chest pain and may remain elevated for 7-10 days
C. Trophonin T increases in non Q wave infarction
D. Rapid releases of Troponin T indicate successful recanalization of infarct related artery

215. Which of the following agents is most suitable for prehospital thrombolysis?
A. Reteplase
B. Streptokinase
C. APSAC
D. Urokinase

216. Which of the following procedures has been associated with increased mortality?
A. Primary PTCA in MI with shock
B. Rescue PTCA in failed thrombolysis in MI
C. Routine empherical use of PTCA following thrombolysis in MI
D. Elective PTCA in AMI when spontaneous or exercise provoked ishcaemia occurs, irrespective of thrombolytic therapy

207 B 208 D 209 A 210 D 211 A 212 B 213 A 214 A 215 A 216 C

217. Regarding Magnesium in AMI, which of the following statements are true?

A. LIMIT II trial showed mortality benefit in Magnesium treated patient

B. ISIS-4 trial did not show any mortality benefit in Magnesium treated patient

C. Both statements are true

D. None of them are true

218. Early use of Beta blocker in MI showed mortality benefit in which of the following trials?

A. ISIS-1

B. ISIS-2

C. ISIS-3

D. ISIS-4

219. In acute MI, which of the following drugs have been shown to cause statistically significant mortality benefits?

A. Nitrates

B. ACE Inhibitors

C. Nifedpine

D. Both nitrates and ACE inhibitors

220. Right ventricular infarction causes:

A. Raised atrial natriuretic factor

B. Steep right atrial Y descent

C. Square root sign in right ventricular pressure tracing

D. All of the above

221. Which of the following oils has the highest concentration of monounsaturated fat?

A. Rapeseed oil

B. Sunflower oil

C. Corn oil

D. Olive oil

222. Following statements are true regarding fatty acids *except:*

A. Best dietary source of poly unsaturated fatty acids are nuts, vegetable oils and oil rich fish

B. Rapeseed oil is rich in monounsaturated fatty acid

C. Margarine contains trans-unsaturated fatty acids

D. Trans-unsaturated fatty acids reduces cholesterol and risk of heart disease

223. Regarding platelet glycoprotein IIb/IIIa receptor antagonists, following statements are true:

A. Reduces post PTCA ischaemic complications at 6 months

B. Reduces mortality in unstable angina

C. Both of the above

D. None of the above

224. First dose hypotension is least common with:

A. Fosinopril

B. Perindopril

C. Quinapril

D. Cizalapril

225. Which of the following statins reduce both cholesterol and triglyceride?

A. Atorvastatin

B. Pravastatin

C. Cerivastatin

D. None of the above

226. Regarding thrombolysis in acute ischaemic stroke, which of the following statements are true:

A. The time window is 6 hours following the onset

B. Streptkinase is the agent of choice

C. Prior MRI scan is mandatory

D. None of the above

227. A history of preinfarction angina in patients with first Q wave infarction is associated with:

A. Higher peak CPK activity

B. Higher incidence of inhospital ventricular tachycardia

C. Lower ejection fraction

D. Lower incidence of pump failure and cardiac mortality

217 C 218 A 219 B 220 D 221 D 222 D 223 C 224 B 225 B 226 C 227 D

228. Mibefradil is a:

A. T-channel calcium antagonist
B. K-channel opener
C. Adenosine A_1 receptor blocker
D. None of the above

229. Which of the following pathogens have the strongest association with atherosclerosis?

A. Cytomegalovirus
B. Chlamydia pneumonia
C. Helicobacter pylori
D. Streptococcus viridans

230. In ESSENCE study, comparing LMW heparin with UF heparin in unstable angina:

A. LMW heparin was superior to UF heparin in mortality reduction
B. Significant fewer patients required revascularization in LMWH group
C. Overall cost was less with LMW heparin group
D. All of the above

231. In failed thrombolysis with streptokinase in AMI, which of the following statements are true?

A. Repeat thrombolysis with streptokinase may be tried
B. Alternative thrombolytic agent (t PA) is preferable
C. Rescue PTCA is an option
D. All of the above

232. Regarding thrombolysis in critical limb ischaemia with tPA, which of the following statement is FALSE?

A. Dose is higher than that is used in MI
B. Produces result equivalent to those of surgery when measured by limb salvage
C. Can take 3 hours to restore the circulation in an ischaemic leg
D. Most successful in occlusions due to embolus

233. Nicorandil:

A. Has balanced arterial vasodilatory and venodilatoy properties
B. Has no negative inotrophic effect
C. Has got direct cardioprotective effect
D. All of the above

234. Nislodipine:

A. Is a dihydropyridine calcium channel antagonist
B. May be used in ischaemic LV dysfunction
C. Both are true
D. None of them are true

235. Compared to medical therapy, carotid artery surgery improves prognosis in which group of patients?

A. Less than 30% carotid artery stenosis
B. 30-69% carotid artery stenosis
C. 70-99% carotid artery stenosis
D. No statistical difference between these three groups.

236. In Paroxysmal AF, following drugs are useful *except:*

A. Flecainide
B. Digoxin
C. Propafenone
D. Amiodarone

237. Commonest microbiology of right sided endocarditis associated with intravenous drug abuse:

A. Staphylococcus aureus
B. Enterococci
C. Fungi
D. Culture negative

238. Commonest organism of prosthetic value endocarditis in first two months of surgery is:

A. Staphylococcus aureus
B. Coagulase negative staphylococcus
C. Fungi
D. Streptococci

228 A 229 B 230 D 231 D 232 B 233 D 234 C 235 C 236 B 237 A 238 B

239. Antibiotic prophylaxis for infective endocarditis is indicated in following conditions *except:*
A. Sclerotherapy for oesophageal varices
B. Esophageal dilatation
C. Bronchoscope with rigid bronchoscope
D. Cardiac catheterization

240. Following drugs increase HDL cholesterol *except:*
A. Oestrogen in postmenopausal women
B. Nicotinic acid
C. Probucol
D. Simvastatin

241. Which of the following drugs may increase triglyceride level?
A. Cholestyramine
B. Nicotinic acid
C. Probucol
D. Lovastatin

242. Which of the following drugs has powerful antioxidant property?
A. Nicotinic acid
B. Colestipol
C. Bezafibrate
D. Probucol

243. In NIDDM, following statements are true *except:*
A. HDL level is low.
B. Elevated level of triglycerides
C. Increased platelet aggregability
D. Chylomicron level does not change appreciably

244. Following are the haemodynamics changes during 2nd trimester of normal pregnancy:
A. Decreased systemic vascular resistance
B. Increased pulse pressure
C. Diastolic BP falls more than the systolic BP
D. All of the above

245. Which of the following is not a major manifestation in rheumatic fever (Jones criteria)?
A. Chorea
B. Erythema marginatum
C. Subcutaneous nodules
D. Prolonged P-R interval

246. Which of the following muscle relaxants have got no appreciable cardiovascular side effects?
A. Tubocurarine
B. Metocurine
C. Vecuronium
D. Pancuronium

247. HRT with oestrogen causes all *except:*
A. Reduction of total cholesterol
B. Reduction of LDL cholesterol
C. Reduction in triglyceride
D. Increase in HDL

248. Arrhythmogenic right ventricular dysplasia is:
A. Common in males
B. May cause sudden death
C. Beta blocker is often helpful
D. All of the above

249. Regarding DDD pacing in hypertrophic obstructive cardiomyopathy:
A. 10% of HCM patients are candidates
B. Gradient is reduced by an average of 50%
C. Both are true
D. None of them are true

250. Risk of sudden death in HOCM is increased with following conditions *except:*
A. Nonsustained VT in 48 hour Holter monitoring
B. Sustained supraventricular arrhythmia
C. Severe functional limitation and symptoms
D. Young age

239 D 240 C 241 A 242 D 243 D 244 D 245 D 246 C 247 C 248 D 249 C 250 C

251. In HOCM, following drugs increase the intensity of gradient and murmur *except:*
- A. Phenylephrine
- B. Digitalis
- C. Isoproterenol
- D. Amyl nitrite

252. In which of the following trials aspirin has been shown to reduce cerebral stroke in atrial fibrillation:
- A. AFASAK
- B. BAATAF
- C. CAFA
- D. SPAF-1

253. Following statements are true regarding high altitude pulmonary oedema *except:*
- A. Usually occurs in elderly population
- B. Chest pain may be the accompanying symptom
- C. Rapid ascent to altitudes in excess of 2500 metre is the main responsible factor
- D. Gradual ascent is preventive

254. Which of the following is a selective beta blocker with ISA activity:
- A. Pindolol
- B. Oxprenolol
- C. Acebutolol
- D. Timolol

255. In isolated systolic hypertension of the elderly:
- A. Diuretics reduces the risk of stroke
- B. Beta blocker also reduces the risk of stroke
- C. Both are true
- D. None of them are true

256. Which of the following drugs is predominantly an arteriolar dilator rather than a balanced arterial and vasodilator?
- A. Nitroprusside
- B. Minoxidil
- C. Alpha blockers
- D. Nitroglycerin

257. Which of the following statements are TRUE?
- A. Carotid sinus baroreceptor are located in the internal carotid artery just above the bifurcation of the common carotid artery
- B. Afferent impulse travel via the sinus nerve of Herring
- C. Vasodepressor variety accounts for 5-10% of cases of carotid sinus hypersensitivity
- D. All of the above are true

258. Batista operation is done in:
- A. Dilated cardiomyopathy
- B. Hypertrophic cardiomyopathy
- C. Arrthymogenic right ventricular dysplasia
- D. None of the above

259. Which of the following drugs does not cause Q-T prolongation?
- A. Amiodarone
- B. Phenytoin
- C. Astemizole
- D. Terfenadine

260. Which of the following statements regarding the BARI trial is true?
- A. It is a comparative study between CABG and PTCA in multivessel coronary artery disease
- B. There was a mortality difference in favour of CABG in diabetic patients
- C. There was no significant mortality difference in the non diabetic patients
- D. All of the above are true

261. Compared to medical therapy, CABG improves survival in which group of patients?
- A. 3 vessel disease with LV dysfunction
- B. 2 vessel disease (right coronary artery and circumflex artery) with normal LV function
- C. 1 vessel disease with normal LV function
- D. All of the above

251 A 252 D 253 A 254 C 255 C 256 B 257 D 258 A 259 B 260 D 261 A

262. Following statements are true regarding IMA graft in CABG:
- **A.** Long term patency rate is highest in LAD
- **B.** Patency rate is higher of LIMA than for RIMA
- **C.** Increased incidence of sternal wound infection after IMA implants
- **D.** All of the above

263. Dressler's syndrome:
- **A.** Extremely rare following thrombolysis
- **B.** May cause constrictive pericarditis
- **C.** Colchicine therapy may be helpful in some cases
- **D.** All of the above

264. Which of the following statements are true?
- **A.** T type calcium channels account for earlier phase of opening of calcium channel.
- **B.** L type calcium channels are involved in calcium induced calcium release
- **C.** Conventional calcium channel antagonists interact with L type calcium channels.
- **D.** All of the above

265. Regarding myocardial stunning following statements are true *except:*
- **A.** Coronary blood flow is reduced
- **B.** Myocardial energy metabolism is normal
- **C.** Duration is in hours to days
- **D.** Full recovery is usual

266. Following drugs improve survival in cardiac failure:
- **A.** Digoxin
- **B.** Carvedilol
- **C.** Enoximone
- **D.** All of the above

267. Clopidogrel:
- **A.** Is a novel antihypertensive
- **B.** Is a new low molecular weight heparin
- **C.** Is a novel antiarrhythmic
- **D.** None of the above

268. Atrial natriuretic peptides:
- **A.** Reduce sympathetic tone in the peripheral vasculature
- **B.** Increase renal blood flow
- **C.** C-type natriuretic peptide is a more potent dilator of veins than the other two peptides.
- **D.** All of the above

269. Following statements are true regarding loop diuretic *except:*
- **A.** Plasma half life of frusemide is prolonged in renal failure
- **B.** Plasma half life of Bumetanide is prolonged in liver disease
- **C.** Ethacrynic acid causes less ototoxicity
- **D.** Torsemide is better absorbed orally than Frusemide

270. Following drugs have been shown to reduce postoperative blood loss significantly following open heart surgery:
- **A.** Aprotinin
- **B.** Tranexamic acid
- **C.** Aminocaproic acid
- **D.** All of the above

271. Regarding aprotinin, following statements are true *except:*
- **A.** Is a polypeptide with molecular weight of 6512 Kda
- **B.** Inhibits Kallikrein
- **C.** Indirectly inhibits the formation of activated factor XII
- **D.** Alters platelet function

272. Regarding stress Echocardiography in hibernating myocardium, following statements are true:
- **A.** Hibernating myocardium contracts in response to low dose of IV dobutamine (5 to 10 mgm/kg/minute)
- **B.** Cardiac function may deteriorate following high dose of dobutamine infusion (upto 40 mgm/kg/minute)
- **C.** Both are true
- **D.** None of them are true

262 D 263 D 264 D 265 B 266 B 267 D 268 D 269 C 270 D 271 C 272 C

273. Which of the following tests is most specific for detection of myocardial viability?
- **A.** Technetium 99m sestamibi imaging
- **B.** Dobutamine echocardiography
- **C.** Thallium 201 stress redistribution imaging
- **D.** Thallium 201 rest-redistribution imaging

274. Following drugs cause increased incidence of myopathy with statins *except:*
- **A.** Fibrates
- **B.** Nicotinic acid
- **C.** Oral anticoagulants
- **D.** Erythromycin

275. Following drugs potentiate the action of oral anticoagulants *except:*
- **A.** Gemfibrozil
- **B.** Bezafibrate
- **C.** Clofibrate
- **D.** Simvastatin

276. Which of the following drugs has been shown to reduce mortality in cardiac failure?
- **A.** Amrinone
- **B.** Milrinone
- **C.** Vesnarinone
- **D.** None of the above

277. Which of the following statements is not true regarding carvedilol?
- **A.** Selective Beta blocker
- **B.** Blocks Alpha 1 receptor
- **C.** Reduces mortality in Ischaemic cardiomyopathy
- **D.** Reduces mortality in dilated cardiomyopathy

278. Dose adjustment of amiodarone is required in:
- **A.** Hepatic dysfunction
- **B.** Renal dysfunction
- **C.** Cardiac failure
- **D.** None of the above

279. Torsades de Pointes may be caused by following drugs *except:*
- **A.** Amiodarone
- **B.** Flecainide
- **C.** Quinidine
- **D.** Sotalol

280. Purple toe syndrome:
- **A.** Is caused by Warfarin
- **B.** Cholesterol emboli has been implicated
- **C.** Both are true
- **D.** None of them are true

281. The anticoagulant action of Warfarin is potentiated by all *except:*
- **A.** Metronidazole
- **B.** Disulfiram
- **C.** Allopurinol
- **D.** Phenytoin

282. Following are the ECG features of tricuspid atresia:
- **A.** Left axis deviation
- **B.** Right atrial enlargement
- **C.** Left ventricular hypertrophy
- **D.** All of the above

283. Following are associations with congenital corrected transposition:
- **A.** Congenital heart block
- **B.** Type B WPW syndrome
- **C.** Ebstein's anomaly
- **D.** All of the above

284. Most common important lesion associated with Ebstein's anomaly is:
- **A.** Ostium primum defect
- **B.** VSD
- **C.** Pulmonary stenosis or atresia
- **D.** PDA

---

273 B 274 C 275 B 276 D 277 A 278 D 279 B 280 C 281 D 282 D 283 D 284 C

285. Following statements are true regarding anomalous pulmonary origin of the coronary artery *except:*

A. Occurs in about 0.4% of patients with congenital cardiac anomalies
B. Usually the left coronary artery arises from the posterior sinus of the pulmonary artery
C. Usually manifested at age of 5-6 years
D. May be temporarily treated by ligation of left coronary artery at its origin

286. In the Nurses Health study, following conditions were associated as risk factor for pulmonary embolism *except:*

A. Smoking
B. High blood pressure
C. Increased body mass index
D. Diabetes mellitus

287. Which of the following conditions is the most common cause of hypercoagulable state leading to venous thrombosis?

A. Homocysteinemia
B. Factor V Leiden mutation
C. Anticardiolipin antibody
D. Antithrombin III deficiency

288. D dimer ELISA test may be positive in:

A. Pulmonary embolism
B. Myocardial infarction
C. Pneumonia
D. All of the above

289. Commotio cordis:

A. Is concussion of heart caused by blunt trauma
B. Usually occurs in young people
C. Death is usually uncommon
D. All of the above

290. Which of the following statement is true regarding VAN QWISH trial?

A. Patients with non Q wave MI, benefit from invasive management with coronary angiography and revascularization.
B. Patients with non Q wave infarction, fare better with conservative ischaemia guided therapy
C. Amiodarone reduces mortality in ischaemic cardiomyopathy
D. None of the above

291. Which of the following is the best method of diagnosing arrhythmogenic right ventricular dysplasia?

A. MRI scan
B. CT scan
C. Echocardiography
D. PET scan

292. MRI scan is very helpful in diagnosing which of the following conditions?

A. Cardiac sarcoidosis
B. Cardiac amyloidosis
C. Cardiac haemochromatosis
D. All of the above

293. Which of the following statement regarding Liddles syndrome is not true?

A. Inherited as autosomal dominant pattern
B. Hypertension is due to apparent mineralo-corticoid excess
C. Hypertension is caused by chronic activity of the channel causing excess Na absorption in the kidney
D. Responds to spironolactone therapy

294. Long term benefits with platelet GbIIb/IIIa inhibitors in patients undergoing PTCA was found in which of the following trials?

A. CAPTURE
B. EPIC
C. PRISM
D. PRISM PLUS

285 C 286 D 287 B 288 D 289 D 290 B 291 A 292 D 293 D 294 B

295. Heart Protection Study: all are true *except:*
- **A.** Involved more than 20,000 patients
- **B.** Follow up of 5 years
- **C.** Compared simvastatin with placebo
- **D.** Included patients with LDL cholesterol >130 mg%

296. All are true about Heart Protection Study *except:*
- **A.** Largest trial till date with long follow up
- **B.** Primary prevention trial
- **C.** Compared simvastatin with placebo
- **D.** Reduced all cause mortality by 13%

297. Heart Protection Study showed all *except:*
- **A.** 18% reduction in risk of coronary death
- **B.** 25% reduction in risk of fatal/nonfatal myocardial infarction, fatal/nonfatal stroke or coronary/noncoronary revascularization
- **C.** Significant reduction in nonvascular death
- **D.** Significant reduction in noncoronary vascular death

298. HPS study showed benefit of statin treatment in all *except:*
- **A.** Patients with coronary artery disease
- **B.** Diabetes mellitus
- **C.** Occlusive disease of non-coronary arteries
- **D.** Man < 40 years

299. In HPS study: all are true *except:*
- **A.** Risk reduction of vascular events was independent of baseline LDL level
- **B.** More benefit was seen in patients with higher baseline LDL
- **C.** Similar benefit was seen in patients with high or low LDL
- **D.** Degree of benefit was directly proportional to extent of LDL lowering

300. REVERSAL trial: all are true *except:*
- **A.** Compared atorvastatin 80 mg with pravastatin 40 mg
- **B.** Trial duration was 18 months
- **C.** Showed that intensive lipid lowering caused no progression of atheroma compared to moderate lowering
- **D.** Showed mortality benefit with intensive lipid lowering

301. REVERSAL trial: all are true *except:*
- **A.** Primary end point was percentage change in atheroma volume
- **B.** Secondary end point was effect on fatal/nonfatal vascular events
- **C.** Change in atheroma volume was assessed by IVUS
- **D.** LDL cholesterol from baseline of 150 mg% was reduced to 110 mg% in pravastatin group vs 77 mg% in atorvastatin group

302. Beneficial effect of statins in acute coronary syndromes was shown by all *except:*
- **A.** MIRACLE
- **B.** PROVE-IT TIMI-22
- **C.** A to Z trial
- **D.** REVERSAL

303. In PROVE IT TIMI-22: all are true *except:*
- **A.** Evaluated intense lipid lowering therapy in patients of acute coronary syndrome
- **B.** Compared atorvastatin 80 mg with pravastatin 40mg
- **C.** Mean follow up was 24 months
- **D.** Benefit of therapy appeared after 6 months

304. In PROVE IT TIMI-22: all are true *except:*
- **A.** 16% reduction in risk of death or MACE
- **B.** 28% reduction in risk of mortality
- **C.** 25% reduction in risk of ischemic stroke
- **D.** Benefit of therapy was seen as early as 30 days

305. The dose of statin producing 30-40% reduction in LDL cholesterol are all *except:*
- **A.** Atorvastatin 10 mg
- **B.** Rosuvastatin 5 mg
- **C.** Simvastatin 20 mg
- **D.** Pravastatin 20 gm

295 D 296 B 297 C 298 D 299 B 300 D 301 B 302 D 303 D 304 C 305 D

306. LDL cholesterol of < 70 mg% should be the target in all *except:*
A. Acute coronary syndrome
B. CAD with metabolic syndrome
C. Coronary artery disease with diabetes
D. Post CABG patients

307. All are diagnostic criteria of metabolic syndrome *except:*
A. Waist circumference > 40 inches in men and > 35 inches in women
B. Triglycerides ≥ 150 mg/dl
C. HDL < 40 mg% in men and < 50 mg/dl in women
D. BP ≥ 140/90 mm Hg

308. Maximum increase in HDL cholesterol is seen with:
A. Niacin
B. Fibrates
C. Statins
D. CETP inhibitors like torcetarib

309. Myopathy is least likely to occur when following fibrate is combined with statin ?
A. Gemfibrogil
B. Bezafibrate
C. Fenofibrate
D. Clofibrate

310. Contrast induced nephropathy is prevented by all *except:*
A. N-acetyl cysteine
B. Fenoldopam
C. Adequate hydration
D. Isosmolar contrast agent

311. Brugada syndrome: all are true *except:*
A. Autosomal dominant
B. Male predominance
C. Due to mutation in SCN5A
D. Arrhythmia occurs at age of 20 years

312. Arrhythmogenic right ventricular dysplasia: all are true *except:*
A. Male predominance
B. Age of presentation is 25-35 years
C. Autosomal dominant inheritance
D. Polymorphic VT is common

313. In Brugada syndrome, all are true *except:*
A. Mutation is seen in chromosome 3
B. SCD occurs during sleep
C. VF preceded by monomorphic VT
D. Age of presentation is between 35-40 years

314. ST segment elevation is right precordial leads is seen in all *except:*
A. Brugada syndrome
B. ARVD
C. Hypocalcemia
D. Normal variant

315. ST elevation in right precordial leads is seen in all of the of the following *except:*
A. Hypercalcemia
B. Hypokalemia
C. Duchenne's muscular dystrophy
D. Freidreich's ataxia

316. ICD therapy has shown mortality benefit in all *except:*
A. Ischemic cardiomyopathy
B. Dilated cardiomyopathy
C. Acute MI with LVEF < 30%
D. Old MI with LV dysfunction

317. Benefit of cardiac resynchronization therapy is seen in all *except:*
A. MYHA class III or IV symptoms
B. QRS interval > 120 msecs
C. Atrial fibrillation
D. PR > 150 msecs

318. Cardiac resynchronization therapy produces all *except:*
A. Improves symptoms
B. Improves exercise capacity
C. Decrease progression of heart failure
D. Decrease mortality

306 D 307 D 308 D 309 C 310 B 311 D 312 D 313 C 314 C 315 B 316 C 317 C 318 D

319. COMPANION trial: all are true *except:*
- **A.** Compared pharmacological therapy with CRT with/without ICD in patient of heart failure
- **B.** Risk of death or hospitalization due to any cause reduced by 20% by CRT with or without ICD
- **C.** Risk of death due to any cause decreased by both CRT and CRT with ICD
- **D.** Risk of death or hospitalization due to heart failure decreased by both CRT and CRT with ICD

320. All are true features of rheumatic myocarditis *except:*
- **A.** Increased troponin I
- **B.** Soft S1
- **C.** S3
- **D.** Mitral regurgitation

321. All are true about rheumatic myocarditis as seen histologically *except:*
- **A.** Inflammatory cells in perivascular connective tissue cells
- **B.** Myocyte necrosis
- **C.** Aschoff nodules
- **D.** Aschoff nodules do not contain cells of myocardial origin

322. SYNERGY trial was characterized by all *except:*
- **A.** Compared efficacy and safety of enoxaprin with heparin
- **B.** Included patients of chronic stable angina and unstable angina
- **C.** Death and myocardial infarction identical at 30 days in both groups
- **D.** Major bleeding complication identical in both groups

323. All the drugs can be used for prehospital thrombolysis *except:*
- **A.** Anistreplase
- **B.** Reteplase
- **C.** Tenecteplase
- **D.** Lanoteplase

324. Once dye-induced renal dysfunction develops, creatinine levels generally peak at ___ days and remain elevated for ___ days:
- **A.** 1 and 7-14
- **B.** 2-3 and 7-14
- **C.** 7 and 14-21
- **D.** 4-5 and 7-14

325. Risk factors for dye-induced nephrotoxicity include all of the following *except:*
- **A.** Baseline hypovolemia
- **B.** Diabetic nephropathy
- **C.** Large contrast load
- **D.** Female patients
- **E.** Impaired left ventricular function

326. Which of the following statements about the coronary collateral circulation is true:
- **A.** Collaterals are often demonstrated by angiography in coronary arteries with 80% stenosis
- **B.** Collaterals usually take several days to manifest angiographically after acute MI
- **C.** Collaterals represent the formation of new vessels as opposed to the utilization of existing blood vessels
- **D.** Coronary collaterals can dilate in response to nitrates and beta-adrenergic agonists and constrict in response to serotonin

327. Which of the following statements about the coronary anatomy is false:
- **A.** The RCA is dominant in about 85% of cases
- **B.** The left main coronary artery trifurcates about 30-40% of the time
- **C.** The ramus intermedius is analogous to a diagonal, usually supplying the free wall of the left ventricle
- **D.** About 20% of LADs fail to reach the diaphragmatic aspect of the left ventricle, terminating before or at the cardiac apex
- **E.** Techniques to preferentially engage the LAD over the left circumflex coronary artery include clockwise rotation of a Left Judkins catheter and selection of a longer curve Judkins catheter

319 C 320 A 321 B 322 B 323 A 324 B 325 D 326 D 327 D

328. Which of the following influences the amount of radiation exposure to the X-ray operator:

A. Length of exposure (time)
B. Patient thickness
C. Distance from the source
D. Kvp and field size
E. All of the above

329. The annual occupational dose limit to an interventionalist's eyes is:

A. 500 millirem
B. 5,000 millirem
C. 15,000 millirem
D. 50,000 millirem

330. Which features are associated with coronary fistula?

A. Confined almost exclusively to the LAD
B. Demonstrates a stenotic segment in systole but not in diastole
C. The most common congenital coronary anomaly resulting in myocardial ischemia
D. Can lead to infective endocarditis, heart failure, myocardial ischemia
E. C and D both

331. Which of the following coronary variants is associated with sudden death?

A. Coronary artery fistula
B. Myocardial bridging
C. Coronary artery aneurysm
D. Left coronary artery from right coronary sinus coursing between the aorta and pulmonary artery
E. Left coronary artery from right coronary sinus coursing anterior to the aorta and pulmonary artery

332. All of the following statements about contrast reactions are true *except:*

A. Previous anaphylaxis carries a recurrence rate of 15% without premedication
B. Asthmatics, especially those with nasal polyps, represent a high-risk group for contrast reactions, with a 6-9 fold increased risk compared to non-asthmatics
C. In using corticosteroids to reduce the risk of contrast reactions, it is important to begin pretreatment at least 6 hours before exposure
D. Contrast-induced renal dysfunction is characterized by creatinine levels that peak in 3-5 days and oliguria in 30%
E. A and C both

333. Reasonable approaches to the management of patients with aspirin-induced anaphylaxis who require percutaneous intervention include all of the following, *except:*

A. Aspirin desensitization
B. Ticlopidine/clopidogrel
C. GpIIb/IIIa receptor antagonist
D. Hydrocortisone 100 mg IV plus ASA 81 mg PO
E. All are correct

334. Which of the following statements regarding contrast agents is false?

A. Nonionic contrast agents may possess thrombogenic properties compared to ionic
B. High osmolar agents are associated with more dye reactions than low osmolar agents
C. Ionic agents have been found to have decreased thrombogenicity compared to nonionic agents in both static and flowing blood
D. Ioxaglate and iohexol are both low-osmolar agents, but with differ in electric charge
E. All iodinated contrast agents can cause acute renal dysfunction following angiography

328 E 329 C 330 E 331 D 332 E 333 A 334 C

335. Which of the following statements about coronary vascular reactivity is true?

A. Acetylcholine causes normal coronary arteries to vasodilate due to a direct effect on smooth muscle
B. Acetylcholine causes vasoconstriction in atherosclerotic coronary arteries
C. Nitrates cause coronary vasodilatation by stimulating production of nitric oxide from endothelial cells
D. Endothelium independent vasodilators include: serotonin, ADP, thrombin, and increased shear stress
E. None of the above

336. Patients receiving continuous heparin prior to PTCA may be resistant to heparin during the procedure:

A. True
B. False
C. Should never be given heparin during the procedure
D. Heparin resistance is not known during PCI

337. Which of following statements is true?

A. Warfarin and heparin inhibit the same factors of the coagulation cascade
B. Tissue factor is the main stimulus to thrombin generation after plaque disruption
C. Aspirin inhibits ADP-induced platelet activation
D. Fibrinopeptide A is a marker of thrombin generation
E. The activated clotting time can reliably measure the effect of warfarin

338. Which of the following statements is true?

A. Stent implantation in a ruptured plaque is followed by elastic recoil.
B. Decreased shear stress is a major predictor of plaque disruption and platelet aggregation
C. Digestion of the fibrous cap is inhibited by local infiltration of monocytes
D. Lipid accumulation in the atherosclerotic plaque increases its elasticity and decreases its propensity for rupture
E. The interface between the lipid-rich core and thicker fibrous layers is the most vulnerable site for plaque rupture

339. In the setting of previous myocardial infarction, the physiologic assessment of a "borderline lesion" is best evaluated by which of the following techniques?

A. Angiography
B. Virtual histology catheter
C. Fractional flow reserve
D. Resting translesional pressure
E. Coronary flow reserve

340. Compared to percutaneous mitral commissurotomy, surgical commissurotomy is:

A. Longer lasting
B. Results in less decline in PA pressure
C. Associated with less mitral regurgitation
D. Not different in long term clinical outcome
E. None of the above

341. Asymptomatic patients with mitral stenosis should be considered for balloon valvuloplasty if:

A. The pulmonary artery systolic pressure at rest is greater than 30 mmHg
B. The pulmonary artery systolic pressure at rest is greater than 40 mmHg
C. The pulmonary artery systolic pressure with exercise is greater than 40 mmHg
D. The pulmonary artery systolic pressure with exercise is greater than 60 mmHg
E. Only if the pulmonary artery systolic pressure at rest is more than 90 mmHg

335 B 336 A 337 B 338 E 339 C 340 D 341 D

342. Which of the following de novo lesions has the highest chance to restenose:
A. A mid-LAD lesion
B. A distal RCA lesion
C. An ostial SVG lesion
D. An OM branch lesion
E. All have the same chance for restenosis

343. Which of the following statements about angiography for the detection of intracoronary thrombus is correct?
A. Sensitivity and specificity are low
B. Sensitivity and specificity are high
C. Sensitivity is low and specificity is high
D. Sensitivity is high and specificity is low
E. The negative predictive value is high

344. Which is the correct order indicating the magnitude of the decrease in the plasma fibrinogen level produced by the following 4 agents?
A. TNK-tPA > tPA > rPA > streptokinase
B. TNK-tPA = tPA = rPA > streptokinase
C. TNK-tPA < tPA < rPA < streptokinase
D. TNK-tPA = tPA = rPA < streptokinase
E. TNK-tPA = tPA < rPA < streptokinase

345. Neointimal hyperplasia inside a Palmaz-Schatz stent is more frequently found at:
A. The edges
B. The body
C. The articulation
D. Edges and articulation
E. Uniformly distributed throughout the stent

346. For patients in cardiogenic shock, the greatest mortality is seen in those patients with the following:
A. Left ventricular failure
B. Right ventricular failure
C. Ventricular septal rupture
D. Mitral regurgitation
E. Tamponade

347. Restenosis after vein graft stenting has been shown to be:
A. Higher for covered stents than for standard stents
B. Reduced by treatment with IIb/IIIa receptor blockade.
C. Less in de novo lesions
D. Significantly reduced by Ir192 brachytherapy
E. C and D both

348. What is the type of energy used for electro-anatomical mapping of the heart (biosense system)?
A. X-ray fluoroscopy
B. Ultrasound
C. Magnetic resonance
D. Electrical potentials
E. Ultra-low magnetic field

349. Which of the following statements about supported angioplasty is true?
A. Severe aortic stenosis is a contraindication to IABP.
B. Significant hemolysis and platelet count decrease to <50,000 are possible complications of IABP.
C. Effective diastolic augmentation requires a stable cardiac rhythm for both IABP and CPS.
D. When percutaneous cardiopulmonary support is used, intravenous heparin should be dosed to maintain the ACT at 300-350 seconds.
E. CPS can be continued up to 10 hours after its initiation

350. A 64-year-old man presented in the ER with recent anterior wall MI (estimated to begin >12 hours from presentation) and was treated with ASA, heparin, and IV nitroglycerin. Although he has become pain free, he is progressively breathless. His heart rate is 110 bpm, his arterial pressure 78/45 mm Hg and his oxygen saturation is 90% on 2 L O_2 supplement. The nitroglycerin was stopped, but hypotension persisted. Cardiac

342 C 343 C 344 C 345 E 346 C 347 E 348 E 349 B

examination reveals a 2/6 systolic murmur, not dissimilar to the one detected on admission. Which of the following statements regarding this patient's condition is true?

A. Echocardiography and right heart catheterization are needed
B. Initiation of oxygen vasopressor therapy should be prompt
C. Administration of tPA and intra-aortic balloon counterpulsation will prolong this patient's survival
D. Vasopressors should not be administered before the performance of right heart catheterization.
E. Immediate coronary angiography and revascularization will result in improved survival

351. The above patient is undergoing cardiac catheterization on day 4 of acute myocardial infarction. Which of the following statements is true?

A. The ventricular septum is ruptured
B. This patient should undergo immediate IABP placement and be referred for cardiac surgery.
C. The pulmonary blood flow is greater than systemic blood flow.
D. All are true

352. All are antithrombotic properties of statins, *except:*

A. Decrease in tissue factor expression
B. Reduced platelet aggregation
C. Increased PAI-1 levels
D. Reduced inflammatory-thrombotic interactions
E. All are correct

353. Clinical characteristics of patients who derive the greatest absolute benefit from adjunctive GP IIb/IIIa antagonist therapy in the setting of an acute coronary syndrome include all of the following *except:*

A. Elevated myocardial enzymes
B. Planned medical therapy
C. Diabetes
D. Planned percutaneous coronary intervention
E. Prior chronic aspirin use

354. A 75-year-old man with chronic CAD on ASA, beta-blockers, and nitrates presents to the ER at 11:00 PM with chest pain after ingestion of 100 mg of sildenafil. His arterial blood pressure is 75/40 mm Hg; you are consulted over the telephone regarding the treatment plan. Which of the following would you recommend?

A. Immediate injection of epinephrine subcutaneously
B. Immediate therapy with IV isotonic fluid bolus plus phenylephrine infusion
C. Immediate therapy with dopamine, with possible addition of dobutamine when the systolic arterial pressure is at least 100 mm Hg
D. Immediate therapy with repeated IV glucose and isotonic fluid boluses plus epinephrine SC
E. Immediate therapy with IV glucose and isotonic fluid followed by right heart catheterization and intra-aortic balloon counterpulsation for hemodynamic support

355. Which of the following agent is a noncompetitive, high-affinity blocker of the GP IIb/IIIa integrin?

A. Abciximab
B. Enoxaparin
C. Eptifibatide
D. Tirofiban
E. Xemilofiban

356. Which of the following is correct regarding diagnostic tests for HIT type II?

A. The standard platelet aggregation assay is highly specific, but only 30%-50% sensitive
B. The serotonin release assay can be performed only in highly specialized centers
C. The enzyme-linked immunosorbent assay for IgG has low specificity
D. The heparin-induced platelet aggregation assay is more sensitive than the standard platelet aggregation
E. All of the above

350 E 351 D 352 C 353 B 354 B 355 A 356 E

357. An ostial, non-thrombotic coronary lesion with length = 16 mm and 40° angulation is classified as:
A. Complex lesions
B. AHA/ACC type A
C. AHA/ACC type B1
D. AHA/ACC type B2
E. AHA/ACC type C

358. All are appropriate first-line medications for a 60-year-old male presenting with rest pain and ST segment depressions *except:*
A. Beta blocker
B. IV NTG
C. Nifedipine-long acting
D. Clopidogrel
E. ACE inhibitor

359. Sinus venosus atrial septal defect is associated with:
A. Earlier heart failure than a secundum or primum ASD
B. Anomalous pulmonary venous return
C. Persistent left superior vena cava to coronary sinus
D. A, B and C
E. B and C only

360. A 35-year-old asymptomatic female is found on physical exam to have an RV heave/thrill, wide fixed splitting of S2, and a soft diastolic flow rumble. CXR reveals enhanced pulmonary vascularity, and EKG shows right axis deviation and an incomplete RBBB. This presentation is most consistent with:
A. Moderate-size PDA with left to right shunting
B. Moderate-size PDA with right to left shunting
C. Small VSD
D. Ostium secundum ASD
E. Ostium primum ASD
F. Tetralogy of Fallot

361. With regard to the randomized trials of bypass surgery versus medical therapy, which of the following are true?
A. Patients over the age of 65 years were included in the majority of trials
B. The majority of patients were treated with aspirin
C. The use of internal mammary bypass grafts was low
D. The efficacy of bypass surgery over medical therapy was documented in all subsets
E. Left ventricular dysfunction was a marker of a reduced benefit from bypass surgery versus medical therapy

362. Which of the following statements about the mechanisms of restenosis after angioplasty or atherectomy is false?
A. Directional atherectomy reduces elastic recoil compared to PTCA
B. Elastic recoil mainly occurs within 30 minutes after balloon deflation
C. Late arterial remodeling is an important mechanism of restenosis after angioplasty
D. The greater the acute gain, the lower the restenosis
E. Abciximab reduces neointimal hyperplasia in humans through inhibition of the vitronectin receptor

363. Predictors of in-stent restenosis include all of the following, *except:*
A. Post-procedure lumen diameter
B. Edge dissection
C. Diabetes mellitus
D. Small reference vessel dimensions
E. Lesion length

364. Risk factors for restenosis include all of the following, *except:*
A. Balloon angioplasty without stenting
B. Dissection
C. Chronic total occlusion
D. Insulin-treated diabetes mellitus
E. Residual stenosis > 30%

357 D 358 C 359 E 360 D 361 C 362 E 363 B 364 B

365. Which of the following factors has been shown to decrease angiographic restenosis after non-stent coronary interventions?
- **A.** Aggressive lipid-lowering
- **B.** Abciximab
- **C.** Aggressive glucose control in diabetics
- **D.** Aggressive Directional atherectomy
- **E.** Rotational atherectomy

366. Which of the following statements about restenosis is false?
- **A.** Recurrent symptoms > 6 months after the procedure have a low positive predictive value for restenosis
- **B.** The main factor for the development of restenosis after angioplasty is neointimal proliferation
- **C.** Exercise testing using thallium-201 scintigraphy, exercise radionuclide angiography, and dobutamine echocardiography have better sensitivity for detecting restenosis than exercise testing without perfusion imaging
- **D.** Functional testing performed within four weeks of PTCA is frequently associated with false positives
- **E.** Directional atherectomy and stenting have been shown to reduce angiographic restenosis compared to PTCA

367. Which of the following statements regarding the activated partial thromboplastin time is true?
- **A.** There is minimal variability among the commercially available thromboplastins used for this test by various laboratories
- **B.** aPTT accurately estimates the anticoagulant effects of enoxaparin
- **C.** aPTT accurately estimated the anticoagulant effect of abciximab
- **D.** aPTT accurately estimates the anticoagulant effects of warfarin
- **E.** There is great disparity between aPTT and activated clotting time values

368. Which statement regarding thrombolytic agents is true?
- **A.** Streptokinase has higher fibrin specificity than t-PA
- **B.** Urokinase has higher fibrin specificity than TNK-t-PA
- **C.** All thrombolytic agents produce platelet activation
- **D.** t-PA is a derivative of the naturally found r-PA
- **E.** Readministration of t-PA can produce significant allergic reaction

369. Which of the following statements is true?
- **A.** Aggressive lipid lowering can produce regression of a 75% stenotic lesion to <30% after 12 months of therapy
- **B.** Macrophage infiltration in the atherosclerotic plaque strengthens the fibrous cap and reduces its propensity to rupture
- **C.** Following plaque rupture, exposure of tissue factor is the major stimulus for endovascular thrombosis
- **D.** Diabetes mellitus predisposes to plaque rupture
- **E.** Plaque rupture invariably manifests as an acute coronary syndrome

370. All of following factors predispose to plaque rupture, *except:*
- **A.** High shear stress
- **B.** High lipid content
- **C.** Increased macrophage accumulation
- **D.** Thin fibrous cap
- **E.** Increased collagen content

371. Which of the following statements regarding the parameter d-Dimer is true?
- **A.** It is produced during fibrin formation
- **B.** High levels of d-Dimer indicate increased thrombin generation
- **C.** Low levels of d-Dimer indicate increased thrombin activity
- **D.** High levels of d-Dimer indicate increased expression of tissue factor
- **E.** Low levels of d-Dimer indicate decreased fibrinolytic activity

365 D 366 B 367 E 368 C 369 C 370 E 371 E

372. All of the following statements are correct, *except:*
A. The majority of acute coronary syndromes are due to disruption of non-stenotic plaques
B. The majority of the non-stenotic plaques do not rupture
C. The calcium content is not predictive of plaque rupture
D. Plaque rupture is considered to be largely asymptomatic
E. A disrupted plaque always contains angiographically apparent thrombus

373. Heparin's anticoagulant effect is limited by:
A. Inability to inactivate clot-bound thrombin
B. Neutralization by platelet factor 4
C. Inactivation by fibrin-II monomers, which are formed by the action of thrombin on fibrinogen
D. None of the above
E. All of the above

374. The life-cycle of a normal cell can be described in how many phases?
A. 2
B. 5
C. 4
D. 3
E. 6

375. Most dominant factor for thrombus formation in experimental models after PTCA and stent is:
A. Fibrin deposition
B. Platelet deposition
C. Coagulation
D. Thrombin

376. Increased temperature in the vessel wall can be detected in:
A. Normal artery
B. Chronic occlusion
C. Unstable plaque
D. Stable plaque
E. None of the above

377. Which type of endovascular intervention is associated with more profound neointimal hyperplasia in experimental animal models?
A. Balloon
B. Laser
C. Stent
D. Directional atherectomy
E. Rotational atherectomy

378. After PTCA and stenting, reendothelialization occurs in 4-6 weeks. What is the source of endothelial cells?
A. Media
B. Intima
C. Adventitia
D. Adjunct endothelium
E. Circulating blood and adjunct endothelium

379. A vulnerable plaque is characterized by:
A. Chronic exertional angina
B. Disruption of the fibrotic cap at the edges of the lipid core
C. Low number of macrophages
D. Decrease metalloproteinase activity
E. Is characterized by low content in lipoprotein(a)

380. Tissue factor pathway inhibitor:
A. Is a potent anticoagulant
B. Inhibits the intrinsic coagulation pathway
C. Possesses antiplatelet properties
D. Is involved in fibrinolysis
E. All of the above

381. Which of the following statements is false?
A. Low-molecular weight heparins have a selective anti-Xa activity
B. Warfarin inhibits coagulation factors II, VII, IX and X
C. Fibrinopeptide A is a marker of thrombin activity
D. Prothrombin fragment F1+2 is a marker of prothrombin generation
E. aPTT is a good measure of the antithrombotic activity of unfractionated heparin

372 E 373 E 374 B 375 B 376 C 377 B 378 E 379 B 380 A 381 D

382. Which of the following statement is false?
- **A.** Aspirin inhibits the cyclo-oxygenase 1 pathway
- **B.** Clopidogrel inhibits the ADP-related platelet activation
- **C.** Clopidogrel is an active substance and undergoes first pass elimination in the liver
- **D.** Aspirin inhibits the synthesis of thromboxane
- **E.** The distribution of ticlopidine and clopidogrel is 98% in plasma proteins

383. All of the following substances produce vasodilation in the presence of both a healthy 20-year old woman and a 50 year-old man with mild atherosclerosis, *except:*
- **A.** Nitroglycerin
- **B.** Nitroprusside
- **C.** Acetylcholine
- **D.** Adenosine
- **E.** All of the above

384. Stenting has greater late loss than balloon angioplasty:
- **A.** This is unrelated to the mechanisms of restenosis
- **B.** This is due to greater late remodeling
- **C.** This is associated by similar net gain
- **D.** This is a false statement; stenting has less late loss than balloon angioplasty
- **E.** This is counterbalanced by a greater acute gain with stenting

385. A 50-year-old man without previous medical problems presented to the hospital with acute myocardial infarction treated with intravenous accelerated t-PA within 3 hours of the onset of pain. He has the following likelihood: the vessel will remain occluded ____ %, or will have suboptimal (TIMI grade < 3) flow ____ %:
- **A.** 10% and 20%
- **B.** 45% and 20%
- **C.** 20% and 45%
- **D.** 45% and 55%
- **E.** 10% and 30%

386. Following IV thrombolytic therapy for acute MI, recurrent ischemia occurs in ____ % and intracranial bleeding in ____ %:
- **A.** 15-30% and 3-5%
- **B.** 30-45% and 0.5-1.5%
- **C.** 15-30% and 0.5-1.5%
- **D.** 30-45% and 2-5%
- **E.** 40-50% and 0.5%

387. Relative contraindication to intravenous thrombolytics includes all of the following, *except:*
- **A.** Age greater than 80 years
- **B.** Patients who present >12 hours after symptom onset
- **C.** Patients with acute MI due to a saphenous vein graft occlusion
- **D.** Patients with anterior ST elevation MI within 3 hours of presentation to the ER
- **E.** Patients with previous stroke within 2 years

388. Which of the following statements about rescue (salvage) PTCA for failed thrombolysis is false?
- **A.** Rescue PTCA may reduce the risk of heart failure, shock, and death in patients with large infarctions
- **B.** The prognosis of patients after successful rescue PTCA is similar to that after successful thrombolysis
- **C.** Patients requiring rescue PTCA are at no higher risk for reocclusion than patients treated with successful primary PTCA or thrombolytic therapy
- **D.** Early mortality is very high if rescue PTCA is unsuccessful
- **E.** Rescue PTCA is associated with higher bleeding complications compared to primary PTCA

382 C 383 C 384 E 385 C 386 C 387 D 388 C

389. Which of the following statements about primary PTCA for acute MI is false?

A. Profound hypotension and bradycardia occur more commonly after PTCA of the right coronary artery (compared to left coronary artery)

B. In-hospital recurrent ischemia occurs in 10-15%

C. The need for blood transfusion after primary PTCA has been associated with thrombolytic agents, bypass surgery, prolonged anticoagulation, and indwelling sheaths

D. In comparison to IV thrombolytics, intracranial bleeding is lower with primary PTCA

E. The use of intracoronary t-PA before PTCA improves the procedural success rate

390. Symptomatic vessel reocclusion after successful primary PTCA occurs in ___ % of patients prior to discharge:

A. 3-5%

B. 8-14%

C. 15-20%

D. 21-25%

E. 26-30%

391. Vessel reocclusion after successful rescue PTCA occurs in ____ % of patients:

A. 3-7%

B. 8-14%

C. 15-20%

D. 21-25%

E. 26-30%

392. By 6-months after successful primary PTCA for acute MI, reocclusion of the infarct-related artery occurs in _______ % and restenosis in _______ %:

A. 30% and 60%

B. 30% and 20%

C. 10% and 40%

D. 10% and 20%

E. 30% and 40%

393. Which of the following statements about PCI for acute MI is true?

A. The routine use of intraaortic balloon pump to reduce reinfarction and reocclusion after primary PTCA is not recommended

B. Intracoronary stenting is indicated (ACC/AHA) for routine use during primary acute MI intervention

C. Rotational atherectomy is recommended for the treatment of calcified lesions in acute MI

D. A platelet IIb/IIIa inhibitor is indicated (ACC/AHA) for routine use during acute MI intervention

E. The combination of stenting and platelet IIb/IIIa inhibitor, provides survival benefit at one-year follow-up after primary acute MI intervention

394. Compared to IV thrombolysis for acute MI, primary (direct) PTCA is associated with all of the following, *except:*

A. Allows immediate definition of coronary anatomy

B. Results in less reocclusion, recurrent ischemia, and reinfarction

C. Results in similar rates of acute vessel patency and TIMI-3 flow

D. Results in better survival in high-risk patients

E. Is associated with a lower risk of intracranial hemorrhage

395. Potential indications for IABP-supported intervention include all of the following, *except:*

A. Target vessel supplies the majority of viable myocardium

B. Ejection fraction < 20%

C. Triple vessel disease with LV ejection fraction of 40%

D. Severe mitral regurgitation

E. Cardiogenic shock and multivessel disease

389 E 390 D 391 E 392 C 393 A 394 C 395 C

396. Which of the following statements about intra-aortic balloon pumping (IABP) is false?
- **A.** IABP decreases myocardial oxygen demand, increases coronary perfusion pressure, and increases cardiac output by 20-40%
- **B.** Significant hemolysis and platelet count decrease to <50,000 are possible complications
- **C.** Complications are more common in females and in patients with pre-existing peripheral vascular disease or diabetes
- **D.** Effective diastolic augmentation requires a stable cardiac rhythm IABP
- **E.** Routine use of IABP in acute MI decreases mortality

397. When percutaneous cardiopulmonary support is used, intravenous heparin should be dosed to maintain the ACT at ____ seconds:
- **A.** 200-250
- **B.** 250-300
- **C.** 300-350
- **D.** 350-400
- **E.** 400

398. Which of the following statement is false?
- **A.** Streptokinase is associated with decrease in fibrinogen and increase in plasmin levels
- **B.** tPA is more fibrin-specific and has greater catalytic activity than rPA in vitro
- **C.** Hepatic clearance of tPA is faster compared to rPA
- **D.** High affinity fibrin binding is attributed to the finger domain of the tPA molecule, which is not present in the rPA molecule
- **E.** TNK-tPA can be given as a bolus because it has longer half-life and is less fibrin specific than tPA

399. Intra-aortic balloon counterpulsation produces:
- **A.** Increase in coronary flow during diastole with subsequent increase in contractility and decrease in preload and afterload
- **B.** Decrease in afterload, but no significant effect on coronary flow beyond significant stenoses
- **C.** Decrease in afterload and preload, with increased coronary flow especially beyond significant stenoses
- **D.** Increase in coronary flow without significant effect on afterload or preload
- **E.** Mild to moderate aortic regurgitation

400. A 63 year old woman sustained an inferior myocardial infarction and was treated with tPA at another hospital 3 days ago. She was transferred to your facility after developing pulmonary edema. On admission, the EKG indicates Q-wave inferior MI with tall R-waves in v1 and v2 leads. Echocardiography reveals the inferolateral walls to be non-cotractile and there is 4+ mitral regurgitation with a ruptured papillary muscle. Her arterial pressure on presentation is 70/40 mmHg and required escalating doses of vasopressor agents during the transfer, her heart rate is 102 bpm, and her oxygen saturation is 88% on 100% FiO_2. Which treatment plan to select?
- **A.** IV metoprolol to decrease the heart rate to 60-70 bpm and IV nitroglycerin for afterload reduction
- **B.** IV metoprolol to decrease the heart rate to 60-70 bpm and IV enalaprilat for afterload reduction
- **C.** Cardiopulmonary support with immediate cardiac catheterization/angiography and evaluation for CABG and mitral valve repair/replacement
- **D.** Intra-aotric balloon counterpulsation and coronary intervention of the culprit artery; the mitral regurgitation should be expected to regress after revascularization
- **E.** Immediate mitral valve surgery

396 E 397 E 398 E 399 B 400 C

401. Which of the following statements is wrong? Cardiogenic shock is typically characterized by:

A. Decreased cardiac output and decreased peripheral vascular resistance
B. Increased pulmonary wedge pressure and left ventricular end-diastolic pressure
C. Evidence of tissue hypoperfusion and oliguria
D. An extensive myocardial infarction
E. Worsening? pre-shock? condition over the intial hours of hospitalization

402. Which of the following statement is true?

A. Cardiogenic shock is mostly due to a mechanical complication of an acute MI
B. The pre-existing left ventricular dysfunction is irrelevant to the development of cardiogenic shock during an acute myocardial infarction
C. Thrombolytic therapy reduces mortality in patients with ST-elevation MI and established cardiogenic shock
D. Stent implantation is superior to balloon angioplasty alone for the treatment of patients with cardiogenic shock
E. Emergency surgery is indicated for the treatment of patients with cardiogenic shock due to a mechanical complication of acute MI

403. A 64 year old man presented in the ER with recent anterior wall MI (estimated to begin >12 hours from presentation) and was treated with ASA, heparin, and IV nitroglycerin. Although he has become pain free, he is progressively breathless. His heart rate is 110 bpm, his arterial pressure 78/45 mmHg and his oxygen saturation is 90% on 2 lt O_2 supplement. The nitroglycerin was stopped, but hypotension persisted. Cardiac examination reveals a 2/6 systolic murmur, not dissimilar to the one detected on admission. Which of the following statements regarding this patient's condition is false?

A. Echocardiography and right heart catheterization are needed
B. Initiation of oxygen vasopressor therapy should be prompt
C. Administration of t-PA and intra-aortic balloon counterpulsation will prolong this patient?s survival
D. Vasopressors should not be administered before the performance of right heart catheterization
E. Immediate coronary angiography and revascularization can result in improved survival

404. 79 year old woman is admitted with cardiogenic shock 6 hours after the onset of crushing chest pain. EKG shows 4 mm ST elevation anterolaterally. Echocardiography in the ER reveals the anterior, septal, and lateral walls to be non-contractile. Right heart catheterization reveals a pulmonary capillary wedge pressure of 25 mm Hg, and a mean right atrial pressure of 8 mm Hg. Despite high doses of vasopressors the systolic blood pressure remains under 80 mmHg. Which of the following statements regarding this patient's management is true?

A. Women have worse outcome than men with cardiogenic shock
B. Age more than 75 years is a criterion to select immediate percutaneous rather than surgical coronary revascularization in this patient
C. An extension of the infarct to the right ventricular myocardium is most likely responsible for the shock state
D. Immediate placement of an intra-aortic balloon pump should be performed

405. Of all major causes of cardiogenic shock, the highest mortality is associated with which etiology?

A. LV failure
B. RV failure
C. Acute severe MR
D. Ventricular septal rupture
E. Tamponade

401 A 402 E 403 E 404 D 405 D

406. You are at a community hospital without a cardiac catheterization laboratory and a 56 year old patient without a contraindication to thrombolytic therapy presents in cardiogenic shock. The ideal therapy should include the following:

A. IABP
B. Thrombolytics
C. Transfer for emergency angiography and early revascularization (angioplasty/stent or CABG)
D. All of the above

407. Which of the following statements is false regarding the thienopyridine class of drugs?

A. This class includes ticlopidine and clopidogrel
B. Both ticlopidine and clopidogrel work by reversibly inhibiting the binding of ADP to its receptor found on the platelet surface
C. Both agents prolong the bleeding time, but neither drug affects the partial thromboplastin time (PTT) or activated clotting time (ACT)
D. Both agents prevent ADP-mediated up-regulation of the platelet glycoprotein IIb/IIIa receptor, and reduce thrombosis from shear stress
E. Both agents are metabolized by the liver to active metabolites and take several days to achieve maximal platelet inhibition

408. Which of the following statement is false regarding the use of aspirin plus ticlopidine in patients undergoing coronary stent placement:

A. On the basis of several randomized trials, aspirin and ticlopidine are more effective at reducing stent thrombosis and other major adverse events than aspirin alone and aspirin combined with coumadin
B. Bleeding is equally frequent with aspirin and ticlopidine as with aspirin and coumadin
C. The most serious side effects of ticlopidine are neutropenia and thrombotic thrombocytopenic purpura (TTP)
D. Treatment with ticlopidine several days prior to coronary stenting appears to result in more complete platelet inhibition and less procedural myocardial infarction
E. Because the risk of stent thrombosis 2 weeks post-implantation is less than the combined incidence of neutropenia and TTP, most stented patients should receive ticlopidine for a period of only 2 weeks after the procedure

409. Which of the following statement is false regarding the role of aspirin in coronary intervention?

A. Aspirin has been shown to reduce the incidence of acute occlusion after PTCA by as much as 50% and is considered essential therapy prior to non-emergent interventions
B. Aspirin allergy is an indication for postponement of elective coronary intervention
C. Aspirin desensitization is considered too dangerous for individuals who have had an anaphylactic reaction to aspirin.
D. Clopidogrel is the antiplatelet treatment of choice in patients intolerant of aspirin
E. The results of the Antiplatelet Trialists' Collaboration, a retrospective meta-analysis of 145 randomized trials of antiplatelet agents, provided clear evidence that an aspirin dose of 75 mg/day is less effective than a dose of 325 mg/day

410. A 65-year-old woman with recent non-Q-wave myocardial infarction is scheduled to undergo coronary intervention. Diagnostic angiography performed 2 days ago revealed a complex 20 mm long lesion of the proximal right coronary artery. She has been on chronic therapy with aspirin and has received ticlopidine 250 mg bid for the past 2 days. She has also been treated with intravenous unfractionated heparin infusion, which is interrupted at the time of sheath insertion. Her weight is 80 Kg and her height 165 cm. Use of weight-adjusted dose of abciximab has been opted. Which of the following statements regarding the appropriate next step for this patient's management is correct?

406 D 407 B 408 B 409 E

A. Abciximab plus 7,000 units of intravenous heparin should be administered immediately after insertion of the femoral sheaths
B. 10,000 units of intravenous heparin should be administered immediately after insertion of the femoral sheaths; abciximab should be administered when the activated clotting time value is 200-300 seconds
C. Abciximab plus 5,600 units of intravenous heparin should be administered immediately after insertion of the femoral sheaths
D. 5,600 units of intravenous heparin should be administered immediately after insertion of the femoral sheaths; abciximab should be administered when the activated clotting time value is 200-300 seconds
E. The activated clotting time should be measured before any heparin bolus is given

411. Medical therapy for unstable angina is associated with in-hospital mortality in ____ % and development of myocardial infarction in ___ %:
A. 1% and 10%
B. 1% and 20%
C. 5% and 10%
D. 5% and 20%
E. 12% and 22%

412. Which of the following statements about adjunctive pharmacological therapy during PCI for unstable angina is false?
A. Aspirin reduces the incidence of acute closure by 30-50%
B. The combination of clopidogrel plus warfarin has been shown to be superior to aspirin plus ticlopidine for the prevention of subacute stent thrombosis
C. Platelet IIb/IIIa inhibition reduces the rate of MI following PCI
D. Intraprocedural heparin dose requirements may be higher in patients with acute ischemic syndromes compared to stable angina
E. In patients undergoing primary PTCA, hirudin reduces early cardiac events during the infusion period compared to unfractionated heparin

413. Which of the following statements about pharmacological therapy of pre-existing thrombus is false?
A. Pretreatment with a 2-14 day course of heparin does not reduce the procedural risk
B. High-dose intravenous heparin (ACT > 350 seconds) may be associated with lower rates of abrupt closure
C. Thrombolytic therapy improves outcome in patients with unstable angina undergoing PTCA
D. Pretreatment with aspirin, heparin and a platelet IIb/IIIa inhibitor decreases the incidence of myocardial infarction both pre and post-PCI
E. Thrombectomy devices do not obviate the need for intense antithrombotic therapy

414. Which of the following statements regarding the use of abciximab in PCI is false?
A. It reduces the incidence of death or MI at 30 days and 6 months
B. It reduces the need for bail-out stenting
C. It does not reduce angiographic restenosis in nondiabetic patients
D. It reduces urgent repeat revascularization within 6 months
E. Its effect in preventing death or MI can be predicted by preintervention characteristics

415. Which of the following statements is false regarding clopidogrel?
A. In the CAPRIE (Clopidogrel versus Aspirin in Patients at Risk of Ischemic Events) trial, over 19,000 patients were randomized into one of three treatment groups: (i) clopidogrel 75 mg once daily, (ii) aspirin 325 mg once daily, or (iii) clopidogrel 75 mg plus aspirin 325mg once daily

410 E 411 A 412 B 413 C 414 E

B. Inclusion criteria for CAPRIE included recent ischemic stroke, recent myocardial infarction (MI), or established peripheral arterial disease
C. Although the results from the trial demonstrated that clopidogrel-treated patients had a reduced incidence of MI, ischemic stroke, or vascular death, the data were not sufficient to recommend that patients currently on aspirin be switched to clopidogrel
D. CAPRIE was a secondary prevention trial
E. A 75 mg/day dose of clopidogrel was chosen because a previous dose-finding study demonstrated that higher doses did not achieve greater steady-state inhibition of platelet aggregation to 5 uM ADP

416. In the management of an 80 kg 60-year-old man with abciximab before elective PCI, which of the following statements is true?
A. Abciximab dose is independent of patient weight
B. Abciximab should be initiated 20 minutes before insertion of the femoral sheath
C. An initial heparin bolus dose of 10,000 U is appropriate
D. An initial heparin bolus dose of 7,000 U should be administered
E. Heparin bolus dose of 5,600 U will achieve the lowest bleeding complication rate and the highest clinical benefit

417. A 45-year-old man was admitted with unstable angina at another hospital. Coronary angiography showed an 80% mid LAD lesion. He was started on enoxaparin and transferred for PCI. Which of the following statements regarding this patient's management is correct?
A. Enoxaparin has been proven to be as effective as abciximab in preventing post-PCI complications
B. Enoxaparin has been shown to be more efficacious than unfractionated heparin in preventing post-PCI complications and CPK-MB elevation
C. The anticoagulant effect of enoxaparin cannot be assessed reliably by the aPTT or the ACT
D. PCI should be performed only after completion of 4 days of enoxaparin therapy
E. After intracoronary stent implantation, enoxaparin can be continued for 4 weeks instead of ticlopidine, as the two drugs have been proven equivalent for the prevention of stent thrombosis

418. Which of the following statements is false?
A. Tirofiban is a competitive inhibitor of the fibrinogen receptor on the platelets
B. Integrilin is a cyclic peptide that inhibits the fibrinogen binding site of the IIb/IIIa receptor
C. Abciximab is a chimeric monoclonal antibody that inhibits fibrinogen binding by a conformational change of the IIb/IIIa receptor molecule
D. The half-life of tirofiban and integrilin is 90-120 min and may be prolonged in patients with renal insufficiency
E. Readministration of abciximab has a 6% incidence of anaphylaxis due to its antigenicity

419. Which of the following statement about aspirin-allergy is false?
A. Desensitization of individuals with aspirin-induced anaphylaxis should not be attempted
B. A previous cutaneous reaction to aspirin places the individual at increased risk for anaphylaxis upon readministration of the drug
C. H1 and H2 histamine receptor antagonists can usually control cutaneous symptoms during the peri-procedural period
D. The absence of previous adverse reactions does not predict continuing tolerance
E. Aspirin sensitivity may appear in over 10% of asthmatics, and over 30% of asthmatics with rhinosinusitis

415 A 416 E 417 D 418 E 419 B

420. Which of the following is correct regarding diagnostic tests for HIT type II?

A. The standard platelet aggregation assay is highly specific but only 30-50% sensitive

B. The serotonin release assay can be performed only in highly specialized centers

C. Enzyme-linked immunosorbent assay for IgG has low specificity

D. Heparin induced platelet aggregation assay is more sensitive than the standard platelet aggregation

E. All of the above

421. Which of the following agent is a concentration (dose) dependent blocker of the GP IIb/IIIa integrin?

A. Abciximab

B. Enoxaparin

C. Eptifibatide

D. Fraxiparin

E. Danaparoid

422. Which of the following trials did not document statistically significant efficacy with treatment in the PCI indication?

A. EPILOG

B. EPISTENT

C. ESPRIT

D. EPIC

E. None of the above

423. The composite endpoints of clinical trials of GP IIb/IIIa inhibition in PCI incorporate multiple components. Which of the following components generally contributes to the greatest number of events to these composite endpoints?

A. Death

B. Myocardial infarction

C. Urgent revascularization

D. Restenosis-related revascularization

424. Which complication of GP IIb/IIIa inhibition is relatively common and should be routinely screened for?

A. Disseminated intravascular coagulation

B. Renal dysfunction

C. Thrombocytopenia

D. Thrombosis

425. Which of the following agents is reversed primarily via renal clearance?

A. Abciximab

B. Eptifibatide

C. Tirofiban

D. A and B

E. B and C

426. Which of the following statements regarding sildenafil is false?

A. Maximum dose is 100 mg daily

B. Its use is contraindicated in nitrate users

C. Lower dosage is recommended in liver and renal dysfunction

D. Overdose can produce profound hypotension

E. Hypotension due to sildenafil-nitrate interaction can be exacerbated by phenylephrine

427. Which of the following statement is correct regarding metformin therapy?

A. It should be discontinued two days before the day of coronary intervention in all patients

B. It may produce profound hypoglycemia in patients with renal insufficiency

C. Lactic acidosis and megaloblastic anemia may occur

D. Renal failure post-intervention should be excluded before resuming metformin

428. Which of the following is true about phenylephrine?

A. Is a pure α-adrenergic agonist

B. Is a pure α-adrenergic blocker

C. Is a pure β-adrenergic blocker

D. Is a pure β-adrenergic agonist

E. None of the above

420 E 421 C 422 E 423 B 424 C 425 E 426 E 427 D 428 A

429. The ESSENCE and TIMI 11B trials:

A. Establish the superiority of enoxaparin vs. unfractionated heparin in reducing ischemic events

B. Establish the superiority of enoxaparin vs. placebo in reducing ischemic events

C. Establishes the superiority of dalteparin vs. placebo in reducing ischemic events

D. Enrolled only patients with non-ST elevation myocardial infarction

E. Options A and D are correct

430. Statements about heparin-induced thrombocytopenia (HIT) are true *except:*

A. Type I HIT is due to heparin's direct platelet aggregating effect and is associated with platelet counts of 50,000 to 150,000/mm2

B. Type II HIT is due to an autoantibody directed against the platelet factor IV-heparin complex and is typically associated with platelet counts < 50,000/mm2

C. Type I HIT is more common that Type II HIT, has a benign clinical course, and often improves even if heparin is continued

D. Type II HIT can be associated with fatal venous and arterial thromboses

E. Type I and Type II HIT require discontinuation of all heparin

431. Which of the following statement regarding activated clotting time (ACT) monitoring for percutaneous coronary intervention (PCI) is false?

A. ACT is inversely associated with abrupt coronary closure

B. ACT is directly associated with bleeding risks

C. No optimal threshold value for ACT has been established

D. ACT measured by Hemotech usually exceeds that by Hemochron

432. The potential advantages of low molecular weight heparin vs. unfractionated heparin do not include which of the following?

A. More stable dose response with more reliable level of anticoagulation

B. Relative resistance to platelet factor IV

C. Lower incidence of thrombocytopenia

D. Lower anti-factor Xa to anti-factor IIa ratio

433. All of the following are causes of constrictive pericarditis *except:*

A. Procainamide

B. Practolol

C. Chloroquine

D. Hydralazine

434. All of the following are causes of CCP *except:*

A. Sarcoidosis

B. Dermatomyositis

C. Sjögren's syndrome

D. Wegner's granulomatosis

435. Increased incidence of pericarditis is seen with all *except:*

A. Sclerotherapy of varices

B. Epicardial pacemakers

C. Thrombolysis in MI

D. Unfractionated heparin in MI

436. Subacute CP is one that occurs after how much time of pericardial insult?

A. 3 weeks to 1 month

B. 1 month to 3 months

C. 3 months to 12 months

D. > 12 months

437. All of the following are true about constrictive pericarditis *except:*

A. Continuously restricts filling from the beginning of diastole

B. Characterized by elevated left atrial pressure

C. Early diastolic filling is at high velocity

D. High atrial pressure as AV valves open

429 A 430 E 431 D 432 D 433 C 434 C 435 D 436 C 437 A

438. Conditions causing increased RA pressure and increase venous pressure are seen in all *except:*
A. RVMI
B. Hypertensive heart disease
C. Acute pulmonary embolism
D. RCMP

439. All are true about CCP *except:*
A. Near equilibration of all cardiac pressure in CP
B. Vigrous diuretic treatment changes equilibrium to unbalanced
C. Stroke volume and heart rate are the major 2 compensatory mechanism
D. Coronary blood flow is reduced but adequate in uncomplicated CP

440. All are true about chest X-ray in CCP *except:*
A. Classically bilateral effusions more common than unilateral
B. SVC and azygos vein dilated
C. Only chamber recognized on chest X-ray is enlarged RA
D. Pericardial calcification is seen in upto 50% cases that are chronic

441. True about MRI in CCP are all *except:*
A. Tube like appearance of ventricles with enlarged LA
B. Sinuous/angulated ventricular septum
C. Any thickening > 3.5 mm differentiates between constriction and restriction
D. Absent myocardium is one of the most important feature ruling out surgery

442. All are true about echo in CCP *except:*
A. Transesophageal echo is better than TTE in showing pericardial thickening
B. Ventricular septal motion may be paradoxical,, anterior or flat
C. Ventricular septal notch coincides with early diastolic abnormality
D. Flat LV posterior wall is almost never seen in CP

443. Which of the following differentiates effuso-constrictive from constrictive pericarditis?
A. Negative atrial waves more common in former
B. X descent > y descent
C. Square root configuration is more prominent in LV
D. Near equalization (= 5 mm Hg0 in all diastolic chamber

444. Common presentations of chronic constrictive pericarditis may include all *except:*
A. Congestive failure
B. Pleural effusion
C. Pulmonary embolism
D. RA thrombosis

445. Clinical features of constrictive pericarditis include all *except:*
A. Central symptoms like dyspnea, fatigue
B. Relatively fixed blood volume
C. Pulsus paradoxus is more than 80% cases
D. Dyspnea on exertion and pleural effusion

446. All of the following may be present in CCP *except:*
A. SAAG > 10 gm/dl
B. Exudative or transudative ascites
C. Proteinuria nephrotic syndrome
D. Pancytopenia is never seen

447. ECG changes in CCP include all *except:*
A. Notched wide p waves
B. Abnormal q waves
C. Thin narrow QRS complexes
D. Low to flat 'T' waves

448. True about elastic constrictive pericarditis include all *except:*
A. Due to thick fluid rich in blood and fibrin
B. Resembles tamponade and mimicked by malignancies
C. Prominent S3 and absent S4
D. Prominent x descent

438 B 439 C 440 C 441 D 442 D 443 B 444 C 445 C 446 D 447 C 448 C

449. True about effuso-constrictive pericardits are all *except:*

A. Can be due to constriction with local tamponade due to loculated effusion

B. 'x' descent > 'y' descent with frequent pulsus paradoxus

C. Drainage causes pericardial pressure to drop to '0'

D. Kussmaul's' sign is suppressed by draining fluid

450. True about pericarditis due to infective endocarditis are all *except:*

A. Due to immune complex deposition

B. Caused by erosion of valve ring abscess and ruptured aortic sinus

C. Strep viridans and staph aureus are most common causes

D. Hemorrhagic effusions are more common than sterile non hemorrhagic effusions

451. Common causes on non-tubercular bacterial pericarditis include all *except:*

A. Streptococcal

B. Staphylococcus

C. Clostridial

D. Pneumococcal

452. PCR for diagnosing tubercular pericarditis: all are true *except:*

A. 100% sensitivity and 70% specificity for active TB

B. Blood in pericardial fluid gives false positive results

C. Only drawback is poor prognostic value in AIDS/HIV with adenopathy

D. Very useful for atypical myocobacterial infections

453. All of the following contribute to diagnostic evaluation of TB pericarditis *except:*

A. Streptodornase antibodies

B. Antimyolemmal antibodies

C. Anti myosin antibodies

D. Adenosine deaminase

454. Most common pericardial affection in heart is in form of:

A. Adhesions

B. Sterile effusions

C. Calcific pericarditis

D. Serofibrinous exudates

455. Which of the following is not a true statement about pericarditis in AIDS?

A. Myocarditis generally accompanies pericarditis

B. Pericarditis occurs in 6 form with effusion as commonest

C. EBV is not associated with neoplastic pericarditis

D. Kaposi's sarcoma and Hodgkin's lumphoma are associated

456. Which of the following does not involve pericardium?

A. W. Bancrofti

B. D. medinensis

C. N. americanus

D. S. strongyloidosis

457. Most common symptom of pericardial malignancy is n:

A. Dyspnea

B. Nonproductive cough

C. Orthopnea

D. Unexplained chest pain

458. All are true about hypothyroid pericarditis *except:*

A. Classically high protein, low cholesterol pericarditis

B. Increased incidence in Down's syndrome

C. Microvoltage ECG

D. Echo shows findings in only 5-30% cases

449 D **450** D **451** C **452** B **453** A **454** B **455** C **456** D **457** C **458** A

459. Features suggestive of pericardial malignancy are all *except:*
A. Large effusion
B. Refractory heart failure
C. Unexplained hepatomegaly
D. Persistent pericardial rub with all 3 components

460. High levels of hyaluronic acid in pericardial fluid is present in:
A. Thymomas
B. Teratomas
C. Mesothelioma
D. Phaeochromocytomas

461. All are true about pericarditis in rheumatic fever *except:*
A. Occurs within 1st week of fever and carditis
B. Some degree of effusion is the rule
C. Discrete fibrotic Epicardial patches with increased fibrin effusion
D. Valvulitis is rarely associated with pericarditis

462. True about MI associated pericarditis are all *except:*
A. Can occur in 2 forms
B. Rub is the only sign in infract pericarditis
C. Infract pericarditis is always associated with transmural infarct
D. Acute pericarditis with non-transmural infarct is most likely post MI syndrome

463. Most common and least specific manifestation of rheumatic fever is:
A. Arthritis
B. Carditis
C. Nodules
D. Rash

464. Which of the following is not caused by milrinone and dopamine in patients of heart failure:
A. Decrease preload
B. Decrease afterload
C. Increase contractility
D. Vasoconstriction

465. All of the following may cause hypotension among patients with inferior wall MI *except:*
A. Tachyarrhthmias
B. Bezold Jarisch reflex
C. LV septal rupture
D. Bradyarrhythmia

466. Which of the following is a stage III change in ECG in a case of pericarditis:
A. ST elevation, upright T waves
B. ST isoelectric, inverted T waves
C. ST elevation, upright to flat T waves
D. ST isoelectric, upright T waves

467. All of the following are criteria for diagnosing Acute MI in presence of LBBB *except:*
A. ST elevation ≥ 1 mm concordant with QRS
B. ST segment depression ≥ 1 mm in lead V_1, V_2 or V_3
C. ST segment elevation ≥ 5 mm discordant with QRS
D. ST segment elevation ≥ 4 mm in V_5-V_6

468. What is the 30 days mortality according to Gusto-1 trial , in patients with different killip haemodynamics class?
A. I, II, III, IV: 5%, 13%, 50%, 80%
B. I, II, III, IV: 5%, 13%, 30%, 57%
C. I, II, III, IV: 10%, 26%, 42%, 70%
D. I, II, III, IV: 10%, 32%, 64%, 90%

469. All of the following form high risk in unstable angina *except:*
A. Positive cardiac biomarkers
B. Angina with LVS3
C. Rest angina > 20 min relieved with sublingual nitrates
D. Rest angina with dynamic ST-T changes

459 D 460 C 461 D 462 C 463 A 464 D 465 A 466 B 467 D 468 B 469 C

470. All of the following are high risk features with exercise electrocardiography *except:*
A. Ischemia at low heart rate (≤ 120 beats/min)
B. Early positive test ≤ 3min
C. Sustained ST depression ≤ 5 minutes after cessation of exercise
D. Inability to complete 6 minutes of Bruce protocol

471. Myocarditis treatment trials used all of the flowing *except:*
A. Cyclophosphamide
B. Corticosteroid
C. Cyclosporine
D. Azathioprine

472. All are true about Yamaguchi's apical cardiomyopathy *except:*
A. Seen in 25% of Japanese population and 2% outside Japan
B. Localised hypertrophy of distal ventricle beyond chordae tendinae
C. Moderate but significant incidence of sudden cardiac death
D. Beta blockers may be helpful

473. Most common genetic defect in HCM is:
A. Beta-myosin heavy chain
B. Cardiac troponin T
C. Alpha-tropomyosin
D. Myosin binding protein C
E. Ventricular myosin regulatory light chain

474. All of the following may be isolated findings in HCM *except:*
A. Q waves in inferolateral leads
B. Normal ECG
C. Right axis deviation
D. Negative precordial T waves

475. In sudden deceleration injuries of heart, which of the following is most commonly injured?
A. Right atrium
B. Left atrium
C. Right ventricle
D. Left ventricle

476. Most common valve involved in cardiac injury:
A. Aortic valve
B. Mitral valve
C. Tricuspid valve
D. Pulmonary valve

477. All of the following can be used for vasodepressor syncope *except:*
A. Disopyramide
B. Methylphenidate
C. Beta blockers
D. Scopolamine

478. In children taking digitalis which of the toxicity is not common:
A. Nausea and vomiting
B. Ventricular ectopics
C. Bradyarrhythmias
D. AV block

479. All of the following are pulmonary vasodilators *except:*
A. Nifedipine
B. NO
C. Hypoxia
D. Hypocarbia

480. A person at sea level breathing 100% oxygen can increase PO_2 upto:
A. 100 mmHg
B. 200 mmHg
C. 400 mmHg
D. 600 mmHg

481. Which of the following arrhythmia is a characteristic of digitalis toxicity?
A. Torsades de pointes
B. Bidirectional VT
C. VT with LAHB + RBBB
D. Accelerated idioventricular rhythm

470 C **471** A **472** C **473** A **474** C **475** A **476** A **477** B **478** B **479** C **480** C **481** B

482. Central obesity is associated with which of the following:
A. Conn's syndrome
B. Cushing's syndrome
C. Pheochromocytoma
D. Hyperthyroidism

483. Myopathy is a side effect of:
A. Lovastatin
B. Nicotinic acid
C. Probucol
D. Clofibrate

484. In primary and secondary prevention trials which of the drug is useful:
A. Lovastatin
B. Nicotinic acid
C. Probucol
D. Clofibrate

485. Gradient between PCWP and LA exists in all *except:*
A. Cortriatriatum
B. Pulmonary vein stenosis
C. LA myxoma
D. MS

486. In a case of AS with LV dysfunction. The severity of AS is estimated by:
A. Gradient across valve
B. LVET
C. Aortic valve area
D. None of the above

487. Suprasystemic pulmonary resistance is seen in all *except:*
A. PPH
B. MS
C. VSD with Eisenmenger's
D. Valvular PS with intact septum

488. Cath data saturation: RV 69%, RA 67%, AO 71% and LA 70% diagnosis is:
A. VSD
B. ASD
C. TGA
D. TAPVC

489. In nonvalvular AF:
A. Rate control is better than rhythm control
B. Rhythm control is better than rate
C. Both strategies equivalent
D. Strategies to be individualised

490. Survival into adulthood is seen in:
A. TAPVC
B. Ebstein's anomaly
C. d-TGA
D. Truncus arteriosus

491. A 35 year old lady with atypical chest pain has abnormal exercise ECG. The next step is:
A. CAG
B. Exercise echocardiography
C. Antianginal therapy
D. None of the above

492. Nitrate tolerance is prevented by all *except:*
A. Once daily dosing
B. K^+ channel opener
C. Eccentric dosing
D. Continuous nitrate patches

493. After operative surgery LV function is most like'y to be improved in:
A. MS with AS
B. MR
C. AS with LV dysfunction
D. AR with LV dysfunction

494. CAD is common in all *except:*
A. Familial hyperlipidemia
B. Kawasaki's disease
C. Supravalvular AS
D. Homocystinuria

482 B 483 B 484 A 485 D 486 C 487 C 488 D 489 C 490 B 491 B 492 D 493 C 494 C

495. In an ECG if lead I is positive lead aVF negative and II is equivocal axis is:
A. -30°
B. -60°
C. -90°
D. +60°

496. Pericarditis is characterized by all *except:*
A. ↑ ESR
B. Pleuritic pain
C. Chest pain ↑ on lying down
D. Convex ST elevation in ECG

497. In a case of MS with AS the gradient across aortic valve is likely to be:
A. Underestimated
B. Overestimated
C. Cannot be estimated
D. None of the above

498. TOF in children differs from TOF in adults by:
A. ↑ systemic resistance
B. ↑ a wave in JVP
C. ↑ perioperative ventricular arrhythmias
D. ↑ WPW syndrome

499. Drug to be avoided in managing NSVT in a patient of HOCM is:
A. Amiodarone
B. Sotalol
C. Beta blocker
D. None of the above

500. The half life of adenosine is:
A. 10 sec
B. 20 sec
C. 30 sec
D. 60 sec

501. The commonest sign in pulmonary embolism is:
A. Tachypnea
B. Tachycardia
C. Chest pain
D. Loud S2

502. In a population having high prevalence of disease, which of the following will be altered:
A. Sensitivity
B. Specificity
C. Predictive value
D. Odds ratio

503. In a clinical trial, a false negative result may be commonly seen if:
A. Randomization of errors
B. If the study is not blind
C. Low sample size
D. Large sample size

504. Radiation treatment may be complicated by all *except:*
A. DCMP
B. Occlusive CAD
C. Pericarditis
D. Myocarditis

505. The following is helpful in primary prevention of CAD:
A. Metoprolol
B. Aspirin
C. Alpha tocopherol
D. Statins

506. Myocardial infarction pattern in the ECG of an infant suggests:
A. HOCM
B. ALCAPA
C. MI
D. PS

507. LVS4 is seen in all *except:*
A. HT
B. HOCM
C. Severe AS
D. Acute MR

495 A 496 D 497 A 498 C 499 B 500 A 501 A 502 C 503 C 504 A 505 D 506 B 507 D

508. Which prosthetic valve is not suitable in children?
A. Starr Edwards valve
B. St Judes valve
C. Bjork Shilley valve
D. Bioprosthetic valve

509. Marantic endocarditis is seen in:
A. Prosthetic valves
B. SLE
C. Malignancy
D. Aorto arteritis

510. Libman sach's endocarditis is seen in:
A. SLE
B. Ankylosing spondylitis
C. RA
D. Polyarteritis nodosa

511. The most common lesion in ankylosing spondylitis is:
A. AR
B. Pericarditis
C. CHB
D. Myocarditis

512. Echo evaluation of ASD is not reliable for:
A. Size
B. Site
C. Velocity of flow
D. Degree of shunting

513. Echo sign which persists after repair of ASD:
A. Dilated RV
B. Paradoxical septal motion
C. Large excursion of TV
D. MVP

514. Supracristal VSD is best diagnosed by:
A. Parasternal short axis view
B. Parasternal long axis
C. Apical 4 chamber
D. Apical 5 chamber

515. Little likelihood of visualization by transthoracic echocardiography is:
A. AV septum
B. Perimembranous septum
C. Supracristal region
D. Aortic dissection of descending thoracic aorta

516. Right and left ventricular diastolic dimension ratio following surgical repair of TOF should not exceed:
A. 0.7
B. 0.65
C. 0.60
D. 0.55

517. Feature not observed in endocardial cushion defect:
A. Paradoxical septal motion
B. Thickened AML
C. Primum ASD
D. Inlet VSD

518. Echo sign: most specific for diagnosis of ischemia:
A. Akinesia
B. Dyskinesia
C. Lack of systolic wall thickening
D. Systolic wall thinning

519. LVPW motion is not increased in:
A. Paradoxical septal motion
B. Vent aneurysm
C. Aortic stenosis
D. MR

520. Echo finding carrying maximum predictive value for existence of pressure gradient in HOCM:
A. ASH
B. SAM of AML
C. Mid systolic closure of AV valve
D. Delayed closure of MV

508 D 509 C 510 A 511 A 512 C 513 B 514 A 515 D 516 A 517 A 518 C 519 A 520 B

521. Most common clinical feature of post MI pericarditis:
A. Rub
B. Chest pain
C. Pleuritic pain
D. Fever

522. Most common cause of death in true LV aneurysm:
A. Arrhythmia
B. CHF
C. Rupture
D. Asystole

523. Most common type of CAD in Unstable angina:
A. Single vessel
B. Double vessel
C. Triple vessel
D. Multiple vessels

524. All of the following can occur in blunt trauma to chest *except:*
A. Ventricular aneurysm
B. VSD
C. Coronary occlusion
D. AR

525. Differential diagnosis of wide QRS tachycardia are all *except:*
A. WPW with orthodromic conduction
B. WPW antidromic conduction
C. SVT with aberrancy
D. Fascicular tachycardia

526. PVR more than SVR in:
A. PS with intact septum
B. VSD with shunt reversal
C. Single ventricle
D. TOF

527. Indication for pacing in Sick sinus syndrome:
A. Symptomatic
B. Asystole for more than 2 seconds
C. Atrial fibrillation without symptoms
D. Asymptomatic

528. Drug of choice in preventing VT in ARVD is:
A. Amiodarone
B. Sotalol
C. Metoprolol
D. Ibutilide

529. Stem cells used for myocardial regeneration are:
A. Fetal cardiomyocytes
B. Embryonal stem cells
C. Skeletal myoblasts
D. Bone marrow cells
E. All of the above

530. Commonest cause of CNS involvement in TOF:
A. Polycythemia
B. Hypoxia
C. Paradoxical embolism
D. Brain abscess

531. Minor criteria important in Indian context in rheumatic fever:
A. Polyarthralgia
B. Increased ESR
C. History of rheumatic fever
D. ↑ PR interval in ECG

532. Microangiopathic haemolytic anemia is seen in:
A. MR
B. MS
C. AS
D. TS

533. S2 splitting following birth is heard after:
A. 48 hrs
B. 24 hrs
C. 72 hrs
D. 96 hrs

521 A 522 B 523 A 524 D 525 A 526 B 527 A 528 B 529 E 530 D 531 A 532 C 533 A

534. Myomectomy most common complication:
A. VSD
B. CHB
C. LV dysfunction
D. Arrhythmias

535. Acute PE with TR without CHF; the pulmonary artery systolic pressure is:
A. 25-50 mm Hg
B. 50-75 mm Hg
C. 10-12 mm Hg
D. 5-10 mm Hg

536. ACE-inhibitors increases serum creatinine in all *except:*
A. Hypotension
B. NIDDM
C. Hypertension
D. CHF

537. Fetal effect of ACE inhibitors are all *except:*
A. Hypertension
B. Polyhydramnios
C. Growth retardation
D. Organ hypoplasia

538. Pulmonary balloon dilatation is least useful in:
A. PS with cyanosis
B. PS with CHF
C. PS with infundibular stenosis
D. PS with VSD

539. Prostaglandin in fetus is used in all *except:*
A. HLHS
B. COA
C. TAPVC
D. Pulmonary atresia

540. Propranolol in fetus causes all *except:*
A. Hypoglycemia
B. Bradycardia
C. Respiratory depression
D. Hypocalcemia

541. In parasternal short axis view; all are seen *except:*
A. Coronary artery
B. Pulmonary artery
C. Left ventricle
D. ASD

542. Upper limit of cardiac output during peak exercise can reach what percentage of basal value?
A. 200%
B. 400%
C. 600%
D. 800%

543. The O_2 saturation in normal LV cavity:
A. 95%
B. 97%
C. 100%
D. 85%

544. Propagation velocity of atrial and ventricular muscle:
A. ≥ 0.05
B. ≥ 0.5 m/s
C. ≥ 1-1.2 m/s
D. 0.3 to 0.4 m/sec

545. The plateau of action potential is due to:
A. Inward $Ca2^+$, outward K^+
B. Inward K^+, outward $Ca2^+$
C. Inward Ca2+, Inward $Ca2^+$
D. Outward k^+, Outward $Ca2^+$

546. The sequence of activation in a normal heart. The last part to be activated is:
A. Apex
B. Upper septum
C. Posterobasal paraseptal region
D. Left free wall

534 B 535 A 536 C 537 A 538 D 539 C 540 D 541 C 542 C 543 B 544 D 545 A 546 C

547. Coronary artery involvement in aortoarteritis is seen in:
A. 5%
B. 10%
C. 15%
D. 20%

548. Energy for electrical activation of heart is:
A. 1%
B. 5%
C. 10%
D. 50%

549. Systemic vascular resistance increases in:
A. Fever
B. Standing
C. Thyrotoxicosis
D. Pregnancy

550. Thrombasthenia is due to defect in:
A. Contractile protein
B. Platelet formation
C. Platelet adhesion
D. Vascular endothelium

551. Post extrasystolic potentiation is due to:
A. Intracellular Calcium overload
B. Increased epinephrine level
C. Decreased intracellular cAMP
D. Increased intracellular cAMP

552. Fastest conduction occurs in:
A. SA node
B. Atrial muscle
C. Purkinje fiber
D. AV node

553. Which does not contribute to S1?
A. Opening of pulmonary valve
B. Force of contraction of LV
C. Mitral valve closure
D. Chordae tendinae vibration

554. AV node is supplied by:
A. RCA
B. LCx
C. LAD
D. OM1

555. Nitrate tolerance can be overcome by:
A. Eccentric dosage
B. Once a day administration
C. K^+ channel opener
D. Patch administration

556. In Poiseuille's equation, the flow is related inversely to which power of radius:
A. 1
B. 2
C. 3
D. 4

557. Commonest tumor of AV nodal region:
A. Fibroma
B. Rhabdomyoma
C. Angioma
D. Myxoma

558. Which is not a contractile protein but a regulatory protein?
A. Actin
B. Tropomyosin
C. Myosin
D. None

559. The formula used calculating mixed venous oxygen saturation is:
A. Dubois's formula
B. Flamm's formula
C. Dexter's formula
D. Antman's formula

560. O_2 consumption is equal to:
A. Arteriovenous oxygen difference
B. PCW oxygen saturation into cardiac output
C. Arteriovenous oxygen difference times stroke volume
D. Cardiac output/AV difference

547 B 548 A 549 B 550 C 551 A 552 C 553 A 554 A 555 D 556 D 557 C 558 B 559 B 560 A

561. Pulmonary vascular resistance in dyne sec cm^{-5}:
A. 20-250
B. 800-1600
C. 1600-3200
D. 250-500

562. Active relaxation of myocardium by:
A. Tropomyosin
B. Troponin I
C. Troponin T
D. Actin

563. Calcium influx in myocardium occurs in:
A. Phase I
B. Phase II
C. Phase III
D. Phase IV

564. Between central and peripheral artery waveform: which is not true?
A. The incisura is replaced by dicrotic notch
B. The dicrotic notch occurs earlier than incisura
C. The ascending limb is steeper in central artery
D. The incisura coincides with aortic valve closure

565. Risk of sudden cardiac death is highest in patients of heart failure who are in NYHA:
A. Class II
B. Class III-a
C. Class III-b
D. Class IV

566. Normal Pericardial fluid:
A. 15 ml
B. 60 ml
C. 70 ml
D. 80 ml

567. RA/RV pressure gradient is increased in inspiration due to:
A. ↓ RV diastolic pressure
B. ↑ RV systolic pressure
C. ↑ RV filling pressure
D. None of the above

568. The hangout interval indicates change over pressure between:
A. Ao-Pa
B. RV-PA
C. LV-RV
D. LV-LA

569. Normal PCWP with pulmonary oedema:
A. High altitude oedema
B. High BP with auscultation
C. Cortriatrum
D. Pulmonary venous HTN

570. TMT termination is indicated in:
A. Ataxia
B. Grade I-II angina
C. ST elevation in non Q leads
D. ST depression >2 mm

571. LV angio: how much contrast has to be given:
A. 30 ml
B. 50 ml
C. 70 ml
D. 90 ml

572. Digital subtraction angiogram: true is:
A. Large amount of contrast is required
B. More detailed analysis of the arterial system
C. Dynamic image
D. Less radiation exposure than conventional angiogram

573. LV angio view for IVS visualisation is:
A. LAO cranial
B. LAO caudal
C. RAO
D. AP

561 A 562 B 563 B 564 B 565 A 566 A 567 A 568 B 569 A 570 C 571 A 572 B 573 A

574. Best assessment of LV contractility:
A. ESPVR
B. VCF
C. Maximum lipidity
D. End systolic wall stress

575. Method of detecting LV mass:
A. 2D echo
B. M mode
C. LV angio
D. All

576. Pulmonary embolism: RV systolic pressure can be calculated by Doppler with the help of:
A. PR Jet
B. TR jet
C. Tricuspid inflow pattern
D. Normal value of E Slope

577. O_2 saturation is lowest in:
A. SVC
B. IVC
C. Coronary sinus
D. Pulmonary artery

578. Mixed venous sample taken from:
A. PA
B. IVC
C. SVC
D. CS

579. Temporary pacing is indicated in all except (in acute MI):
A. Newly developed RBBB
B. Newly developed LBBB
C. RBBB-LPHB
D. All the above

580. Ambulatory – BP monitoring is done in all *except:*
A. Sick sinus syndrome
B. Adverse effects of drugs
C. Pacemaker syndrome
D. Carotid sinus hypersensitivity

581. TMT after 4 weeks of inferior wall MI–Lack of SBP response is due to most commonly:
A. Effect of drugs
B. Physical deconditioning
C. LMC disease (left main)
D. Myocardial stunning

582. Fetal echo: best time to assess structural anomalies of heart:
A. Between 16-29 weeks
B. 29-26 weeks
C. 26-28 weeks
D. 28-30 weeks

583. Earliest enzyme to elevate in acute MI:
A. CK-MB
B. CK-MM
C. Troponin-T
D. Myoglobin

584. Patient with MI coming on 8th day, which enzyme is beneficial in diagnosis:
A. SGOT
B. CPK
C. Troponin T
D. Myoglobin

585. In a patient following MI (<4 weeks), tread-mill will not be useful before coronary angiogram in which situation:
A. Inferior wall MI
B. Angina
C. LV dysfunction
D. Mitral regurgitation

586. Which of the following is not indicative of multivessel disease in exercise test?
A. Crescendo angina
B. ST depression in multiple leads
C. Hypotension
D. Unifocal VPC >20/mt

574 A **575** A **576** B **577** C **578** A **579** A **580** A **581** A **582** A **583** D **584** C **585** B **586** D

587. Which is not useful to determine myocardial viability?
A. 99mTc
B. Contrast Echo
C. Th 201
D. Dobutamine echo
E. All of the above

588. Thallium 201 is suggestive of LV dysfunction by:
A. Reversible thallium defect
B. Low lung uptake
C. Post stress LV dilation
D. Defect in single arterial region

589. Endomyocardial biopsy is the gold standard for:
A. EMF
B. DCMP
C. Cardiac transplant rejection
D. Sarcoidosis

590. 35 year old male with atypical chest pain, TMT negative: next step will be:
A. Coronary angiography
B. Stress echo
C. Treatment of chest pain
D. Thallium-201 stress test

591. Blood flow by PET scan: all are used *except:*
A. 13 NH3
B. 18 FDG
C. 82 Rb
D. 18 H_2O

592. Pulmonary anatomy best delineated by:
A. Standard CT
B. Cine MRI
C. Multiplanar MRI
D. Ultra fast CT

593. Tech ^{99m} pyrophosphate scans in AMI:
A. 1st day of infarct
B. 7 days of infarct
C. 2-3 days of infarct
D. 10 days of infarct

594. In a 70 year 40kg male 1 MET:
A. 3.5 ml/kg/min
B. 1.5 ml/kg/min
C. 1 ml/kg/min
D. 2 ml/kg/min

595. Contrast echocardiography is useful in:
A. L → R shunt
B. R → L shunt
C. Both
D. None

596. MVP: most specific echo view:
A. Apical 4 chamber
B. Parasternal long axis
C. 2 chamber
D. Short axis

597. Mitral EPSS normal:
A. <6 mm
B. <10 mm
C. <12 mm
D. <14 mm

598. On TMT, least associated with bad prognosis:
A. 1 mm ST depression
B. Ventricular ectopic
C. Angina during exercise
D. Hypotension

599. TMT is contraindicated in:
A. Compensated CCF
B. Recent onset chest pain <48 hr
C. Asymptomatic, non critical AS
D. Congenital CHB

600. T sign on echo is seen in:
A. ASD
B. PDA
C. RSOV
D. Tricuspid atresia

587 B 588 C 589 C 590 D 591 B 592 C 593 C 594 A 595 C 596 B 597 A 598 B 599 B 600 A

601. O_2 consumption in a patient of 42 kgs performing 20 METS is:
A. 245 ml
B. 1400 ml
C. 700 ml
D. 2100 ml

602. In TMT, specific sign of reversible ischaemia is:
A. T inversion
B. T flattening
C. U inversion
D. Inverted T becoming upright

603. Positive TMT is:
A. 1 mm flat depression
B. Appearance of ventricular bigeminy
C. 2 mm of down sloping ST depression
D. Increased QRS duration

604. Specific sign of acute myocardial ischaemia during TMT:
A. Angina
B. Hypotension
C. ST changes
D. NSVT

605. Most specific for viability of myocardium:
A. PET
B. Stress echo
C. Thallium 201 stress test
D. CAG

606. EPSS is increased in:
A. DCMP
B. AR
C. RCM
D. CP

607. EF slope: normal value is:
A. <15 m/sec
B. 25-35 m/sec
C. 35-50 m/sec
D. >50 m/sec

608. Contrast echocardiography useful in:
A. ASD
B. VSD
C. A-P window
D. All

609. Gooseneck on contrast ventriculography is seen in:
A. d-TGA
B. AV canal defect
C. A-P window
D. Tricuspid atresia

610. Egg on side appearance on Chest X-ray is seen in:
A. d-TGA
B. DORV
C. TAPVC
D. TOF

611. Earliest X-ray sign of pulmonary venous HTN:
A. Peribronchial cuffing
B. Kerley B sign
C. Perihilar plethora
D. Cephalization or redistribution of PV blood flow

612. Square root sign in LV pressure tracing is seen in all *except:*
A. HOCM
B. Tamponade
C. Constriction
D. MS

613. Step up at atrial level occurs in all *except:*
A. ASD
B. PDA
C. Coronary sinus RA fistula
D. PAPVC

601 D 602 C 603 C 604 B 605 A 606 A 607 D 608 D 609 B 610 A 611 D 612 B 613 B

614. Dexter's criteria is used to assess:
A. Pulmonary vascular resistance
B. Significance of left to right shunt
C. Systemic vascular resistance
D. Qp/Qs

615. For TMT, the resistance of skin electrode surface should be less than:
A. 5000 Ω
B. 10000 Ω
C. 20000 Ω
D. 15,000 Ω

616. Doppler (CW) measurement of velocity, the factors considered are all *except:*
A. Received frequency
B. Transmitted frequency
C. Cosine of the angle
D. Doppler frequency shift

617. Highly sensitive investigation for detecting arrhythmia in MVP:
A. Holter
B. Echo
C. Treadmill
D. ECG

618. For stress echo, which of the following is used?
A. Agitated saline
B. Urograffin
C. 82Rb
D. $18H_2O$

619. In hypertension, which of the following will not decrease B.P:
A. Alcohol supplementation
B. Magnesium
C. K supplementation
D. Ca supplementation

620. Antihypertensive therapy reduce cardiovascular mortality by:
A. 10%
B. 14%
C. 30%
D. 60%

621. 35 year old lady taking oral contraceptive produces hypertension due to:
A. Essential
B. Renal parenchymal disease
C. Renovascular disease
D. All of the above

622. All of the following are indications of surgery in Ebstein's anomaly *except:*
A. CT ratio > 65%
B. Cyanosis
C. Functional class II
D. Recurrent PSVT

623. Myxedema associated with all *except:*
A. Low QRS voltage
B. Type III hyperlipidemia
C. Preexcitation syndrome
D. Sinus bradycardia

624. Regarding NTG: which is a true statement?
A. May cause chest pain in HOCM
B. Primary mechanism is by increase vasodilation
C. Commonly causes Methemoglobinaemia
D. Prolonged use increase in receptors density

625. Aortic root angio leading to opacities in pulmonary artery is least likely in:
A. RSOV to RV
B. RSOV to LV
C. RSOV to RA
D. RSOV to PA

626. BP difference of greater than 5mmHg in upper limbs is seen in all *except:*
A. PDA
B. Subvalvular AS
C. Origin of SCA from descending thoracic aorta
D. Coarctation of aorta

614 B 615 A 616 A 617 A 618 A 619 A 620 C 621 D 622 C 623 C 624 B 625 B 626 B

627. **Interstitial nephritis is associated with all *except:***
A. Hyperkalemia, hypercholoremic acidosis
B. Increased ammonia production and excretion
C. Fanconi's syndrome
D. leucocyturia

628. **Increase chance of aortic dissection is seen in all *except:***
A. ASD
B. CoA
C. PDA
D. Cong AS (6%)

629. **Barter's syndrome: all are seen *except:***
A. Hypertension
B. Metabolic alkalosis
C. Hypokalemia
D. Response to NSAIDS

630. **Drug contraindicated during pregnancy:**
A. Enalapril
B. Digoxin
C. Propanalol
D. Heparin

631. **Large tongue is seen in all *except:***
A. Hyperthyroidism
B. Amyloidosis
C. Down's syndrome
D. Hurters syndrome

632. **Pompe's disease: all are seen *except:***
A. Type II glycogen storage disease
B. HCMP
C. Phytanic acid storage
D. Acid maltase deficiency

633. **Suprasystemic RV pressure is seen in:**
A. PS with intact IVS
B. Eisenmengers syndrome
C. TOF
D. PA

634. **Aortic oxygen saturation-98% & PA oxygen saturation-58% is suggestive of:**
A. Low cardiac output state
B. High output state
C. Right to left shunt
D. Left to right shunt

635. **PA saturation greater than aortic saturation is seen in all *except:***
A. Taussig Bing anomaly
B. DORV with doubly committed VSD
C. TGA
D. Pulmonary atresia

636. **Lipoprotein A all are true *except:***
A. Bell shaped distribution in population
B. Independent risk factor for population
C. Niacin can be used for Rx
D. Easily standardised assays

637. **Square wave pattern in right heart is seen with valsalva in all *except:***
A. ASD B. VSD
C. CCF D. CCP

638. **Features suggestive of impaired LV function in TMT is:**
A. Failure of BP to rise
B. ST depression
C. Inadequate rise of heart rate
D. NSVT

639. **Which of the following is not seen in obesity?**
A. Decreased oxygen consumption
B. Increased EDV
C. LVH
D. Increased QTc

640. **H wave is seen in all *except:***
A. Restrictive CMP
B. CP
C. Right ventricular infarction
D. Pulmonary embolism

627 B 628 A 629 A 630 A 631 A 632 C 633 A 634 A 635 D 636 D 637 B 638 A 639 A 640 D

641. Right heart border is formed by all *except:*
A. SVC
B. RA
C. IVC
D. PA

642. Rarest type of RSOV is:
A. Into RA
B. Into LV
C. Into RV
D. Into PA

643. I/V propanalol decreases oxygen consumption by:
A. Decreasing HR
B. Decreasing EDV
C. ↓ SV
D. ↑ coronary blood flow

644. Suprasystemic PA pressure can be seen in patients of Eisenmenger's syndrome due to reversal of shunt of:
A. ASD
B. VSD
C. PDA
D. AP window

645. Syndrome X is associated with all *except:*
A. Normal coronaries
B. Normal coronary reserve
C. Angina
D. More in women

646. WPW syndrome is significant because of:
A. Associated with SCD
B. Paroxysmal atrial tachycardia
C. Ebstein's anomaly
D. HOCM

647. AF with fast ventricular rate all are useful *except:*
A. Digoxin
B. Disopyramide
C. Diltiazem
D. Verapamil

648. Most useful to diagnose supraventricular arrhythmia:
A. Carotid massage
B. Holter monitoring
C. Oesophageal ECG
D. Multiple ECG lead

649. AV nodal re-entrant tachycardia–radio frequency ablation done to abolish:
A. Fast pathway
B. Slow pathway
C. Both pathways
D. AV nodal ablation

650. Mechanism of atrial flutter:
A. Right atrial re-entry current near tricuspid valve cusp
B. Left atrial re-entry current near pulmonary vein
C. Ectopic focus near SVC
D. Ectopic focus near PV

651. AF with MS: first heart sound is loud in:
A. Mild MS
B. Moderate
C. Severe MS
D. All

652. TR murmur true is:
A. Holosystolic if RVSP normal (right ventricular systolic pressure)
B. In expiration murmur intensity decreases
C. In failure Carvallo's sign absent
D. All of the above

653. MI is least common in which chamber of heart:
A. LA
B. RA
C. RV
D. LV

641 D 642 B 643 A 644 A 645 B 646 A 647 B 648 C 649 B 650 A 651 D 652 C 653 A

654. **Maximum chance of infective endocarditis:**
A. VSD
B. Bicuspid aortic valve
C. ASD
D. PS

655. **IE is likely in:**
A. Eisenmenger's VSD
B. MVP with MR
C. PAPVC
D. PDA with PA pressure equally systemic pressure

656. **Right sided IE; all are true *except:***
A. Common in post partum period
B. In drug abusers
C. Staph aureus
D. Good prognosis

657. **Pseudoejection sound can be heard in all *except:***
A. HOCM
B. MVP
C. Ebstein's anomaly
D. Valvular PS

658. **60 year old lady of RHD with endocarditis due to enterococci on treatment with Ampicillin/gentamicin; Azotaemia is caused by:**
A. Renal tubular damage by gentamicin
B. Membranous nephropathy due to enterococci
C. Focal glomerulonephritis
D. Renal infraction

659. **In infective endocarditis, false statement regarding Janeway lesions is:**
A. Tender
B. Hemorrhagic areas in sole hand
C. 4-10 mm
D. Septic embolic causes if

660. **Infective endocarditis prophylaxis is needed in:**
A. Rigid bronchoscopy
B. Hysteroscopic biopsy
C. Flexible bronchoscopy
D. Percutaneous liver biopsy

661. **Most common finding on light microscopy of renal biopsy in a patient of infective endocarditis is:**
A. Focal and segmental proliferative GN
B. RPGN
C. Diffuse proliferation GN
D. Crescentric GN

662. **Huge vegetation is seen in:**
A. Q fever
B. Streptococcal viridians
C. Staphylococcus
D. Neisseria meningitides

663. **Treatment of choice for elderly with SVT:**
A. Adenosine
B. Digoxin
C. Verapamil
D. Amiodarone

664. **WPW with QRS widening–drug not given is:**
A. Amiodarone
B. Quinidine
C. Procainamide
D. Verapamil

665. **Pacemaker syndrome is seen in all *except:***
A. AAI
B. VVI
C. DDD
D. DDDR

666. **Pacemaker sounds are due to:**
A. Diaphragmatic and intercostal muscle stimulation by the electrode
B. Perforation by the lead
C. Fracture of the pacemaker lead
D. Insulation failure

654 A 655 B 656 D 657 D 658 A 659 A 660 A 661 A 662 D 663 A 664 D 665 B 666 A

667. AV dissociation rules out the diagnosis of:
A. AV nodal re-entrant tachycardia
B. Intra atrial re-entry
C. SA nodal re-entry
D. AVRT

668. Primary VF incidence:
A. 10%
B. 1%
C. 20%
D. 30%

669. Primary VF in MI: true is:
A. Occur in 30% of cases
B. More common in anterior area
C. More common in inferior area
D. Is a predictor of increased mortality

670. LBBB best way to evaluate for ischemia is MR:
A. Stress echo
B. Pacing
C. TMT
D. Isotonic exercise

671. LVH in elderly is a good predictor of mortality in:
A. Men
B. Women
C. Men with strong family h/o CAD
D. Women with strong family h/o CAD

672. In elderly, control of both stroke & CAD is achieved best by:
A. Reduction in SBP
B. Reduction in DBP
C. Homocysteinemia
D. Hypertriglyceridemia

673. T wave alternans with prolonged QT is due to:
A. Beat to beat variation of action potential duration of M cells
B. Left sympathetic over activity
C. Right sympathetic over activity
D. Hypokalemia

674. Left axis deviation (-30 to –90) is seen in:
A. Hypocalcemia
B. Hypomagnesaemia
C. Hypokalemia
D. Hyperkalemia

675. Non-compaction leads to:
A. ARVD
B. WTW
C. CKB in child
D. LBBB in adults

676. Brugada syndrome: mechanism is:
A. Re-entry
B. Triggered activity
C. ↑ automaticity
D. Anisotropy

677. Digitalis toxicity, psychiatric manifestations appear in elderly in:
A. Levels >2 ng/ml
B. Therapeutic levels
C. Subtherapeutic levels
D. Suicidal dose

678. CHF at one year:
A. d-TGA
B. HLHS
C. TOF
D. Ebstein's anomaly

679. Restrictive cardiomyopathy from constrictive pericarditis is best differentiated by:
A. AV valve inflow velocities
B. Pulmonary artery pressure
C. Equalization of chamber pressure
D. Square root sign

680. Acute MR all are indicated *except:*
A. Diuretics
B. Vasodilators
C. Digoxin
D. IABP

667 D 668 A 669 C 670 A 671 A 672 A 673 A 674 A 675 D 676 A 677 B 678 D 679 A 680 C

681. All are given in hypertension *except:*
A. Digoxin
B. Diuretics
C. Vasodilator
D. Calcium channel blocker

682. Causes of MI in child less than 10 weeks:
A. Familial hypercholesterolemia
B. ALCAPA
C. HLHS
D. HOCM

683. Which of the following statement is incorrect?
A. Acute MI can occur in the absence of total occlusion
B. Majority of MI have <50% of coronary occlusion
C. Females have more unstable angina than males
D. PTCA is of no use in cardiogenic shock

684. Sudden cardiac death occurs in:
A. CHF
B. Amyloidosis
C. MS
D. Atrial flutter

685. Syncope is seen in:
A. Prinzmetal's angina
B. Atrial myxoma
C. Hypoglycemia
D. Hypercalcemia

686. IABP causes all *except:*
A. Increase cardiac output
B. Decreases ischaemia
C. Increase coronary flow
D. Improves mortality

687. Congenital heart block is associated with all *except:*
A. Anti Ro antibodies
B. CTGA
C. Viral infection
D. Anti ds DNA

688. Favourable lipid profile is seen with all *except:*
A. ACE inhibitor
B. β blocker
C. Prazosin
D. Clonidine

689. Pericardial window is useful for treating effusions secondary to:
A. Malignancy
B. Connective tissue disease
C. Uremia
D. Constrictive pericarditis

690. Precapillary pulmonary hypertension is seen in:
A. Pulmonary embolism
B. Eisenmenger's syndrome
C. Primary pulmonary hypertension
D. HIV

691. QRS axis in a patient with ECG showing pure 'R' wave in aVR and aVL:
A. +0 to +60
B. +60 to +120
C. -60 to -120
D. -30 to -60

692. Which of the following is thrombogenic at endothelial level?
A. Activated C protein
B. Thrombomodulin
C. Antithrombin III
D. Thrombospondin

693. LV contraction coincides with:
A. M_1
B. QRS complex
C. Carotid upstroke
D. Initiation of apex cardiogram

681 A 682 B 683 D 684 B 685 B 686 D 687 D 688 B 689 A 690 C 691 C 692 D 693 B

694. Paradoxical splitting of both S1 and S2 seen in:
A. HOCM
B. AS
C. LBBB
D. All of above

695. Accessory pathways are found in:
A. Ebstein's anomaly
B. Hypoplastic left heart syndrome
C. c-TGA
D. All of the above

696. Increased pulmonary blood flow with normal LA pressure:
A. TAPVC
B. Truncus arteriosus
C. VSD
D. AR

697. In a trained athlete which is not seen:
A. Increased CO_2 by 5 times
B. O_2 consumption increased by 10 times
C. Increased stroke volume by 3 times
D. Increased heart rate by 3 times

698. METS indicate:
A. Myocardial O_2 consumption
B. O_2 consumption corrected for body weight
C. Skeletal muscular O_2 consumption
D. Cerebral O_2 consumption

699. SAECG (Late potentials):
A. Very low frequency signal
B. Correspond with descending limb of T wave
C. Higher amplitude associated with greater chance of VT
D. All of above
E. None of above

700. Eccentric LV hypertrophy is seen characteristically with:
A. AS
B. Chronic AR
C. HOCM
D. DCMP

701. Exposure to Chest X ray results in exposure of:
A. 0.1 rad
B. 0.3 rad
C. 0.5 rad
D. 1 rad

702. Max APD is seen in:
A. SA node
B. AV node
C. Atrium & Ventricle
D. Purkinje cells

703. Max rate of rise of voltage (dv/dt) is seen in:
A. Phase 0 of AP
B. Phase 1 of AP
C. Phase 2 of AP
D. Phase 3 of AP

704. Regarding Valsalva maneuvre, which is true?
A. 40 mmHg for 15 sec
B. 40 mmHg for 25 sec
C. 25 mmHg for 15 sec
D. 25 mmHg for 25 sec
E. 40 mmHg for 40 sec

705. Not seen in RV is:
A. Tendon of Todaro
B. Papillary muscles
C. Moderator band
D. Trabecular septum

706. HAPE true is:
A. Aggravated by exertion at high altitude
B. Seen more in elderly than in young
C. Seen at height of more than 3000m
D. Not occur in people living at high altitude who had descended to ground level for long time

707. Treatment of cyclosporine induced hypertension is:
A. ACE inhibitors
B. Diuretics
C. Calcium channel blockers
D. Beta blockers

694 C 695 D 696 A 697 D 698 B 699 E 700 B 701 A 702 D 703 A 704 A 705 A 706 A 707 C

708. In a case of acute MI with LVF, LA pressure is equal to:
A. Mean PAP
B. Diastolic PAP
C. RVEDP
D. RA mean pressure

709. Regarding Cardiac tamponade, which is true?
A. PA pressure > RA pressure
B. Blunt 'x' descent
C. ↑ RA filling with inspiration
D. All above

710. Regarding digoxin which is true:
A. Mean plasma half life of Ouabain is < 6 hrs
B. Major product of digitalis is digoxin
C. Bioavailability of digitoxin is better than digoxin
D. Plasma half life of digoxin > digitoxin

711. All are digoxin induced arrhythmia *except:*
A. Accelerated junctional rhythm
B. Wide QRS complex tachycardia
C. Atrial tachycardia with block
D. AV dissociation

712. Normal sinus P wave is likely to be seen in:
A. VT
B. AVRT
C. AVNRI
D. Ectopic atrial tachycardia

713. Least venodilator effect:
A. NTG
B. Hydralazine
C. Captopril
D. Prazosin

714. β blocker acts on RAS system by:
A. ↓ renin release from JG apparatus
B. ↓ conversion of prorenin to rennin
C. ↓ conversion from AT1 to ATII
D. Block the effect of ATII

715. Most common cause of IE in young:
A. Strep viridans
B. Strep pyogenes
C. Enterococcus
D. Staph aureus

716. IE is most likely to affect:
A. AS
B. MS
C. PS
D. TS

717. Peripheral pulmonary artery stenosis seen with:
A. Rubella
B. Noonan
C. Williams
D. Holt Orain syndrome

718. Holt Oram is associated with:
A. OP ASD
B. OS ASD
C. AV canal septal defect
D. SV ASD

719. Which is true about hard exudate?
A. Old protein leak
B. S/o ischemia
C. Mostly seen near optic disc and radiation from centre
D. Seen in nerve layer of retina

720. Pregnancy is associated with:
A. ↑ CO
B. ↑ SV
C. ↑ HR
D. None
E. All of above

721. Anemia is associated with all *except:*
A. ↓ A-V O_2 diff
B. ↓ SVR
C. ↑ CO
D. ↓ ESM at the base of the heart

708 B 709 C 710 C 711 B 712 A 713 B 714 A 715 A 716 A 717 A 718 B 719 A 720 E 721 A

722. ↑ Alveolar to arterial O_2 gradient is seen in:
A. Hyperventilation
B. Hypoventilation
C. R-L shunt
D. High altitude

723. Pulmonary venous desaturation is seen with:
A. Pulmonary AV fistula
B. ARDS
C. Hypoventilation
D. High altitude

724. Patient with PPI having normal sinus 'p' wave followed by each pacing spike followed by ventricular capture: type of pacemaker:
A. VVI
B. AAI
C. VDD
D. DVI
E. AAIR

725. Lactic acid conc. in shock is:
A. 0.1 mmol/L
B. 1.5 mmol/L
C. 10 mmol/L
D. 15 mmol/L

726. Regarding Pompe's disease true is:
A. Mucopolysaccharidoses
B. Associated with DCMP
C. Concentric LVH on ECG
D. Long PR interval

727. Regarding Fabry's disease: true are:
A. Stroke
B. HTN
C. Cataract
D. MI
E. All

728. Valsalva during strain phase: failure to rise BP due to:
A. Sympathetic failure
B. Parasympathetic failure
C. None
D. All

729. All are correctly matched contraindications *except:*
A. β blocker - COPD
B. Reserpine - psychosis
C. Thiazide - Diabetes
D. ACEI - Pregnancy

730. All are correctly matched *except:*
A. B-T shunt: SCA with PA
B. Potts shunt: Descending aorta with LPA
C. Glenn shunt: SVC with ascending aorta
D. Waterstons shunt: Ascending Ao to right pulmonary artery

731. CoA with rib notching involving 3-8 rib on left side:
A. Pre CoA
B. Juxtaductal CoA with narrowing of left subclavian artery ostium
C. CoA with → SCA distal to CoA
D. Post SCA CoA with → SCA distal to CoA

732. Angiokeratoma seen in which:
A. Fabry's disease
B. Von Gierke's disease
C. Marfan syndrome
D. Pompe's disease

733. Most common benign tumor of heart in childhood:
A. Myxoma
B. Fibroma
C. Rhabdomyoma
D. Hemangioma

734. Exercise increases blood flow to:
A. Heart
B. Skin
C. Kidney
D. Liver

722 C 723 A 724 C 725 C 726 C 727 E 728 C 729 C 730 C 731 D 732 A 733 C 734 A

735. Thiazide: all true *except:*
A. Metabolic acidosis
B. ↑ blood sugar concentration
C. ↑ Uric acid
D. ↑ PG

736. Cysticercosis is caused by:
A. T. Saginata
B. T. solium
C. Echinocochus
D. Strongyloids

737. Filariform larva occurs in:
A. Ascaris
B. Ancylostoma duodenale
C. E. vermicularis
D. N. americans

738. Chorioretinitis in perinatal period is caused by:
A. Toxoplasmosis
B. CMV
C. Rubella
D. Herpes simplex

739. All are correctly matched *except:*
A. Vibro cholerae - Enterotoxin
B. Cl. Difficle - Cytotoxin
C. Staph aureus - performed toxin
D. Shigella - preformed toxin

740. All are correctly matched *except:*
A. Quinoline - (-) DNA synthesis
B. Sulfonamide - (-) Cell metabolism
C. Penicillin - Cell wall synthesis
D. Erythromycin - Cell wall synthesis

741. Galactosemia: all are true *except:*
A. Hypertonia
B. Cataract
C. Hypoglycemia
D. Vomiting & Diarrhoea with milk
E. AR

742. Gastrinoma: all are true *except:*
A. Associated with MEN-1
B. Benign
C. 40% presents with diarrhoea
D. Most of them occur in pancreas

743. Somatostatin is present in:
A. Posterior pituitary
B. Locus cerulius
C. GIT
D. Respiratory tract
E. Kidney

744. Carcinoid syndrome: all are true *except:*
A. Hypertension
B. Flushing
C. Diarrhoea
D. Fibrosis of endocardium.
E. Head ache

745. Perimenopausal hot flashes are seen due to:
A. ↓ estrogen
B. ↑ FSH/LH
C. ↓ Progesterone
D. All
E. None

746. Lenticular cataract is seen with all *except:*
A. Hypoparathyroidism
B. Myotonic dystrophy
C. Galactosemia
D. ↑ Chlorpromazine
E. Hemochromatosis

747. During hemodialysis, which drug is least likely to cause unpredictable changes in blood pressure?
A. Minoxidil
B. Prazosin
C. Metoprolol
D. Amlodipine

735 A 736 B 737 D 738 B 739 D 740 D 741 A 742 B 743 C 744 E 745 D 746 E 747 A

748. Brownish blue spot on ear:
A. Raynaud's
B. Alkaptonuria
C. Addison's disease
D. Cataract

749. Hypokalemia is seen with all *except:*
A. Metabolic alkalosis
B. Steroid
C. Cushing syndrome
D. RTA- Type II
E. Cyclosporine

750. Sphingomyelinase deficiency is seen in:
A. Nieman's pick disease
B. Variegate porphyria
C. Morquio disease
D. Ataxia telangiectasia

751. PNH is associated with all *except:*
A. Venous thrombosis
B. 15-30% incidence of aplastic anemia
C. Pancytopenia
D. Haemoglobinuria is usually present
E. Serum lysis test

752. IV hemolysis produces all *except:*
A. ↑ bilirubin
B. ↑ haptoglobin
C. ↑ LDH
D. Haemoglobinaemia

753. Iron deposition in following site is benign:
A. Liver
B. Reticuloendothelial cells
C. Pancreas
D. Brain

754. Chronic hepatitis is rare with which hepatitis virus:
A. Hepatitis B
B. Hepatitis C
C. Hepatitis D
D. Hepatitis E

755. Diabetes mellitus is associated with all *except:*
A. Amyloidosis
B. Myotonic dystrophy
C. Friedrichs ataxia
D. Hemochromatosis
E. MEN-IIb syndrome

756. ATN is seen in all *except:*
A. Hypovolemia
B. Immune complex
C. Rhabdomyolysis
D. Haemoglobinuria

757. Which drug ↑ prolactin release?
A. Dopamine
B. Levodopa
C. Bromocriptine
D. Morphine

758. Isolated systolic hypertension is seen in:
A. Elderly
B. Eclampsia
C. All of the above
D. None

759. Regarding respiratory volume: all are true *except:*
A. Total capacity – vital capacity = RV
B. TLC – IC = FRC
C. ERV + RV = FRC
D. IRV + ERV = VC

760. Smoking increases the level of:
A. Carboxy Hb
B. Sulfhemoglobin
C. Met Hb
D. HBF

761. With alcohol following drug interacts:
A. Metronidazole
B. Digoxin
C. Sulfonamide
D. Erythromycin

748 B 749 E 750 A 751 D 752 B 753 B 754 D 755 E 756 B 757 D 758 A 759 D 760 A 761 A

762. P-450 depression is caused by:
- **A.** Cimetidine
- **B.** Ranitidine
- **C.** Phenobarbitone
- **D.** Phenytoin

763. Fabry's disease: all are true *except:*
- **A.** Autosomal recessive
- **B.** Peripheral neuropathy
- **C.** Renal dysfunction
- **E.** Stroke

764. All are true about malarial parasite *except:*
- **A.** Duffy negative phenotype makes RBC resistant to plasmodium vivax
- **B.** Trophozoite are present in RBC
- **C.** Sporozoits are introduced by mosquito into blood
- **D.** Plasmodium malaraie preferentially affects younger RBC's

765. Unilateral delay of contrast I suggestive of:
- **A.** ATN
- **B.** RAS
- **C.** ARF
- **D.** CGN

766. ARDS in baby: all are true *except:*
- **A.** Ventilation with PEEP
- **B.** Inverse ratio ventilation
- **C.** NO
- **D.** Steroid

767. Neurocardiogenic syncope: all are true *except:*
- **A.** Mydriasis
- **B.** Bradycardia
- **C.** Hypotension
- **D.** Tilt table testing positive

768. Hypertrichosis:
- **A.** Minoxidil
- **B.** Diazoxide
- **C.** Hydralazine
- **D.** Captopril

769. Myocardial perfusion is most likely to be affected by:
- **A.** Single artery from RCA
- **B.** ALCAPA
- **C.** LCA from right coronary sinus
- **D.** RCA for (L) coronary sinus

Match the following

770. Recurrent infection	A. Ataxia telangiectasia
771. Corneal clouding	B. Morquio's sign
772. Photosensitivity	C. Variegate porphyria
773. Cherry red spot	D. GM2 Gangliosidoses
774. Blue sea histiocytosis	E. Nieman Pick disease

775. In patients of rheumatic heart disease with chronic AF:
- **A.** Rate control is better than rhythm control
- **B.** Rhythm control is better than rate
- **C.** Both strategies equivalent
- **D.** Strategies to be individualised

776. DINAMIT trial: false is:
- **A.** Included patients of acute MI within 40 days
- **B.** LV ejection fraction < 35% were included
- **C.** Primary end point was cardiac mortality
- **D.** ICD does not reduce overall mortality in high-risk patients who have recently had a myocardial infarction unlike MADIT-II

777. In patients of DCMP cell that should be transplanted is:
- **A.** Skeletal myoblast
- **B.** Bone marrow cells
- **C.** Circulating endothelial progenitor cells
- **D.** Embryonic stem cells

762 A 763 A 764 D 765 B 766 D 767 A 768 A 769 B 770 A 771 B 772 C 773 D 774 E
775 B 776 C 777 A

C. [illegible]
D. [illegible]

769. [illegible] may be affected by:
A. [illegible]
C. [illegible]
D. [illegible]

A. [illegible]

770. [illegible]

771. [illegible]

772. [illegible]

773. [illegible]

774. [illegible]

775. In patients of [illegible]
A. [illegible]
B. [illegible]
C. Both [illegible]
D. [illegible]

776. [illegible]
A. [illegible]
B. [illegible]
C. [illegible]
D. [illegible]

777. [illegible] should be transplanted [illegible]
A. [illegible]
B. [illegible]
C. [illegible]
D. [illegible]

765. [illegible] disease is caused by
A. [illegible]
B. [illegible]
C. [illegible]
D. [illegible]

[illegible]
A. [illegible]
B. [illegible]
C. [illegible]
D. [illegible]

[illegible]
A. [illegible]
B. [illegible]
C. [illegible]
D. [illegible]

[illegible]
A. [illegible]
B. [illegible]
C. [illegible]
D. [illegible]

766. [illegible]
A. [illegible]
B. [illegible]
C. [illegible]
D. [illegible]

767. [illegible] all are true except
A. [illegible]
B. [illegible]
C. [illegible]
D. [illegible] positive

768. [illegible]
A. [illegible]
B. [illegible]

[illegible]